Medical Terminology in a FLASH!

SECOND EDITION

Medical Terminology in a FLASH!

SECOND EDITION

A Multiple Learning Styles Approach

Sharon Eagle, RN, MSN
Nursing Educator, Nursing Program
Wenatchee Valley College
Wenatchee, Washington

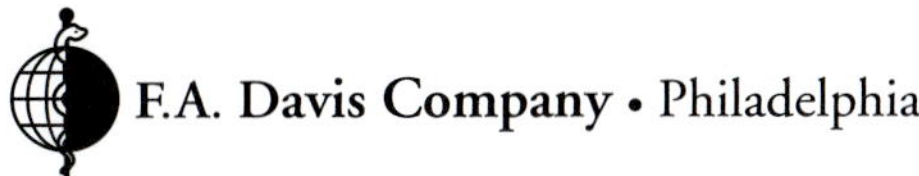
F.A. Davis Company • Philadelphia

F. A. Davis Company
1915 Arch Street
Philadelphia, PA 19103
www.fadavis.com

Printed in the United States of America

Last digit indicates print number: 10 9 8 7 6 5 4 3 2 1

Senior Acquisitions Editor: T. Quincy McDonald
Manager of Content Development: George W. Lang
Developmental Editor: Joanna Cain
Art and Design Manager: Carolyn O'Brien

As new scientific information becomes available through basic and clinical research, recommended treatments and drug therapies undergo changes. The author(s) and publisher have done everything possible to make this book accurate, up to date, and in accord with accepted standards at the time of publication. The author(s), editors, and publisher are not responsible for errors or omissions or for consequences from application of the book, and make no warranty, expressed or implied, in regard to the contents of the book. Any practice described in this book should be applied by the reader in accordance with professional standards of care used in regard to the unique circumstances that may apply in each situation. The reader is advised always to check product information (package inserts) for changes and new information regarding dose and contraindications before administering any drug. Caution is especially urged when using new or infrequently ordered drugs.

Library of Congress Cataloging-in-Publication Data

Eagle, Sharon.
Medical terminology in a flash! : a multiple learning styles approach / Sharon Eagle. -- 2nd ed.
p. cm.
Includes bibliographical references and index.
ISBN 978-0-8036-2566-2 (alk. paper)
1. Medicine--Terminology. I. Title.
R123.E25 2011
610.1'4--dc22

2011000942

ISBN-10: 0-8036-2566-9

ISBN-13: 978-0-8036-2566-2

DEDICATION

To Mom, Brian, Nicole, Brad, and Mel, all of whom have supported me with unending patience and encouragement.

To Georgie, who understands what true support looks like.

To Gabe and Seth, who came into the world and made me a grandma while I was busy writing the first edition. You bring me so much joy.

PREFACE

Have you ever found yourself confused or intimidated by someone who used medical terms you didn't understand? If so, you are not alone. This is a common occurrence. Health-care providers, be they doctors, nurses, therapists, or others, tend to get so comfortable with medical terminology that it becomes a natural way for them to speak. Unfortunately, they sometimes forget that the listener may not understand what they are saying. As a result, important information gets lost in the process, and you may walk away wondering what in the world was said.

If you've ever wondered why it sounds like these people are speaking "Greek," it's because they are doing just that. Most medical terms are derived from the Greek or Latin languages. So it's not your imagination. This really is a foreign language. In a sense, once you have mastered medical terminology, you may consider yourself to be bilingual.

As intimidating as medical terminology can be, the happy fact is that anyone can learn to understand and use it. It involves just a few simple steps that will be described in this book.

Let's get started. To begin, there is good news, and there is bad news. Let's deal with the bad news first. The key to developing a good understanding of medical terminology is memorization. It's safe to say that 90% of your work will involve memorizing the meanings of word parts. I won't kid you. This can be a lot of work. Remember, I said this would be *simple*, but I didn't say it would necessarily be *easy*. It will require that you invest a certain amount of time and effort. For some of you, memorization may come easily. If you are one of these lucky few, then you will very likely sail through this course with little difficulty. However, if you are one of the many who struggle with memorization, then you may be considering throwing this book into the garbage about now. Before you do that, please allow me to describe a plan that will help you to be successful.

Plan for Success

Built into this plan are a variety of strategies that will make the task of learning and memorizing word parts much easier.

Textbook

This textbook has many features to support your learning:

- **Learning style icons** with corresponding **Learning Style Tip(s)** help you learn and retain new information based on your specific learning style.

- **A workbook format** supports your learning by allowing you to write directly in the book. The act of writing actively engages your brain in a way that reading alone does not. This will enhance your learning.
- **Chapter exercises** allow you to practice translating, creating terms, and using word parts in a variety of ways.
- **An answer key** at the end of the book allows you to check your work. This immediate feedback provides positive reinforcement or immediate correction, both of which will help you learn.
- **Full-color anatomical illustrations of body systems** are included. Body parts are labeled with correct terms, and combining forms are listed. This is reinforced later in each chapter by an exercise that requires you to write in the correct word part associated with each term. This exercise will begin your introduction to human anatomy and will reinforce your association of medical terms to the correct body parts.
- **Color coding of word parts** reinforces learning. You will notice that ***prefixes*** are coded ***green, suffixes*** are coded ***blue, combining forms*** (word root + a vowel) are coded ***teal, abbreviations*** are coded ***orange,*** and ***pathology terms*** are coded ***purple***. This color coding directly corresponds with the color-coded flash cards (described below). Three hundred ten (310) of these flash cards are included for free in the back of the textbook. An additional 200+ cards, including many of the cards with pathology terms, are available to be downloaded for free from the DavisPlus website for this text.

Web Exercises

If you go to http://davisplus.fadavis.com/, you will have access to several student resources, including:

- Audio glossary
- Interactive audio exercises
- Listening exercises
- Labeling exercises
- Memory games
- Concentration games
- Interactive flash cards
- Printable flash cards
- Practice quizzes

These varied resources will ensure that you learn medical terminology in an engaging and effective way.

By completing the fun exercises on the website that accompanies this book, you will review medical terms in a variety of ways. Furthermore, you will have the opportunity to practice spelling medical terms, hear terms pronounced, and complete word-building and deciphering exercises.

Flash Cards

Color-coded flash cards that correspond to the word parts in this textbook are available for your use. Most of these cards contain visual cues as well.

- Be sure to practice with the flash cards after you complete each related section of the book. Each day, select a few cards to take with you in your purse or pocket, and review them during otherwise "wasted" moments during the day.

- If you review 5 to 10 different flash cards several times each day in the manner suggested, you can easily memorize 35 to 70 new terms each week without using your "official" study time. Over 10 weeks, that adds up to 350 to 700 new terms! For more ideas on how to use your flash cards, see the following section on Flash Card Games.
- Repetition is the key to memorization; flash cards make repetition easy.
- Because the flash cards are color-coded, you will not only memorize the meanings of the word parts but will also memorize whether the word parts are prefixes, suffixes, combining forms, or pathology terms, without even making a conscious effort!
- The flash cards have terms with the same or similar meanings grouped together. Therefore you will easily memorize two, three, or more terms in the same time it would normally take to memorize just one.

Flash Card Games

- **Partner Flash/2 Players:** Need: 1 set of flash cards. Give selected cards to a partner. The partner will flash each card in front of you, one at a time. You will agree on a preset amount of time to name the correct meaning (5 seconds or less). Run through the cards until you can name each of them within the designated time limit. This is a good exercise to use when your partner does not know medical terminology (such as a family member).
- **Memory Game/1 to 2 Players:** Need: 2 sets of flash cards. Combine two sets of flash cards (or selected terms from two sets). Shuffle the cards, and lay them out face down in rows. Each partner will take a turn flipping over two cards to try to create a "match" (such as two cards that both say "gastr/o"). In order to get credit for the match, the player must pronounce the term and be able to name the correct English translation (stomach). The player keeps all cards correctly matched and translated. The winner is the player with the most cards at the end of the game. This game can be adapted for just one player. The player simply collects matches one at a time until all cards are used.
- **Speed/2 Players:** Need: At least 6 sets of flash cards. Each partner selects designated cards from three sets (such as pathology terms for the respiratory system). Partners will shuffle their cards and, when ready, will begin laying down cards near each other (each in a separate pile) at the same time. When partners happen to lay down identical cards, the first one to correctly say the term and name the correct definition takes the matching cards from both piles and puts them aside. Matches will be infrequent at the beginning but will occur more and more frequently as cards are eliminated from play. The game continues until all cards are out of play. The winner is the one who collects the most pairs.
- **Score Four/3 or More Players:** Need: 1 set per player. Each player contributes a set of designated cards related to one or more body systems. All cards are shuffled together, and four are dealt to each player. Remaining cards are placed in a "draw" pile in the center of the table. The object of the game is to collect all four cards of a term. Because the cards have identifying data on both sides, the players will have to hold the cards so that no one else can see them. Players take turns asking one other player for cards with a specific term. For example, Player 1 already has two cards with the term "gastr/o" and wants to collect the other two. On her turn, she may name one other player and ask for all cards with the term

"gastr/o." At the same time, Player 1 must correctly pronounce the term and give the correct translation (stomach) in order to "earn" the cards. Player 2 must hand over all cards with that term. If Player 2 does not have that card, then Player 1 must draw a card from the draw pile. Once a player has collected all four cards, the player may lay them on the table and must again name the term and the correct translation. If the player forgets these steps when laying down the cards, another player may claim the cards by stating the magic words "Score Four!" and must then pronounce the term and identify the correct translation. If the player is unable to name the correct translation (without looking), the original player keeps control of the cards. The winner of the game is the one with the most four-card matches when all cards have been played.

REVIEWERS

MICHELLE BLESI, CMA (AAMA), AA, BA
Program Director, Instructor
Medical Assisting
Century College
White Bear Lake, MN

CAROLYN BRAUDAWAY, MS, RN
Assistant Professor
Nursing
Columbia Union College
Takoma Park, MD

ELIZABETH T. BRYAN, PT, OCS, CWCE, CKTP, ACCE
Instructor and Academic Coordinator
Physical Therapy Assistant
Linn State Technical College
Jefferson City, MO

ABIGAIL G. GORDON, PT, DPT
Clinical Assistant Professor
Physical Therapy
Howard University
Washington, DC

MALENA KING-JONES, MS, RN, ONC
Assistant Professor
Nursing
D'Youville College
Buffalo, NY

ABIGAIL MITCHELL, DHED, MSN, RN
Professor
Nursing
D'Youville College
Buffalo, NY

PAULA A. OLESEN, RN, MSN
Program Director
Nursing
South Texas College
McAllen, TX

ROBERT RICHMAN, MD
Instructor
Allied Health
Eastern Arizona College
Thatcher, AZ

SHIRLEY J. SHAW, BA, MA, AA
Professor Emeritus
Business Career and Technical Education Division
Northland Pioneer College
Holbrook, AZ

DIANA M. SMITH, RN
Instructor
Health Care
Lancaster County Career and Technology Center
Willow Street, PA

PAMELA URMANN
Instructor
Nursing
San Juan Basin Technical College
Mancos, CO

CAROL YODER, MSN, RN
ESL Advisor
Nursing and Allied Health
Norwalk Community College
Norwalk, CT

MICHELE YOUAKIM, PHD
Clinical Assistant Professor
Rehabilitation Science
State University of New York
Buffalo, NY

ACKNOWLEDGMENTS

To many wonderful people at the F.A. Davis Company I owe a huge debt of gratitude. A heartfelt thanks to Quincy McDonald, Senior Acquisitions Editor, for your belief in me and for helping to create the vision. You always seemed to know just when I most needed encouragement and guidance and provided both more times than I can count. Special thanks also to George Lang, Manager of Content Development, Health Professions/Medicine; Elizabeth Stepchin, Developmental Associate; Erin Leigh Peick and Joanna Cain, RN, Developmental Editors, of Auctorial Pursuits, Inc. I can't imagine attempting such a huge project without your knowledge and expertise.

Thanks to my students for challenging me with their questions and curiosity and renewing me with their energy and idealism. Ultimately, they are the reason for this book. My hope is that it will serve as a portal into the fascinating world of health care for others like them and provide a good start on a long and rewarding journey.

Finally, my thanks to the reviewers, who took on the time-intensive task of reading through part or all of the manuscript in its various stages and provided valuable feedback and suggestions.

CONTENTS IN BRIEF

CONTENTS

INTRODUCTION

Learning Styles

All people have learning "styles" but no two people are exactly alike. Understanding more about your own unique learning style will aid you in choosing study techniques that will be most effective for you. But how do you identify your style? Read through the descriptions that follow and see which style seems most familiar to you. Most people are actually a combination of styles, but one tends to be dominant.

Solitary Learners

Solitary learners prefer to study alone. They find the conversation of others to be distracting rather than helpful. They should avoid study groups.

Study Strategies for Solitary Learners

- Find a quiet, isolated place to study, such as a corner of the library or a quiet room in your house.
- Work through all of the exercises in each chapter of this book, and be sure to use the answer key to get immediate correction and feedback.
- Complete the exercises on the CD that correspond to the chapter you are studying.
- Be sure to use the flash cards as directed in the book.
- Select and take 5 to 10 flash cards with you each day, and review them when time allows. You will get the greatest benefit by using them in the following way:
  - Review them several times, reading the medical term side. Pause and see if you can remember the correct translation on your own. Then flip the card over to see if you are correct.
  - Now review them several more times, reading the English translation side. Pause and see if you remember the correct medical term. Then flip the card over to check yourself.

Social Learners

Social learners are just the opposite of solitary learners. When they try to study alone, their minds tend to wander, and they are easily distracted. They need to talk with other people and discuss issues in order to "think out loud." Exchanging ideas with others helps them to process the information and gain deeper understanding.

Study Strategies for Social Learners

- Try to identify other social learners in your class with the same needs.
- Make arrangements to study with a partner or in a group.
- Take turns "running" the flash cards with one another.
- Quiz one another using exercises or terms from the book.
- Take turns looking up terms in this book or in your medical dictionary. Practice pronouncing terms and discussing their meanings.
- Persuade family members or roommates to help you by doing some of the same activities described above.
- Be sure to attend class because you need the social interaction. Having the chance to ask questions and participate in discussions will help you immensely.

Auditory Learners

Auditory learners need to hear the spoken word. When they try to read or study silently, they may notice that their mind wanders. Few people are strong auditory learners, yet nearly everyone can benefit from adding an auditory component to their study techniques.

Study Strategies for Auditory Learners

- Study with others (see suggestions for social learners).
- Listen to others pronounce the terms, and participate in discussions.
- If you must study alone, try reading out loud so that you can listen to your own voice.
- Repeat the terms out loud after you read them or after you hear them. When you first do this, you may feel silly, but you will be amazed at how helpful it is to hear a voice (even your own) speak the terms and translations. Your brain will process and remember the information much better.
- Speak out loud when reviewing the flash cards (for the same reason as described above).
- Listen to the audio CD. It is extremely helpful in learning the terms and the correct pronunciation.

Be sure to attend class. The class structure provides numerous opportunities to listen to the instructor and classmates pronounce and discuss the medical terms.

Visual Learners

Visual learners must see the information with their own eyes. Hearing it just isn't enough. For these people, listening to a dull lecture without the benefit of interesting visuals is equivalent to taking a sleeping pill. They find their mind wandering and cannot understand why they have such a hard time paying attention. Most adults are strong visual learners.

Study Strategies for Visual Learners

- Read this book.
- Take time to review all of the illustrations and tables. It will be time well invested.
- Use the flash cards. They were developed especially for you. Along with the term, they provide a pronunciation guide, strong visual cues, and the English translation.

- The CD also presents information in a visually appealing manner, so be sure to make full use of it.
- Use colored highlighters on key terms as you read the text. You may even enjoy using highlighters of different colors to "code" or highlight information of different categories.
- Draw pictures, arrows, diagrams, or any other illustrations that help you make connections and understand concepts.

Kinesthetic Learners

Kinesthetic learners need "hands-on" interaction to learn. Sitting still and listening for long periods drives these people nuts. Observing others is not enough. Kinesthetic learners must *do* for themselves. They can't wait to get up and get moving. They love hands-on activities. Most adults are kinesthetic learners.

Study Strategies for Kinesthetic Learners

- You will benefit from many of the same strategies as the social learners. The more interaction you have with others, the better.
- Play learning games with the flash cards.
- Completion of learning activities is critically important for you. This includes the book activities, CD exercises, and group exercises.
- Attend class so you can do all of the above.

Most adults are predominantly visual/kinesthetic learners, yet possess some of the traits of all of these styles. However, you may be the exception. If you are unsure what your style is, try all of these techniques to see what works best for you.

Whatever your learning style, you are sure to find that mastering medical terminology is well worth the effort. Your reward will be the new understanding and insights that you gain. What was once a confusing and mysterious realm will now open its doors to you. You will begin to understand the language and the world of health and medicine.

LEARNING STYLES 1

Overview

Learning style theory suggests that individuals learn information in different ways according to their unique abilities and traits. Therefore, while all humans are similar, the ways in which you perceive, understand, and remember information may be somewhat different from other people's.

In truth, all people possess a combination of styles. You may be especially strong in one style and less so in others. You may be strong in two or three areas or may be equally strong in all areas. No style is inherently good or bad; they simply indicate how you most effectively perceive and process new information. As you learn about the styles described in this chapter and come to identify your own, you will then be able to modify your study activities accordingly. This will aid you in making the very most of your valuable study time, will enhance your learning, and will support you in doing your very best in future classes.

Sensory Learning Styles

Experts have identified a number of learning styles and given them a variety of names. Some are described in an abstract and complex manner, while others are relatively simple and easy to grasp. For ease of understanding, this book uses the simpler learning styles. This is done so you can quickly come to understand the basic elements of learning style theory and, more importantly, identify and understand your own style.

When learning, there are several ways to perceive and grasp new information. You may use your senses to see it and hear it. You may use touch and manipulation or your sense of taste or smell. You may find it useful to think aloud as you discuss the new information with someone else. Because the senses are so often involved in the acquisition of new information, many learning styles are named accordingly: visual, auditory, kinesthetic (hands-on or tactile), and so on.

Visual Learners

Most people are strongly visual learners. To most accurately and quickly grasp new information, these people need to see it represented visually. The more complex the data, the more this is true. Visual learners especially like data that are colorful and visually striking. Visual information can be presented in many ways. Examples include:

- Written words
- Diagrams

- Shapes
- Patterns
- Colors
- Symbols
- Illustrations
- Graphs
- Photos
- Tables
- Flowcharts
- Time lines
- Maps
- Handouts
- Posters
- Flash cards
- PowerPoint presentations
- Internet data
- Videos
- Live demonstrations

If you are a visual learner, you may have already noticed that you are drawn to visual information. Unless you are also an auditory learner, you may have some difficulty remembering information that is shared only verbally. Consequently you may ask others to repeat themselves, or better yet, to write it down. When looking through books, magazines, or instruction manuals, you are especially drawn to photos and any visual illustrations because they help you to more accurately see what is being discussed. Within the classroom, you prefer instructors who use written outlines and lots of visual aids.

Visualization is a powerful tool for you. In your health-care program you will very likely learn specific skills and procedures. Examples may include injecting, drawing blood, and recording a patient's electrocardiogram. The first time you do this with a real patient you will likely feel nervous. You can use visualization to help you prepare. Find a quiet place such as a break room or even a supply closet. Close your eyes. Take a deep breath and exhale slowly to relax. Now visualize approaching the patient and performing the procedure. Picture each step exactly as you will perform it; be sure to visualize yourself using any necessary equipment. Not only will this process help you mentally rehearse the procedure, but it will also allow you to make a supply list as you note each of the needed items. This form of mental rehearsal is nearly as good as the real thing and will allow you to enter the patient's room feeling calmer, more clearheaded, and more prepared to competently perform the procedure.

As a visual learner, you find writing notes helpful, and you often like to study alone where you can occasionally close your eyes and see in your mind's eye the situation or circumstances being studied. When learning tasks or procedures, you like to have written instructions. You are also able to close your eyes and mentally rehearse through the process of visualization because you can picture everything clearly. During exams you recall information by "seeing" it in your mind's eye, whether it is an actual picture or diagram or a fragment of written text. During conversations or discussions you tend to use visual words such as "see," "look," and "picture." Examples include:

- Let me see if I understand.
- Let's look at this.
- See what you think of this.

- I see what you mean.
- I'm trying to picture it.

You generally have a good sense of direction, rarely get lost, and can easily interpret and use maps. Your office and home may be littered with lists and notes that you've written to organize yourself and to remember things. You love self-adhesive note pads. You find listening to a lecture without stimulating visuals to be boring and tedious. You need to take notes, draw, or doodle to keep from falling asleep. In fact, you may appear to other people as if you are distracted or daydreaming when doodling on paper. However, you know that it actually helps you listen better. Your work and hobbies include activities that make use of color, shapes, and design or visual art. Just a few examples are drawing, painting, quilting, photography, and scrapbooking.

Study Strategies for Visual Learners

If you are a visual learner, try using any study or memory technique that aids you in visually seeing and recalling information. You may find **mnemonics** (memory aids) especially helpful for remembering lists or sequenced pieces of information. Generally speaking, the more creative, whimsical, funny, or absurd they are, the better you will remember them. There are many different types of mnemonics. Some examples are:

- Children use the well-known alphabet song, a musical mnemonic, to learn their ABCs.
- Students in anatomy classes use one of several mnemonic variations to remember the 12 cranial nerves (olfactory, optic, oculomotor, trochlear, trigeminal, abducens, facial, acoustic, glossopharyngeal, vagus, spinal accessory, and hypoglossal). One example is "On old Olympus' tower tops, a Finn and German viewed some hops." Note that the first letter of each word is the same as the first letter of each cranial nerve's name.
- Most people use this spelling mnemonic to remember where to place the I and E: "I before E, except after C."

Another form of commonly used mnemonics is the **acronym**. An acronym is an abbreviation created by using the first letters or word parts in names or phrases. Examples of acronyms include:

LASER—**L**ight **a**mplification by **s**timulated **e**mission of **r**adiation
INTERPOL—**Inter**national Criminal **Pol**ice Organization
FAQ—**F**requently **a**sked **q**uestions
CD-ROM—**C**ompact **d**isc **r**ead-**o**nly **m**emory
PIN—**P**ersonal **i**dentification **n**umber
OLD CART—**O**nset, **l**ocation, **d**uration, **c**haracter, **a**ggravating factors, **r**elieving factors, **t**reatments
VS—**V**ital **s**igns

The seven warning signs of cancer can be remembered in the acronym CAUTION:

Change in bowel or bladder habits
A sore throat that does not heal
Unusual bleeding or discharge
Thickening or a lump in the breast or other area
Indigestion or difficulty swallowing
Obvious change in a mole or wart
Nagging cough or hoarseness

And finally, the warning signs of malignant melanoma are shown by the acronym ABCD:

Asymmetry—One half of the mole does not match the other half.
Border—The edges of the mole are irregular or blurred.
Color—The color varies throughout, including tan, brown, black, blue, red, or white.
Diameter—The mole is larger than 6 millimeters.

Auditory Learners

Many people are auditory (or aural) learners. In order to most accurately and quickly grasp new information, these people need to hear it spoken. The more complex the data, the more this is true. The most common example of auditory information sharing is during a classroom lecture; however, there are other ways to hear information. Examples include audiotapes, videotapes, computer tutorials (with audio content), and oral discussions.

If you are an auditory learner, you may have already noticed that you are drawn to information presented aloud. Unless you are also a visual learner, you may have some difficulty remembering written information without some verbal discussion or review. You may often ask others to elaborate on details orally or to repeat themselves so you can hear it again. When recalling events, you can sometimes hear how someone else speaks. You notice subtle inflections that convey meaning. Chances are you enjoy music and have a good sense of rhythm. You may play an instrument or sing. At the very least, you are an avid appreciator of music and may prefer the radio or stereo to television at least part of the time. Music evokes emotion in you. For example, you notice that you feel energized, joyous, or melancholy in response to certain music. You may also notice that songs or jingles pop into your head and stay there for hours. Your work and your hobbies often involve sound. Examples include playing musical instruments, attending concerts, composing music, or working as a sound engineer or even a band or orchestra conductor.

During conversations or discussions you tend to use auditory words such as "sound" and "hear." Examples include:

- That sounds like...
- Music to my ears.
- This rings a bell.
- I hear what you're saying.
- You are coming through loud and clear.
- I'm tuned in.

Study Strategies for Auditory Learners

If you are an auditory learner, try using any study or memory techniques that allow you to hear information aloud, whether it is the spoken word or data set to music or any other auditory format. Auditory learners are also usually verbal learners as well. If this is true for you, then you learn best when you have the chance for a verbal exchange. This allows you to speak to and listen to others. For this reason, you are probably a social learner and often prefer studying with a partner or in a study group. You find mnemonics helpful, especially if they include rhymes or are catchy and fun to say out loud. A common example is the following mnemonic used to help people remember the number of days in each month:

Thirty days hath September,
April, June, and November;

All the rest have thirty-one,
Excepting February alone:
Which has twenty-eight, that's fine,
Till leap year gives it twenty-nine.

Another example of a mnemonic that relates to health care is the acronym MONA. Nurses and other health-care workers often use this mnemonic when providing emergency care for patients experiencing possible myocardial infarction (heart attack):

Morphine
Oxygen
Nitrates
Aspirin

Verbal Learners

It is sometimes said that some people must think (first) in order to speak. For verbal learners the reverse may be true: They feel compelled to speak in order to think. What this means is that speaking aloud helps them to process information and think things through. This is especially true when the information is complex or the situation feels stressful. These people often talk to themselves. Such individuals may state that doing so helps to slow down their brain in order to help them focus and think more clearly.

Many people are verbal learners. This includes use of the spoken and the written word.

If you are a verbal learner, you may seek out a trusted friend to act as a sounding board. You do not expect this person to solve your problem; rather, you need him to listen as you think aloud and bounce things off him. This friend may offer no advice at all, yet you usually find these sessions enormously helpful. Most likely, you love to read and enjoy some type of writing. This could take a professional form such as becoming an author or personal forms such as writing poetry for your own enjoyment or simply writing in a private journal. You enjoy learning new words and incorporating them into your vocabulary. You find rhymes and tongue twisters entertaining. You may enjoy reading poetry aloud because speaking it is more enjoyable than silently reading it. Your occupation or hobbies may include public speaking, writing, or politics. You enjoy a lively discussion or even a debate, as well as interactive social activities such as playing games or simply visiting, because this includes verbal exchange. During conversations you tend to use verbal words such as "talk," "spell," and "word." Examples include:

- Let's talk about this.
- I will spell it out.
- In other words...
- The best word to describe...

Study Strategies for Verbal Learners

If you are a verbal learner, try using any study or memory techniques that allow you to speak aloud in order to recite data or explain concepts. Like auditory learners, you find mnemonics helpful, especially if they are fun to say or include rhyming. You may also find writing to be very helpful. Writing down important data such as outlines, summaries, and vocabulary helps you remember the content. You are very likely a social learner who benefits from studying with a partner or in a study group. This provides ample opportunity for discussion. You especially benefit from explaining challenging concepts or "teaching" your study partners about a given topic. For example, the members of your study group may decide to teach one another about the four major joint types in the body: hinge, ball-and-socket, pivot, and gliding. Each person describes the appearance and function of a type of joint and gives an example. One person may compare a hinge joint like those found in the knee and elbow to a door hinge. As she does so, she describes how it moves back and forth like a door that swings open and shut. The next person may compare a pivot joint, such as the one in the neck, to a chair that turns back and forth in a 180-degree half circle. Other students go on to teach about their assigned joints and give examples. To maximize the value of this exercise for verbal learners, you can add a requirement that all members of the group must verbally repeat key information or phrases after the "teacher."

Kinesthetic Learners

Most people have some kinesthetic (tactile) aspects to their learning style even though it may not be their most dominant style. People who are strong kinesthetic learners need to use their bodies as they learn. They like to touch and manipulate objects. This is especially important when learning physical skills. When assembling things they may forgo reading the instructions and just assemble the product based on feel and instinct. They are usually successful, but if not, they may check the instructions, which will now make much more sense to them since they have become physically acquainted with the parts. Examples of physical learning include:

- Demonstrations
- Simulations
- Practicing a skill

If you are a kinesthetic learner, you may have already noticed that you are eager to get your hands on objects and do things yourself. When the information being learned is theoretical, you are still eager to move your body somehow, even if it is to draw a diagram or fidget in your chair. Sitting through lengthy lectures feels tedious and almost painful to you. You like to touch things, and very likely have hobbies that include manipulating objects or making things with your hands, such as woodworking, gardening, baking, assembling puzzles, putting models together, sewing, playing a musical instrument, and sculpting. You notice textures and like how they feel. Your most productive thinking time occurs when you are on the move in activities such as biking, hiking, walking, or even running on a treadmill. You get restless if you sit around too long, and feel eager to do something. You are very physical when communicating and may use big hand and arm gestures. You may enjoy dancing, sports, and other physical activities. During conversations or discussions, you tend to use physical action or sensation words like "feel" and "touch." Examples include:

- This doesn't feel right.
- I follow you.
- Get a grip.
- Keep in touch.
- This just doesn't sit right.
- I feel it in my gut.
- I need to get a handle on this.
- I'm trying to get a feel for...

Study Strategies for Kinesthetic Learners

If you are a kinesthetic learner, try using any study or memory techniques that allow you to move your body or touch objects. When learning skills or procedures, your best strategy is to actually get your hands on the needed supplies and practice the procedure. For example, consider again the study group in which you and your friends are each describing major types of body joints. In addition to verbally describing the joints and giving examples, add a requirement that each person must somehow act out or physically mimic the joint movement—something like a charades game with talking allowed. The person describing the hinge joint now must physically get up and find a door to open and shut while she describes its function. Better yet, she might play the part of the door herself and move her body back and forth. The next person compares a pivot joint, such as the one in his neck, to a chair that turns back and forth in a 180-degree half circle. As he describes this, he literally turns his head back and forth and then turns the chair back and forth in a 180-degree circle. After each person performs a physical demonstration, other members of the group must perform the same movement. This gives everyone full kinesthetic value from the activity.

When actual physical practice of a skill is not possible, visualization is a great alternative. It gives you the chance to "practice" skills in your mind and even move your body, arms, and hands as you would when performing the actual skill. When the content is theoretical, you still benefit from physical movement. Play learning games, use flash cards, complete activities included in your textbook, use the student activity disc that accompanies many textbooks (including this one), and interact with a study partner or group.

Social Preferences

In addition to your sensory learning style, you also have a social preference for learning. If you notice that interacting with others helps you to grasp and understand information, you are most likely a social learner. On the other hand, if you do your best when working alone without the distraction of others, you are very likely a solitary learner.

Social Learners

Many people are social learners. They learn most effectively when they are able to interact with other people. They enjoy group **synergy** (the enhanced action of two or more agents working together cooperatively) and are able to think things through with the verbal exchange that occurs during a lively discussion. Examples of social learning include:

- Discussions about specific topics
- Question-and-answer sessions
- Group projects
- Group games

If you are a social learner, you may have already noticed that you are drawn to social situations and don't like to study alone. You communicate and interact well with others. You enjoy listening to and helping others. You may also be a verbal-auditory learner and may enjoy discussions and bouncing ideas off other people. You are drawn to social situations and may stay after class to talk with others. If you are athletic, you may prefer group sports to solo activities. You also enjoy social activities such as dancing and board games. You like working through problems with a partner or a group. Work activities may include teaching, coaching, or working in a people-oriented setting such as a restaurant or retail store. During conversations or discussions, you tend to use social wording which includes "we" and "let us." Examples include:

- If we work cooperatively...
- Let's work it out.
- Let's explore this.
- We should get together and...

Study Strategies for Social Learners

If you are a social learner, you may find that you feel restless and have difficulty staying focused when you try to study alone. You need to seek out opportunities to study with one or more additional people. If there isn't a study group available, consider starting one. Group activities can include discussion, learning games, role-playing, and creating mnemonics together. Your study group will be most effective if you set and adhere to some ground rules that provide structure. It's your group, so the rules are up to you, but here are some suggestions:

- Identify a group leader—preferably someone with some knowledge or experience in the subject being studied.
- Have the group complete specified readings or assignments prior to each meeting.
- Have the group members agree to stay on task so the group doesn't deteriorate into a social group or complaint session.
- Set and follow time limits.
- Encourage all members to contribute.

Solitary Learners

Many people are solitary learners. They learn most effectively when they are able to study alone without distraction from others. They are often somewhat private, and enjoy time alone to ponder and reflect. They are strongly independent and know what works for them; trying to conform to the group can be a source of frustration.

There are many ways that solitary learners study. The important thing is that they do it alone. They may read, review notes, and listen to recorded lectures (if they are also auditory), or they may incorporate any number of other strategies. During conversations or discussions, they tend to use solitary "me" or "I" language. Examples include:

- I need to think this over.
- Let me ponder it.
- I'll get back to you.
- I'll let you know what I decide.

Study Strategies for Solitary Learners

If you are a solitary learner, you may feel frustrated trying to study with a partner or a group. You may feel like they are wasting your time and believe you would do better by yourself. You focus and concentrate best when alone. You are somewhat analytical and goal oriented. You are also a self-starter and don't need anyone else to prompt you or to provide structure. You have learned to enjoy your own company and enjoy solitude. Many people, especially your social friends, may find this difficult to understand, since they may not like being alone. You may be known to travel alone, dine out alone, and go to movies or concerts alone. You don't feel that you are missing out when you do this; in fact, you may prefer it because you don't have to negotiate with anyone else about what to do or where to go. You may enjoy solitary hobbies and may work for yourself or dream of working for yourself one day. You are self-reflective and interested in personal improvement. Strong solitary learners often end up in jobs where they work independently. Examples include writing, farming, forestry, or other outdoor occupations.

Global versus Analytical Preferences

In addition to the styles described above, most people tend to initially grasp information either as a whole, looking at the "big picture," or in a more sequential fashion in which the individual parts are studied first to comprehend the whole. If you are in the first group, you are a global learner; if you are in the second group, you are an analytical learner.

Global Learners

Global learners, sometimes called *holistic* learners, generally see the big picture first and later pay more attention to details. For example, when studying the human body, global learners first see it as a whole, complete organism. With that picture in mind, they are then able to begin studying the parts. This is true even when studying individual body systems, such as the cardiovascular system. Global learners first grasp the big picture of the entire system as it circulates blood throughout the body. With further study and thought, they appreciate how the system delivers oxygen and nutrients and eliminates waste through a complex network of vessels including veins, arteries, and capillaries.

If you are a global learner, your primary learning style may be a mix of visual and auditory. You are also probably a social learner. If you are a global learner, you often respond based on intuition or emotion and are able to grasp symbolism. You may be able to accept rules, such as a math equation, without necessarily understanding how the steps work. You may be more interested in general themes than little details and are good at paraphrasing ideas and concepts. Along the same lines, you are good at recognizing relationships and reading between the lines. You are flexible and do well with multitasking. When studying new concepts, you usually compare them with concepts you already understand. For example, when first learning about the lymphatic system, you may think, "This is very similar to what I know about the vascular system. They both have a complex network of vessels that convey fluid through the body." As you study the lymphatic system in detail, you then begin to distinguish the important differences.

All learning styles provide benefits as well as potential challenges. If you are a global learner, you may experience periods of frustration relieved by moments of insight when the "light comes on" and you suddenly "get it." When reading, you desire to know the main point or bottom line. When you encounter a term or concept you don't understand, you may skim over it, hoping that it will make sense as you continue on. This strategy sometimes works for you, but you risk missing important details. You may not like being asked to explain details to others or to write out how you achieved your final answer. You may resist accepting critical feedback and may often be late to class or work. You usually feel a need to know the whys before you commit your enthusiasm and energy to a project.

Study Strategies for Global Learners

If you are a global learner, you are probably also a visual-auditory learner. Therefore, be sure to try the study and memory techniques previously described for those styles. If you find studying details to be tedious and boring, try to find other, more creative and fun ways to learn the same material. For example, you may prefer drawing your own colorful diagrams or may enjoy using audiovisual tutorials or other activities that are often on the student discs that accompany textbooks or are available online.

Use your strengths. You are flexible. You are a multitasker. Don't be afraid to mix it up a bit to make your study efforts more lively and enjoyable. You are good at seeing the big picture and recognizing relationships; therefore, begin each study session by identifying the relationship between what you are currently studying and your future career ambitions.

Here is a study activity that may help you connect current studies with future career goals. Meet with a group of fellow students or with a study partner. In addition to verbalizing or explaining terms and concepts, add an additional requirement: Give a hypothetical example of a time in your future career when knowing this information will be necessary. For example, imagine that today your group is studying the structure and function of the neurological system, in particular the structure of the basic neuron. As a global learner, you are more interested in whether the human body works as it should, and you may be less attuned to details. Furthermore, you wish to get on with learning about your role as a future medical assistant, nurse, or whatever occupation you are pursuing.

As you study the structure of the neuron today, you are challenged with seeing the value of such detailed trivia in your future role and career. Consider the important function of that little neuron in transmitting signals, and the way each of its structural parts supports that function. Then ask yourself what might happen if some of the protective coating (myelin sheath) begins to erode. How might that affect the function of the body? And how might that lead the person to show up in the clinic or hospital in which you will be working? How might your understanding of that little neuron help you to understand your patient, her symptoms, her diagnosis, and her needs? One day you may be responsible for providing care to a patient with multiple sclerosis or another degenerative neuromuscular disorder. Keep this in mind as you study the neurological system today. Then challenge yourself to get the maximum value from your investment of time and energy.

Beware your tendency to overlook details. You can compensate with strategies that help you identify and remember details of significance. While reading, make note of terms, concepts, or sections that you skipped over or did not understand. You can do this by highlighting these areas in a specific color or by writing notes in the margins. Once you've completed your initial read-through, force yourself to return to each of these areas and investigate them further. When deciding how much time and energy to devote to each one, ask yourself the following questions:

- Is there a learning objective in the syllabus that pertains to this content?
- Might this content impact my understanding of the whole?
- How likely is the instructor to include a test question on this content?
- How relevant is this content to the remainder of this class, to future classes, or to my future career?

Analytical Learners

Analytical learners, sometimes called *logical, linear, sequential,* or *mathematical* learners, generally need to see the parts before fully comprehending the whole. For example, when studying the human body, analytical learners prefer to study in a methodical fashion beginning with the smallest parts and working up to the whole. Such people will prefer to take classes such as chemistry and cellular biology before taking classes like anatomy and physiology. As they continue learning about each of the body systems, they begin to appreciate how each relates to the others and constitutes the whole organism.

Analytical learners readily identify patterns and like to group data into categories for further study. They love to create and follow agendas, make lists with items ranked by priority, and approach problem-solving in a logical, methodical manner. They like to create and follow procedures and may grow impatient with others who do not. Analytical learners are often linear and orderly in their thinking and seek to quantify things whenever possible. They often pursue careers in accounting, sciences, computer technology, engineering, law enforcement, and mathematics.

If you are an analytical learner, your primary learning style may be verbal. If this is true, then you process information verbally, which means you sometimes talk to yourself and think aloud. You may also have a visual dimension to your style, since this lends itself so well to grouping information into categories and drawing connections. However, you could be a mix of any of the styles previously described. Because you are so methodical, you may also be a solitary learner and prefer a quiet environment. Working with others who are not analytical may frustrate you. You tend to respond to problems logically rather than emotionally. This serves you well in some cases but may cause you to be labeled by others as cold and unfeeling. On the other hand, you have an eye for detail, and are organized and forward thinking. Most work teams need at least one person with your skills to ensure accuracy and quality. Your logical mind makes you especially good at noting errors or flaws in other people's reasoning; however, those people may not always appreciate this. You are especially good at mathematics or any pursuit that requires logic and strategy. You may enjoy brainteasers such as sudoku, or games of strategy like chess and certain computer games. However, your less-analytical friends may grow weary of playing games with you, since you nearly always win.

Some of the same qualities that are your strengths can, at times, become a source of frustration. For example, you may get stuck in "analysis paralysis" as you study details. This can stall forward movement and impair decision-making. Some may accuse you of being stubborn, rigid, or inflexible. You may also struggle in fast-paced, stressful environments where quick decisions are required. You may also feel frustrated when other people issue personal opinions as facts. To you, facts are only facts when they are indisputably accurate and supported by reliable data. In turn, other people may become frustrated by your need to gather more data and process information in detail (often verbally). In most cases, they really don't want to hear all of your logic and rationale, and instead wish you would just get to the point.

Study Strategies for Analytical Learners

If you are an analytical learner, use your style to maximize learning, but take care not to get stuck in analysis paralysis or sidetracked with insignificant detail. Try the study and memory techniques previously described that are relevant to your basic style. Put your organizational talent to work to make your study efforts productive: Make an agenda or create a list of topics to be studied. Prioritize topics to ensure that you address the most important things first. This is your "Must Know" list. Set and follow time limits, but don't over analyze your plan. It is most important to get busy studying. Rather than getting sidetracked with interesting (but low-priority) items, make another list of topics as you go along titled "It Would Be Nice to Know." Come back to this list later if—and only if—time permits. Use your gift for identifying patterns by noting patterns within the material you are studying. This can be useful when you prepare for exams, because test questions often focus on features that are similar and those that are different. For example, a myocardial infarction (MI) and angina both cause chest pain. In both cases, the pain is caused by inadequate blood supply to the heart. These are two important and similar features when comparing these disorders—chest pain and lack of oxygen. On the other hand, an MI causes actual death of heart muscle tissue, while angina does not. This is an important difference.

As an analytical learner, you may not be able to hear new information while you are focusing on and processing other information. Consequently, you may often feel like the instructor moves too quickly during lecture. However, you must remember that if she speaks slowly enough for you to hear, write, and process the data, your global-learner classmates will grow uninterested and restless. They may perceive the class as boring and may believe the instructor moves too slowly. Therefore, your best bet is to use multiple strategies that allow you to get good class notes, identify important details, and delay much of your detailed information-processing until a later time. This might mean that you focus on writing during class and record the lecture (with your instructor's permission) so you can hear it later. Such a plan keeps you from missing significant details. This should lower your stress and allow you to enjoy class more. Another option is to get notes at a later time from a classmate, so you can devote your in-class energy to listening. If you do this, be sure to select someone who is a very thorough and accurate note taker.

To make the most of some study strategies, you must give yourself permission to be illogical or even silly. If a technically "inaccurate" mnemonic or silly song will help you remember something, then why not use it? Your global-learner classmates can help you with this if you will let them.

You are a good reflective thinker and are able to evaluate your own performance. However, this can also become a flaw, since you are probably a perfectionist and may be too hard on yourself. You must learn to let the small stuff go, not let other people bug you, and give yourself permission to be less than perfect. If other students distract or annoy you with their behaviors or chosen study tactics, try to ignore them. You may need to physically separate yourself from them to do so. You need to do your "analytical thing" and allow them to do their "global thing." You will both achieve the same goals in different ways. The exception is when you must work with others as part of a group assignment. This can be challenging for students of different styles, but this mirrors real life. In fact, this is the main reason instructors assign group work: It gives you the opportunity to practice communication and teamwork skills. In this case, it will help if everyone on the team begins by sharing information about their individual styles, including strengths, flaws, and needs. Group roles and tasks can be divided according to each person's style and strengths.

As an analytical learner, you may sometimes feel overwhelmed by unstructured environments and unexpected events. For this reason, you must think carefully about your career choice. The same abilities that serve you very well in some settings could hold you back in others. Since you are reading this book, you may be embarking on a career in health care. Fortunately there are many paths within this arena. Be sure to select one that allows you to use your talents to their fullest. It is for you to decide what this might be. However, someone with your ability to methodically process and analyze data, ensure accuracy, and work independently might do especially well in certain settings, such as medical coding, research, laboratory technology, quality control, or utilization review. On the other hand, you generally do not like unpredictability or group work. Therefore trying to work in a fast-paced, unpredictable environment might prove frustrating for you and your team. Examples might include roles in which you must provide patient care in an emergency department, urgent care center, or other medical units with very ill patients.

Identifying Your Style

How do you identify your learning style? In reading through this chapter you may have recognized yourself in one or more of the styles described. Remember that nobody has one style exclusively. Your style may have a combination of some or all of these but may be especially strong in one or two areas. Identifying the dominant aspects of your learning style will help you understand yourself better. It will also help you to identify study strategies that will be most effective for you. This allows you to make the most of your valuable and limited study time. It will help you to be more successful in this course than you might have otherwise been. It will also help you to be more successful in any future classes that you take. Therefore, taking a few minutes now to clearly identify your style will pay off in the long run.

Learning Styles and Medical Terminology

Any course in medical terminology requires students to learn and remember a huge amount of information. As you learn various terms and their meanings, you must find a way to commit this knowledge to memory. In other words, you must *memorize* a lot of data. There is no way around it; you are learning a foreign language, and to become fluent in this language you must develop a large, accurate vocabulary and must know how to use it.

So how does learning style theory apply to learning medical terminology? By having a clear understanding of your style, you will be able to use your strengths and abilities to their fullest. Knowing what *not* to do becomes as important as knowing what to *do*. Because learning and remembering memorized data are key to this course, understanding how memory works will help you to accomplish this.

Memory

Human memory is the process by which people store, retain, and retrieve information (see Fig. 1-1). Perceiving, processing, and storing information are complex processes that involve many parts of your brain. It is beyond the scope of this book to describe the process in detail. However, a few key points are worth mentioning.

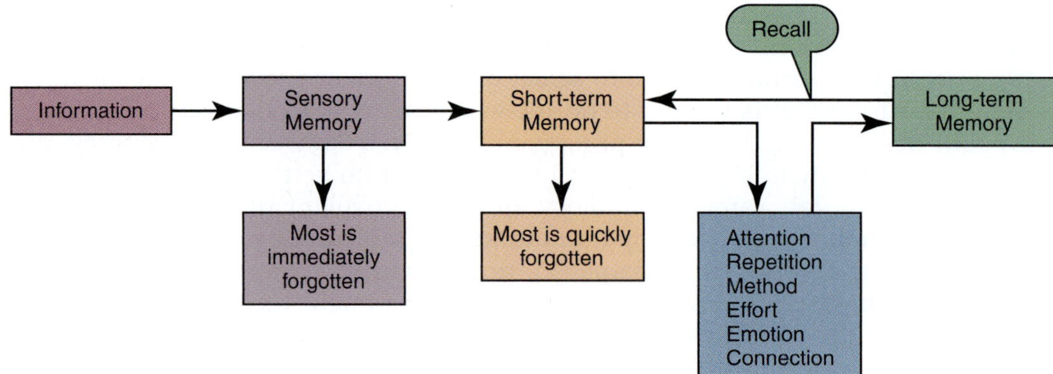

FIGURE 1-1 **Memory**

Sensory memory involves the first brief impression during which your brain registers patterns, sounds, smells, or other sensory data. You then almost immediately forget it, although you do store some data for later retrieval.

Perception and storage of information requires a complex combination of electrical and chemical functions within the nervous tissue of your brain, usually in your **short-term memory**. This allows you to retrieve it for a very short span of time, usually several seconds to several minutes. In general, most people are able to retrieve four to seven items of information from short-term memory. This capability is increased if the data is clustered into groups; this is known as **chunking**. For example, you may have noticed that it is easier to remember a string of numbers, such as a telephone number, if you chunk the numbers, such as in 233-467-9012 rather than 2334679012.

Memorization is a method that allows you to recall data through a process known as rote learning. It can be an effective strategy for you if you use it in the right way. It has been shown that most people's ability to retain memorized information is enhanced if they rehearse the data intermittently over an extended period of time rather than using last-minute cram-and-forget method. In other words, cramming may or may not get you through the next exam, but it certainly will not support your long-term success in future classes or your future career. To get important memorized data into your **long-term memory** you must do more than cram. Long-term memory is capable of storing an infinite amount of data for an indefinite period of time, perhaps for a lifetime. However, getting the information you wish to remember into your long-term memory is sometimes challenging. A number of factors are required, among them healthy functioning of several parts of the brain and sufficient quantity and quality of sleep. Others include:

- Attention (the extent to which you consciously attend to and focus on the data)
- Repetition (rehearsal of the data over and over)
- Information-processing method (strategies used to analyze and remember data; examples include chunking or other means of organizing data and using creative tricks such as mnemonics and acronyms)
- Study effort (the time and energy you devote; the greater your effort, the better your recall)

- Emotional relationship (relating the information being studied to strong emotional feelings or significant events)
- Connection (relating new information to a prior experience or previously learned information)

Some activities hamper your ability to store and recall information in both your short-term and long-term memory banks. Examples include:

- Interference (stimuli that hamper your ability to attend to information as you learn)
- Cramming (extensive memorization of a large amount of data over a short period of time; cramming results in very poor recall and may displace other data in short-term memory)

Some general measures can help you in this process. General self-care activities that enhance memory include healthy nutrition, stress-reduction activities, regular exercise, socialization activities, and regular, good-quality sleep.

Plan for Success

To ensure your success in this course, you must take a bit of time now to do a self-assessment. It won't take long and the information you gather will pay off big-time. Completing the chapter activities below will guide you in this process. Once you've identified your own style, then you can proceed through this book. You will notice specific *Learning Style Tips* scattered throughout all chapters (see Fig. 1-2). They are targeted to specific styles, so be sure to read all of those relevant to your style. Specific icons have been placed next to each tip to identify which learning style it applies to. This allows you to read only those most relevant to you. However, you may wish to read them all; your style is probably a blend of the various styles, and you may want to consider trying all of the tips to find the ones that fit you best.

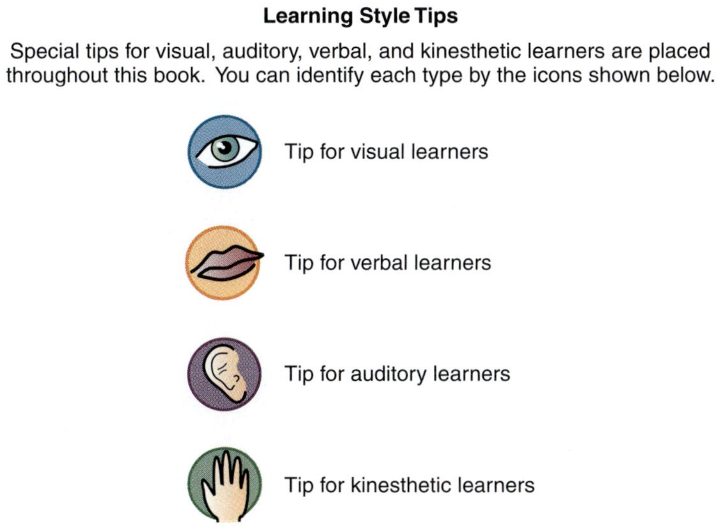

Learning Style Tips

Special tips for visual, auditory, verbal, and kinesthetic learners are placed throughout this book. You can identify each type by the icons shown below.

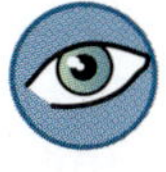
Tip for visual learners

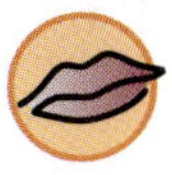
Tip for verbal learners

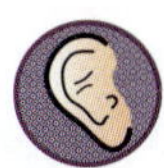
Tip for auditory learners

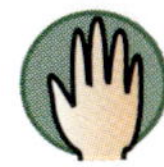
Tip for kinesthetic learners

FIGURE 1-2 **Learning style tips**

Chapter Activities

1. **Visit the websites listed to take their free self-assessment tests.**
   - http://vark-learn.com/english/index.asp
   - http://www.edutopia.org/multiple-intelligences-learning-styles-quiz

   Describe your results.

2. **Now that you know what your dominant style is, read again the sections of this chapter that pertain to your style. Briefly describe the type of study strategies most likely to be effective for you.**

3. **Describe the plan that you believe will help you to be most effective in this course. Include approximate study times and techniques and whether they will be solitary or social in nature.**

4. **Describe the activities you plan to employ to transfer as much medical terminology data as possible into your long-term memory.**

As you continue through this book, you will find study tips included in every chapter. These tips suggest study techniques for all learning styles. Keep an open mind as you move forward and be willing to try any that you believe may be helpful. Make notes as you do so about what did and did not work well, and anything you might do differently next time. By the end of this course, you will have developed a good working knowledge of medical terminology. You will also have learned more about yourself and your learning style than you know now. Both of these things will serve you extremely well in your future classes and career.

Websites

Please visit the F.A. Davis website at http://davisplus.fadavis.com/eagle/medterm to view an extensive list of websites to aid you in your studies.

Practice Exercises

Matching

Match the following terms with the correct description. Each answer is used once. Check Appendix G for the correct answers.

Exercise 1

1. _______ Visual
2. _______ Auditory
3. _______ Verbal
4. _______ Kinesthetic
5. _______ Social
6. _______ Solitary

a. Prefers to study alone
b. Needs to see data with their eyes
c. Needs to speak in order to think
d. Needs to hear the spoken word
e. Enjoys group synergy and lively discussions
f. Needs to touch and manipulate things

True or False

Decide whether the following statements are true or false. Check Appendix G for the correct answers.

Exercise 2

1. True False Most people have only one or two predominate learning styles.
2. True False The more complex data are, the more important it is for visual learners to see it.
3. True False Written text is an example of visual data.
4. True False Most auditory learners are also solitary learners.
5. True False Kelly enjoys meditation and traveling alone. She is probably a solitary learner.

Multiple Choice

Select the one best answer to the following multiple-choice questions. Check Appendix G for the correct answers.

Exercise 3

1. Colors, tables, and live demonstrations all appeal to which type of learners?
   a. Visual
   b. Auditory
   c. Kinesthetic
   d. Verbal
2. Visual learners are most likely to make which of the following statements?
   a. "That sounds like an experience I had."
   b. "This doesn't feel right to me."
   c. "I see what you mean."
   d. "Let's cooperate on this project."
3. Which of the following is the best example of an auditory way to get information?
   a. Reviewing flash cards
   b. Watching a PowerPoint presentation
   c. Listening to a lecture
   d. Asking a question
4. Jonathon loves music and is always humming, whistling, or singing something. In a recent conversation he told his friend, "I hear you loud and clear." Jonathon is most likely:
   a. A visual learner
   b. A social learner
   c. An auditory learner
   d. A kinesthetic learner
5. Brian fidgets in the classroom and struggles to get through lectures, yet when he is in the laboratory, he does very well and enjoys learning. His dominant learning style is most likely:
   a. Auditory
   b. Solitary
   c. Kinesthetic
   d. Verbal

6. Which of the following statements is true regarding global learners?
   a. They are usually very good at mathematical calculations.
   b. They often get immersed in details.
   c. They like to know the whys before committing enthusiasm and energy to a project.
   d. They are usually very punctual.
7. All of the following statements are true regarding analytical learners **except**:
   a. They are sometimes called holistic learners.
   b. They like to take a methodical approach to studying.
   c. They readily identify patterns and like to group data into categories for further study.
   d. They love to create and follow agendas and make lists with items ranked by priority.
8. Which of the following statements is true regarding analytical learners?
   a. They are probably social learners.
   b. They often respond to problems emotionally.
   c. They are often described as flexible and versatile.
   d. They have an eye for detail.
9. All of the following words of advice are specifically appropriate for analytical learners **except**:
   a. Make an agenda to plan your studies.
   b. Identify patterns within the material you are studying.
   c. Give yourself permission to be illogical or even silly.
   d. Try studying with a group of people with various styles.
10. Which of the following statements about memory is true?
   a. Sensory memory involves the first brief impression during which the brain registers sensory data such as patterns, sounds, or smells.
   b. Short-term memory allows you to retrieve data in a very short span of time, usually several seconds to several minutes.
   c. Chunking is a technique that increases the number of items one can recall.
   d. All of these.

True or False

Decide whether the following statements are true or false. Check Appendix G for the correct answers.

Exercise 4

1. True False Many learning styles are named according to the special senses.
2. True False Few people are strongly visual learners.
3. True False Visual learners prefer data to be presented simply in black and white.
4. True False *Auditory* and *aural* have similar meanings.
5. True False Kinesthetic learners like to touch and manipulate objects.

Multiple Choice

Select the one best answer to the following multiple-choice questions. Check Appendix G for the correct answers.

Exercise 5

1. Diagrams, shapes, and patterns are examples of which type of data?
   a. Kinesthetic
   b. Visual
   c. Solitary
   d. Verbal
2. Posters, flash cards, and PowerPoint presentations all appeal to:
   a. Kinesthetic learners
   b. Visual learners
   c. Auditory learners
   d. Social learners
3. Which of the following statements is true regarding visual learners?
   a. They can recall information by "seeing" it in their mind's eye.
   b. During conversations they use visual words such as "touch" and "feel."
   c. They like to bounce things off their friends.
   d. None of these.

4. All of the following techniques are helpful to visual learners **except**:
   a. Mnemonics
   b. Acronyms
   c. Group discussion
   d. Rhymes

5. Oral discussions appeal to students with which learning style?
   a. Verbal
   b. Auditory
   c. Social
   d. All of these

6. Which of the following statements are true regarding global learners?
   a. They are sometimes called sequential learners.
   b. They like to analyze details.
   c. Their learning styles may be a mix of visual and auditory.
   d. They approach problem-solving in a very logical manner.

7. All of the following words of advice are specifically appropriate for global learners **except**:
   a. You are a multitasker, so don't be afraid to mix it up a bit and make your study efforts more lively and enjoyable.
   b. Begin each study session by identifying the relationship between what you are currently studying and your future career ambitions.
   c. Beware of your tendency to get stuck in analysis paralysis.
   d. While reading, make note of terms or concepts that you skipped over and later take time to look them up.

8. All of the following statements are true regarding analytical learners **except**:
   a. They approach problem-solving in a logical, methodical manner.
   b. They dislike following official procedures.
   c. They seek to quantify things whenever possible.
   d. They often pursue careers in accounting, sciences, and engineering.

9. All of the following words of advice are specifically appropriate for analytical learners **except**:
   a. Prioritize items of importance for studying.
   b. Consider seeking work in an area that allows you to process and analyze data.
   c. Consider recording lectures.
   d. All of these.

10. Which of the following statements about memory is true?
    a. Most data moves easily from short-term to long-term memory.
    b. Emotional feelings affect whether some information is stored in long-term memory.
    c. Cramming is an effective method of transmitting data into long-term memory.
    d. All of these.

MEDICAL WORD ELEMENTS 2

Word Parts

Most medical words derive from Greek or Latin and therefore may look and sound odd to you. However, once you have taken the time to learn the meanings of the word parts, you will be able to understand most of the medical terms you encounter, regardless of how big or complex they appear. There are three types of word parts and two classes of words that you need to know. The three types of word parts are combining forms (created by joining a *word root* to a *combining vowel*), prefixes, and suffixes. The two classes of words are abbreviations and pathology terms.

Combining Forms

The ***combining form (CF)*** is created by joining a ***word root (WR)*** with a ***combining vowel (CV)***. A word root is the main stem of the word. An example using a nonmedical term is the word *walked.* The main stem or root of this word is *walk.*

walked main stem or root word

CF = WR + CV

The purpose of a combining vowel is to make the medical term easier to pronounce. You could say that it makes medical terms more "user friendly" for the tongue. In nearly all cases, the combining vowel is an ***o***, although there are a few exceptions. The combining vowel has no impact on the meaning of the term; it is placed between word parts to link them together. For example, consider the root *therm,* which means *heat.* If this word root is combined with an *o* (CV), the result is the ***combining form therm/o.*** Combining vowels are typically used to link word parts together regardless of whether the following part is a suffix or another combining form.

Flashpoint

The combining vowel doesn't change the word's meaning, but it does make it easier to pronounce.

When to Use a Combining Vowel

To determine the need for a combining vowel, notice whether the following word part begins with a consonant or a vowel. If it begins with a consonant, as in the word *therm/o/meter,* then a combining vowel (often *o*) is usually needed. However, if the next word part begins with a vowel (*a, e, i, o, u*), then a combining vowel is usually not needed. This is because the vowel at the beginning of the next word part serves as the combining vowel. For example, when the root *arthr,* which means *joint,* is combined with the suffix *-itis,* which means *inflammation,* no combining vowel is needed. The *i* in *-itis* serves as the combining vowel. The new term *arthr/itis* is created, which means *inflammation of a joint.* This term may already be familiar to you.

> **Flashpoint**
> When a term is created by using a combining vowel to link two word parts together, the emphasis nearly always shifts to the syllable containing the combining vowel. The vowel, when an *o*, also changes to a short "ah" sound. See the following examples:
>
> thermometer:
> pronounced
> thĕr-MŎ-mĕ-tĕr
> gastroscopy:
> pronounced
> găs-TRŎS-kō-pē

Prefixes

A ***prefix*** is a word part that comes at the beginning of the word. For example, again consider the word root *therm.* If it is joined with the prefix ***hypo-*** (*beneath or below*) and the suffix *-ia* (*condition*), then a new word is created: ***hypo****/therm/ia*, a condition of low heat. As you may already know, this term is used in reference to a condition of low body temperature.

> **Flashpoint**
> *Pre* means *before,* so it makes sense that prefixes are located at the beginnings of words.

Suffixes

A ***suffix*** is a word part that comes at the end of the word. If the suffix ***-meter*** (*instrument used to measure*) is added to the combining form *therm/o*, the result is the creation of the word *therm/o/****meter***, an instrument used to measure heat.

The terms we have been using are diagrammed below so that you can clearly see how the word parts fit together, as well as when and why combining vowels are used.

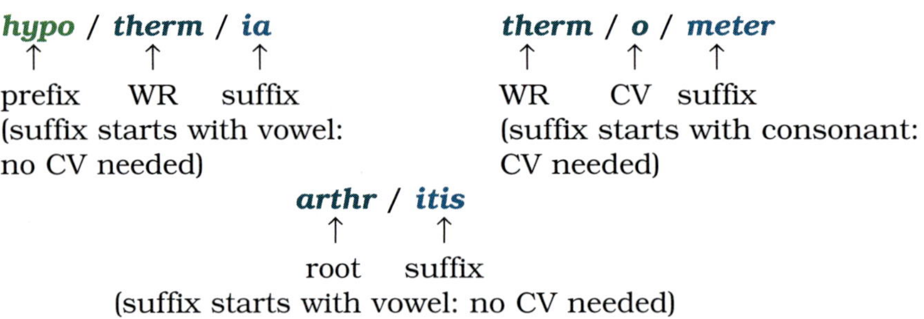

> **Flashpoint**
> Suffixes are located at the ends of words.

Three Simple Steps

There are just three simple steps to follow as you begin deciphering medical terms:

1. Translate the *last* word part first.
2. Translate the *first* word part next.
3. Translate *following* word parts in order.

It's that simple. Here is an example: Consider the term **esophagogastroduodenoscopy**. This term is quite a mouthful and may seem rather intimidating. However, we will follow the three simple steps described above, and you will see how easy it can be to decipher its meaning. You may find it helpful to put slashes between the word parts: esophag/o/gastr/o/duoden/o/scopy. After practicing these steps a few times, you won't need to do this anymore.

Step 1

-Scopy is a ***suffix*** that means *visual examination.*

Step 2
Esophag/o is a ***combining form*** that means *esophagus.*

Step 3
Gastr/o is a ***combining form*** that means *stomach.*
Duoden/o is a ***combining form*** that means *duodenum,* which is the first part of the small intestine.

Now put it all together. The final translation of esophagogastroduodenoscopy: **visual examination of the esophagus, stomach, and duodenum,** also known as an **upper endoscopy**.

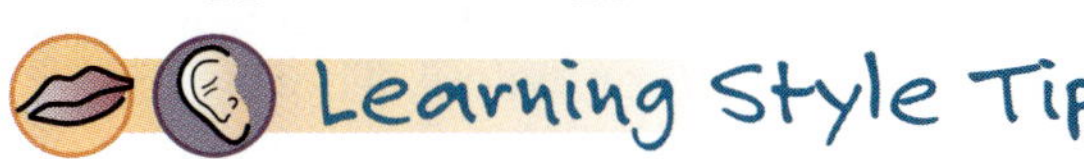

Give note cards with terms and definitions to friends and family members. Ask them to quiz you every time they see you (or chat with you on the phone).

Flashpoint
It may help you to remember the order in which to complete these steps if you consider the order in which you write your name on most legal forms: last, first, middle.

Abbreviations

Abbreviations are used extensively in health care because there are so many terms that are lengthy and difficult to pronounce. Abbreviations save time and simplify the speaking and writing of such terms. However, it is very important that you only use abbreviations that are commonly recognized and have been approved by the facility in which you work. Making up your own abbreviations or using ones not recognized by your facility can lead to communication errors and can potentially jeopardize patient well-being. Two examples of commonly used abbreviations are ***CAD***, which stands for *coronary artery disease,* and ***EGD***, which is the abbreviation for the large term you just learned, *esophagogastroduodenoscopy.* As you continue through this book, you will notice that each chapter contains a table of abbreviations that pertain to the body system you are studying.

Flashpoint
Abbreviations save time and are much easier to say and write than large terms.

Pathology Terms

Pathology terms are used extensively in health care; they refer to diseases and disorders of all body systems. An example is ***multiple sclerosis***, a chronic disease in which nerves lose the ability to transmit messages to the muscles. Students sometimes struggle with these terms because the three-step deciphering process that you just learned often does not work with these terms. Learning and remembering pathology terms requires study and memorization. However, this book includes some helpful tips to assist you with this process. The pathology terms are presented in color-coded sections of each chapter and are included in the learning exercises at the end of each chapter. There are also color-coded flash cards for many of the pathology terms from each chapter.

Closer Look

Let's take a closer look at the concepts mentioned previously.

Prefixes

Prefixes are always located at the beginnings of words, and they always modify the meaning of the word in some way. As an example, let's take another look at the word *hypothermia.* The prefix ***hypo-*** means *beneath* or *below.* Therefore, this term indicates *a condition of heat that is below normal.* A common cause of hypothermia is exposure to cold weather without adequate clothing.

Now let's see what happens when we change the prefix to ***hyper-***, which means *excessive* or *above.* The newly created word, *hyperthermia,* means *a condition of excessive heat.* This term refers to high body temperature. As you can see, changing the prefix can drastically change the meaning of the term. Hyperthermia might refer to a fever caused by an illness such as the flu. Another example of hyperthermia is heatstroke, a life-threatening condition caused when a person becomes too hot and dehydrated. This typically occurs when a person is exposed to a hot, humid environment and does not use adequate cooling measures.

Flashpoint
Prefixes always change the meaning of the term.

This chapter introduces you to a large number of prefixes. They have been grouped according to several general categories. Table 2-1 includes prefixes that indicate size, quantity, or number. In some cases the term is quite specific: For example, the prefix *tri-* means *three,* and the prefixes *quadri-* and *tetra-* mean *four.* In other cases the terms are less specific and refer to general amounts. Examples are the terms *multi-*, which means *many,* and *poly-*, which means *much.* Other terms such as *a-* and *an-* indicate the absence of something. The term *anuria,* for example, indicates *absence of urine,* and the term *anacusia* indicates *absence of hearing.* To begin familiarizing yourself with these prefixes, read through the following tables and answer the questions in the exercises that follow them. Note that the prefixes are generally arranged in alphabetical order; however, where there are two or more terms with the same or very similar meanings, they are grouped together. This will make them easier for you to learn. Don't worry about word building yet. Just focus on learning and memorizing these prefixes. To help you with this process, study these tables using the following steps:

1. Read the prefix in the first column.
2. Practice pronouncing the prefix correctly by using the guide in the second column.
3. Read the meaning aloud in the third column.
4. Write the prefix in the fourth column as you again pronounce it aloud.

Note that most of these prefixes will be reviewed again throughout the following chapters.

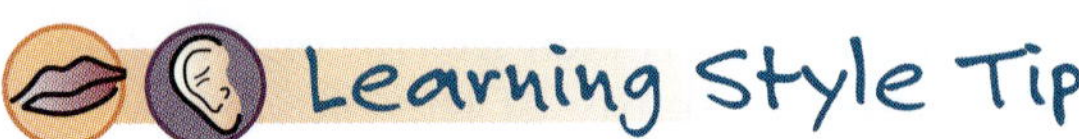

Reading the terms aloud helps verbal and auditory learners. If you are a verbal learner, you need to say them. If you are an auditory learner, you need to hear them, even if it is in your own voice.

TABLE 2-1
PREFIXES THAT INDICATE SIZE, QUANTITY, OR NUMBER

Prefix	Pronunciation Guide	Meaning	Write the Prefix
a-, an-, in-	ā, ăn, ĭn	without, not, absence of	
ambi-	ăm-bē	both, both sides, around, about	
bi-	bī	two	
di-	dī	twice, two, double	
hemi-, semi-	hĕm-ē, sĕm-ē	half	
iso-	ī-sō	same, equal	
macro-	mă-krō	large	
micro-	mī-krō	small	
mono-, uni-	mŏ-nō, ū-nĭ	one, single	
multi-	mŭl-tē	many	
poly-	pŏ-lē	much	
oligo-	ō-lĭ-gō	deficiency	
pan-	păn	all	
quadri-, tetra-	kwŏ-drĭ, tĕ-tră	four	
tri-	trī	three	

Practice Exercises

Fill in the Blanks

Fill in the blanks below using prefixes from Table 2-1. Check Appendix G for the correct answers.

Exercise 1

1. Prefixes that mean *one* are ______________ and ______________.
2. The prefix that means *deficiency* is ______________.
3. The prefix that means *small* is ______________.
4. Prefixes that mean *without, not,* or *absence of* are ______________, ______________, and ______________.
5. Prefixes that mean *four* are ______________ and ______________.

6. Prefixes that mean *half* are ______________________ and ______________________.

7. The prefix that means *both* or *both sides* is ______________________.

8. The prefix that means *large* is ______________________.

9. The prefix that means *much* is ______________________.

10. The prefix that means *same* or *equal* is ______________________.

True or False

Decide whether the following statements are true or false. Check Appendix G for the correct answers.

Exercise 2

1.	True	False	The prefix *ambi-* means *half.*
2.	True	False	The prefix *macro-* means *small.*
3.	True	False	The prefix *iso-* means *same* or *equal.*
4.	True	False	The prefix *pan-* means *none* or *zero.*
5.	True	False	The prefix *tri-* means *three.*
6.	True	False	The prefixes *bi-* and *di-* mean *three.*
7.	True	False	The prefix *micro-* means *small.*
8.	True	False	The prefixes *quadri-* and *tetra-* mean *two.*
9.	True	False	The prefix *multi-* means *many.*
10.	True	False	The prefixes *semi-* and *hemi-* mean *half.*

Learning Style Tip

Use the flash cards every day. They were created especially for you! Read both sides and be sure to note the visual cues on most of them.

Prefixes That Indicate Location, Direction, or Timing

The prefixes in Table 2-2 indicate location, direction, or timing. For example, the prefix *epi-* in *epigastric* indicates a physical location *above* the stomach. The prefix *circum-* in *circumoral* indicates a physical location *around* the mouth. The prefixes *brady-* and *tachy-* are commonly used to indicate timing or speed. *Bradykinesia* indicates *slow movement* and *tachycardia* indicates *rapid heartbeat.* Other terms may indicate direction. For example, the prefix *ab-* in *abduction* indicates movement *away from* the body and the prefix *ad-* in *adduction* indicates movement *toward* the body.

TABLE 2-2
PREFIXES THAT INDICATE LOCATION, DIRECTION, OR TIMING

Prefix	Pronunciation Guide	Meaning	Write the Prefix
ab-	ăb	away from	
ad-	ăd	toward	
anti-	ăn-tē	against	
brady-	bră-dē	slow	
con-	kŏn	together, with	
contra-	kŏn-tră	against, opposite	
circum-	sĕr-kŭm	around	
dia-, trans-	dī-ă, trănz	through, across	
ec-, ecto-	ĕk, ĕk-tō	out, outside	
en-, end-, endo-, in-, intra-	ĕn, ĕnd, ĕn-dō, ĭn, ĭn-tră	in, within, inner	
epi-	ĕ-pĭ	above, upon	
eso-	ĕs-ō	inward	
ex-, exo-, extra-	ĕks, ĕk-sō, ĕk-stră	away from, outside, external	
hyper-, super-, supra-	hī-pĕr, soo-pĕr, soo-pră	excessive, above	
hypo-, infra-, sub-	hī-pō, ĭn-fră, sŭb	below, beneath	
inter-	ĭn-tĕr	between	
para-, peri-	pă-ră, pĕr-ĭ	beside, near	
post-	pōst	after, following	
pre-	prē	before	
pro-	prō	before, forward	
re-, retro-	rē, rĕ-trō	behind, back	
tachy-	tăk-ē	rapid	
ultra-	ŭl-tră	beyond	

Practice Exercises

Fill in the Blanks

Fill in the blanks below using prefixes from Table 2-2. Check Appendix G for the correct answers.

Exercise 3

1. The prefix that means *beyond* is ____________________.
2. The prefix that means *away from* is ____________________.

3. Prefixes that mean *across* or *through* are ______________ and ______________.

4. Prefixes than mean *in, within,* or *inner* are ______________, ______________, ______________, ______________, and ______________.

5. The prefix that means *toward* is ______________.

6. The prefix that means *slow* is ______________.

7. The prefix that means *above* or *upon* is ______________.

8. Prefixes that mean *out* or *outside* are ______________ and ______________.

9. Prefixes than mean *away from, outside,* or *external* are ______________, ______________, and ______________.

10. The prefix that means *around* is ______________.

True or False

Decide whether the following statements are true or false. Check Appendix G for the correct answers.

Exercise 4

1. True False The prefix *anti-* means *against.*
2. True False The prefix *tachy-* means *rapid.*
3. True False The prefixes *re-* and *retro-* mean *behind* or *back.*
4. True False The prefix *epi-* means *below.*
5. True False The prefix *con-* means *together* or *with.*
6. True False The prefix *contra-* means *against* or *opposite.*
7. True False The prefix *eso-* means *outward.*
8. True False The prefixes *hyper-*, *super-*, and *supra-* mean *excessive* or *above.*
9. True False The prefixes *para-* and *peri-* mean *beside* or *near.*
10. True False The prefix *pro-* means *between.*

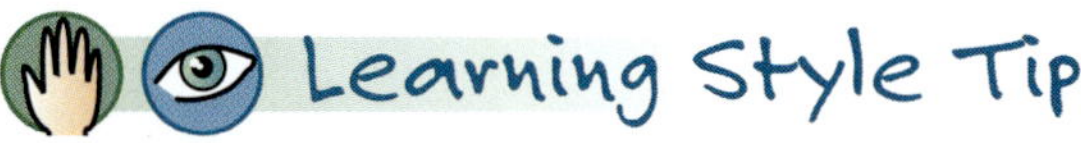

Physically holding and flipping through flash cards (while reading them, of course) helps kinesthetic and visual learners learn and remember.

TABLE 2-3
OTHER PREFIXES

Prefix	Pronunciation Guide	Meaning	Write the Prefix
auto-	aw-tō	self	
dys-	dĭs	bad, painful, difficult	
eu-	ū	good, normal	
mal-	măl	bad, inadequate	
neo-	nē-ō	new	
tox-	tŏks	poison, toxin	

Other Prefixes

Table 2-3 includes prefixes that indicate a variety of other meanings.

Practice Exercises

Fill in the Blanks

Fill in the blanks below using prefixes from Table 2-3. Check Appendix G for the correct answers.

Exercise 5

1. The prefix that means *poison* is ____________________.
2. The prefix that means *good* or *normal* is ____________________.
3. Thc prcfix that mcans *new* is ____________________.
4. The prefix than means *bad, painful,* or *difficult* is ____________________.
5. The prefix that means *self* is ____________________.

True or False

Decide whether the following statements are true or false. Check Appendix G for the correct answers.

Exercise 6

1. True False The prefix *mal-* means *against.*
2. True False The prefix *neo-* means *new.*
3. True False The prefix *tox-* means *try.*

4. True False The prefix *auto-* means *car.*

5. True False The prefix *dys-* means *self.*

STOP HERE.
Select the Prefix Flash Cards and run through them at least three times before you continue.

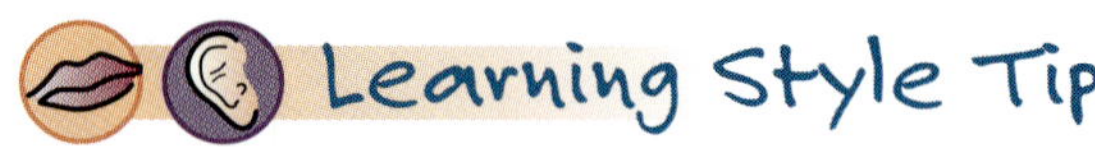

Study with a partner so you can take turns quizzing each other. Verbalizing terms and definitions helps verbal learners; listening to each other helps auditory learners.

Suffixes

Suffixes are word parts that appear at the ends of words and modify the meaning in some way. Consider the combining form *appendic/o,* which means *appendix.* If the suffix ***-itis*** (*inflammation*) is added, the term *appendic/itis* is created. As you may already know, this term means *inflammation of the appendix.*

> **Flashpoint**
> Suffixes always change the meaning of the term.

This chapter introduces you to a large number of suffixes. They have been grouped according to several general categories. Note that the suffixes are generally arranged in alphabetical order; however, where there are two or more suffixes with the same or similar meanings, they are grouped together. This will make them easier for you to learn. Don't worry about word building yet. Just focus on learning and memorizing these suffixes. To help you with this process, study the suffix tables using the following steps:

1. Read the suffix in the first column.
2. Practice pronouncing the suffix correctly by using the guide in the second column.
3. Read the meaning aloud in the third column.
4. Write the suffix in the fourth column as you again pronounce it aloud.

Table 2-4 shows suffixes that indicate medical specialty and Table 2-5 contains suffixes that indicate surgeries, procedures, or treatments. Note that these suffixes will be reviewed again throughout the following chapters.

Practice Exercises

Fill in the Blanks

Fill in the blanks using suffixes from Tables 2-4 and 2-5. Check Appendix G for the correct answers.

TABLE 2-4
SUFFIXES THAT INDICATE MEDICAL SPECIALTY

Suffix	Pronunciation Guide	Meaning	Write the Suffix
-iatrics, -iatry	ī-ă-trĭks, ī-ă-trē	field of medicine	
-iatrist, -ician, -ist	ī-ă-trĭst, ĭ-shŭn, ĭst	specialist	
-logist, -ologist	lō-jĭst, ŏl-ō-jĭst	specialist in the study of	
-logy, -ology	lō-jē, ŏl-ō-jē	study of	

TABLE 2-5
SUFFIXES THAT INDICATE SURGERIES, PROCEDURES, OR TREATMENTS

Suffix	Pronunciation Guide	Meaning	Write the Suffix
-centesis	sĕn-tē-sĭs	surgical puncture	
-cidal, -cide	sī-dăl, sīd	destroying, killing	
-desis	dē-sĭs	surgical fixation of bone or joint, binding, tying together	
-dilation	dī-lā-shŭn	widening, stretching, expanding	
-ectomy	ĕk-tō-mē	excision, surgical removal	
-graphy	gră-fē	process of recording	
-metry	mĕ-trē	measurement	
-pexy	pĕk-sē	surgical fixation	
-plasty	plăs-tē	surgical repair	
-rrhaphy	ră-fē	suture, suturing	
-scopy	skō-pē	visual examination	
-therapy	thĕr-ă-pē	treatment	
-tomy	tō-mē	cutting into, incision	
-tripsy	trĭp-sē	crushing	

Exercise 7

1. Suffixes that mean *field of medicine* are ______________________ and ______________________.

2. Suffixes that mean *specialist in the study of* are ______________________ and ______________________.

3. The suffix that means *surgical repair* is ______________________.

4. Suffixes that mean *destroying* or *killing* are ______________________ and ______________________.

5. The suffix that means *process of recording* is ____________________.

6. The suffixes *-logy* and *-ology* mean ____________________.

7. The suffix *-desis* means ____________________.

8. The suffix *-ectomy* means ____________________.

9. The suffix *-metry* means ____________________.

10. The suffix *-scopy* means ____________________.

True or False

Decide whether the following statements are true or false. Check Appendix G for the correct answers.

Exercise 8

1.	True	False	The suffix *-graphy* means *measurement.*
2.	True	False	The suffix *-dilation* means *widening, stretching,* or *expanding.*
3.	True	False	The suffix *-plasty* means *surgical repair.*
4.	True	False	The suffix *-therapy* means *treatment.*
5.	True	False	The suffix *-ician* means *technician.*
6.	True	False	The suffix *-pexy* means *pain.*
7.	True	False	The suffix *-rrhaphy* means *suture* or *suturing.*
8.	True	False	The suffix *-tomy* mean *cutting into* or *incision.*
9.	True	False	The suffix *-tripsy* means *treatment.*
10.	True	False	The suffix *-centesis* means *centimeter.*

Objective and Subjective Data

When documenting information in a patient's medical record, health-care providers often categorize it as either objective or subjective data. Objective data includes information that can be observed, measured, or quantified in some way. An example is a patient's temperature measured with a thermometer. Even observations made about a patient's behavior are objective. Examples include descriptions of body posture, movement, and verbal statements. In contrast, information about how a patient is feeling is a classic example of subjective data; it does not lend itself to measurement or observation. Examples of subjective information include physical sensations such as pain or nausea and emotional feelings such as anger, sadness, or happiness. You may find this confusing, since no doubt you have observed people's behavior and concluded they were happy, sad, mad, or ill. However, what you observed was their behavior, not their actual physical sensations or emotional feelings. Perhaps this will seem clearer when you consider a time when you assumed someone was feeling a certain way only to learn that you were mistaken. Your assumption was based upon your interpretation of the behavioral clues you saw. However, the only way to ever know for sure how another person feels is for them to tell you.

Suffixes That Indicate Sensation, Feeling, Action, or Movement

Table 2-6 includes suffixes that indicate sensory experience, sensation, or subjective feeling. Table 2-7 includes suffixes that indicate action or movement. Some refer to conscious actions an individual takes, such as speech (*-phasia*). Others indicate action within the body that is involuntary (*-spasm*). Note that many of these suffixes will be reviewed again throughout the following chapters.

Flashpoint

An easy way to remember the difference between subjective and objective is that **s**ubjective data is based on what the patient **s**ays. **O**bjective data is based on what you **o**bserve.

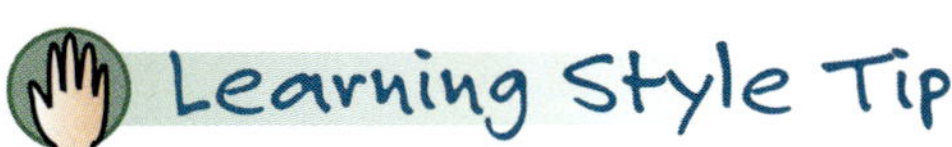

Kinesthetic learners need to move. So imagine you are playing charades—or really play—and challenge yourself to act out each of the terms as you study them.

TABLE 2-6

SUFFIXES THAT INDICATE SENSORY EXPERIENCE, SENSATION, OR SUBJECTIVE FEELING

Suffix	Pronunciation Guide	Meaning	Write the Suffix
-acusia, -acusis, -cusis	ă-koo-zē-ă, ă-koo-sĭs, koo-sĭs	hearing	
-algesia, -algesic, -algia, -dynia	ăl-jē-zē-ă, ăl-jē-zĭk, ăl-jē-ă, dĭ-nē-ă	pain	
-dipsia	dĭp-sē-ă	thirst	
-esthesia	ĕs-thē-zē-ă	sensation	
-opia, -opsia, -opsis, -opsy	ō-pē-ă, ŏp-sē-ă, ŏp-sĭs, ŏp-sē	vision, view of	
-osmia	ŏz-mē-ă	smell, odor	
-phobia	fō-bē-ă	fear	
-phoria	fō-rē-ă	feeling	

TABLE 2-7

SUFFIXES THAT INDICATE ACTION OR MOVEMENT

Suffix	Pronunciation Guide	Meaning	Write the Suffix
-clasis, -clast	klăs-ĭs, klăst	to break	
-ectasis	ĕk-tă-sĭs	dilation, expansion	
-emesis	ĕm-ĕ-sĭs	vomiting	
-gen, -genesis, -genic, -genous	jĕn, jĕn-ĕ-sĭs, jĕn-ĭk, jēn-ŭs	creating, producing	
-kinesia, -kinesis	kĭ-nē-zē-ă, kĭ-nē-sĭs	movement	

Continued

TABLE 2-7
SUFFIXES THAT INDICATE ACTION OR MOVEMENT—cont'd

Suffix	Pronunciation Guide	Meaning	Write the Suffix
-lysis	lĭ-sĭs	destruction	
-pause, -stasis	pawz, stă-sĭs	cessation, stopping	
-phage, -phagia	fāj, fā-jē-ă	eating, swallowing	
-phasia	fā-zē-ă	speech	
-rrhage, -rrhagia	rĭj, ră-jē-ă	bursting forth	
-rrhea	rē-ă	flow, discharge	
-rrhexis	rĕk-sĭs	rupture	
-spasm	spă-zŭm	sudden involuntary contraction	
-uresis	ū-rē-sĭs	urination	

Practice Exercises

Fill in the Blanks

Fill in the blanks below using suffixes from Tables 2-6 and 2-7. Check Appendix G for the correct answers.

Exercise 9

1. Suffixes that mean *hearing* are ____________________, ____________________, and ____________________.

2. Suffixes that mean *vision* or *view of* are ____________________, ____________________, ____________________, and ____________________.

3. The suffix that means *feeling* is ____________________.

4. The suffix that means *smell* or *odor* is ____________________.

5. Suffixes that mean *creating* or *producing* are ____________________, ____________________, ____________________, and ____________________.

6. Suffixes that mean *bursting forth* are ____________________ and ____________________.

7. Suffixes that mean *eating* or *swallowing* are ____________________ and ____________________.

8. The suffix that means *vomiting* is ______________________.

9. The suffix that means *destruction* is ______________________.

10. The suffix that means *rupture* is ______________________.

True or False

Decide whether the following statements are true or false. Check Appendix G for the correct answers.

Exercise 10

1. True False The suffixes *-acusia*, *-acusis*, and *-cusis* mean *pain.*
2. True False The suffix *-dipsia* means *feeling.*
3. True False The suffixes *-opia*, *-opsia*, *-opsis*, and *-opsy* mean *vision* or *view of.*
4. True False The suffix *-osmia* means *sound.*
5. True False The suffix *-esthesia* means *sensation.*
6. True False The suffixes *-algesia*, *-algesic*, *-algia*, and *-dynia* mean *pain.*
7. True False The suffix *-phobia* means *fear.*
8. True False The suffixes *-clast* and *-clasis* mean *cessation.*
9. True False The suffix *-pause* means *relaxation.*
10. True False The suffix *-phasia* means *eating* or *swallowing.*

Suffixes That Indicate Diseases, Disorders, or Conditions

Many suffixes in the medical language indicate diseases, disorders, or conditions; these are demonstrated in Table 2-8. Some terms, such as *-derma* (*skin*),

Flashpoint
Many suffixes provide clues about the nature or location of the disorder.

TABLE 2-8
SUFFIXES THAT INDICATE DISEASES, DISORDERS, OR CONDITIONS

Suffix	Pronunciation Guide	Meaning	Write the Suffix
-cele	sēl	hernia	
-constriction	kŏn-strĭk-shŭn	narrowing	
-cytosis	sī-tō-sĭs	a condition of cells	
-derma	dĕr-mă	skin	
-edema	ĕ-dē-mă	swelling	
-emia	ē-mē-ă	a condition of the blood	

Continued

TABLE 2-8

SUFFIXES THAT INDICATE DISEASES, DISORDERS, OR CONDITIONS—cont'd

Suffix	Pronunciation Guide	Meaning	Write the Suffix
-gravida	gră-vĭ-dă	pregnant woman	
-ia, -ism	ē-ă, ĭz-ŭm	condition	
-iasis	ī-ă-sĭs	pathological condition or state	
-itis	ī-tĭs	inflammation	
-lepsy, -leptic	lĕp-sē, lĕp-tĭk	seizure	
-lith	lĭth	stone	
-malacia	mă-lā-sē-ă	softening	
-megaly	mĕg-ă-lē	enlargement	
-necrosis	nĕ-krō-sĭs	tissue death	
-oid	oyd	resembling	
-oma	ō-mă	tumor	
-osis	ō-sĭs	abnormal condition	
-oxia	ŏk-sē-ă	oxygen	
-paresis	pă-rē-sĭs	slight or partial paralysis	
-partum, -tocia	pārt-ŭm, tō-sē-ă	childbirth, labor	
-pathy	pă-thē	disease	
-penia	PĒ-nē-ă	deficiency	
-pepsia	pĕp-sē-ă	digestion	
-phonia	fō-nē-ă	voice	
-plasia, -plasm	plā-zē-ă, plăz-ŭm	formation, growth	
-plastic	plăs-tĭk	pertaining to formation or growth	
-plegia	plē-jē-ă	paralysis	
-plegic	plē-jĭk	pertaining to paralysis	
-pnea	nē-ă	breathing	
-pneic	nē-ĭk	pertaining to breathing	
-ptosis	tō-sĭs	drooping, prolapse	
-salpinx	săl-pĭnks	uterine (fallopian) tube	
-sclerosis	sklĕ-rō-sĭs	hardening	
-static	stă-tĭk	not in motion, at rest	
-stenosis	stĕ-nō-sĭs	narrowing, stricture	
-thorax	thōr-ăks	chest	
-trophy	trō-fē	nourishment, growth	
-uria	ū-rē-ă	urine	

-emia (*a condition of the blood*), and *-thorax* (*chest*), provide specific clues about the body part involved. Other terms, such as *-constriction* (*narrowing*), *-edema* (*swelling*), and *-itis* (*inflammation*), provide clues about the nature of the disease or disorder. Note that many of these suffixes will be reviewed again throughout the following chapters.

Practice Exercises

Fill in the Blanks

Fill in the blanks below using suffixes from Table 2-8. Check Appendix G for the correct answers.

Exercise 11

1. The suffix that means *pregnant woman* is ______________________.
2. The suffix that means *stone* is ______________________.
3. Suffixes that mean *seizure* are ______________________ and ______________________.
4. The suffix that means *hernia* is ______________________.
5. The suffix that means *softening* is ______________________.
6. The suffix that means *voice* is ______________________.
7. The suffix that means *not in motion* or *at rest* is ______________________.
8. The suffix that means *narrowing* or *stricture* is ______________________.
9. The suffix that means *tumor* is ______________________.
10. The suffix that means *resembling* is ______________________.

True or False

Decide whether the following statements are true or false. Check Appendix G for the correct answers.

Exercise 12

1. True False The suffix *-lith* means *little.*
2. True False The suffixes *-ia* and *-ism* mean *condition.*
3. True False The suffix *-derma* means *down.*

4. True False The suffix *-megaly* means *motion.*

5. True False The suffix *-necrosis* means *tissue death.*

6. True False The suffixes *-partum* and *-tocia* mean *person.*

7. True False The suffix *-osis* means *oxygen.*

8. True False The suffix *-trophy* means *nourishment* or *growth.*

9. True False The suffix *-thorax* means *chest.*

10. True False The suffix *-rrhea* means *flow or discharge.*

Other Suffixes

There are literally thousands of medical instruments, used for countless procedures and treatments. Many are categorized according to their general purpose. Cutting instruments go by various names, many ending with the suffix *-tome.* Recording instruments also have many different names; however, many of them end with the suffix *-graph.* Many instruments used for measurement end with the suffix *-meter,* and many of those used for viewing various parts of the body end with the suffix *-scope.* These terms are listed in Table 2-9. Another group of commonly used suffixes all mean *pertaining to* (see Table 2-10). Still other suffixes not easily categorized are listed in Table 2-11. Table 2-12 lists the rules for changing the endings of some terms from the singular to the plural form.

TABLE 2-9

SUFFIXES THAT INDICATE INSTRUMENTS

Suffix	Pronunciation Guide	Meaning	Write the Suffix
-graph	grăf	recording instrument	
-meter	mĕ-tĕr	measuring instrument	
-scope	skōp	viewing instrument	
-tome	tōm	cutting instrument	

TABLE 2-10

SUFFIXES THAT MEAN "PERTAINING TO"

Suffix	Pronunciation Guide	Meaning	Write the Suffix
-ac, -al, -ar, -ary, -eal, -ial, -ic, -ical, -ory, -ous, -tic*, -tous*	ăk, ăl, ăr, ār-ē, ē-ăl, ē-ăl, ĭk, ĭ-kăl, ō-rē, ŭs, tĭk, tŭs	pertaining to	

*-tic, a variation of -ic is sometimes used; -tous, a variation of -ous is sometimes used.

TABLE 2-11
OTHER SUFFIXES

Suffix	Pronunciation Guide	Meaning	Write the Suffix
-cyte, -cytic	sīt, sīt-ĭk	cell	
-gram	grăm	record	
-ole, -ule	ōl, ūl	small	
-prandial	prăn-dē-ăl	meal	
-stomy	stō-mē	mouthlike opening	

TABLE 2-12
PLURAL ENDINGS

Singular Form	Plural Form	Rule	Singular Example	Plural Example
-a	-ae	retain -a and add -e	vertebra	vertebrae
-ax	-aces	drop -x and add -ces	thorax	thoraces
-is	-es	drop -is and add -es	diagnosis	diagnoses
-ix, -ex	-ices	drop -ix or -ex and add -ices	appendix	appendices
-um	-a	drop -um and add -a	diverticulum	diverticula
-us	-i	drop -us and add -i	thrombus	thrombi
-y	-ies	drop -y and add -ies	ovary	ovaries

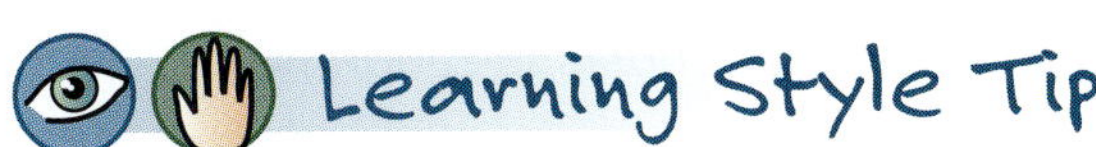

Use brightly colored highlighters to color-code categories of information such as prefixes, suffixes, and combining forms.

Flashpoint
The suffixes of many instrument names provide clues about their purpose or function.

Practice Exercises

Fill in the Blanks

Fill in the blanks below using Tables 2-9 through 2-12. Check Appendix G for the correct answers.

Exercise 13

1. The suffix that means *recording instrument* is ____________________.
2. The suffix that means *cutting instrument* is ____________________.
3. The suffix that means *measuring instrument* is ____________________.

4. The suffix that means *viewing instrument* is ______________________.

5. Suffixes that mean *cell* are ______________________ and ______________________.

6. The suffix that means *meal* is ______________________.

7. Suffixes that mean *small* are ______________________ and ______________________.

8. The suffix that means *mouthlike opening* is ______________________.

9. The suffix that means *deficiency* is ______________________.

10. The suffix that means *record* is ______________________.

True or False

Decide whether the following statements are true or false. Check Appendix G for the correct answers.

Exercise 14

1.	True	False	The suffixes *-al, -ial, -tic,* and *-tous* mean *pertaining to.*
2.	True	False	The suffixes *-ole* and *-ule* mean *pertaining to.*
3.	True	False	The suffixes *-cyte* and *-cytic* mean *small.*
4.	True	False	The plural form of the word *appendix* is *appendixes.*
5.	True	False	The plural form of the word *diagnosis* is *diagnoses.*
6.	True	False	The suffixes *-ac, -ar, -ory,* and *-ous* mean *pertaining to.*
7.	True	False	The plural form of the word *thrombus* is *thrombuses.*
8.	True	False	The suffixes *-y, -um,* and *-ex* mean *pertaining to.*
9.	True	False	The suffixes *-ary, -ical, -ic,* and *-eal* mean *pertaining to.*
10.	True	False	The plural form of the word *diverticulum* is *diverticula.*

Deciphering Terms

Occasionally you will find a word made up of only a prefix and a suffix. Some examples are listed below. Write the correct meaning of these medical terms. Check Appendix G for the correct answers.

Exercise 15

1. bilateral ____

2. hypoxia ____

3. euphoria ______________________________

4. anacusis ______________________________

5. anosmia ______________________________

6. hemiplegia ______________________________

7. polyuria ______________________________

8. bradykinesia ______________________________

9. postpartum ______________________________

10. neoplasm ______________________________

Pronunciation

It often takes a considerable amount of practice before the pronunciation of medical terms comes easily and naturally. It will help if you develop good habits right from the start. Carefully review the pronunciation guidelines in Table 2-13. These guidelines will help you learn correct pronunciation.

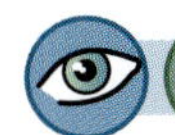 **Learning Style Tip**

Use a white board to write colorful notes or draw diagrams and funny pictures of important data.

TABLE 2-13
PRONUNCIATION GUIDE

Letters	Guidelines	Examples
ae and oe	pronounce only the *e*	pleurae (PLOO-rē)
-es	when located at the end of a word, may be pronounced as a separate syllable	nares (NĀR-ēz)
g and c	pronounce as *j* and *s* before *e, i,* and *y*	generic (jĕ-NĔR-ĭk) gelatin (JĔL-ă-tĭn) cycle (SĪ-kĭl) cytology (sī-TŎ-lō-jē)
g and c	pronounce as *g* and *k* before other letters	gait (gāt) gastric (GĂS-trĭk) caffeine (kă-FĒN) calcium (KĂL-sē-ŭm)
-i	when located at the end of a word, generally indicates a plural; pronounce as *ī* or *ē*	alveoli (ăl-VĒ-ō-lī) bronchi (BRŎNG-kī)
pn-	pronounce only the *n*	pneumonia (nū-MŌ-nē-ă) pneumatic (nū-MĂT-ĭk)
ps-	pronounce only the *s*	psoriasis (sō-RĪ-ă-sĭs) psychology (sī-KŎL-ō-jē)

STOP HERE.
Select the Suffix Flash Cards and run through them at least three times before you continue.

Practice Exercises

Deciphering Terms

Occasionally you will find a word made up of only a prefix and a suffix. Some examples are listed below. Write the correct meaning of these medical terms. Check Appendix G for the correct answers.

Exercise 16

1. toxic ______________________________
2. autograph ______________________________
3. polyphobia ______________________________
4. anesthesia ______________________________
5. atrophy ______________________________
6. multigravida ______________________________
7. tetraplegia ______________________________
8. hyperemesis ______________________________
9. postprandial ______________________________
10. dyspnea ______________________________

Multiple Choice

Select the one best answer to the following multiple-choice questions. Check Appendix G for the correct answers.

Exercise 17

1. Which of the following prefixes is matched with the correct definition?
   a. *Ambi-*: against
   b. *An-*: with
   c. *Pan-*: without
   d. *Bi-*: two

2. The prefixes *hemi-* and *semi-* mean:
   a. Both, both sides
   b. Twice, two, double
   c. Half
   d. Whole
3. Which of the following prefixes is matched with the correct definition?
   a. *Infra-*: above
   b. *Pro-*: beyond
   c. *Re-*: behind, back
   d. *Ultra-*: after
4. Which of the following prefixes means *bad* or *inadequate*?
   a. *Mal-*
   b. *Eu-*
   c. *Tox-*
   d. *Auto-*
5. The prefix *auto-* means:
   a. New
   b. Poison
   c. Self
   d. None of these
6. The suffix *-pexy* means:
   a. Widening, stretching, expanding
   b. Surgical fixation
   c. Surgical puncture
   d. Measurement
7. Which of the following suffixes is matched with the correct definition?
   a. *-Phoria*: fear
   b. *-Phobia*: feeling
   c. *-Dynia*: pain
   d. *-Algia*: sound

8. Which of the following suffixes is matched with the correct definition?
   a. *-Edema*: eating
   b. *-Lith*: loosening
   c. *-Malacia*: softening
   d. *-Megaly*: measurement

9. Which of the following suffixes is matched with the correct definition?
   a. *-Paresis*: pregnancy
   b. *-Partum*: partial
   c. *-Plegia*: pain
   d. *-Pnea*: breathing

10. All of the following suffixes mean *pertaining to* **except**:
    a. *-Ar*
    b. *-Ory*
    c. *-Itis*
    d. *-Tic*

11. All of the following prefixes mean *without, not,* or *absence of* **except**:
    a. *An-*
    b. *In-*
    c. *Uni-*
    d. *A-*

12. Which of the following prefixes means *all?*
    a. *Pan-*
    b. *Ambi-*
    c. *Multi-*
    d. *Micro-*

13. The prefix *di-* means:
    a. Diagonal
    b. Diagram
    c. Dilate
    d. None of these

14. The prefixes *a-*, *an-*, and *in-* all mean:

    a. Both, double

    b. Without, not, of

    c. Many, much

    d. None of these

15. Which of the following prefixes is matched with the correct definition?

    a. *Mono-*: one, single

    b. *Multi-*: twice

    c. *A-*: with

    d. *Hemi-*: whole

16. Which of the following prefixes is matched with the correct definition?

    a. *Neo-*: new

    b. *Eu-*: good, normal

    c. *Dys-*: bad, painful

    d. All of these

17. Which of the following prefixes means *bad, painful,* or *difficult?*

    a. *Tox-*

    b. *Eu-*

    c. *Dys-*

    d. *Neo-*

18. The prefix *neo-* means:

    a. Self

    b. Bad

    c. New

    d. None of these

19. The suffix *-ician* means:

    a. Field of medicine

    b. Study of

    c. Specialist

    d. Physician

20. Which of the following suffixes is matched with the correct definition?
    a. *-Lysis*: flow, discharge
    b. *-Cele*: pregnant woman
    c. *-Kinesia*: movement
    d. *-Uresis*: eating, swallowing

21. Which of the following suffixes is matched with the correct definition?
    a. *-Ology*: study of
    b. *-Opsy*: vision, view of
    c. *-Cidal*: destroying, killing
    d. All of these

22. Which of the following suffixes is matched with the correct definition?
    a. *-Iasis*: illusion
    b. *-Necrosis*: tissue death
    c. *-Oma*: hernia
    d. *-Oxia*: air

23. All of the following suffixes mean *pain* **except**:
    a. *-Algesic*
    b. *-Dynia*
    c. *-Phobia*
    d. *-Algia*

24. Which of the following terms has been correctly changed to the plural form?
    a. Thorax: thoraces
    b. Diagnosis: diagnoses
    c. Diverticulum: diverticula
    d. All of these

25. Which of the following prefixes means *in, within, or inner?*
    a. *Endo-*
    b. *Contra-*
    c. *Super-*
    d. *Trans-*

LEVELS OF ORGANIZATION 3

Overview

The human body is arranged in a complex, yet orderly fashion (see Fig. 3-1). Therefore a systematic approach to studying it is helpful. Chemistry courses typically study the human body at the atomic and molecular levels. Some biology courses, such as cellular biology, study the body at the cellular level. Other courses such as anatomy and physiology and medical terminology generally study the body at the organ and organ-system levels. This will be our approach.

Cell Level

Cells are the structural units that form all body tissues. Their functions are consistent with the functions of the tissues they comprise. Their walls are composed of a membrane made up of lipids (fats), proteins, and other components that selectively allow certain substances, such as nutrients, to enter and other substances, such as wastes, to leave. Within the cell is a gelatinous substance called cytoplasm. It surrounds a variety of tiny structures called organelles that are important to cellular function. The largest of these is the nucleus. Contained within the nucleus is deoxyribonucleic acid (DNA), which is the genetic material that makes up the blueprint for your body. It includes information that determines your gender, skin, hair and eye colors, and numerous other features.

Flashpoint
There are many different specialized cell types in the human body. Just a few categories are muscle cells, bone cells, and nerve cells (neurons).

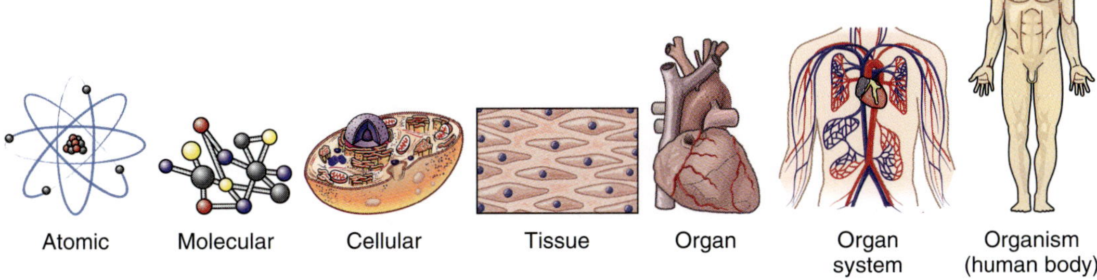

FIGURE 3-1 Levels of organization

Tissue Level

Tissue is composed of a group of similar cells that perform a specific function. The types of tissue are epithelial, connective, nervous, and muscle tissues.

Epithelial tissue forms the epidermis (top layer of the skin) and surface layer of the membranes. It may be composed of a single layer (simple), or of several layers (stratified). It is also classified according to the cell shape: squamous (flat), cuboidal (cube shaped), or columnar (cylindrical) (see Fig. 3-2). Epithelial tissue has many functions, including protection, absorption, and secretion. Because of its location and the large amount of wear and tear it undergoes, it has an amazing ability to replace itself, sometimes as often as every 24 hours.

Flashpoint

Epithelial tissue has an amazing ability to replace itself.

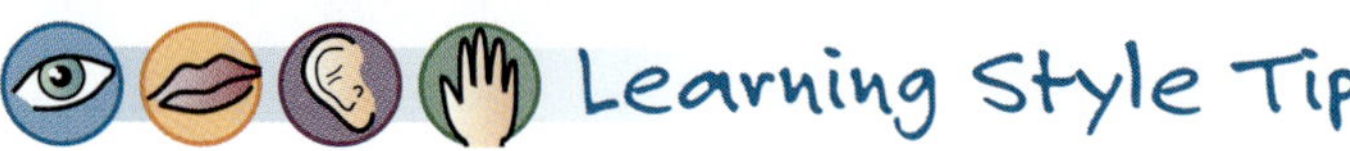

Sketch simple drawings of the three cellular shapes with colorful markers and label them. Speak aloud as you do this. Kinesthetic learners will remember this even better if they make models of cells out of clay.

Simple Squamous Cells

Simple squamous cells are flat in shape.

Simple Cuboidal Cells

Simple cuboidal cells are cube shaped.

Simple Columnar Cells

Simple columnar cells are cylindrical in shape.

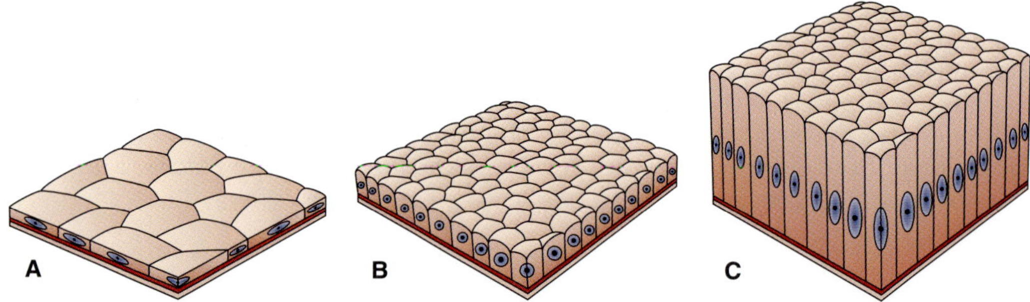

FIGURE 3-2 **Common cell shapes: (A) Squamous cells, (B) Cuboidal cells, (C) Columnar cells**

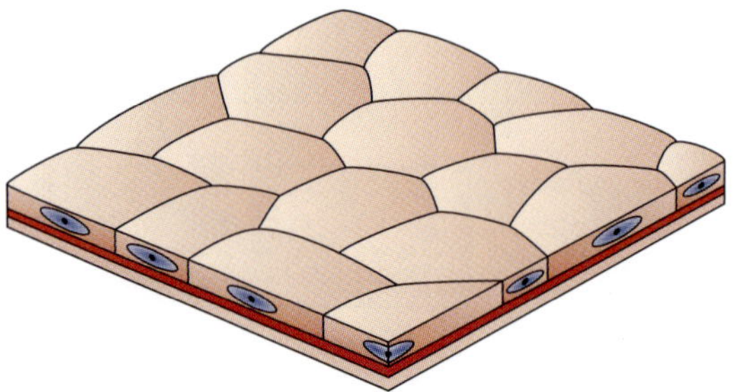

FIGURE 3-3 **Simple squamous cells**

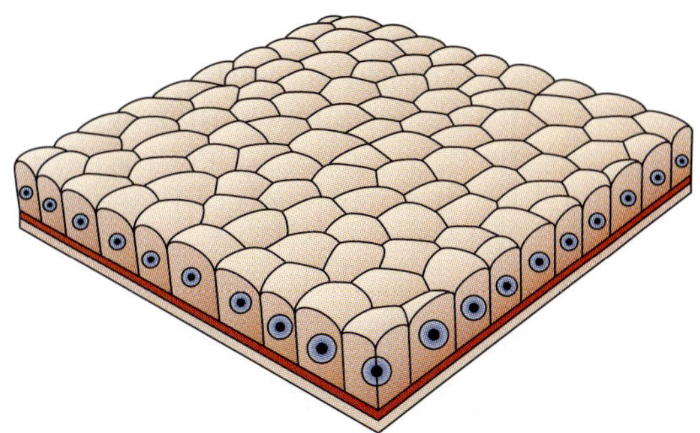

FIGURE 3-4 **Simple cuboidal cells**

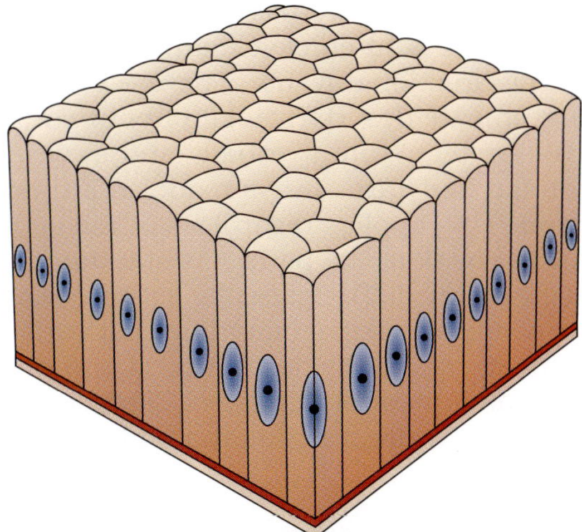

FIGURE 3-5 **Simple columnar cells**

Connective Tissue

Connective tissue acts to connect and support other body tissues. There are various types of connective tissue, including cartilage, adipose (fat), bone, elastic fiber, and even blood.

Flashpoint

Connective tissue does just what its name suggests: It connects and supports other body tissues.

Nervous Tissue

Nervous tissue is composed of nerve cells called neurons, which function to transmit nerve impulses by the release of chemicals called neurotransmitters. Nervous tissue comprises the brain, spinal cord, and nerves for the entire body.

Muscle Tissue

Muscle tissue comprises cells called contractile fibers. As each muscle cell contracts or relaxes, it shortens or lengthens. Consequently, the muscle also shortens or lengthens. Muscles help you move your body, make your heart beat, help many of your internal organs function, and maintain your blood pressure.

Organ and Organ-System Level

Organs are structures made up of two or more types of tissue that perform specialized functions. For example, the heart is composed of cardiac muscle tissue, various types of membranes, and special nervous tissue. Many organs and related structures function together as organ systems to accomplish a specific purpose. For example, the heart acts as a pump; along with a complex network of arteries, veins, and capillaries, it comprises the cardiovascular system. This system circulates blood throughout your body for your entire lifetime. There are many other organ systems as well. You will learn about each of these as you read this book.

Directional Terms and Anatomical Position

Accurate communication is critically important in the world of health care. To ensure that this occurs, all health-care workers must speak the language of medical terminology, in a clear and efficient manner. You will begin learning this language by learning directional terms. The use of these terms will enable you to accurately communicate descriptive data about your patient to other members of the health-care team, both verbally and in writing.

References to the human body are always made as if the patient is standing in the **anatomical position**. This applies regardless of the actual position of the patient. In the anatomical position, the patient is standing upright, with arms at the side and palms facing forward. The patient's legs are straight and the toes are pointing forward. The midline is an imaginary line that runs from the head to the feet and through thc umbilicus and divides the body into right and left halves. The midline is often used as a point of reference. Table 3-1 includes commonly used directional terms and provides a list of anatomical orientations.

Flashpoint
Having a good command of directional terms will enable you to communicate accurately with others, whether you are speaking verbally or writing in the medical record.

Body Planes

Body planes are imaginary slices or cuts through the body that divide it vertically or horizontally. They are used as points of reference. To visualize this, imagine a person standing in an upright position. Now imagine dissecting this person with imaginary vertical and horizontal planes. The **sagittal** plane runs vertically from front to back and divides the body into right and left halves. The **frontal** plane runs vertically from left to right and divides the body into front and back portions. The **transverse** plane is horizontal and divides the body into upper and lower portions.

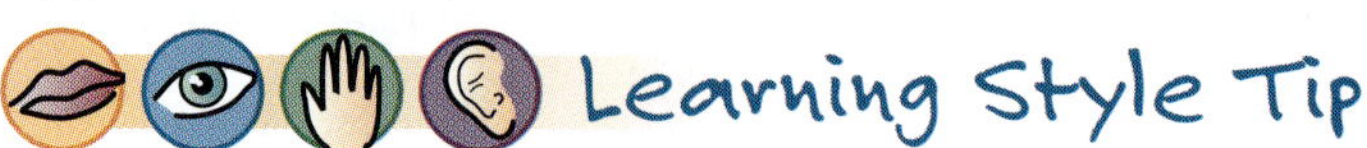

Study with several classmates or enlist the help of family or friends. Identify one person as your patient. Write directional terms on pieces of tape and take turns placing them on the appropriate parts of the patient's body. For the midline, use one long piece of tape; for the planes, pretend to slice the patient into sections. Speak aloud throughout the activity to achieve the full verbal and auditory benefit.

Body Cavities, Regions, and Quadrants

The body is divided into a dorsal cavity and a ventral cavity (see Fig. 3-6). The dorsal cavity is located on the posterior or back part of the body. It is further

TABLE 3-1
DIRECTIONAL TERMS AND ANATOMICAL ORIENTATIONS

Term	Combining Form	Meaning	Term	Combining Form	Meaning
abduction		movement away from the body	adduction		movement toward the body
anterior	anter/o	toward or near the front; ventral	posterior	poster/o	toward or near the back; dorsal
base		the lower or supporting part of any structure	apex		the pointed tip of a conical structure
deep		further into the body	superficial		near the surface of the body
medial	medi/o	toward the midline; nearer to the middle	lateral	later/o	away from the midline; toward the side
proximal	proxim/o	nearer to the origin or point of attachment	distal	dist/o	further from the origin or point of attachment
superior	super/o	above or nearer to the head	inferior	infer/o	beneath or nearer to the feet
supine		lying horizontally facing upward	prone		lying horizontally facing downward
ventral	ventr/o	front; anterior	dorsal	dors/o	back; posterior

divided into the cranial cavity, which contains the brain, and the vertebral cavity, which contains the spinal column. The ventral cavity, located on the anterior or front side of the body, consists of the thoracic and abdominopelvic cavities. The thoracic cavity contains the lungs, heart, great vessels, trachea, and thymus. The abdominopelvic cavity is one large cavity, but an imaginary line is sometimes drawn to create a boundary between the abdominal and pelvic cavities. The abdominal cavity contains the stomach, pancreas, liver, gallbladder, and large and small intestines. The kidneys lie at the back of the abdomen in an area called the retroperitoneal space, just lateral to (to the side of) the spinal column. The pelvic cavity contains the sigmoid colon, rectum, bladder, and—in females—the uterus, fallopian tubes, and ovaries.

Two systems are commonly used to visually divide the abdominopelvic cavity for communication and documentation purposes. The nine-region system divides it into nine approximately equal sections, much like a tic-tac-toe grid. The four-quadrant system divides it into four equal sections, which intersect at the umbilicus (see Fig. 3-7). The midline is an imaginary parallel line that runs through the umbilicus and divides the body into right and left halves.

Flashpoint
The nine regions divide the abdomen into a tic-tac-toe-like grid.

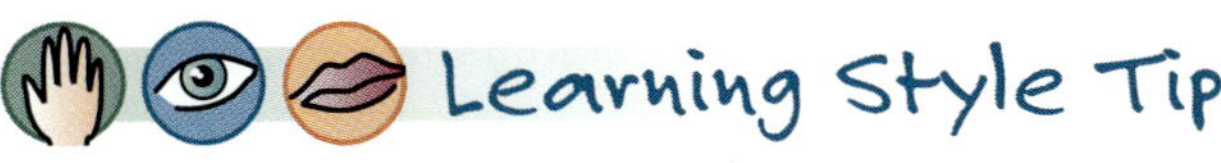

Study with several classmates or enlist the help of family or friends. Identify two people to serve as the patients. Use strips of tape to divide one patient's abdomen into quadrants and the other patient's abdomen into regions. Next add pieces of tape with the correct names to label each quadrant or region.

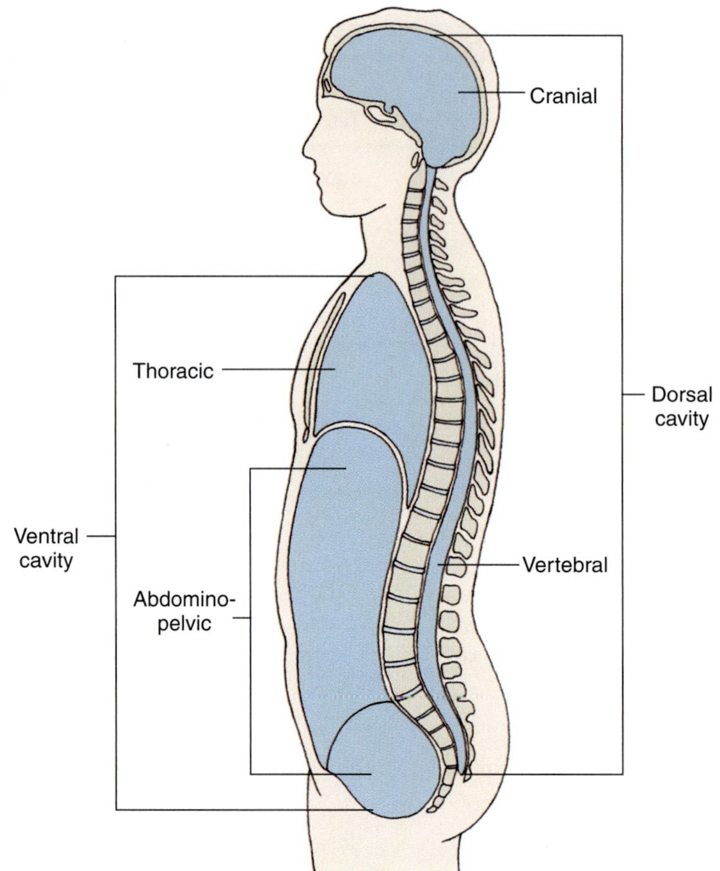

FIGURE 3-6 **Body cavities**

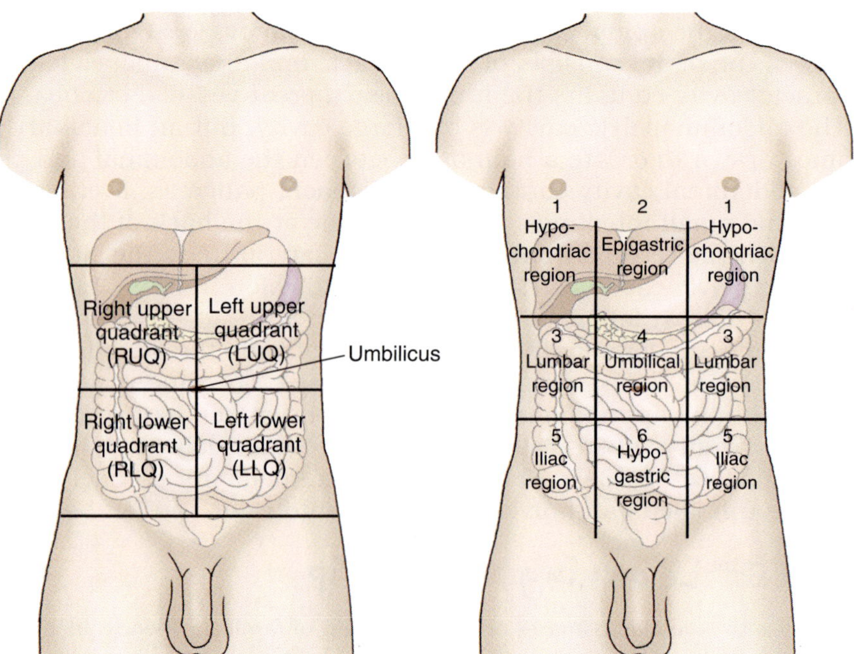

FIGURE 3-7 **Abdominal quadrants and regions**

TABLE 3-2

ABBREVIATIONS

AP	anteroposterior	PA	posteroanterior
LAT	lateral	RLQ	right lower quadrant
LE	lower extremity	RUQ	right upper quadrant
LLQ	left lower quadrant	UE	upper extremity
LUQ	left upper quadrant		

Abbreviations

Table 3-2 lists some of the most common abbreviations related to body organization, as well as others often used in medical documentation.

Practice Exercises

Directional Terms

Complete the following practice exercises using Tables 3-1 and 3-2. Check Appendix G for the correct answers.

Exercise 1

1. **Fill in the blanks in Figure 3-8 with the correct names of the body cavities.**

2. **Fill in the blanks in Figure 3-9 with the correct names of the abdominal quadrants and regions.**

Multiple Choice

Select the one best answer to the following multiple-choice questions. Check Appendix G for the correct answers.

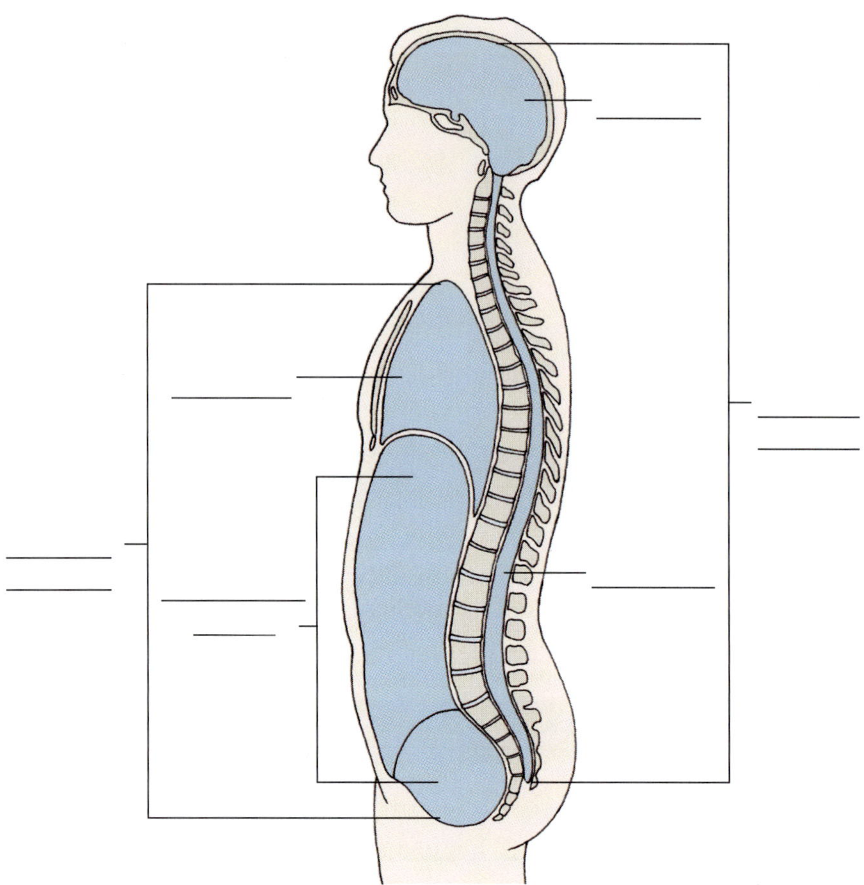

FIGURE 3-8 Body cavities with blanks

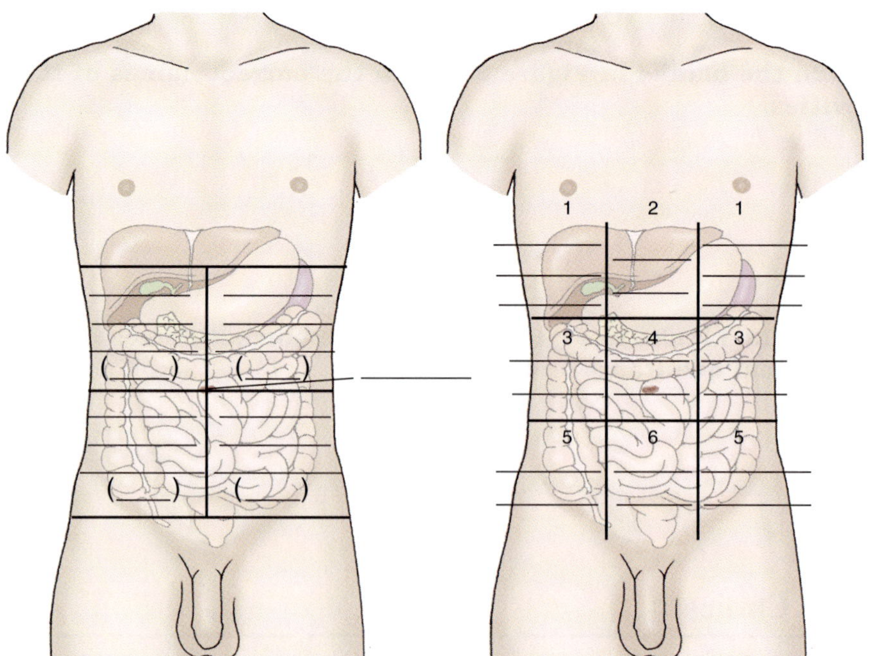

FIGURE 3-9 Abdominal quadrants and regions with blanks

Exercise 2

1. What term describes the position of the elbow relative to the wrist?
   a. Anterior
   b. Distal
   c. Lateral
   d. Superior
2. Levels of organization of the human body from smallest to largest are:
   a. Molecular, tissue, atomic, cellular, organ, organ system, human body
   b. Atomic, molecular, cellular, tissue, organ, organ system, human body
   c. Tissue, cellular, atomic, molecular, organ, organ system, human body
   d. None of these
3. What term describes the position of the fingers relative to the wrist?
   a. Superior
   b. Medial
   c. Distal
   d. Anterior
4. All of the following are types of tissues in the human body **except**:
   a. Staphylococci
   b. Connective
   c. Nervous
   d. Muscle
5. Movement away from the body is known as:
   a. Adduction
   b. Abduction
   c. Addiction
   d. Transverse

Locating Body Parts Using Directional Terms

Place the following letters at the specified locations on Figure 3-10. Check Appendix G for the correct answers.

Exercise 3

1. **Place the letter A just superior to the right elbow on the anterior surface of the arm.**
2. **Place the letter B on the anterior, superior surface of the head.**

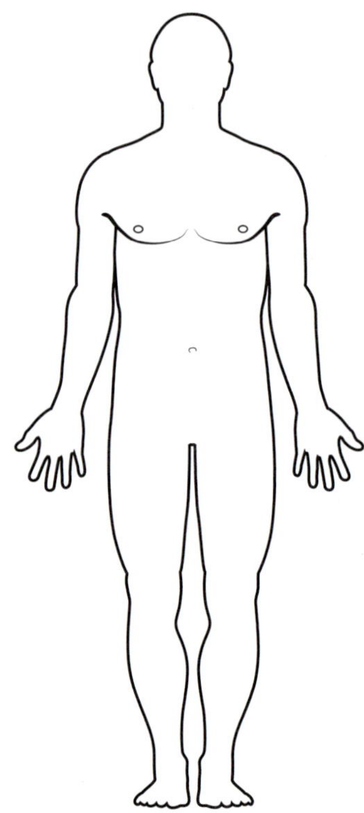

FIGURE 3-10 **Human body illustration**

3. **Place the letter C on the distal portion of the left arm on the anterior surface, just proximal to the wrist.**
4. **Place the letter D slightly inferior to the umbilicus.**
5. **Place the letter E just inferior to the right knee.**
6. **Place the letter F on the anterior chest wall, lateral to the sternum (center) on the left.**
7. **Place the letter G lateral to the umbilicus on the right.**
8. **Place the letter H proximal to the left knee.**

Fill in the Blanks

Fill in the blanks below. Check Appendix G for the correct answers.

Exercise 4

1. The abbreviation *LAT* stands for ________________________.
2. The pointed tip of the heart is the ________________________.
3. The abbreviation *UE* stands for ________________________.
4. A person who is lying down and facing upward is in the ________________________ position.
5. The abbreviation *RLQ* stands for ________________________.

6. Pain located near the body surface is said to be ________________________.

7. The abbreviation *PA* stands for ________________________.

8. A person who is lying facedown is in the ________________________ position.

9. The abbreviation *LUQ* stands for ________________________.

10. The bottom of the right lung may be described as the ________________________.

Multiple Choice

Select the one best answer to the following multiple-choice questions. Check Appendix G for the correct answers.

Exercise 5

1. Which of the following statements is true?
   a. The arrangement of the human body is simple.
   b. Chemistry courses typically study the body at the cellular level.
   c. Cellular biology courses study the body at the chemical level.
   d. Medical terminology generally studies the body at the organ and organ-system levels.

2. What term describes the position of the mouth relative to the nose?
   a. Superior
   b. Dorsal
   c. Proximal
   d. Inferior

3. Which of the following statements is true regarding cells?
   a. They are composed of body tissues.
   b. Their walls protect them by not allowing any substances to enter or leave.
   c. The fluid within cells is called plasma.
   d. The genetic blueprint of the body is contained within the cell nucleus.

4. Where is the right lung, in reference to the heart?
   a. Anterior
   b. Proximal
   c. Lateral
   d. Ventral

5. Which of the following statements is true?
   a. Squamous cells are cube shaped.
   b. Cuboidal cells are cylindrical in shape.
   c. Columnar cells are cube shaped.
   d. None of these.

INTEGUMENTARY SYSTEM

4

Structure and Function

You may not think of the skin as an organ, but it is actually the largest organ of the body. Let's take a look at the structure and function of the integumentary system.

The skin consists of three layers (see Fig. 4-1). The **epidermis** is the thin outer layer that is constructed mostly of nonliving, keratinized cells. It is waterproof and provides protection for the deeper layers. The epidermis is thickest on the soles of the hands and feet. The base of this layer, aptly named the **basement membrane**, is where new, living epidermal cells are produced. These cells are pushed upward as even newer cells form beneath them. Eventually they rise to the top, away from blood vessels and nerve endings, and die, thus

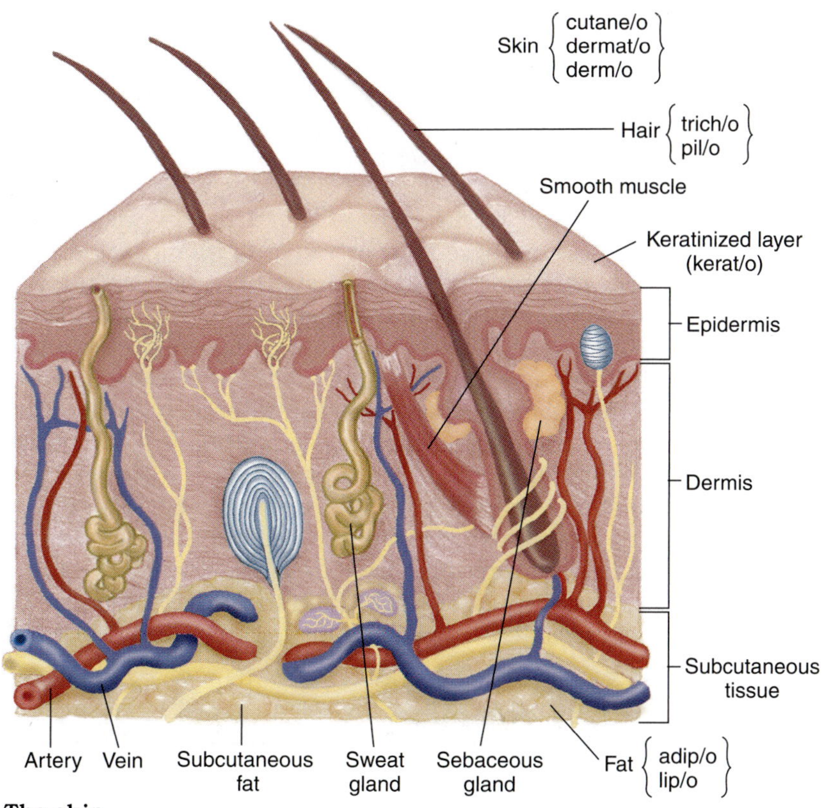

FIGURE 4-1 The skin

becoming keratinized (hardened) tissue. This is why cells on the top layer of your skin can be scraped away without causing pain.

Flashpoint
The prefix *epi-* means *above* or *upon;* so the name *epidermis,* which means *above or upon the dermis,* tells you exactly where it is located.

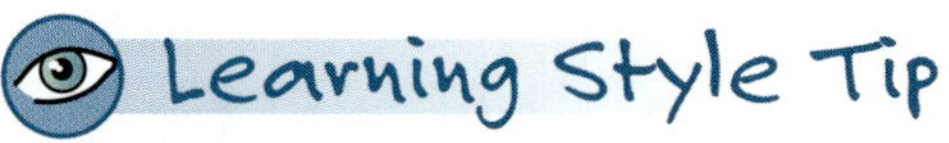

Visual learners should look carefully at the illustrations and photos in this book. They were created especially for you.

The **dermis** lies just beneath the epidermis and is much thicker. It is made up of fibrous connective tissue containing elastin, which provides elasticity, and collagen, which provides strength. It also contains a good blood supply and numerous other structures, including hair follicles, nerves, sweat glands, oil glands, and sensory receptors.

Beneath the dermis is the **subcutaneous layer**. This layer contains fat tissue as well as deeper blood vessels, nerves, the lower part of hair follicles, elastin, and collagen. The subcutaneous layer provides insulation for deeper structures.

Accessory structures of the skin include the **sudoriferous (sweat) glands, sebaceous (oil) glands,** hair, and nails. Sudoriferous glands are located throughout the body but are more concentrated in some areas, such as the soles of the feet and palms of the hands. Sebaceous glands are found at the base of hair follicles all over the body; they secrete an oily substance called sebum.

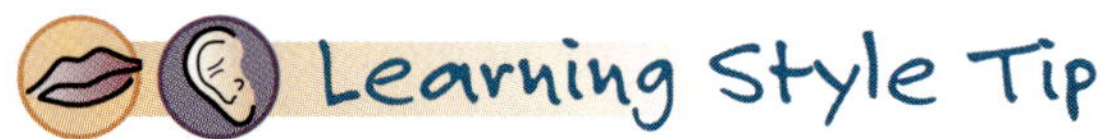

Verbal and auditory learners should remember that you need to *speak* and *hear* the information. Additionally, you may be a social learner—so find a study buddy or join a study group whenever possible.

The skin (and its accessory structures) serves several important functions in the body. Its major functions are protection and temperature regulation. It protects your body from bacteria and other microorganisms, damaging ultraviolet light from the rays of the sun, and extreme temperatures. Because the outer layer of your skin is waterproof, it keeps pathogens (tiny disease-causing organisms) from entering even when it gets wet, unless there is a break in the skin. Sebum discourages bacterial growth; it also lubricates your skin to keep it soft and supple. If pathogens do get in through a ***laceration*** (a cut or tear in the flesh) or an ***abrasion*** (an area where skin or mucous membranes are scraped away), infection may occur. However, as the tissue becomes irritated, a natural inflammatory response occurs. When this happens, the body increases circulation of blood to the injured area. This is responsible for the ***edema*** (swelling) and ***erythema*** (redness) that appear. Increased numbers of **leukocytes** (white blood cells) arrive to fight off the invaders and, quite literally, gobble them up. The increased circulation also helps speed the process of healing, as debris is cleared away and healthy new cells fill in the injured area, along with scar tissue.

The skin also contains **melanocytes**, which are pigment-producing skin cells. The pigment they produce, melanin, gives skin its colors. In response to ultraviolet light from the sun, melanocytes produce more melanin, causing a suntan. Melanin helps filter ultraviolet light and protect the skin from further damage. The amount of melanin in your skin varies depending on your heredity and ethnicity.

Flashpoint
Melanin in the skin turns dark to create a suntan.

Temperature and Pain Perception

Because the skin contains a number of different specialized nerves and sensory receptors, it plays a vital role in our ability to perceive cold and heat as well as pressure and pain. These messages signal us to take measures to increase physical comfort, such as putting on a coat for warmth. In addition, they also provide an important protective function: If you accidentally touch a very hot surface, your heat and pain receptors immediately send a message to your central nervous system, and you respond by pulling your hand away. Such a response is a protective **reflex**, which happens so quickly that you don't have time to think about it.

The integumentary system also plays an important role in body-temperature regulation. It provides insulation to keep you warm when the external environment is too cold. As your environment becomes colder, your hands and fingers become pale in color, because the blood vessels near your skin's surface constrict in order to give off less heat and thus conserve it for deeper organs. The opposite also occurs: When your environment is too hot, these same blood vessels dilate (expand) in order to give off more heat. This response may cause you to have a flushed appearance. In addition, your sweat glands secrete moisture, which evaporates on your skin's surface and provides even more cooling.

Hair and Nails

Hair and **nails** are also accessory structures of the integumentary system. Hair is found on most parts of the body and is especially prominent on the head, in the nose and ears, and on the face as eyebrows and eyelashes. It serves a protective function, as it filters out dust and debris from the air. The part of the hair that you can see is the hair shaft. The part buried in the skin is the hair follicle, which contains the root. Hair is made up of a protein called keratin; it gets its color from melanin. With aging, the amount of melanin may decrease, leading to graying of hair. As new cells are formed in the hair root, older keratinized cells are pushed up and become part of the hair shaft.

Nails help to protect the ends of our fingers and toes. The nail forms in the nail root and is made up of keratinized squamous epithelial cells. As nails grow in a flattened shape, they slide very slowly over a layer of epithelial tissue called the nail bed. The area at the base of the nail, sometimes called the half-moon, is the lunula. This is where new growth occurs. Figure 4-2 shows the structure of the nail.

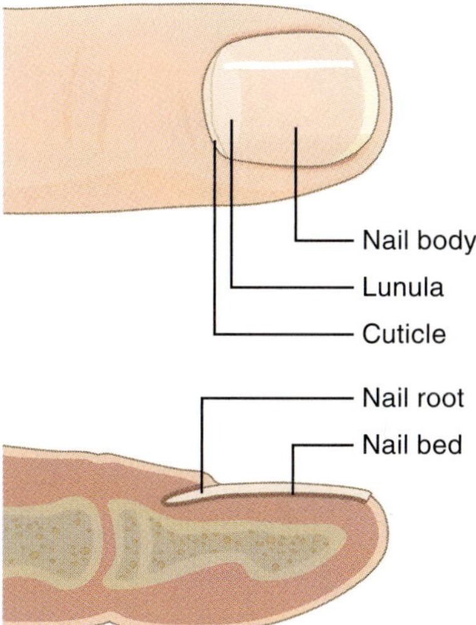

FIGURE 4-2 **Nail structure**

Flashpoint
Sensory receptors in the skin help to protect us from harm by signaling heat, cold, pressure, and pain.

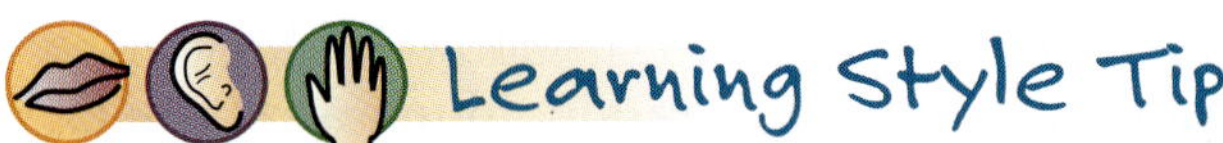

If you are a verbal and auditory learner, be sure to recite these new combining forms aloud so you benefit from saying and hearing them. Kinesthetic learners can have fun being overly dramatic with your expressions, pronunciation, and body movements as you say the terms. You may feel silly doing this, but you will remember the terms better later on.

Combining Forms

Table 4-1 lists combining forms that pertain to the integumentary system. Table 4-2 lists combining forms related to color.

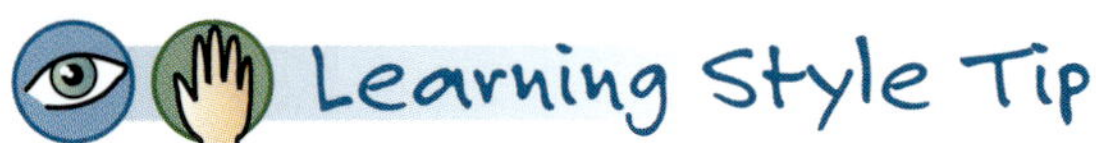

Visual and kinesthetic learners may use colored markers or pens to highlight or underline terms with their associated colors (e.g., highlight *cyan/o* in blue) and draw silly pictures to associate with any others that you can think of (e.g., draw a wrinkly face next to *rhytid/o*).

STOP HERE.
Select the Combining Form Flash Cards for Chapter 4 and run through them at least three times before you continue.

TABLE 4-1
COMBINING FORMS RELATED TO THE INTEGUMENTARY SYSTEM

Combining Form	Meaning	Example (Pronunciation)	Meaning of New Term
adip/o	fat	adipoid (Ă-dĭ-poyd)	resembling fat
lip/o		lipoma (lĭ-PŌ-mă)	tumor of fat
cutane/o	skin	cutaneous (kū-TĀ-nē-ŭs)	pertaining to the skin
derm/o		dermoplasty (DĔR-mō-plăs-tē)	surgical repair of the skin
dermat/o		dermatologist (dĕr-mă-TŎ-lō-jĭst)	specialist in the study of the skin
cyt/o	cell	cytology (sī-TŎ-lō-jē)	study of cells
eti/o	cause	etiology (ē-tē-Ŏ-lō-jē)	study of causes

TABLE 4-1
COMBINING FORMS RELATED TO THE INTEGUMENTARY SYSTEM—cont'd

Combining Form	Meaning	Example (Pronunciation)	Meaning of New Term
hidr/o	sweat	hidrosis (hī-DRŌ-sĭs)	abnormal condition of sweat
hydr/o	water	hydrotherapy (hī-drō-THĔR-ă-pē)	water therapy
idi/o	unknown, peculiar	idiopathic (ĭd-ē-ō-PĂTH-ĭk)	pertaining to an unknown disease
kerat/o	keratinized tissue, cornea	keratotomy (kĕr-ă-TŎ-tō-mē)	cutting into or incision of the cornea
morph/o	shape	morphology (mōr-FŎ-lō-jē)	study of shapes
myc/o	fungus	mycosis (mī-KŌ-sĭs)	abnormal condition of fungus
necr/o	dead	necrosis (nĕ-KRŌ-sĭs)	abnormal condition of dead (tissue)
onych/o	nail	onychomalacia (ŏn-ĭ-kō-mă-LĀ-sē-ă)	softening of the nail
path/o	disease	pathologist (pă-THŎ-lō-jĭst)	specialist in the study of disease
pil/o	hair	depilous (DĔP-ĭl-ŭs)	absence of hair
trich/o		trichopathy (trĭk-ŎP-ă-thē)	disease of the hair
rhytid/o	wrinkle	rhytidectomy (rĭt-ĭ-DĔK-tō-mē)	surgical removal of wrinkles
scler/o	hardening, sclera	sclerosis (sklĕ-RŌ-sĭs)	abnormal condition of hardening
seb/o	sebum	seborrhea (sĕ-bō-RĒ-ă)	flow or discharge of sebum
son/o	sound	sonogram (SŎ-nō-grăm)	record of sound
xer/o	dry	xeroderma (zēr-ō-DĔR-mă)	dry skin

TABLE 4-2
COMBINING FORMS RELATED TO COLOR

Combining Form	Meaning	Example	Meaning of New Term
albin/o	white	albinism (ĂL-bĭ-nĭ-zum)	condition of whiteness
leuk/o		leukorrhea (loo-kō-RĒ-ă)	white flow or discharge

Continued

TABLE 4-2

COMBINING FORMS RELATED TO COLOR—cont'd

chromat/o	color	chromatic (krō-MĂ-tĭk)	pertaining to color
cirrh/o	yellow	cirrhosis (sĭ-RŌ-sĭs)	abnormal condition of yellowness
xanth/o		xanthoderma (zăn-thō-DĔR-mă)	yellow skin
cyan/o	blue	cyanosis (sī-ă-NŌ-sĭs)	abnormal condition of blueness
erythem/o	red	erythematous (ĕr-ĭ-THĒM-ăt-us)	pertaining to redness
erythr/o		erythrocyte (ĕ-RĬTH-rō-sīt)	red (blood) cell
melan/o	black	melanoma (mĕ-lă-NŌ-mă)	black tumor

Practice Exercises

Fill in the Blanks

Fill in the blanks below using Tables 4-1 and 4-2. Check Appendix G for the correct answers.

Exercise 1

1. condition of whiteness ______________________
2. surgical removal of wrinkles ______________________
3. yellow skin ______________________
4. black tumor ______________________
5. abnormal condition of blueness ______________________
6. study of causes ______________________
7. white flow or discharge ______________________
8. pertaining to redness ______________________

9. red (blood) cell _______________

10. study of shapes _______________

11. specialist in the study of disease _______________

12. pertaining to color _______________

13. dry skin _______________

14. flow of sebum _______________

15. resembling fat _______________

16. abnormal condition of hardening _______________

17. tumor of fat _______________

18. absence of hair _______________

19. water therapy _______________

20. disease of the hair _______________

21. pertaining to the skin _______________

22. specialist in the study of the skin _______________

23. study of cells _______________

24. incision into the cornea _______________

25. surgical repair of the skin _______________

26. abnormal condition of fungus _______________

27. abnormal condition of dead (tissue) _______________

28. softening of the nail _______________

29. abnormal condition of yellowness _______________

30. abnormal condition of sweat _______________

31. record of sound _______________

32. pertaining to an unknown disease _______________

33. **Fill in the blanks in Figure 4-3 with the appropriate combining forms.**

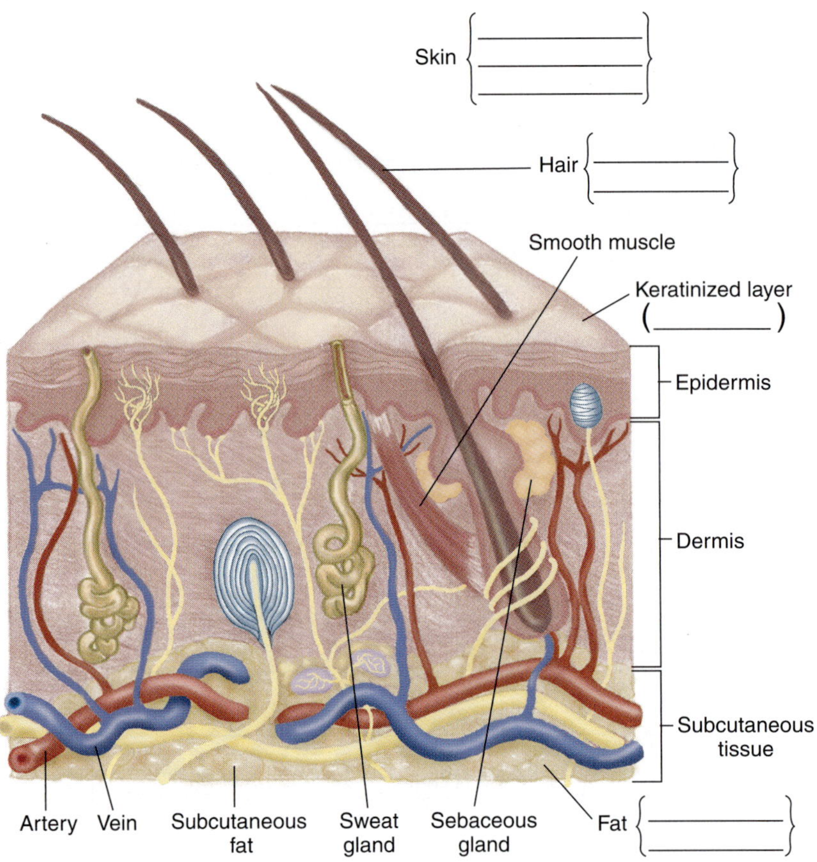

FIGURE 4-3 **Skin with blanks**

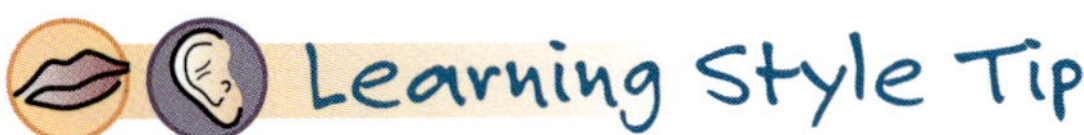

Learning Style Tip

If you are a verbal and auditory learner and are self-conscious about speaking aloud while studying, then find a private, secluded area like the back corner of the library, an empty classroom, or even your car.

Abbreviations

Abbreviations are used extensively in the world of health care. The primary reason is to save time in both written and verbal communications. As you will see, some medical terms are quite lengthy and difficult to pronounce. This is yet another reason for the use of abbreviations. Imagine having to say **endoscopic retrograde cholangiopancreatography** more than once in a conversation!

Table 4-3 lists some of the most common abbreviations pertaining to the integumentary system, as well as some that are commonly used for documentation or medication orders.

Flashpoint

Using abbreviations can save you time and lengthy documentation; but to avoid miscommunication, be sure to only use accurate, approved abbreviations.

STOP HERE.

Select the Abbreviation Flash Cards for Chapter 4 and run through them at least three times before you continue.

TABLE 4-3
ABBREVIATIONS

BCC	basal cell carcinoma	IV	intravenous
Bx, bx	biopsy	MM	malignant melanoma
C&S	culture and sensitivity	OTC	over-the-counter
decub	decubitus ulcer; also called *pressure ulcer*	PE	physical examination
derm	dermatology	SCC	squamous cell carcinoma
FH	family history	SubQ, Sub-Q	subcutaneous
Hx	history	Sx	symptom(s)
I&D	incision and drainage	Tx	treatment
ID	intradermal (injection)	ung	ointment

Pathology Terms

Table 4-4 lists many of the pathology terms that pertain to the integumentary system.

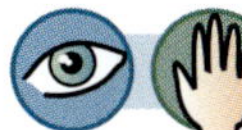
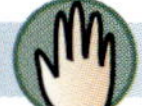

Learning Style Tip

Visual and kinesthetic learners may collect photos and illustrations of pathological conditions from journals, Internet image search engines, and other sources to create a poster or collage. Be sure to write the name of each disorder and a brief description next to each image. Tape the poster somewhere that you will see it daily, and review the information on it at least once each day.

STOP HERE.

Select the Pathology Term Flash Cards for Chapter 4 and run through them at least three times before you continue.

TABLE 4-4
PATHOLOGY TERMS

abrasion (ă-BRĀ-zhŭn)	scraping away of skin or mucous membranes
acne (ĂK-nē)	disease of the sebaceous (oil) glands and hair follicles in the skin, marked by plugged pores, pimples, cysts, and nodules on the face, neck, chest, back, and other areas
actinic keratosis (ăk-TĬ-nĭk kĕr-ă-TŌ-sĭs)	precancerous condition in which rough, scaly patches of skin develop, most commonly on sun-exposed areas such as the scalp, neck, face, ears, lips, hands, and forearms; also known as *solar keratosis*

Continued

TABLE 4-4

PATHOLOGY TERMS—cont'd

alopecia (ă-lō-PĒ-shē-ă)	autoimmune disease that results in loss of hair; alopecia areata causes patchy hair loss from the scalp; alopecia totalis causes total scalp hair loss; alopecia universalis causes total body hair loss (see Fig. 4-4)

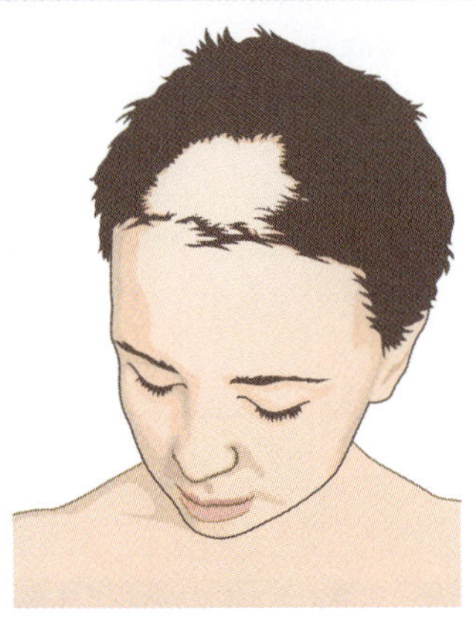

FIGURE 4-4 **Alopecia**

basal cell carcinoma (BĀ-săl sĕl kăr-sĭ-NŌ-mă)	common type of skin cancer that typically appears as a small, shiny papule and eventually enlarges to form a whitish border around a central depression or ulcer that may bleed
bulla (BŬ-lă)	large blister or skin vesicle filled with fluid
burn (bŭrn)	type of thermal injury to the skin caused by a variety of heat sources; classified according to severity as first-degree (superficial), second-degree (partial-thickness), and third-degree (full-thickness) (see Fig. 4-5)

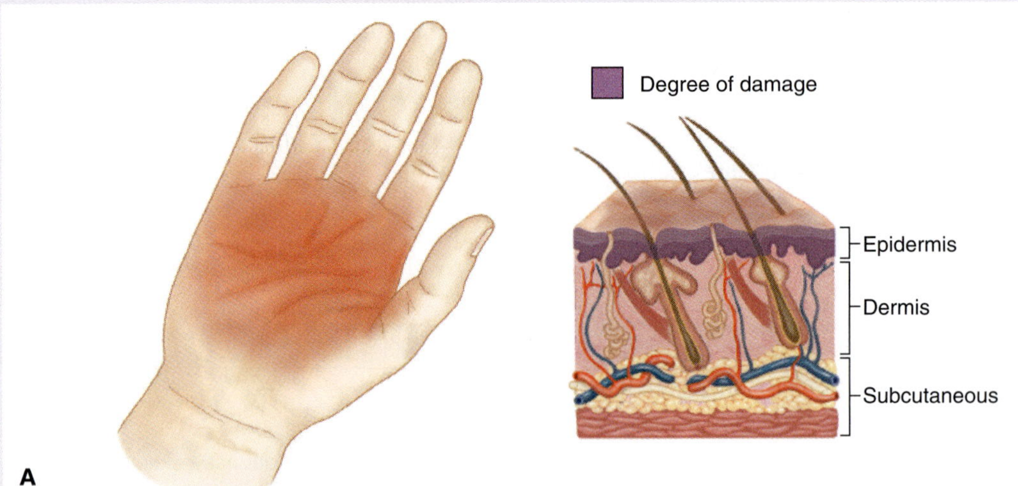

FIGURE 4-5 **(A) First-degree burn**

TABLE 4-4

PATHOLOGY TERMS—cont'd

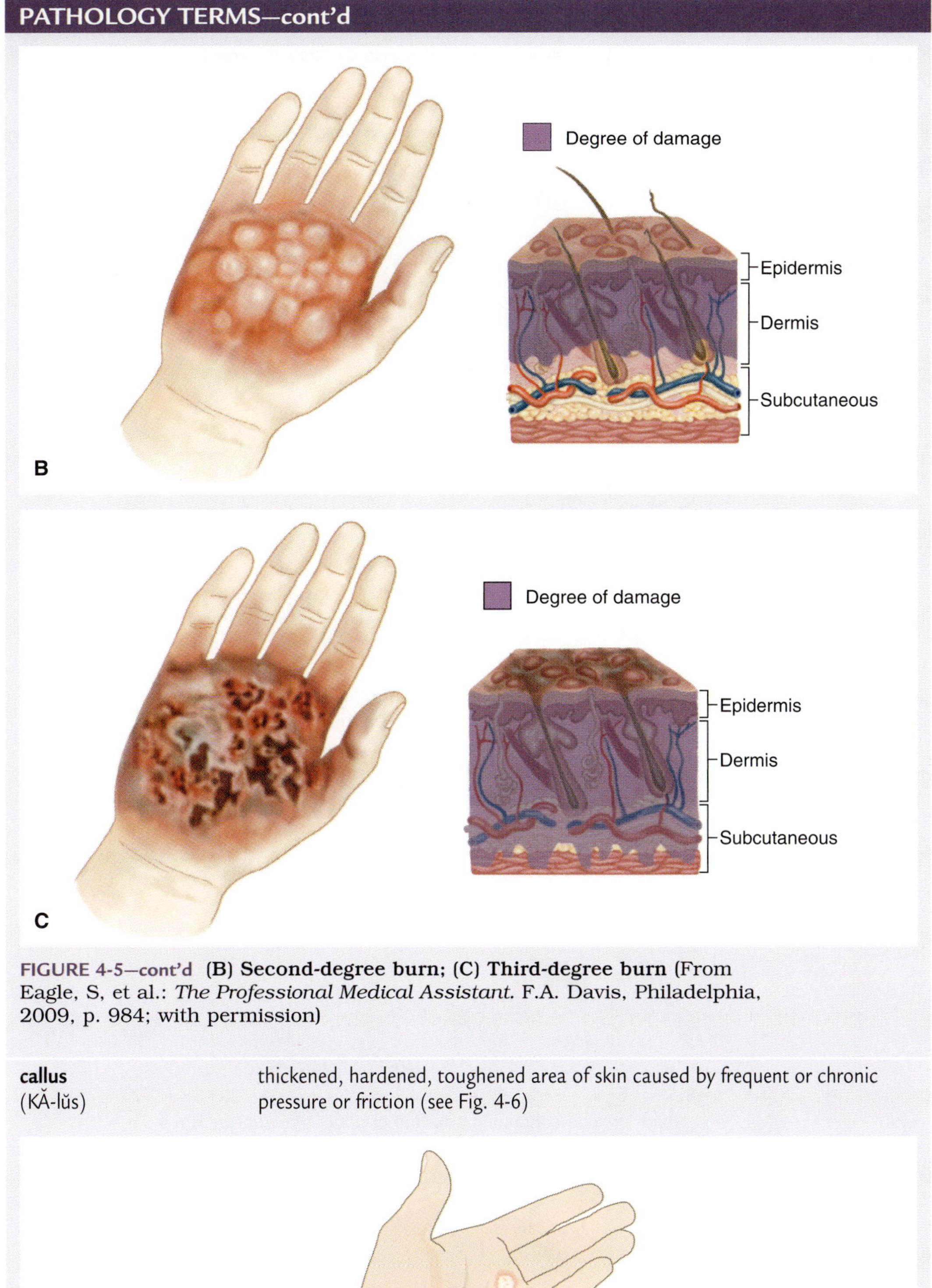

FIGURE 4-5—cont'd (B) **Second-degree burn**; (C) **Third-degree burn** (From Eagle, S, et al.: *The Professional Medical Assistant.* F.A. Davis, Philadelphia, 2009, p. 984; with permission)

callus (KĂ-lŭs)	thickened, hardened, toughened area of skin caused by frequent or chronic pressure or friction (see Fig. 4-6)

FIGURE 4-6 **Callus**

Continued

TABLE 4-4

PATHOLOGY TERMS—cont'd

carbuncle (KĂR-bŭng-kul)	very large furuncle or cluster of connected furuncles (see Fig. 4-7)
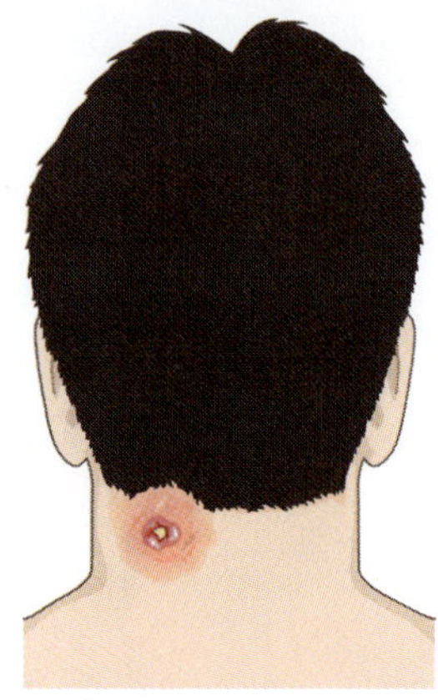 FIGURE 4-7 Carbuncle	
cellulitis (sĕl-ū-LĪ-tĭs)	potentially serious bacterial skin infection marked by pain, redness, edema, warmth, and fever
comedo (KŎ-mē-dō)	blackhead
corn (kōrn)	small callus that develops on smooth, hairless skin surfaces, such as the backs of fingers or toes, in response to pressure and friction; hard corns typically develop on the sides of feet and tops of toes; soft corns usually develop between toes (see Fig. 4-8)
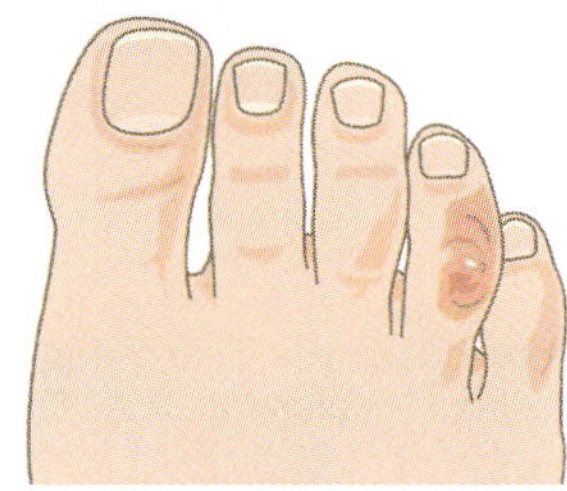 FIGURE 4-8 Corn	
cyst (sĭst)	fluid- or solid-containing pouch in or under the skin (see Fig. 4-9)
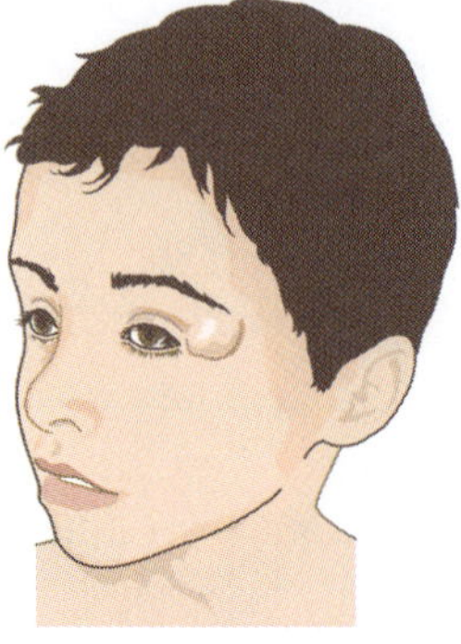 FIGURE 4-9 Cyst	

TABLE 4-4

PATHOLOGY TERMS—cont'd

decubitus ulcer (dē-KŪ-bĭ-tŭs ŬL-sĕr)	area of injury and tissue death caused by unrelieved pressure which impedes circulation in the skin and underlying tissues; also called *pressure ulcer* or *bedsore* (see Fig. 4-10)
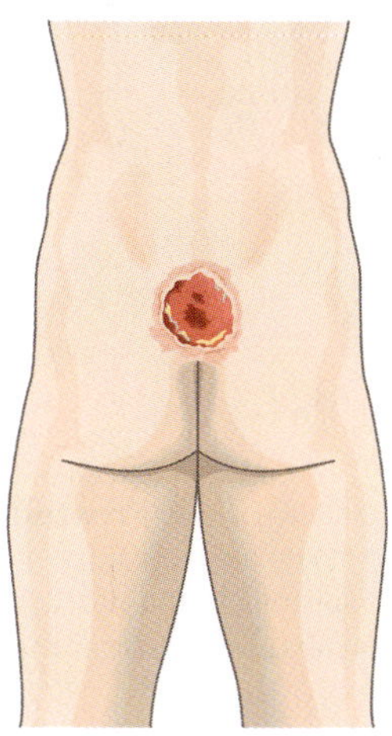 FIGURE 4-10 **Decubitus ulcer**	
ecchymosis, contusion (ĕ-kĭ-MŌ-sĭs, kŏn-TOO-zhŭn)	discoloration of the skin, bruise
eczema (ĔK-zĕ-mă)	inflammatory skin condition marked by red, hot, dry, scaly, cracked, and itchy skin, or blisters
epidermoid cyst (ĕ-pĭ-DĔR-moyd sĭst)	small sac or pouch below the skin surface containing a thick, cheesy substance; appears pale white or yellow, but can be darker in dark-skinned people
fissure (FĬSH-ūr)	small, cracklike break in the skin (see Fig. 4-11)
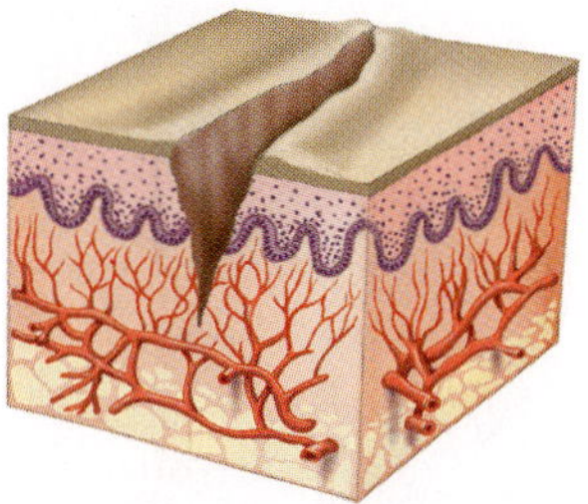 FIGURE 4-11 **Fissure**	
folliculitis (fō-lĭ-kū-LĪ-tĭs)	inflammation of hair follicles, marked by rash with small red bumps, pustules, tenderness, and itching; common on the neck, armpit, and groin area
frostbite (FRŎST-bīt)	injury that occurs when skin tissues are exposed to temperatures cold enough to cause them to freeze (see Fig. 4-12)

Continued

TABLE 4-4

PATHOLOGY TERMS—cont'd

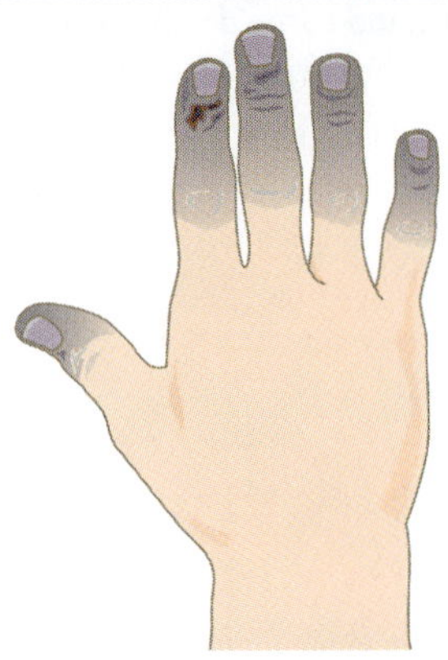

FIGURE 4-12 **Frostbite**

furuncle (FŪR-ŭng-kul)	infection of a hair follicle and nearby tissue, also called a *boil*; more invasive than folliculitis because it involves the sebaceous gland (see Fig. 4-13)

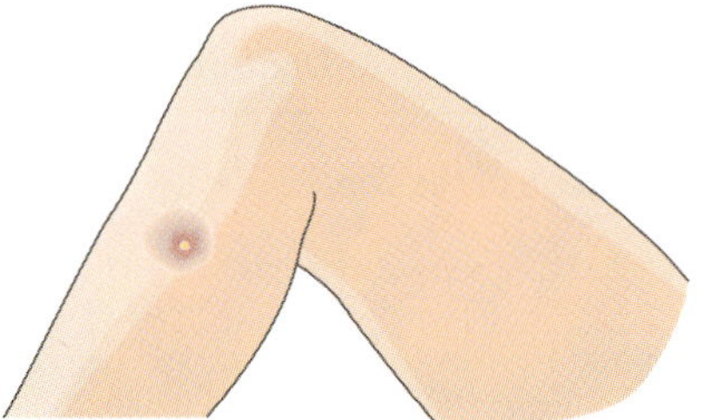

FIGURE 4-13 **Furuncle**

impetigo (ĭm-pĕ-TĪ-gō)	bacterial skin infection marked by yellow to red weeping, crusted, or pustular lesions; common in children (see Fig. 4-14)

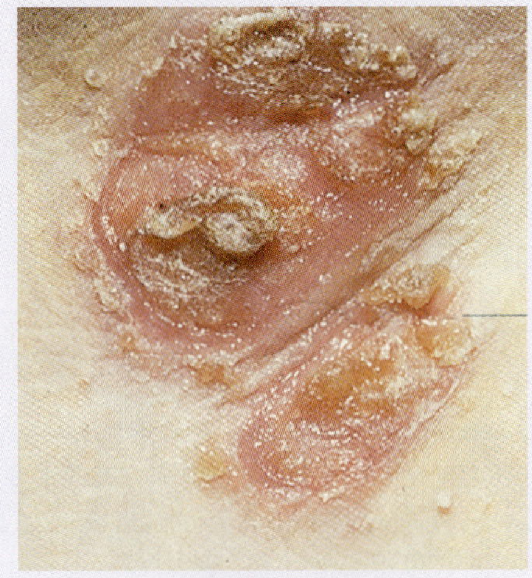

FIGURE 4-14 **Impetigo**

TABLE 4-4

PATHOLOGY TERMS—cont'd	
incision (ĭn-SĬ-zhŭn)	surgical cut in the flesh
laceration (lăs-ĕ-RĀ-shŭn)	cut or tear in the flesh
Lyme disease (līm dĭ-ZĒZ)	bacterial infection transmitted by ticks, marked by erythema migrans, a circular rash that slowly expands and enlarges; untreated disease causes multisystem symptoms
macule (MĂ-kūl)	flat, discolored spot on the skin, such as a freckle (see Fig. 4-15)
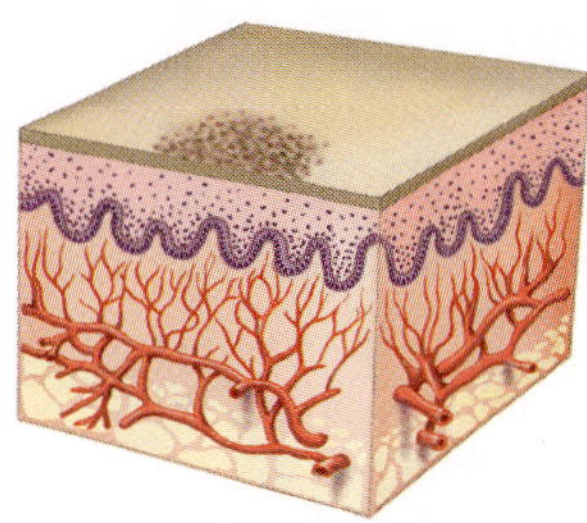 FIGURE 4-15 **Macule**	
malignant melanoma (mă-LĬG-nănt mĕ-lă-NŌ-mă)	aggressive form of skin cancer that often begins as various-colored, asymmetrical lesions larger than 6 mm in diameter
melasma (mĕ-LĂZ-mă)	development of irregular areas of darker-pigmented skin on the forehead, nose, cheek, and upper lip; also called *chloasma* or the *mask of pregnancy*
papule (PĂP-ūl)	small, raised spot or bump on the skin, such as a mole (see Fig. 4-16)
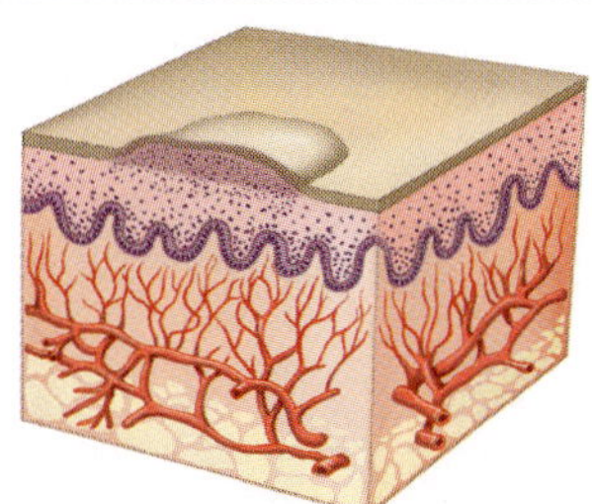 FIGURE 4-16 **Papule**	
paronychia (păr-ō-NĬK-ē-ă)	acute or chronic infection of the margins of the finger- or toenail, marked by warmth, erythema, edema, pus, throbbing, pain, or tenderness; causes the nail to become discolored and thickened
pediculosis (pĕ-dĭk-ū-LŌ-sĭs)	infestation of head, body, or pubic lice, marked by itching, the appearance of lice on the body, and eggs (nits) attached to hair shafts
petechiae (pĕ-TĒ-kē-ē)	tiny red or purple hemorrhagic spots (singular *petechia*) (see Fig. 4-17)

Continued

TABLE 4-4
PATHOLOGY TERMS—cont'd

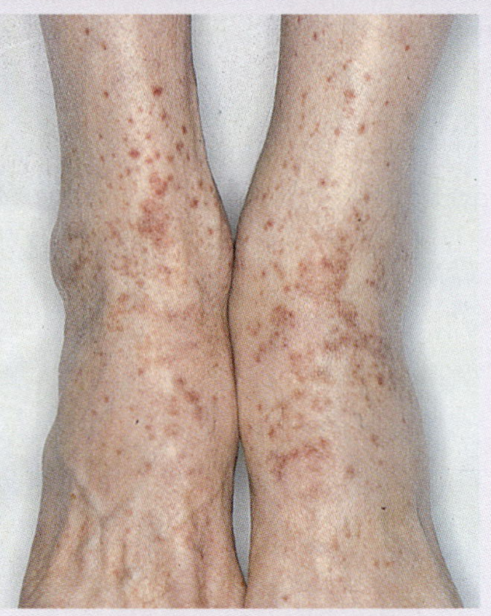

FIGURE 4-17 **Petechiae** (From Goldsmith, L, et al: *Adult & Pediatric Dermatology.* F.A. Davis, Philadelphia, 1997, p. 61; with permission)

psoriasis (sō-RĪ-ă-sĭs)	chronic, inflammatory skin disorder marked by the development of silvery-white scaly plaques or patches with sharply defined borders and reddened skin beneath (see Fig. 4-18)

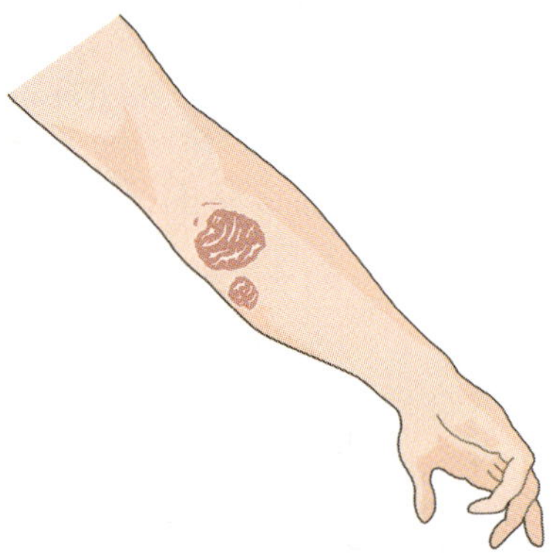

FIGURE 4-18 **Psoriasis**

puncture (PŬNGK-chūr)	hole or wound made by a sharp, pointed instrument
pustule (PŬS-tūl)	small, pus-filled blister (see Fig. 4-19)

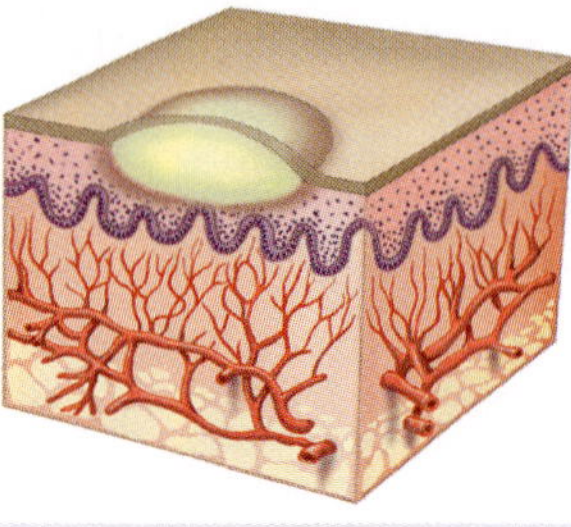

FIGURE 4-19 **Pustule**

TABLE 4-4

PATHOLOGY TERMS—cont'd

Term	Definition
rosacea (rō-ZĀ-sē-ă)	chronic condition that causes flushing and redness of the face, neck, and chest (see Fig. 4-20)

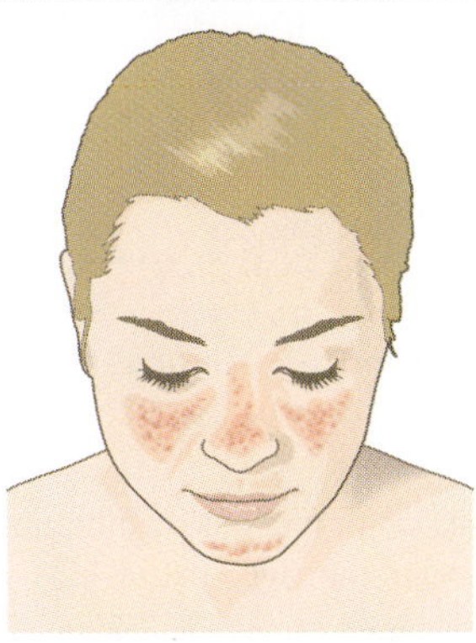

FIGURE 4-20 **Rosacea**

Term	Definition
scabies (SKĀ-bēz)	contagious skin disease transmitted by the itch mite, with symptoms of itching, scaly papules, insect burrows, and secondary infected lesions most prevalent in skin folds at the wrists and elbows, between the fingers, under the arms, in the groin, and under the beltline
scales (skālz)	area of skin that is excessively dry and flaky (see Fig. 4-21)

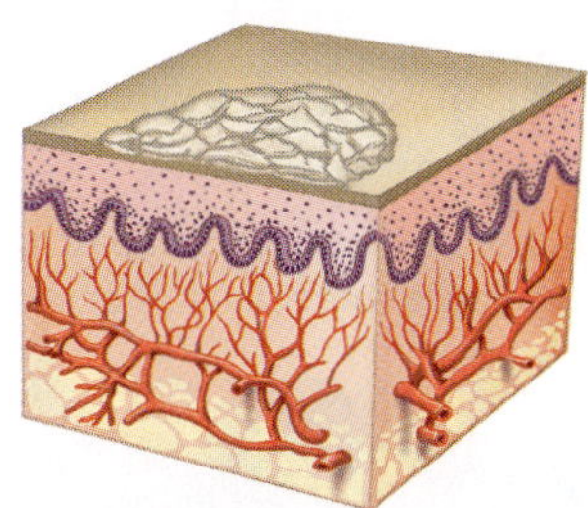

FIGURE 4-21 **Scales**

Term	Definition
sebaceous cyst (sē-BĀ-shŭs sĭst)	small sac or pouch below the skin surface filled with a thick fluid or semisolid oily substance called sebum
seborrheic keratosis (sĕ-bō-RĒ-ĭk kĕr-ă-TŌ-sĭs)	benign, flat, irregularly shaped skin growths of various colors with a warty, waxy, "stuck-on" appearance
squamous cell carcinoma (SKWĀ-mŭs sĕl kăr-sĭ-NŌ-mă)	type of cancer that usually appears in the mouth, esophagus, bronchi, lungs, or vagina and uterine cervix, marked by a firm, red nodule or a scaly appearance; may ulcerate
tinea (TĬ-nē-ă)	fungal skin disease occurring on various parts of the body, also called *dermatophytosis* or *ringworm*; forms include tinea capitis (scalp), tinea corporis (trunk), tinea cruris (genital area; also called *jock itch*), tinea nodosa (mustache and beard), tinea pedis (feet; also called *athlete's foot*), and tinea unguium (nails) (see Fig. 4-22)

Continued

TABLE 4-4

PATHOLOGY TERMS—cont'd

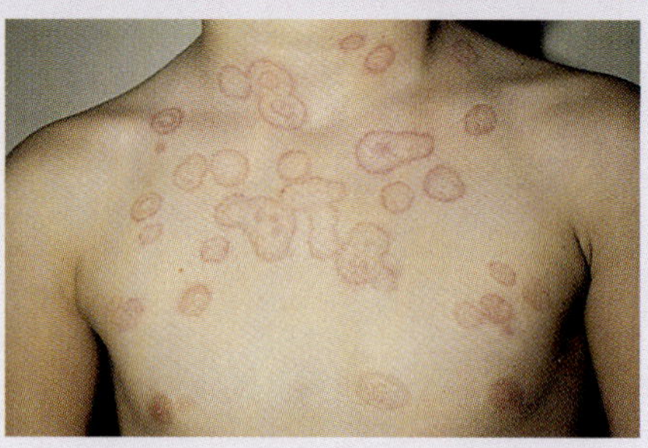

FIGURE 4-22 **Tinea** (From *Taber's Cyclopedic Medical Dictionary*, ed. 20. F.A. Davis, Philadelphia, 2005, p. 2192; with permission)

ulcer (ŬL-sĕr)	lesion of the skin or mucous membranes, marked by inflammation, necrosis, and sloughing of damaged tissues
vesicle (VĔS-ĭ-kul)	clear, fluid-filled blister (see Fig. 4-23)

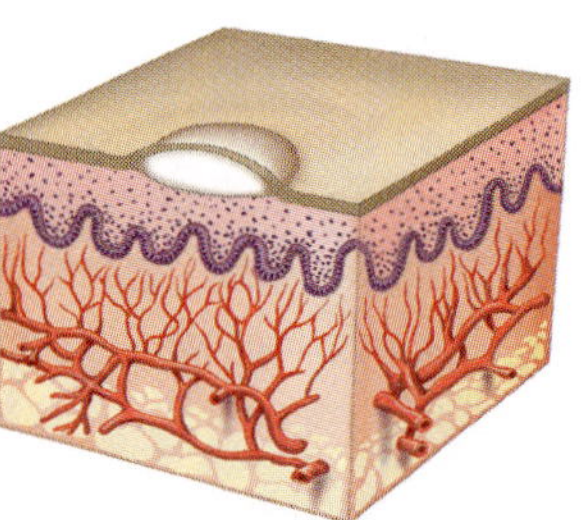

FIGURE 4-23 **Vesicle**

vitiligo (vĭt-ĭl-Ī-gō)	chronic skin disease that results in patchy loss of skin pigment; may also affect hair color and cause white patches or streaks (see Fig. 4-24)

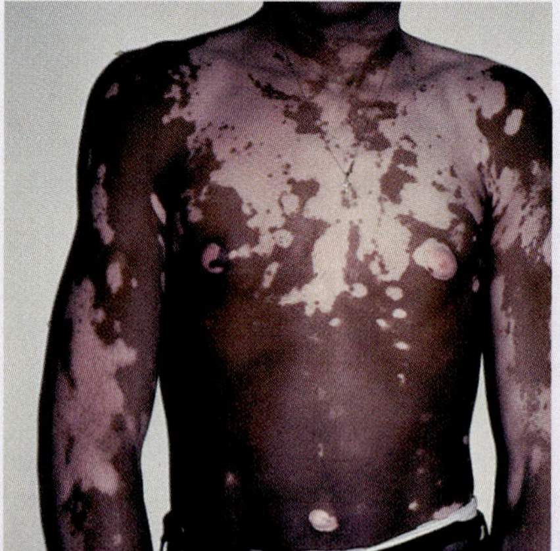

FIGURE 4-24 **Vitiligo** (From Goldsmith, LA, et al.: *Adult and Pediatric Dermatology*. F.A. Davis, Philadelphia, 1997, p. 121; with permission)

wart (wōrt)	small, benign skin tumor caused by various strains of the human papilloma virus (HPV); appearance varies from tiny to moderate-sized bumps or cauliflower-shaped growths
wheal (hwēl)	rounded, temporary elevation in the skin, white in the center with a red-pink periphery and accompanied by itching

Common Diagnostic Tests and Procedures

Biopsy: Removal of a tissue sample for microscopic examination

Cosmetic Enhancement Procedures

Dermabrasion: Removal of small scars, nevi (moles), tattoos, or fine wrinkles with a wire brush or burr impregnated with diamond particles, leaving a smoother surface

Dermaplaning: Removal of small scars, nevi (moles), tattoos, or fine wrinkles with a dermatome (a device resembling an electric razor), leaving a smoother surface

Microdermabrasion: Similar to dermabrasion but less invasive, involving multiple treatments of gentle abrasion; useful in reducing fine lines, nevi (moles), age spots, and acne scars

Chemical peel: Application of a chemical solution to the skin to improve appearance by removing blemishes, fine wrinkles, uneven pigmentation, scars, and tattoos

Laser resurfacing: Use of short pulses of light to remove fine lines and damaged skin, and to minimize scars and even out areas of uneven pigmentation; sometimes called a *laser peel*

Botox: Injection of a small amount of botulinum toxin into selected muscles of the face; interferes with muscle contraction, thereby reducing the appearance of wrinkles

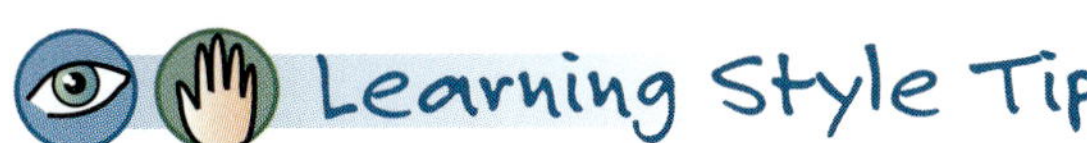

Visual and kinesthetic learners may locate images from journals or websites and glue them to 3-by-5-inch cards to make flash cards for any pathological condition or procedure for which you don't have cards. Review them daily.

Flashpoint

An easy way to remember the difference between a papule and a macule is that you can **p**alpate (touch or feel) a **p**apule, but not a macule.

CASE STUDY

Read the case study and answer the questions that follow. Most of the terms are included in this chapter. Refer to the glossaries (Appendixes B and G) or to your medical dictionary for the other terms.

Cellulitis

Herbert Marshall is a 56-year-old man admitted to the hospital with a severe case of cellulitis. Mr. Marshall has a history of chronic tinea pedis, which he usually treats with OTC medications. When he awoke yesterday, his left foot was erythematous, hot, and tender. He applied an OTC antifungal cream, hoping that would improve his condition. However, today he presented at the clinic complaining of throbbing pain in his foot. The Sx of inflammation have worsened, including increased erythema and edema of the foot and lower leg. After completing a PE, the physician made a diagnosis of cellulitis and admitted Mr. Marshall to the hospital for IV antibiotic Tx.

Cellulitis is an infection of the skin, usually caused when streptococcal or staphylococcal bacteria enter through a break in the skin. Common symptoms include erythema, heat, edema, and tenderness. Treatment for mild cases is oral antibiotics. Severe cases usually require IV antibiotic therapy. Surgical débridement, medical removal of dead tissue, may also be necessary.

Case Study Questions

1. Mr. Marshall's foot has become more:
   a. Blue
   b. Red
   c. Dry
   d. Yellow
2. Mr. Marshall's foot has also become:
   a. Swollen
   b. Hardened
   c. Bruised
   d. Scaly
3. The physician performed a:
   a. Biopsy
   b. Treatment
   c. Physical examination
   d. Incision and drainage
4. Mr. Marshall was admitted to the hospital for:
   a. Treatment
   b. A biopsy
   c. Surgery
   d. A subcutaneous injection
5. The antibiotics will be administered to Mr. Marshall by:
   a. Subcutaneous injection
   b. Intradermal injection
   c. Intramuscular injection
   d. Intravenous injection
6. Mr. Marshall has a history of chronic:
   a. Dry, flaky skin
   b. Blackheads
   c. Loss of skin pigmentation
   d. Athlete's foot
7. The abbreviation Sx stands for:
   a. Symptom(s)
   b. Biopsy
   c. Treatment
   d. Injection
8. Cellulitis is usually an infection of the:
   a. Hair
   b. Skin
   c. Finger- or toenails
   d. Glands
9. Cellulitis is caused by:
   a. A virus
   b. Poor hygiene
   c. Bacteria
   d. Exposure to cold temperatures

10. Cellulitis may be treated by:
- **a.** Oral antibiotics
- **b.** Intravenous antibiotics
- **c.** Surgery
- **d.** All of these

Answers to Case Study Questions

1. b
2. a
3. c
4. a
5. d
6. d
7. a
8. b
9. c
10. d

Websites

Please go to the F.A. Davis website at http://davisplus.fadavis.com/eagle/medterm to view resource websites for the integumentary system.

Practice Exercises

Deciphering Terms

Write the correct meaning of these medical terms. Check Appendix G for the correct answers.

Exercise 2

1. cyanoderma ____________________
2. sclerotic ____________________
3. hyperkeratosis ____________________
4. leukocytopenia ____________________
5. hypodermic ____________________
6. erythrocyte ____________________
7. dermatology ____________________
8. melanocyte ____________________
9. trichomycosis ____________________

10. hypertrophy ______________________________

11. xeroderma ______________________________

12. xanthoma ______________________________

13. lipolysis ______________________________

14. adiposis ______________________________

15. onychoma ______________________________

Fill in the Blanks

Fill in the blanks below using pathology terms from Table 4-4. Check Appendix G for the correct answers.

Exercise 3

1. The term that means *scraping away of skin* is ____________________.
2. Terms that means *discoloration of the skin* or *bruise* are ____________________ and ____________________.
3. The term that means *tiny hemorrhagic spot* is ____________________.
4. ____________________ is a skin infection marked by yellow to red crusted or pustular lesions.
5. ____________________ causes patchy loss of skin pigmentation.
6. A ____________________ is a clear, fluid-filled lesion, such as a blister.
7. A ____________________ is a small, pus-filled blister.
8. The medical name for a blackhead is ____________________.
9. ____________________ is a contagious skin disease transmitted by the itch mite.
10. A small raised spot or bump, such as a mole, is a ____________________.
11. ____________________ results in loss of body hair.
12. A ____________________ is a cut or tear in the flesh.
13. A ____________________ is a small, cracklike break in the skin.
14. ____________________ is an inflammatory skin disease that causes redness, itching, and blisters.

15. A ______________________ is a flat, discolored spot on the skin, such as a freckle.

16. A bacterial skin infection marked by pain, redness, edema, warmth, and fever is called ______________________.

17. The medical name for the fungal infection of the skin commonly known as ringworm is ______________________.

18. ______________________ describes an area of the skin that is excessively dry and flaky.

19. A ______________________ is a fluid- or solid-containing pouch in or under the skin.

20. A ______________________ is a thickened, hardened, toughened area of skin caused by frequent or chronic pressure or friction.

Multiple Choice

Select the one best answer to the following multiple-choice questions. Check Appendix G for the correct answers.

Exercise 4

1. Which of the following terms is **not** paired with the correct meaning?
   a. Erythr/o: red
   b. Xanth/o: white
   c. Melan/o: black
   d. Cyan/o: blue

2. Which of the following abbreviations is **not** paired with the correct meaning?
   a. Bx: biopsy
   b. Tx: treatment
   c. PE: physical examination
   d. FA: family history

3. Which of the following pathology terms is **not** paired with the correct meaning?
   a. Abrasion: scraping away of skin or mucous membranes
   b. Contusion: bruise
   c. Macule: small, raised spot or bump on the skin
   d. Cellulitis: bacterial skin infection

4. Which of the following pathology terms is **not** paired with the correct meaning?
   a. Comedo: blackhead
   b. Cyst: fluid- or solid-containing pouch in or under the skin
   c. Pustule: small, pus-filled blister
   d. Fissure: surgical cut in the flesh

5. Which of the following pathology terms is **not** paired with the correct meaning?
   a. Eczema: inflammatory skin disease with redness, itching, and blisters
   b. Scabies: contagious skin disease transmitted by the itch mite
   c. Impetigo: patchy loss of skin pigmentation
   d. Tinea: fungal skin disease occurring on various parts of the body

Word Building

*Using **only** the word parts in the lists provided, create medical terms with the indicated meanings. Check Appendix G for the correct answers.*

Exercise 5

Prefixes	Combining Forms	Suffixes
circum-	adip/o	-al
epi-	albin/o	-cyte
hypo-	cyan/o	-derma
	cyt/o	-ectomy
	dermat/o	-emia
	derm/o	-ic
	erythr/o	-ism
	kerat/o	-oid
	leuk/o	-oma
	lip/o	-osis
	melan/o	-penia
	myc/o	-tic
	necr/o	
	onych/o	
	trich/o	
	scler/o	
	xanth/o	
	xer/o	

1. resembling fat ____________________
2. pertaining to dry skin ____________________
3. condition of whiteness ____________________
4. abnormal condition of yellowness ____________________

5. pertaining to the skin ______________________

6. pertaining to above or upon the skin ______________________

7. abnormal condition of skin fungus ______________________

8. deficiency of red (blood) cells ______________________

9. abnormal condition of blueness of the skin ______________________

10. hardening of the skin ______________________

11. abnormal condition of hair fungus ______________________

12. abnormal condition of keratinized tissue ______________________

13. white (condition of) blood ______________________

14. abnormal condition of nail fungus ______________________

15. black tumor ______________________

16. pertaining to death ______________________

17. pertaining to beneath the skin ______________________

18. surgical removal of fat ______________________

19. fat cell ______________________

20. dry skin ______________________

True or False

Decide whether the following statements are true or false. Check Appendix G for the correct answers.

Exercise 6

1. True False **Laser resurfacing** involves the use of short pulses of light to remove fine lines and damaged skin and to minimize scars.

2. True False In **dermaplaning**, a surgeon scrapes away the outermost layer of skin using a wire brush or burr impregnated with diamond particles.

3. True False In **Botox**, a small amount of toxin is injected into selected muscles of the face.

4. True False A **biopsy** involves the removal of a tissue sample for microscopic examination.

5. True False The abbreviation for **biopsy** is BSY.

6. True False The abbreviation **ID** stands for *incision and drainage.*

7. True False The abbreviation for **physical examination** is Px.

8. True False The abbreviation **Tx** stands for *treatment.*

9. True False The abbreviation **FH** stands for *family history.*

10. True False The abbreviation **SubQ** stands for *sclerosis.*

Deciphering Terms

Write the correct meaning of these medical terms. Check Appendix G for the correct answers.

Exercise 7

1. hidrotic ____________________
2. morphogenesis ____________________
3. hydrous ____________________
4. mycoid ____________________
5. cirrhotic ____________________
6. chromatogram ____________________
7. leukopenia ____________________
8. sonography ____________________
9. rhytidoplasty ____________________
10. pathophobia ____________________

Multiple Choice

Select the one best answer to the following multiple-choice questions. Check Appendix G for the correct answers.

Exercise 8

1. Which of the following terms is matched with the correct definition?
   - a. Adip/o: acne
   - b. Cutane/o: cell
   - c. Necr/o: dead
   - d. Myc/o: macule

2. Which of the following terms is matched with the correct definition?
   a. Seb/o: sweat
   b. Son/o: shape
   c. Cyan/o: cause
   d. Xanth/o: yellow
3. Which of the following terms is matched with the correct definition?
   a. Dermat/o: dead
   b. Cyt/o: cell
   c. Idi/o: cause
   d. Leuk/o: large
4. Which of the following terms is matched with the correct definition?
   a. Xer/o: white
   b. Albin/o: hardening
   c. Chromat/o: cornea
   d. Erythr/o: red
5. Which of the following terms is matched with the correct definition?
   a. Hidr/o: water
   b. Morph/o: malignant
   c. Onych/o: nail
   d. Rhytid/o: hair
6. Which of the following terms is matched with the correct definition?
   a. SCC: subcutaneous
   b. Bx: treatment
   c. ID: incision and drainage
   d. Ung: ointment
7. Which of the following terms is matched with the correct definition?
   a. Cirrh/o: blue
   b. Xer/o: dry
   c. Melan/o: malignant
   d. Trich/o: treatment
8. Which of the following terms is matched with the correct definition?
   a. PE: probable etiology
   b. Sx: treatment
   c. FH: hair fungus
   d. MM: malignant melanoma

9. Which of the following terms is matched with the correct definition?
   a. Lip/o: skin
   b. Eti/o: unknown
   c. Hydr/o: sweat
   d. Pil/o: hair

10. Which of the following terms is matched with the correct definition?
   a. Kerat/o: cyst
   b. Dermat/o: skin
   c. Path/o: papule
   d. Scler/o: scales

11. Which of the following terms means *abnormal condition of nail softening*?
   a. Cyanoderma
   b. Onychomycosis
   c. Hyperhidrosis
   d. None of these

12. The term *hyperrhytidosis* means:
   a. Disease of the skin
   b. Abnormal condition of excessive wrinkles
   c. Dry skin
   d. None of these

13. A patient is most likely to visit a dermatologist to undergo dermaplaning for which of the following disorders?
   a. Acne
   b. Alopecia areata
   c. Carbuncle
   d. Cyst

14. Which of the following is a malignant condition?
   a. Actinic keratosis
   b. Bulla
   c. Folliculitis
   d. Basal cell carcinoma

15. Which of the following is the result of accidental injury?

a. Callus
b. Melasma
c. Paronychia
d. Abrasion

16. All of the following skin problems are related to excess pressure **except**:

a. Corn
b. Callus
c. Fissure
d. Decubitus ulcer

17. All of the following are infections of the skin **except**:

a. Petechiae
b. Furuncle
c. Impetigo
d. Pustule

18. All of the following procedures involve removal of tissue **except**:

a. Biopsy
b. Dermaplaning
c. Dermabrasion
d. Botox

19. Which of the following helps to remove fine lines or wrinkles?

a. Laser resurfacing
b. Microdermabrasion
c. Dermaplaning
d. All of these

20. Which of the following is done to aid in diagnosis?

a. Microdermabrasion
b. Botox
c. Biopsy
d. None of these

5 NERVOUS SYSTEM

Structure and Function

The nervous system plays a key role in maintaining **homeostasis**, the state of dynamic equilibrium in the internal environment of the body. More complex than the most advanced computer, the nervous system is capable of storing vast amounts of data as well as receiving and sending thousands of messages throughout the body instantly and simultaneously.

While the nervous system functions as a total system, you may find it more easily understood if we divide it into its two major parts: the **central nervous system (CNS)** and the **peripheral nervous system (PNS)**. However, we first begin by looking at the most essential element: the neuron.

Flashpoint

Your brain is something like a very complex computer with infinite data-storage capabilities.

A nerve cell, known as a **neuron**, is illustrated in Figure 5-1. Neurons vary in size and shape, but have the following key parts: **cell body, axon,** and **dendrites.** The cell body houses all of the microscopic structures that keep the cell energized and functioning. The dendrites, which resemble the branches of a tree, are responsible for gathering information from the internal and external environment and sending this information to the cell body. The axon carries electrical impulses and transmits signals to other cells. The axon may be short or quite long, and is sometimes covered in a special protective layer called the **myelin sheath**.

Learning Style Tip

Trace the illustration with your fingertip, naming the various parts aloud and describing their functions as you do so. This tip is useful for visual, auditory, verbal, and kinesthetic learners.

The central nervous system comprises the brain and spinal cord (see Fig. 5-2). This is where data storage and information processing occurs. The brain is made up of three major divisions: the cerebrum, which makes up the largest portion; the cerebellum; and the brainstem. The surface of the cerebrum, called the *cortex,* is characterized by deep folds and shallow grooves, which increase its surface area and maximize function. It is full of neurons as well as specialized support cells called **glia**. It is involved in sensory perception, emotions, and muscle control. The cerebrum is divided into two hemispheres connected by a structure called the corpus callosum. The cerebellum is sometimes called the "little brain." It is located inferior and posterior to the rest of the brain. It is about the size of your fist and is shaped like a walnut. It also has folds and grooves, similar to the cerebrum. It is responsible for posture, balance, and coordination. The brainstem sits anterior to the cerebellum and includes the medulla oblongata and the

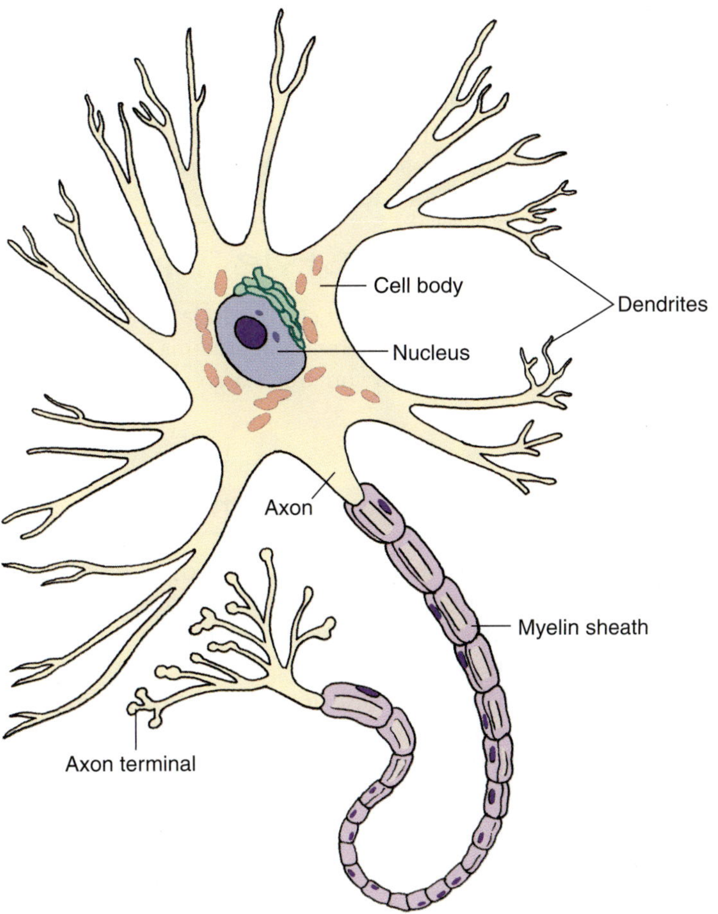

FIGURE 5-1 **Neuron**

pons. It is an essential pathway that conducts impulses between the brain and spinal cord. The brain is enclosed and protected by the hard bones of the skull, known as the **cranium**. The spinal cord extends from the base of the brain down to the second lumbar vertebra, and is surrounded and protected by the vertebral column. It is divided into sections that correspond to the vertebrae and paired spinal nerves. It provides the pathway for sensory impulses to the brain from the rest of the body, and motor impulses from the brain to the rest of the body.

Protecting both the brain and the spinal cord are three membranes called the **meninges**. The meninges provide a supportive structure for many small blood vessels on the brain's surface. They also provide protection to the brain and spinal cord, housing cerebrospinal fluid that continuously circulates and provides a cushion against injury from impact and sudden movement.

A nerve cell in the human body functions somewhat similarly to an electrical cord that might be found in your home. In an electrical cord, the wires are protected by a rubber coating of insulation; so too, your nerves are protected by the myelin sheath. The electrical cord sends electricity from the energy source to the refrigerator, television, or other device so that it can operate. Your nerve cells send electrical impulses down the axon to muscles, organs, or other tissues in the periphery so that they can function. When the insulating layer of an electrical extension cord becomes frayed or otherwise damaged, the cord may "short out"; as a result, signal transmission may be temporarily or permanently lost, and the device may no longer work. Similarly, if the myelin sheath on the axon degenerates or is damaged, the electrical impulse may be temporarily or permanently lost. As a result, the organ or muscle that it innervates may not function properly. This explains some of the symptoms caused by degenerative neuromuscular diseases such as ***multiple sclerosis***.

Flashpoint
Nerve cells in your body are somewhat similar to complex electrical cords.

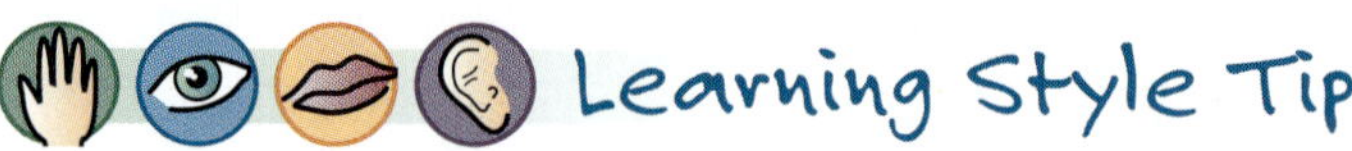

Create a 3-D model of the brain out of clay. Include the key parts as described in this chapter and make each out of a different color. Name them and describe their function aloud as you make them. It's OK if you aren't a great sculptor—the point is to learn and remember!

Central and Peripheral Nervous Systems

The *central* nervous system (brain and spinal cord) is located in the middle, or most *central*, part of the body. The *peripheral* nervous system is located outside of, or *peripheral* to, the CNS, and includes the nerves on either side of the spinal cord and in the arms and legs.

The PNS includes 31 pairs of spinal nerves, 12 cranial nerves, and nerves in the arms and legs. Some nerves are purely sensory and some are purely motor. Sensory nerves gather information such as air temperature from the external

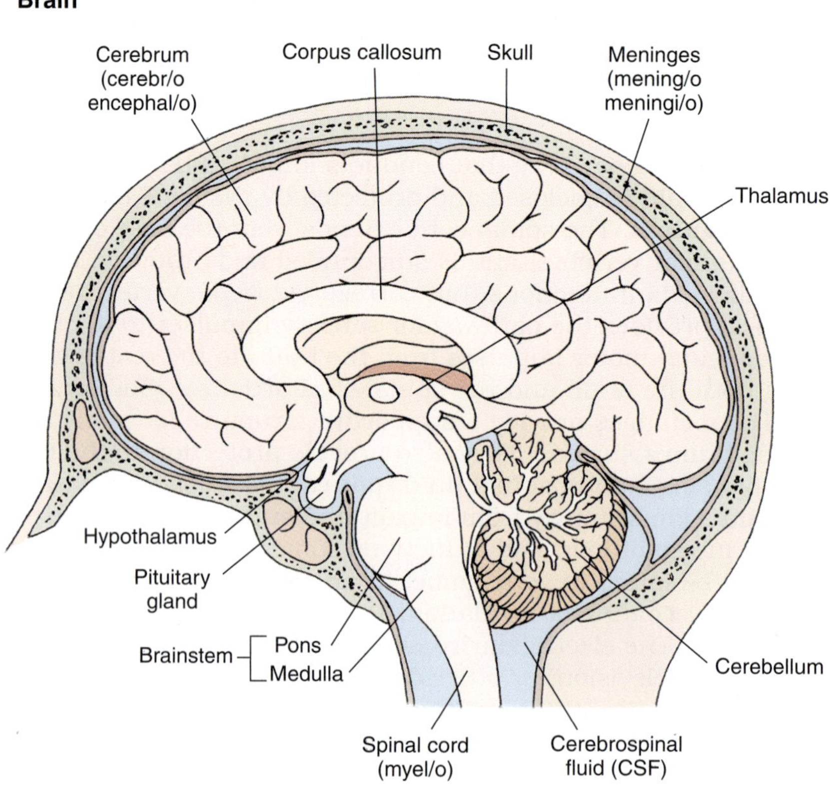

FIGURE 5-2 Central nervous system: (A) brain

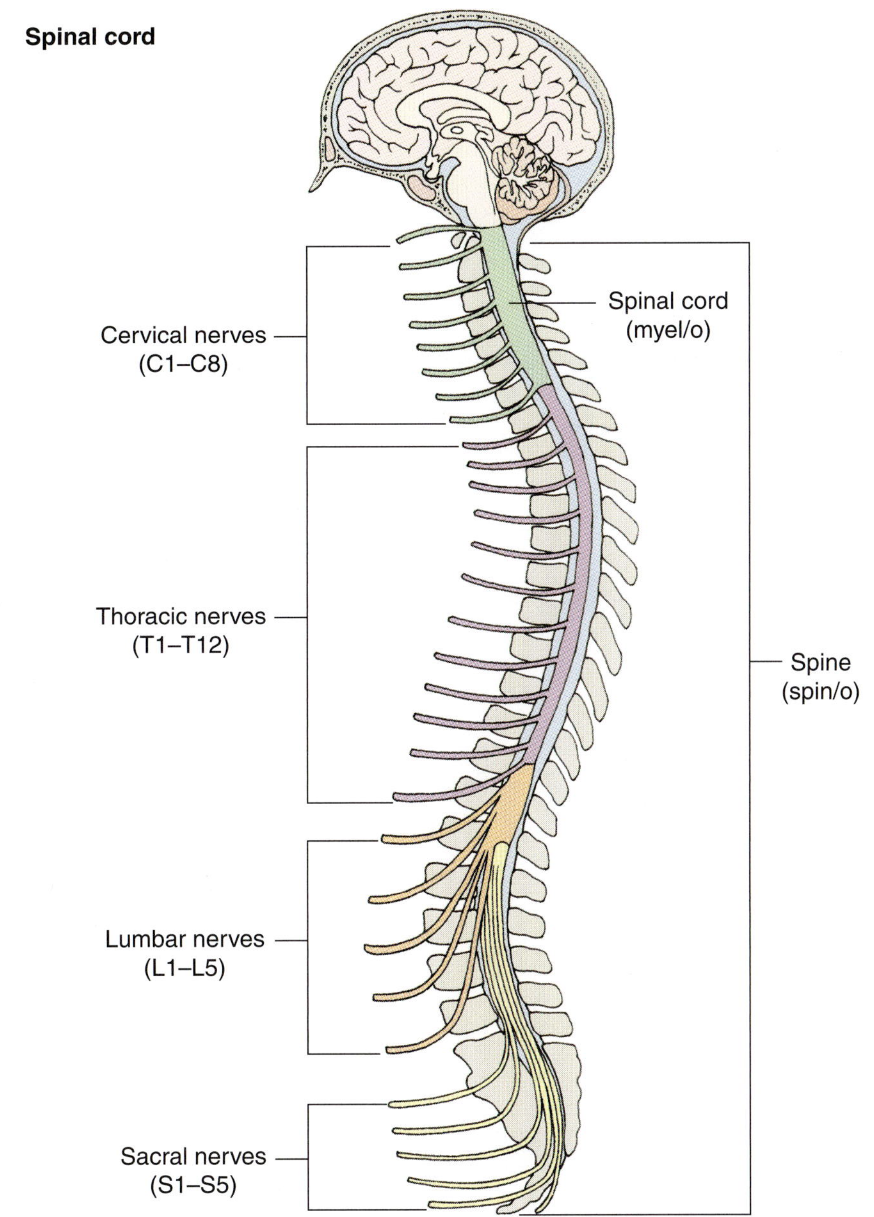

FIGURE 5-2—cont'd **(B) spinal cord**

environment. They also note your response to the environment, such as the sensation of discomfort from feeling cold. This information is sent to the brain, and the brain responds to the information by sending messages back out to the body via the motor nerves, which control body movement. The message may be a conscious one that prompts you to action such as putting on a coat, or it may be unconscious, perhaps causing you to yawn or breathe faster and more deeply to meet your body's need for more oxygen. A key function of the 31 pairs of spinal nerves is innervation of the skin and muscles of the limbs. Specific areas of the skin associated with specific spinal nerves are called *dermatomes* (see Fig. 5-3). *Dermatome* has two meanings. As you learned in Chapter 4, a dermatome is a surgical instrument that produces thin slices of skin. Dermatome is also an area of skin associated with specific spinal nerves. In

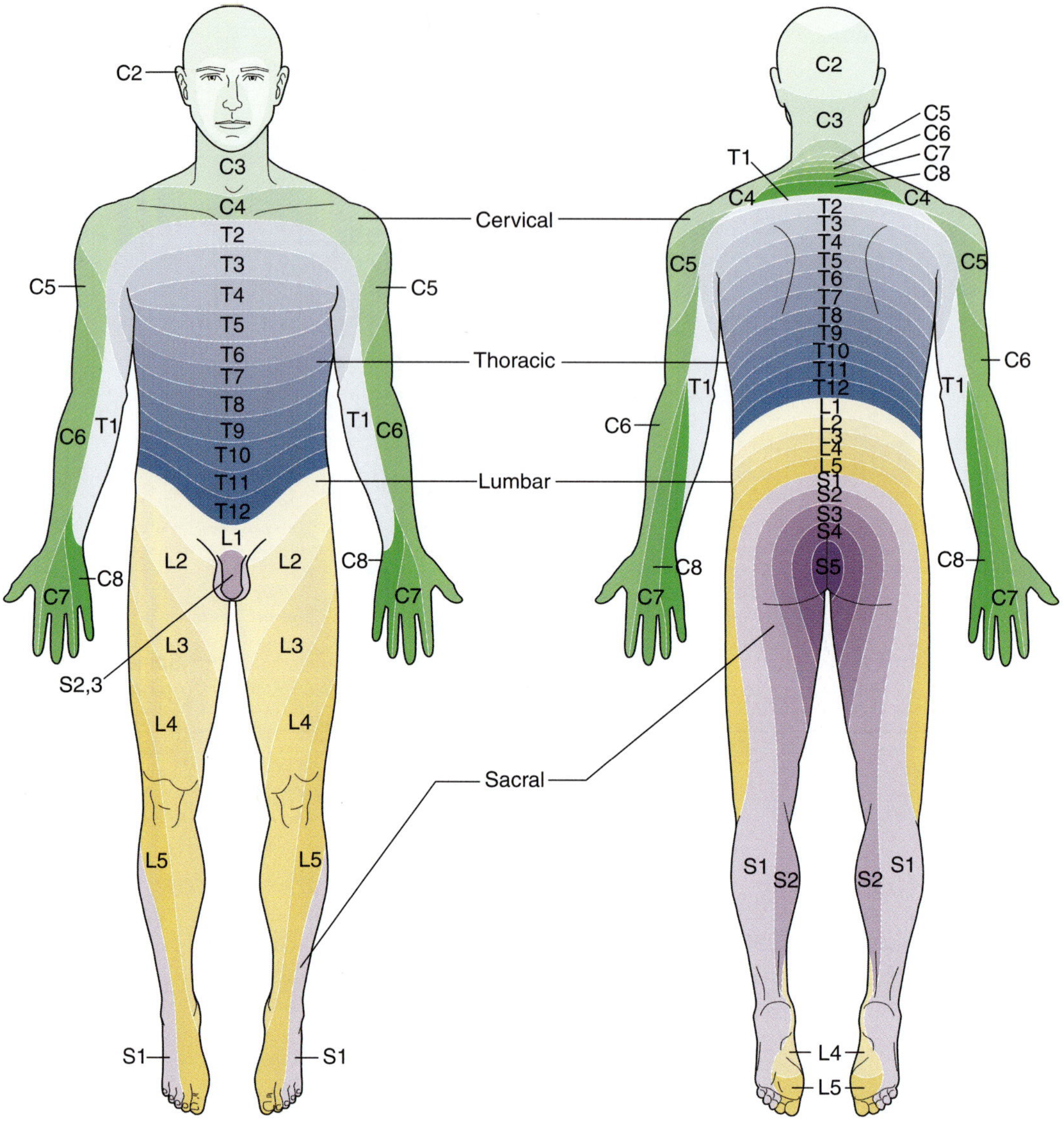

FIGURE 5-3 **Dermatomes** (From Eagle, S, et al.: *The Professional Medical Assistant*. F.A. Davis, Philadelphia, 2009, p. 441; with permission)

some disorders, pain or other sensations caused by spinal-nerve injury are felt along the associated dermatome rather than at the actual site of injury. Thus, if you suffer from compression of a spinal nerve root, you may feel **referred pain** or other symptoms in your arms or legs rather than in your back.

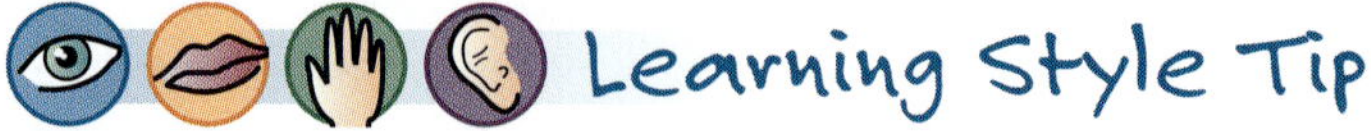

Using masking tape and a marker, label the dermatomes on a study partner. Name them aloud as you do so. Then change roles and let your partner do the same with you.

An important part of the PNS is the autonomic nervous system (ANS), which controls involuntary functions. It consists of motor nerves to smooth muscle, cardiac muscle, and glands such as sweat glands and salivary glands. It is further divided into the sympathetic and parasympathetic nervous systems (see Fig. 5-4). The sympathetic nervous system is responsible for the survival

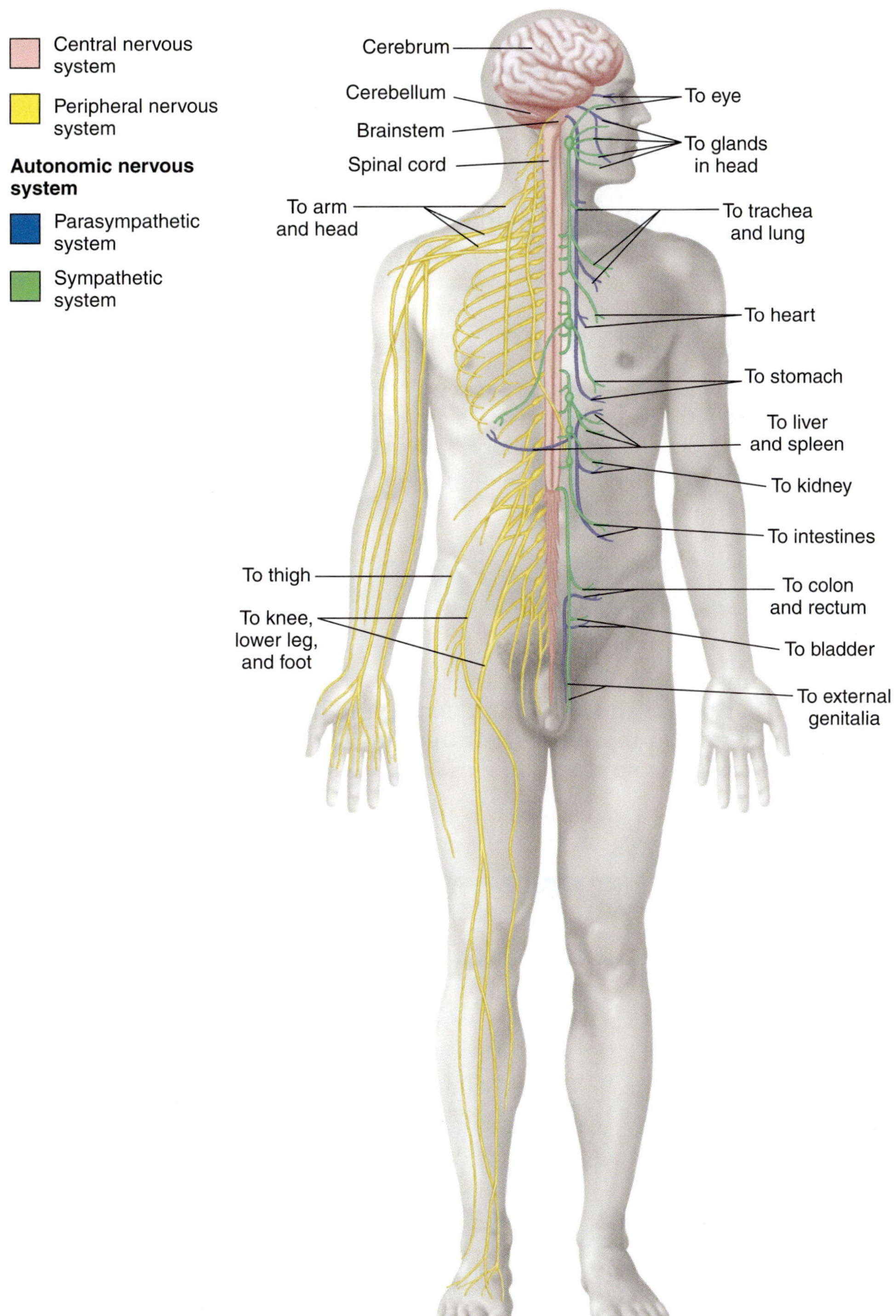

FIGURE 5-4 **Central and peripheral nervous systems, along with the autonomic nervous system** (From Eagle, S, et al.: *The Professional Medical Assistant.* F.A. Davis, Philadelphia, 2009, p. 438; with permission)

response known as the *fight-or-flight response.* This response prcpares a person for action, whether it is to fight in self-defense or to run from danger. Physical changes within the body caused by this response include increased heart rate and force, increased blood pressure and glucose levels, bronchodilation, and decreased intestinal peristalsis. These changes provide the body with increased energy and oxygen while slowing some functions (such as digestion) which are less important at the time. The parasympathetic nervous system essentially creates an opposite response, and dominates during nonstressful times. Some of its effects include decreased heart rate, bronchoconstriction, and increased peristalsis.

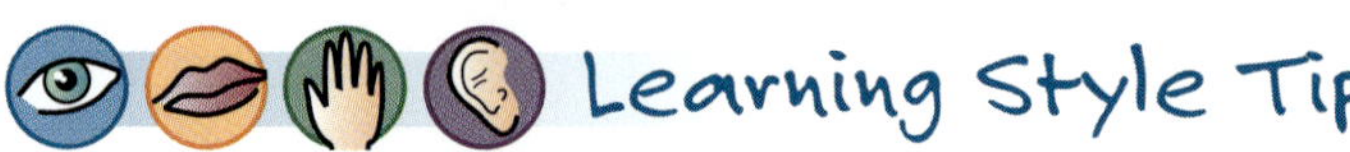

Create your own colorful flowchart on a whiteboard or poster that illustrates the various branches of the nervous system. Doing this yourself will help to clarify the information in your mind and in your memory. Speak aloud as you do so to benefit from verbalizing and hearing the information.

Flashpoint
To remember the functions of the autonomic nervous system, think *autonomic = automatic.*

Combining Forms

Table 5-1 contains combining forms that pertain to the nervous system, examples of terms that utilize the combining form, and a pronunciation guide. Read aloud to yourself as you move from left to right across the table. Be sure to use the pronunciation guide so that you can learn to say the terms correctly.

TABLE 5-1
COMBINING FORMS RELATED TO THE NERVOUS SYSTEM

Combining Form	Meaning	Example	Meaning of New Term
cephal/o	head	cephalalgia (sĕf-ă-LĂL-jē-ă)	pain of the head
cerebell/o	cerebellum	cerebellitis (sĕr-ĕ-bĕ-LĪT-ĭs)	inflammation of the cerebellum
cerebr/o	brain	cerebrovascular (sĕ-rĕ-brō-VĂS-kū-lăr)	pertaining to the brain and vessels
encephal/o		encephalocele (ĕn-SĔF-ă-lō-sēl)	hernia of the brain
gangli/o	ganglion	ganglioma (găng-glē-Ō-mă)	tumor of a ganglion
gli/o	glue, gluelike	glioma (glī-Ō-mă)	gluelike tumor
lex/o	word, phrase	dyslexia (dĭs-LĔK-sē-ă)	bad, painful, or difficult words or phrases
mening/o	meninges	meningitis (mĕn-ĭn-JĪT-ĭs)	inflammation of the meninges
meningi/o		meningioma (mĕ-nĭn-JĒ-ō-mă)	tumor of the meninges

TABLE 5-1
COMBINING FORMS RELATED TO THE NERVOUS SYSTEM—cont'd

Combining Form	Meaning	Example	Meaning of New Term
myel/o	spinal cord, bone marrow	myelography (mī-ĕ-LŎG-ră-fē)	process of recording the spinal cord or bone marrow
narc/o	sleep, stupor	narcolepsy (NĂR-kō-lĕp-sē)	seizure of sleep or stupor
neur/o	nerve	neurocytoma (nūr-ō-sī-TŌ-mă)	tumor of a nerve cell
phas/o	speech	aphasia (ă-FĀ-zē-ă)	absence of speech
psych/o	mind	psychiatry (sī-KĪ-ă-trē)	field of medicine of the mind
radicul/o	nerve root	radiculopathy (ră-dĭ-kū-LŎ-pă-thē)	disease of a nerve root
spin/o	spine	spinal stenosis (SPĪ-năl stĕ-NŌ-sĭs)	abnormal condition of narrowing or stricture of the spinal cord
sthen/o	strength	myasthenia (mī-ăs-THĒ-nē-ă)	condition of absence of muscle strength
thalam/o	thalamus	thalamotomy (thăl-ă-MŎT-ō-mē)	cutting into or incision of the thalamus
ton/o	tension, tone	tonometer (tō-NŎM-ĕt-ĕr)	measuring instrument for tension
ventricul/o	ventricle	ventriculoscopy (vĕn-trĭk-ū-LŎS-kō-pē)	visual examination of a ventricle

STOP HERE.
Select the Combining Form Flash Cards for Chapter 5 and run through them at least three times before you continue.

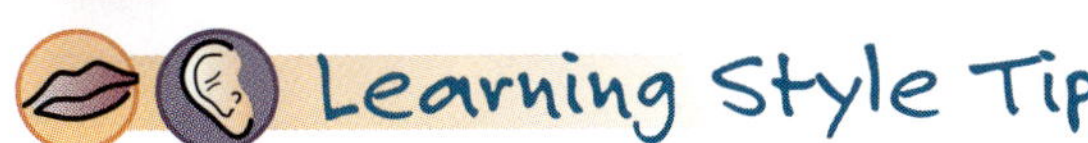

Try this silly exercise: Study with a group or a friend and take turns "selling" each other combining forms. Here's an example of a sales pitch: "Have I got a deal for you! A handy, dandy, multipurpose combining form by the name of ***neur/o***. This versatile little combining form is useful if you happen to have nerve pain (neuralgia) caused by nerve inflammation (neuritis), and you need to see a doctor (neurologist) who specializes in disorders pertaining to the nerves (neurology). If you need an operation (neurosurgery), then you'll need a special doctor (neurosurgeon). And if none of that is true, but you are simply feeling neurotic (pertaining to nerves)—well, it's handy for that too."

Practice Exercises

Fill in the Blanks

Fill in the blanks below using Table 5-1 and Figure 5-2. Check Appendix G for the correct answers.

Exercise 1

1. pain of the head ______________________________
2. tumor of the meninges ______________________________
3. cutting into or incision of the thalamus ______________________________
4. gluelike tumor ______________________________
5. pertaining to the brain and vessels ______________________________
6. inflammation of the meninges ______________________________
7. visual examination of a ventricle ______________________________
8. inflammation of the cerebellum ______________________________
9. process of recording the spinal cord or bone marrow ______________________________
10. tumor of a nerve cell ______________________________
11. measuring instrument for tension ______________________________
12. bad, painful, or difficult words or phrases ______________________________
13. tumor of a ganglion ______________________________
14. seizure of sleep or stupor ______________________________
15. disease of a nerve root ______________________________
16. condition of absence of muscle strength ______________________________
17. hernia of the brain ______________________________
18. absence of speech ______________________________
19. abnormal condition of narrowing or stricture of the spinal cord ______________________________
20. field of medicine of the mind ______________________________
21. **Fill in the blanks in Figure 5-5 with the appropriate anatomical terms and combining forms.**

22. **Fill in the blanks in Figure 5-6 with the appropriate anatomical terms.**

Abbreviations

Table 5-2 lists some of the most common abbreviations related to the nervous system, as well as others often used in medical documentation.

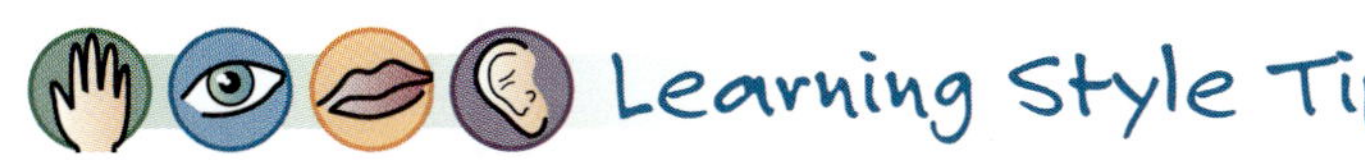

Write out definitions of pathology terms and abbreviations. Read them aloud several times as you do so.

STOP HERE.
Select the Abbreviation Flash Cards for Chapter 5 and run through them at least three times before you continue.

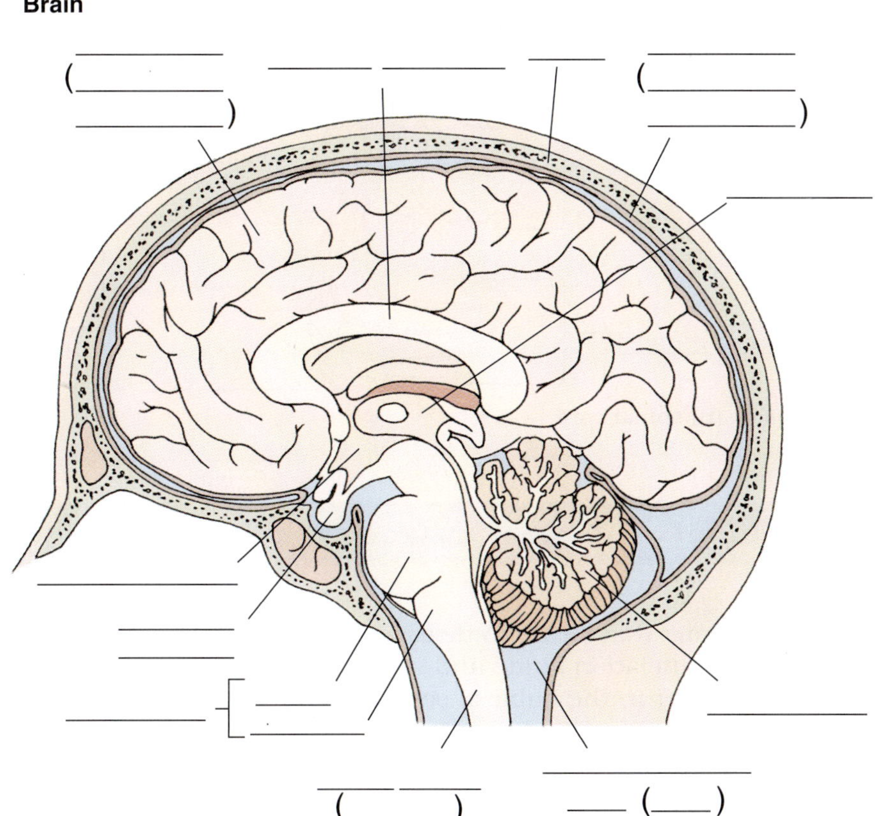

FIGURE 5-5 Central nervous system, with blanks: (A) brain

(continued)

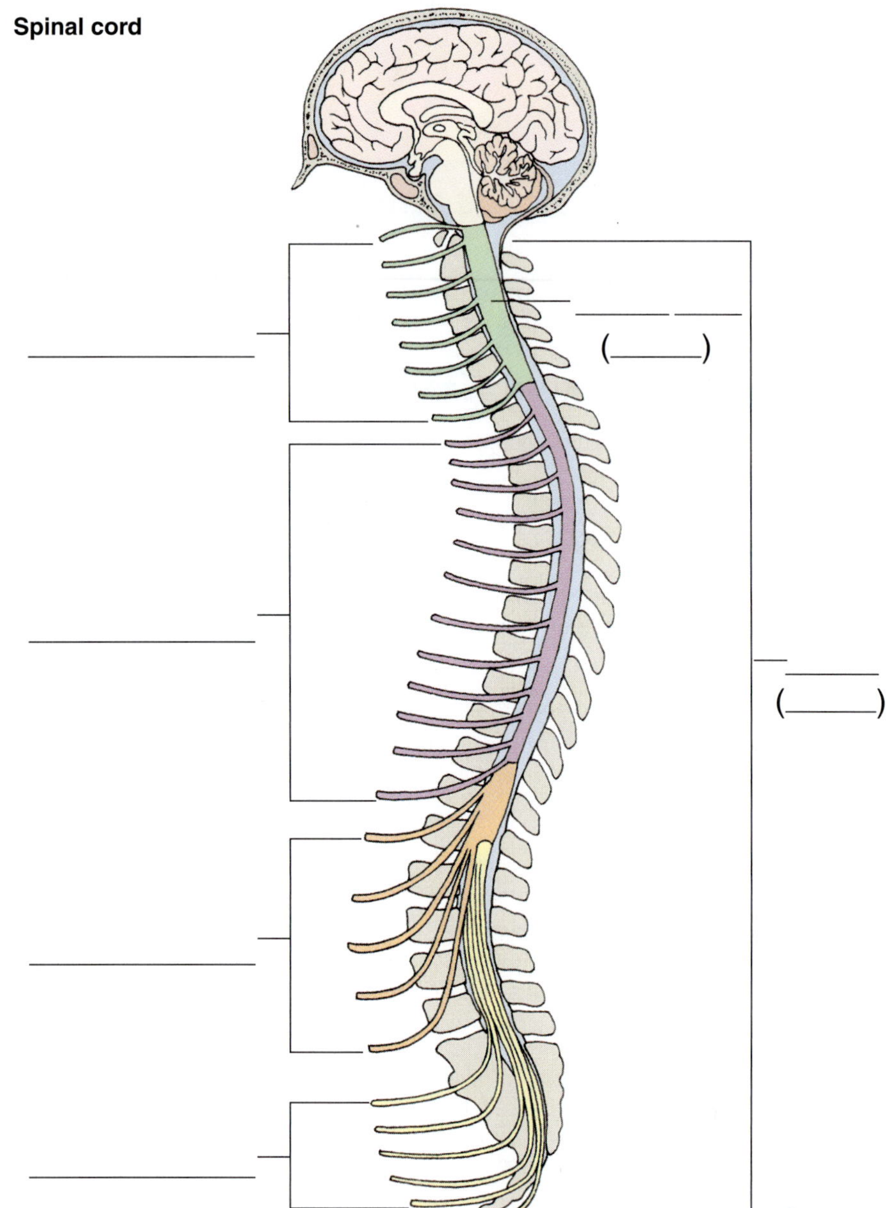

FIGURE 5-5—cont'd (B) spinal cord

Pathology Terms

Table 5-3 lists terms that relate to diseases or abnormalities of the nervous system. Use the pronunciation guide and say the terms out loud as you read them. This will help you get in the habit of saying them properly.

STOP HERE.
Select the Pathology Term Flash Cards for Chapter 5 and run through them at least three times before you continue.

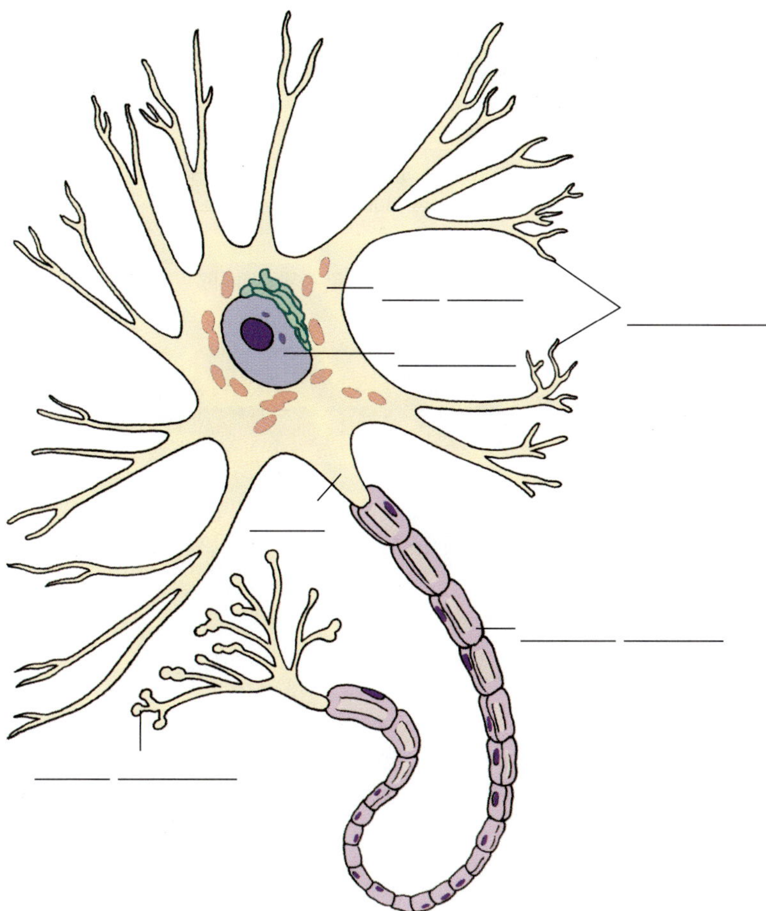

FIGURE 5-6 **Neuron with blanks**

TABLE 5-2
ABBREVIATIONS

ADHD	attention-deficit hyperactivity disorder	ICP	intracranial pressure
ALS	amyotrophic lateral sclerosis (Lou Gehrig disease)	LOC	level of consciousness, loss of consciousness
ANS	autonomic nervous system	LP	lumbar puncture
CNS	central nervous system	MRI	magnetic resonance imaging
CP	cerebral palsy	MS	multiple sclerosis
CSF	cerebrospinal fluid	OCD	obsessive-compulsive disorder
CT	computed tomography	PNS	peripheral nervous system
CVA	cerebrovascular accident	SCI	spinal cord injury
EEG	electroencephalography	TGA	transient global amnesia
EMG	electromyogram	TIA	transient ischemic attack
GBS	Guillain-Barré syndrome	TN	trigeminal neuralgia

TABLE 5-3

PATHOLOGY TERMS

Alzheimer disease (ĂLTS-hī-mĕr dĭ-ZĒZ)	form of chronic, progressive dementia caused by the atrophy of brain tissue
amyotrophic lateral sclerosis (ALS) (ă-mī-ō-TRŌ-fĭk LĂ-tĕr-ăl sklĕ-RŌ-sĭs)	chronic, progressive, degenerative neuromuscular disorder that destroys motor neurons of the body; also called *Lou Gehrig disease*
Bell palsy (bĕl PAWL-zē)	form of facial paralysis, usually unilateral and temporary (see Fig. 5-7)

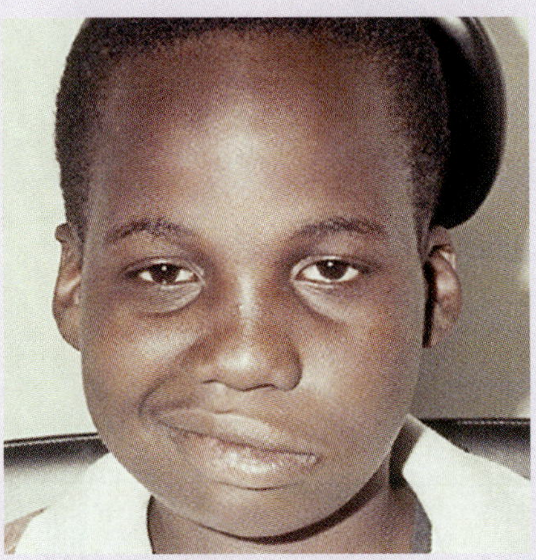

FIGURE 5-7 **Bell palsy** (From Dillon, PM: *Nursing Health Assessment.* F.A. Davis, Philadelphia, 2008, p. 218; with permission. Courtesy of Wills Eye Hospital)

brain abscess (brān ĂB-sĕs)	collection of pus anywhere within the brain
brain attack (brān ă-TĂK)	damage or death of brain tissue caused by interruption of blood supply due to a clot or vessel rupture; also known as *stroke* or *cerebrovascular accident (CVA)* (see Fig. 5-8)

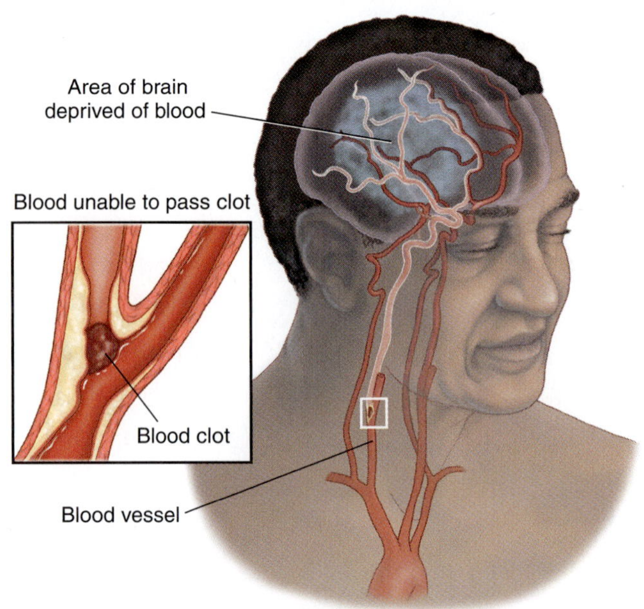

FIGURE 5-8 **Cerebrovascular accident (CVA)** (From Eagle, S, et al.: *The Professional Medical Assistant.* F.A. Davis, Philadelphia, 2009, p. 444; with permission)

TABLE 5-3

PATHOLOGY TERMS—cont'd

brain tumor (brān TŪ-mŏr)	any type of abnormal mass growing within the cranium
cerebral concussion (sĕ-RĒ-brăl kŏn-KŬ-shŭn)	vague term referring to a brief loss of consciousness or brief episode of disorientation or confusion following a head injury
cerebral contusion (sĕ-RĒ-brăl kŏn-TOO-zhŭn)	bruising of brain tissue (see Fig. 5-9)

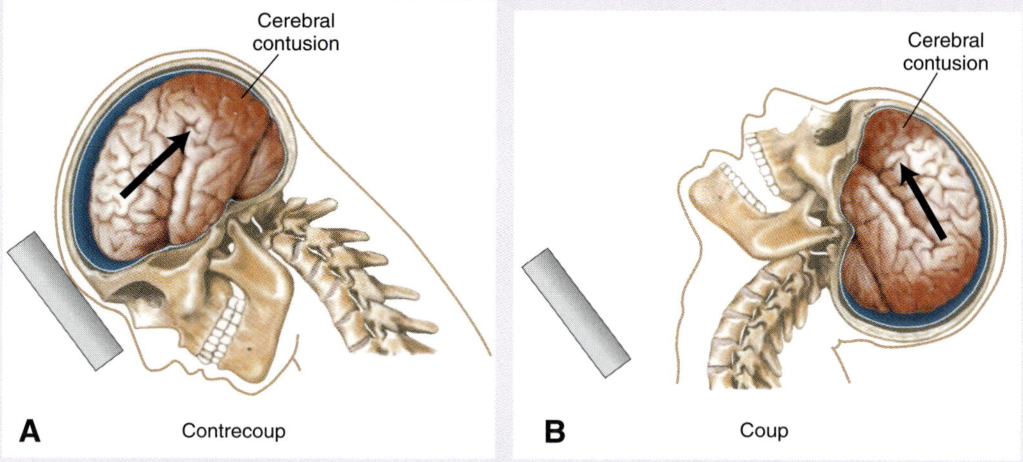

FIGURE 5-9 **Cerebral contusion** (From Eagle, S, et al.: *The Professional Medical Assistant.* F.A. Davis, Philadelphia, 2009, p. 448; with permission)

cerebral palsy (CP) (sĕ-RĒ-brăl PAWL-zē)	group of motor-impairment syndromes caused by lesions or abnormalities of the brain arising in the early stages of development
delirium (dĕ-LĬR-ē-ŭm)	acute, reversible state of agitated confusion, marked by disorientation, hallucinations, or delusions
dementia (dē-MĔN-shē-ă)	progressive neurological disorder, with numerous causes, in which an individual suffers an irreversible decline in cognition due to disease or brain damage; sometimes called *senility*
depression (dē-PRĔSH-ŭn)	mood disorder marked by loss of interest or pleasure in living
encephalitis (ĕn-sĕf-ă-LĪ-tĭs)	inflammation of the brain; often combined with meningitis and then called *encephalomeningitis*
epidural hematoma (ĕp-ĭ-DŪR-ăl hē-mă-TŌ-mă)	collection of blood between the dura mater and the skull
epilepsy (ĔP-ĭ-lĕp-sē)	chronic disorder of the brain marked by recurrent seizures, which are repetitive abnormal electrical discharges within the brain
Guillain-Barré syndrome (GBS) (gē-YĂ-băr-RĀ SĬN-drōm)	acute inflammatory disorder that causes rapidly progressing paralysis (which is usually temporary) and sometimes also sensory symptoms; also known as *acute inflammatory demyelinating polyneuropathy*
Huntington disease (HUN-ting-tun dĭ-ZĒZ)	hereditary, progressive, degenerative nervous disorder that leads to bizarre, involuntary movements and dementia
meningitis (mĕn-ĭn-JĪT-ĭs)	infection and inflammation of the meninges, the spinal cord, and CSF, usually caused by an infectious illness; often combined with encephalitis and then called *encephalomeningitis*

Continued

TABLE 5-3
PATHOLOGY TERMS—cont'd

migraine headache (MĪ-grān HED-āk)	familial disorder marked by episodes of severe throbbing headache that is commonly unilateral and sometimes disabling
multiple sclerosis (MS) (MŬL-tĭ-pul sklĕ-RŌ-sĭs)	disease involving progressive myelin degeneration, which results in loss of muscle strength and coordination
neural tube defect (NUR-ul TŪB dē-fekt)	incomplete closure of the spinal canal, which may allow protrusion of the spinal cord and meninges at birth, leading to paralysis (see Fig. 5-10); also known as *spina bifida*

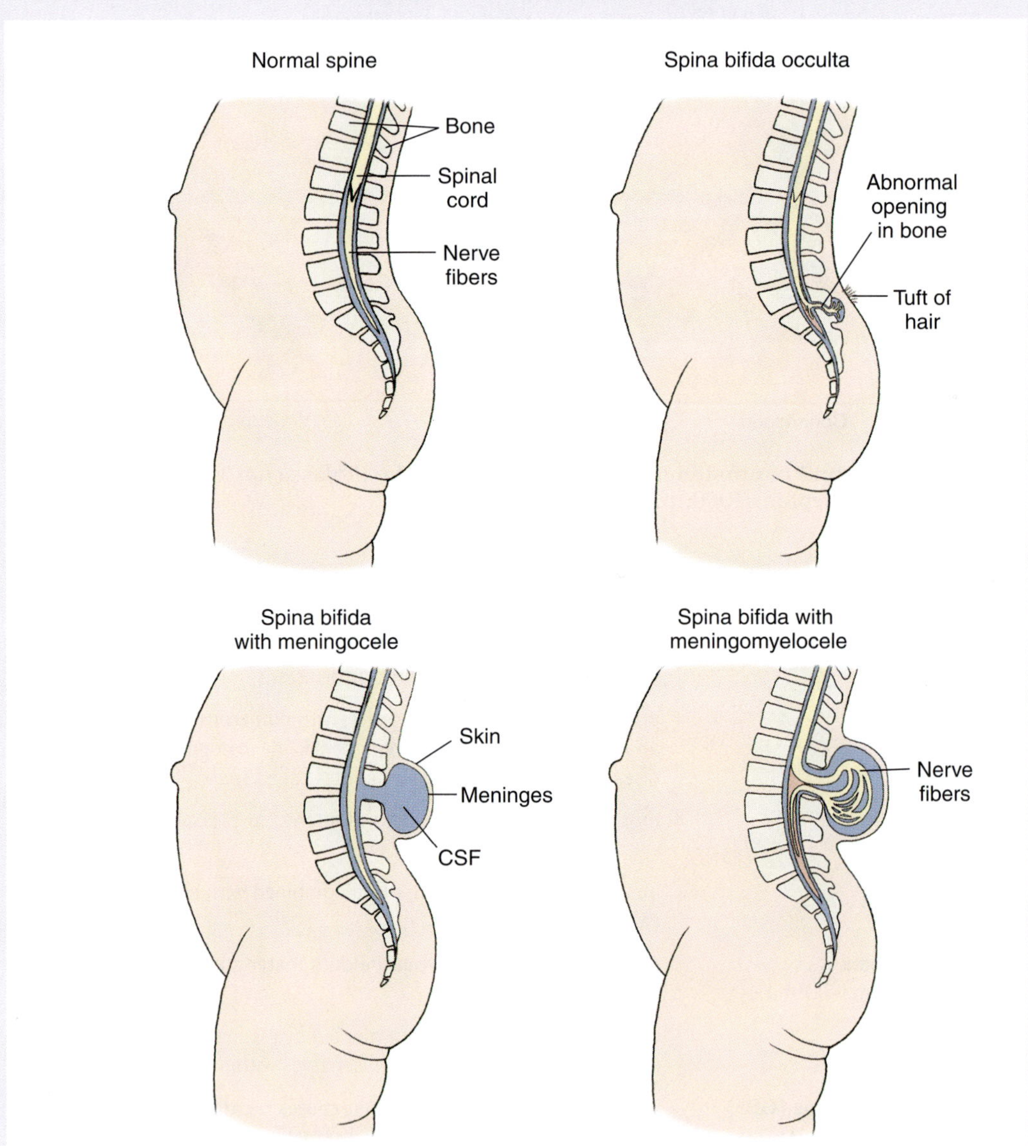

FIGURE 5-10 **Neural tube defect (spina bifida)**

TABLE 5-3

PATHOLOGY TERMS—cont'd

Parkinson disease (PĂR-kĭn-sŏn dĭ-ZĒZ)	progressive, degenerative disorder that results in tremors, gait changes, and occasionally dementia
peripheral neuropathy (pĕr-ĬF-ĕr-ăl nū-RŎP-ă-thē)	dysfunction of nerves that transmit information to and from the brain and spinal cord, characterized by pain, altered sensation, and muscle weakness
poliomyelitis (pōl-ē-ō-mī-ĕl-Ī-tĭs)	inflammation of the spinal cord, caused by a virus, which may result in spinal and muscular deformity and paralysis
Reye syndrome (rī SĬN-drōm)	serious disease associated with aspirin use by children with viral illnesses, which may result in permanent brain damage or even death
sciatica (sī-ĂT-ĭ-kă)	pain, numbness, weakness, or tingling that is felt from the lower back along the pathway of the sciatic nerve into the legs (see Fig. 5-11)

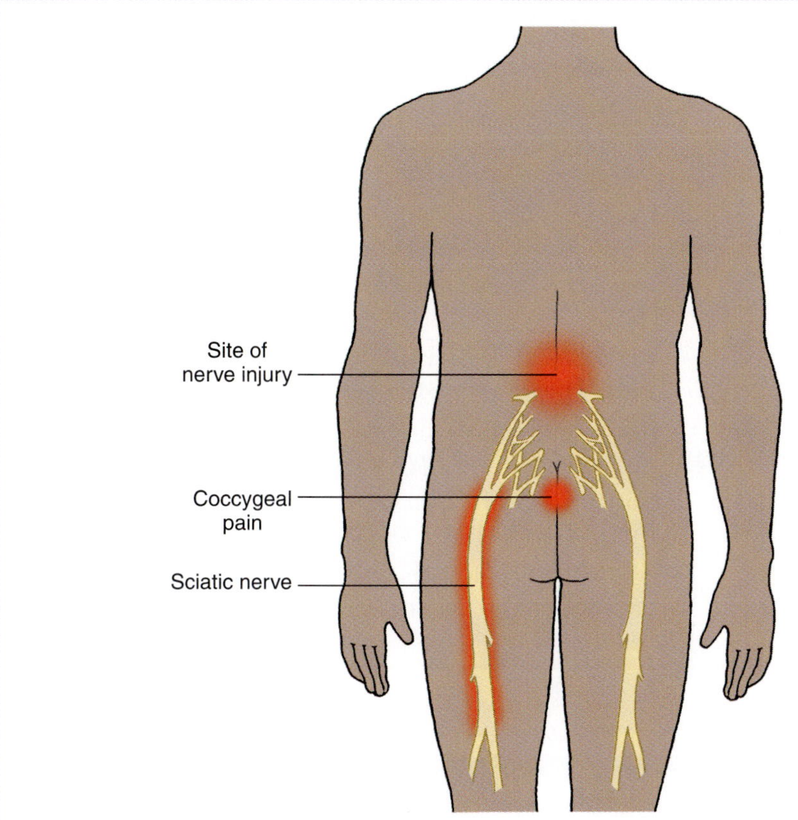

FIGURE 5-11 **Sciatica**

Continued

TABLE 5-3

PATHOLOGY TERMS—cont'd	
shingles (SHĬNG-gulz)	unilateral painful vesicles occurring on the upper body, caused by the herpes zoster virus (see Fig. 5-12)
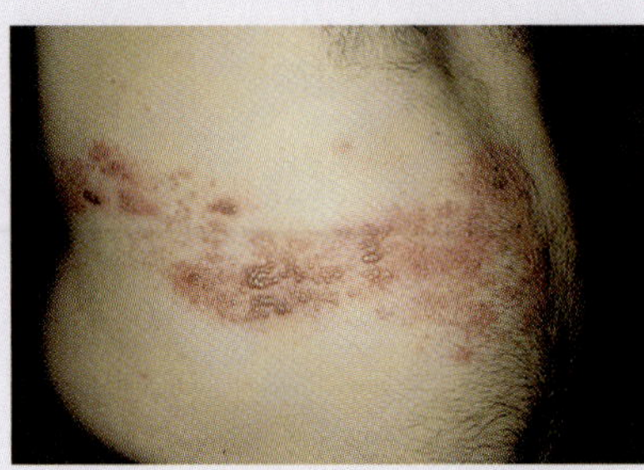 FIGURE 5-12 **Shingles** (From Goldsmith, LA, et al.: *Adult and Pediatric Dermatology.* F.A. Davis, Philadelphia, 1997, p. 307; with permission)	
spinal cord injury (SCI) (SPĪ-năl kord IN-jă-rē)	traumatic bruising, crushing, or tearing of the spinal cord
spinal stenosis (SPĪ-năl stĕ-NŌ-sĭs)	narrowing of an area of the spine that puts pressure on the spinal cord and spinal nerve roots
subdural hematoma (sub-DUR-ul hē-mă-TŌ-mă)	collection of blood between the dura and the arachnoid layer (middle or second layer of the meninges)
tension headache (TĔN-shŭn HED-āk)	nonmigraine headache in which pain is felt in all or part of the head
tetanus (TĔT-ă-nŭs)	noncontagious illness marked by severe, prolonged spasm of skeletal muscle fibers; also known as *lockjaw*
transient global amnesia (TGA) (TRĂNZ-ē-ĭnt GLŌ-băl ăm-NĒ-zē-ă)	rare disorder, not caused by a neurological event or injury, that causes sudden, temporary loss of recent memory
transient ischemic attack (TIA) (TRĂNZ-ē-ĭnt ĭs-KĒ-mĭk ă-TĂK)	temporary strokelike symptoms caused by a brief interruption of blood supply to a part of the brain
trigeminal neuralgia (TN) (trī-JĔM-ĭn-ăl nū-RĂL-jē-ă)	neurological disorder that causes severe, episodic facial pain along the pathway of the fifth cranial (trigeminal) nerve; also called *tic douloureux*

Common Diagnostic Tests

Cerebrospinal fluid (CSF) analysis: Analysis of CSF for blood, bacteria, and other abnormalities

Computed tomography (CT): Study of the brain and spinal cord using radiology and computer analysis

Electroencephalography (EEG): Study of electrical activity of the brain

Electromyogram (EMG): Record of muscle activity from electrical stimulation

Lumbar puncture (LP): Puncture of subarachnoid layer at the fourth intervertebral space to obtain CSF for analysis (see Fig. 5-13)

Magnetic resonance imaging (MRI): Use of an electromagnetic field and radio waves to create visual images on a computer screen

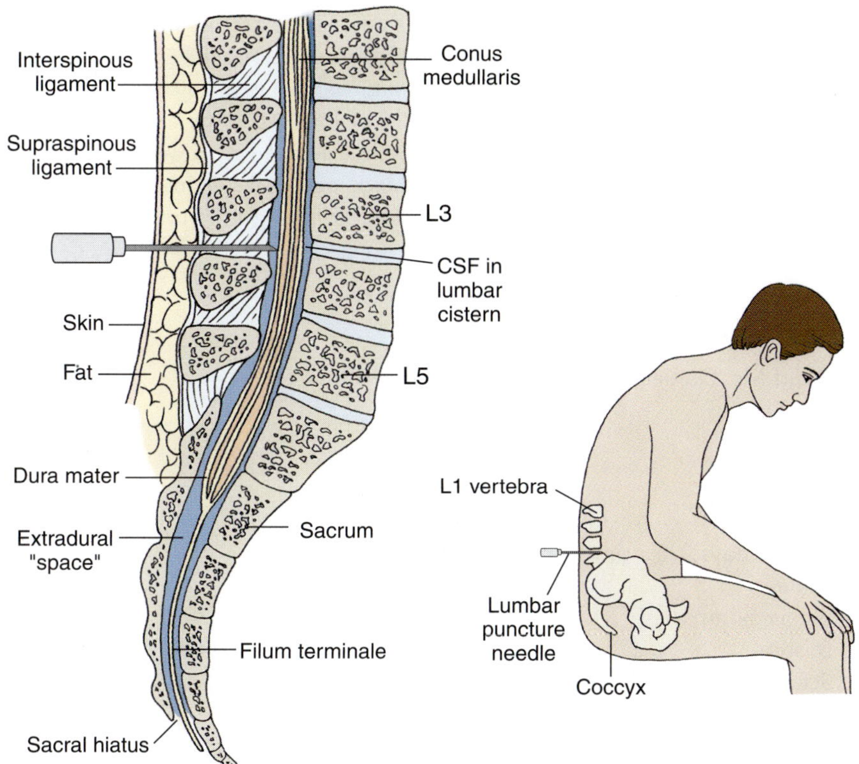

FIGURE 5-13 **Lumbar puncture**

Myelography: Radiography of the spinal cord and associated nerves after intrathecal injection (into the spinal canal) of a contrast medium

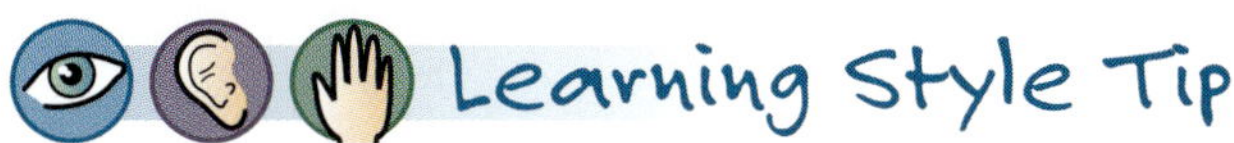

Take the time to view assigned videos: They provide great audiovisual information. And be sure to complete interactive disc activities. They also provide audiovisual content, and usually require hands-on activity completion as well.

Case Study

Read the case study and answer the questions that follow. Most of the terms are included in this chapter. Refer to the glossaries (Appendixes B and G) or to your medical dictionary for the other terms.

Shingles

Nicole Daniels is an 18-year-old female who developed a rash several days ago. She described it as a narrow strip of "tiny bumps" on the right side of her chest. Initially she noticed pruritus. Today she presented with a strip of herpetic vesicles that she describes as "exquisitely painful," with a sensation like a "fiery itch." She complained of sensitivity so severe that wearing clothing was painful because she could barely tolerate anything touching her skin. After completing a Hx and PE, her physician diagnosed her with shingles. He prescribed acyclovir to reduce the viral shedding and neuralgia. He also gave Ms. Daniels a prescription for acetaminophen with codeine to help relieve her pain.

Shingles is caused by the reactivation of the herpes varicella-zoster virus years after an initial outbreak of chickenpox. A painful eruption of vesicles occurs along the course of a segment of a spinal or cranial peripheral nerve. The lesions are nearly always unilateral. The trunk is most often affected, but the face and head may also be involved. After an outbreak of chickenpox, the virus lies dormant in the nerve cells. Individuals with a weakened immune system (from AIDS, cancer, etc.) are more vulnerable to outbreaks. Pain may continue for months after the lesions heal; this is known as *postherpetic neuralgia*. Fortunately, recurrent outbreaks of shingles are rare.

Case Study Questions

1. What did Ms. Daniels first notice on the side of her chest?
   a. Papules
   b. Scales
   c. Macules
   d. Vesicles
2. After a few days, the "tiny bumps" turned into:
   a. Scales
   b. Bigger bumps
   c. Blisters
   d. Scabs
3. Ms. Daniels has neuralgia, which is:
   a. Itching
   b. Nerve pain
   c. Fatigue
   d. Nerve paralysis
4. Chickenpox is caused by:
   a. The herpes varicella-zoster virus
   b. A bacterial infection from chickens
   c. AIDS
   d. A fungus
5. The pattern of the outbreak is usually unilateral. This means that it is:
   a. On both sides of the body
   b. On one side of the body
   c. All over the body
   d. On the upper half of the body
6. People who are most vulnerable to shingles outbreaks are:
   a. Those with strong immune systems
   b. Those with weakened immune systems
   c. Those who have had rubella
   d. Those who have had measles
7. Are recurrences of shingles outbreaks common?
   a. Yes
   b. No

Answers to Case Study Questions

1. d
2. c
3. b
4. a
5. b
6. b
7. No

Websites

Please go to the F.A. Davis website at http://davisplus.fadavis.com/eagle/medterm to view resource websites for the nervous system.

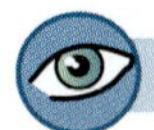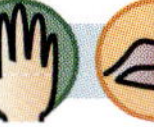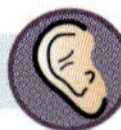 Learning Style Tip

Completing chapter activities gives you the chance to review information in a way that uses your visual and kinesthetic senses. Reading questions aloud helps verbal and auditory learners comprehend and process them better; consequently, you will be more likely to get them correct.

Practice Exercises

Deciphering Terms

Write the correct meaning of these medical terms. Check Appendix G for the correct answers.

Exercise 2

1. cerebrospinal ____________________
2. neuropathy ____________________
3. myeloma ____________________
4. meningitis ____________________
5. encephalography ____________________
6. gliocyte ____________________
7. cerebrosclerosis ____________________
8. hemiplegia ____________________
9. paraplegic ____________________
10. quadriparesis ____________________

Fill in the Blanks

Fill in the blanks below using Table 5-3. Check Appendix G for the correct answers.

Exercise 3

1. The term that refers to a seizure disorder is ____________________.
2. A form of facial paralysis that is usually unilateral and temporary is ____________________.

3. A ______________________ results in the death of brain cells.

4. Incomplete closure of the spinal canal is known as ______________________.

5. A ______________________ causes mild, temporary strokelike symptoms.

6. ______________________ is a hereditary nervous disorder that results in bizarre, involuntary movements and dementia.

7. A ______________________ is defined as bruising of brain tissue.

8. ______________________ is a serious disease, associated with aspirin use by children with viral illnesses, which may result in permanent brain damage or even death.

9. ______________________ is an acute, reversible state of agitated confusion marked by disorientation, hallucinations, or delusions.

10. ______________________ is a collection of blood between the dura mater, also known as the outermost covering of the brain, and the skull.

Multiple Choice

Select the one best answer to the following multiple-choice questions. Check Appendix G for the correct answers.

Exercise 4

1. Mrs. Fritz was hospitalized with a CVA. She is currently comatose and unresponsive. To determine whether she still has meaningful brain activity, the physician will most likely order:
   - a. An EMG
   - b. An LP
   - c. A CFS
   - d. An EEG

2. Ms. Yee sustained a brain attack. Because of this, she currently has diminished sensation and movement on only the right side of her body. Ms. Yee is experiencing:
   - a. Quadriplegia
   - b. Aphasia
   - c. Hemiplegia
   - d. Quadriparalysis

3. Mr. Stutzman is recovering from a stroke but still has difficulty speaking. The proper term for this is:
   - a. Dysphasia
   - b. Dysphagia
   - c. Aphasia
   - d. Aphagia

4. Mrs. Villanueva is recovering from a CVA but is still struggling with swallowing. The proper term for this is:
   - a. Dysphasia
   - b. Dysphoria
   - c. Euphagia
   - d. Dysphagia

5. Mr. Washington was brought to the emergency department with a high fever, confusion, and a headache. The physician wants to obtain a specimen of cerebrospinal fluid to study it for the presence of blood, bacteria, or other abnormalities. What procedure is the physician most likely to perform?
   - a. MRI
   - b. LP
   - c. EMG
   - d. CT

Word Building

*Using **only** the word parts in the lists provided, create medical terms with the indicated meanings. Check Appendix G for the correct answers.*

Exercise 5

Prefixes	**Combining Forms**	**Suffixes**
hemi-	electr/o	-al
infra-	encephal/o	-algia
iso-	gli/o	-cele
para-	mening/o	-ic
poly-	myel/o	-itis
quadri-	neur/o	-oma
	spin/o	-ous
		-paresis
		-pathy
		-plegia

1. much nerve inflammation ______________________________

2. pertaining to positioned beneath the spine ____________________

3. herniation of the spinal cord and meninges ______________________

4. inflammation of the brain and meninges ______________________

5. pertaining to near the spine ______________________

6. tumor of nerve glue ______________________

7. pertaining to the same electricity ______________________

8. partial paralysis of half (the body) ______________________

9. paralysis of four (extremities) ______________________

10. paralysis of two (extremities) ______________________

True or False

Decide whether the following statements are true or false. Check Appendix G for the correct answers.

Exercise 6

1. True False **CT** stands for *craniothoracic.*

2. True False **CNS** stands for *central nervous system.*

3. True False **Epilepsy** is a brain disorder characterized by recurrent seizures.

4. True False A form of facial paralysis affecting one or both sides of the face, which is usually temporary, is known as **Bell palsy**.

5. True False A **transient ischemic attack (TIA)** causes death of the affected brain cells.

6. True False A **shingles** outbreak is caused by the herpes varicella-zoster virus.

7. True False A **CVA** is also known as a brain attack.

8. True False **Sciatica** causes nerve pain in the buttocks and legs.

9. True False **Spina bifida**, or neural tube defect, may cause paralysis.

10. True False **Huntington disease** causes inflammation of the spinal cord by a virus that may result in spinal and muscle deformity and paralysis.

Deciphering Terms

Write the correct meaning of these medical terms. Check Appendix G for the correct answers.

Exercise 7

1. myelomeningocele ______________________
2. myelosclerosis ______________________
3. cerebrospinal ______________________
4. myasthenic ______________________
5. cerebroventricular ______________________
6. narcosis ______________________
7. thalamotomy ______________________
8. myelogram ______________________
9. neurotomy ______________________
10. gliocytic ______________________

Multiple Choice

Select the one best answer to the following multiple-choice questions. Check Appendix G for the correct answers.

Exercise 8

1. Which of the following terms is matched to the correct definition?
   a. Cephal/o: brain
   b. Gangli/o: glue, gluelike
   c. Narc/o: nerve
   d. Ton/o: tension

2. Which of the following terms is matched to the correct definition?
   a. Thalam/o: strength
   b. Myel/o: meninges
   c. Phas/o: speech
   d. Cerebr/o: cranium

3. Which of the following terms is matched to the correct definition?
   a. Lex/o: word, phrase
   b. Radicul/o: reflex
   c. Mening/o: brain
   d. Ventricul/o: vertebrae

4. Which disorder is caused by lesions or abnormalities of the brain arising in the early stages of development?
   a. ALS
   b. Bell palsy
   c. Huntington disease
   d. Cerebral palsy

5. Which of the following causes progressive confusion?
   a. Delirium
   b. Dementia
   c. TIA
   d. Cerebral concussion

6. Which of the following causes an acute form of progressive paralysis?
   a. GBS
   b. Bell palsy
   c. Huntington disease
   d. Spinal stenosis

7. A chronic, progressive, degenerative neuromuscular disorder that destroys motor neurons of the body is:
   a. ALS
   b. MS
   c. Parkinson disease
   d. Spina bifida

8. Which of the following causes temporary memory loss?
   a. MS
   b. TIA
   c. TGA
   d. OCD

9. Delirium is:
   a. An acute, reversible state of agitated confusion marked by disorientation, hallucinations, or delusions
   b. A mood disorder marked by loss of interest or pleasure in living
   c. A progressive neurological disorder that causes irreversible decline in cognition due to disease or brain damage
   d. None of these

10. A collection of blood between the dura and the arachnoid is known as:
    a. A cerebral concussion
    b. A subdural hematoma
    c. A cerebral contusion
    d. Spina bifida

11. A serious disease associated with aspirin use by children with viral illnesses is:
    a. Trigeminal neuralgia
    b. Tetanus
    c. Reye syndrome
    d. Cerebral palsy

12. Which of the following abbreviations refers to a diagnostic procedure?
    a. CVA
    b. ICP
    c. LP
    d. LOC

13. All of the following abbreviations indicate diagnostic procedures **except**:
    a. CT
    b. EEG
    c. EMG
    d. PNS

14. Which of the following terms means *brain tumor?*
    a. Cephaloma
    b. Encephaloma
    c. Ganglioma
    d. Meningioma

15. Which of the following terms means *pertaining to a seizure (episode) of sleep or stupor?*
    a. Narcoleptic
    b. Tonic
    c. Glial
    d. Neuralgia

16. Which of the following terms means *bad, painful, or difficult speech?*
    a. Dysphagia
    b. Euphasia
    c. Dysphasia
    d. Aphasia

17. The term *radiculitis* indicates inflammation of the:
    a. Ganglion
    b. Brain
    c. Thalamus
    d. Nerve root

18. A term that indicates a condition of muscle weakness is:
    a. Myasthenia
    b. Myalgia
    c. Myosclerosis
    d. None of these

19. A term that indicates hardening of the brain is:
    a. Cerebroma
    b. Encephalotome
    c. Cephalodynia
    d. None of these

20. A term that indicates inflammation of the brain and meninges is:
    a. Cerebritis
    b. Neuroencephalitis
    c. Cerebellitis
    d. Encephalomeningitis

CARDIOVASCULAR SYSTEM

6

Structure and Function

The key structure of the cardiovascular system is the heart, which pumps blood throughout your entire body. The circulatory system includes a complex network of arteries, veins, and capillaries.

The heart is a hollow, muscular organ about the size of a closed fist that pumps oxygen-rich blood and nutrients to the trillions of cells of your body. To accomplish this, it beats an average of 60 to 100 times a minute for your entire lifetime. This adds up to 104,000 times per day, and 38,000,000 times per year (see Fig. 6-1). Your heart is located in the center of your chest, slightly to the left, in an area called the mediastinum. It has three layers: the outer lining, called the **epicardium**; the middle muscular layer, called the myocardium; and the inner lining, called the **endocardium**. The heart is enclosed in a fibrous membrane called the **pericardium**, or **pericardial sac**, which also contains a small amount of **pericardial fluid**. This fluid acts as a lubricant that reduces friction as the heart repeatedly contracts and relaxes. Occasionally, inflammation may develop within the pericardial sac. This condition is called ***pericarditis***.

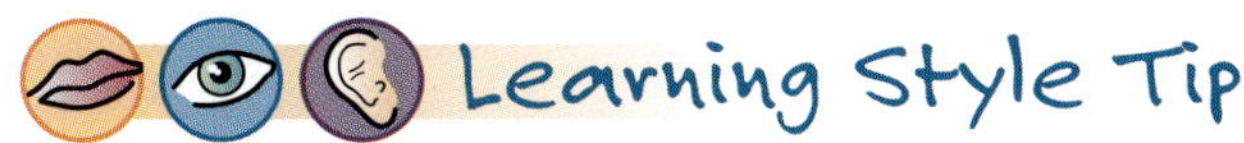

Verbally describe photos or illustrations in this book to a real or imaginary friend who cannot see them. Provide all of the details they need to accurately visualize what you are describing.

Flashpoint
The average person's heart beats 38,000,000 times every year!

The heart has two upper chambers, the right and left **atria**, which perform about 30% of the work, and two larger, lower chambers, the right and left **ventricles**, which perform the other 70% of the work. The left ventricle is the largest and most muscular chamber, because it works harder than the others. The right and left sides of the heart are divided by a thick layer of muscle tissue called the **septum**.

There are four valves in your heart. The **tricuspid valve** exits the right atrium into the right ventricle and the **mitral**, or **bicuspid valve**, exits the left atrium into the left ventricle. The **pulmonary valve** exits the right ventricle into the pulmonary arteries, and the **aortic valve** exits the left ventricle into the aorta.

The largest part of your heart, the lower left area, is known as the **apex**. This site is best for auscultating (listening to) sounds from the mitral valve and is where the **apical pulse** is best heard. Listening to the apical pulse for one full minute is considered the most accurate method of measuring heart rate, and is the preferred method in situations where accuracy is very important.

Blood flows through both sides of heart at the same time. Blood that is low in oxygen (**O_2**) but high in carbon dioxide (**CO_2**) returns from the body to the right

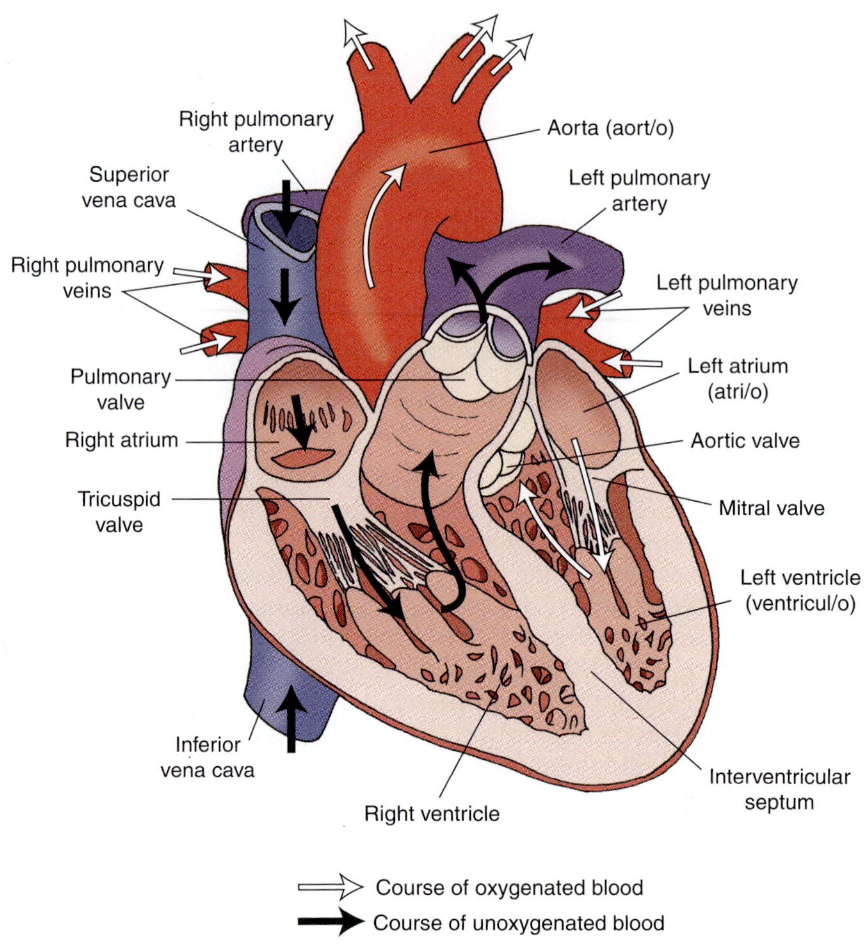

FIGURE 6-1 **The heart**

atrium via the inferior and superior venae cavae. As both atria contract at the same time, they each pump blood to a different area. The right atrium pumps blood downward through the tricuspid valve into the right ventricle. As the right ventricle contracts, it forces blood up and out through the pulmonary valve into the pulmonary arteries. The pulmonary arteries lead to the lungs, where CO_2 is exchanged for O_2. The pulmonary arteries are unique in that they are the only arteries in the body that transport oxygen-poor blood. As the blood circulates through your lungs, it gets rid of CO_2 and picks up O_2. Blood that is now oxygen rich returns through the pulmonary veins to the left atrium. The pulmonary veins are unique in that they are the only veins in the body that transport oxygen-rich blood. As the left atrium contracts, it forces blood downward through the mitral valve into the left ventricle. From there the blood is pumped by the left ventricle upward and out through the aortic valve into the aorta and out to various parts of the body.

Flashpoint

The left ventricle has the largest job of all the heart chambers, since it must pump blood out to the entire body.

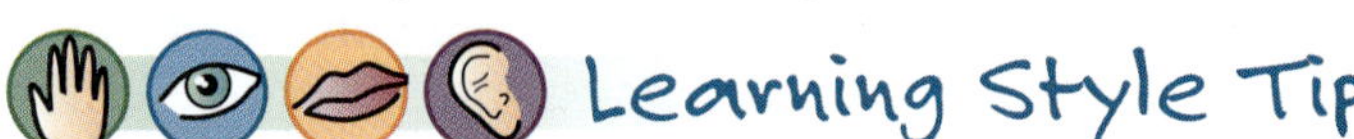

Learning Style Tip

With a study group or a study buddy, use sidewalk chalk to draw a giant illustration of the heart on cement or pavement outdoors. Make it as colorful and as accurate as you can. Label and verbally identify all the heart structures. Draw arrows to indicate the direction of blood flow. When the drawing is complete, take turns walking along the circulatory route through the right side of the heart, to the lungs, back through the left side of the heart, out to the body, and then back to where you started. As you follow this route, identify whether you are simulating the path of oxygen-rich or oxygen-poor blood and why.

The heart has its own network of coronary vessels that keep it supplied with oxygen and nutrients. Occasionally, ***arteriosclerosis*** develops in these vessels and they become narrowed and hardened due to a number of factors, including ***hypertension*** (high blood pressure). In addition, a fatty, plaquelike substance composed of **cholesterol** may build up on the inside surfaces of the coronary vessels, causing further narrowing or even blockage. This is known as ***atherosclerosis***, and contributes to the development of ***coronary artery disease (CAD)***. It is also sometimes called *atherosclerotic heart disease (ASHD)*. If a vessel becomes completely **occluded** (blocked), then the heart muscle downstream dies from a lack of oxygen. This is known as a ***myocardial infarction (MI)*** or a *heart attack*.

As oxygen-rich blood is pumped from the heart, it travels to all parts of the body through an intricate network of arteries (see Fig. 6-2). The arteries vary in size, from the very large **aorta** to very tiny **arterioles**. From the arterioles, blood enters numerous microscopic-sized **capillaries** with walls that are just one cell thick. This allows O_2 and nutrients to easily leave the capillaries and enter the tissues and cells. It also allows waste products and CO_2 to easily move from the cells and tissues back into the capillaries. Blood that is now low in O_2 and high in CO_2 and waste leaves the capillaries and enters microscopic-sized **venules** (tiny veins). As it continues on its return journey, the blood travels through larger and larger veins until it reaches the heart. Blood is drained from the head and upper body via the **superior vena cava** and from the lower body via the **inferior vena cava**. Venous blood travels under much less pressure than arterial blood. Because of this, it cannot easily flow against gravity to ascend the legs and return to the heart. Fortunately, veins contain one-way valves that facilitate circulation by preventing the backflow of blood. The pumping action created by the contraction and relaxation of leg muscles also helps to propel the blood upward.

Have you ever wondered what makes your heart beat? Your heart has its own special pacemaker that has been working since before you were born (see Fig. 6-3). A cluster of specialized cells in your right atrium called the **sinoatrial (SA) node** serves as a natural pacemaker for the heart, initiating an electrical impulse about 60 to 100 times per minute. Each of these impulses is transmitted throughout all the muscle cells of your heart, resulting in an electrical charge called **depolarization**. When this occurs, the inside of the cardiac muscle cells becomes electrically positive in relation to the outside. In response, all of the individual cardiac muscle cells in your atria contract in unison. The name given to the normal rhythm of the heart is *normal sinus rhythm*, named for the SA node (see Fig. 6-4).

Flashpoint
The walls of the capillaries are extremely thin, which allows gases, nutrients, and wastes to easily cross back and forth.

Flashpoint
The sinoatrial node is the heart's natural pacemaker.

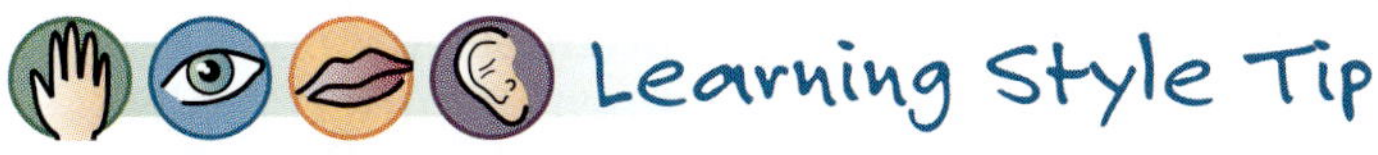

Trace the conduction pathway of the heart with your finger as you verbally identify all of its structures and describe their function.

Within the floor of the right atrium is another pacemaker, the **atrioventricular (AV) node**. It is sometimes thought of as a backup pacemaker. It receives the impulse from the SA node and transmits it downward to both ventricles via

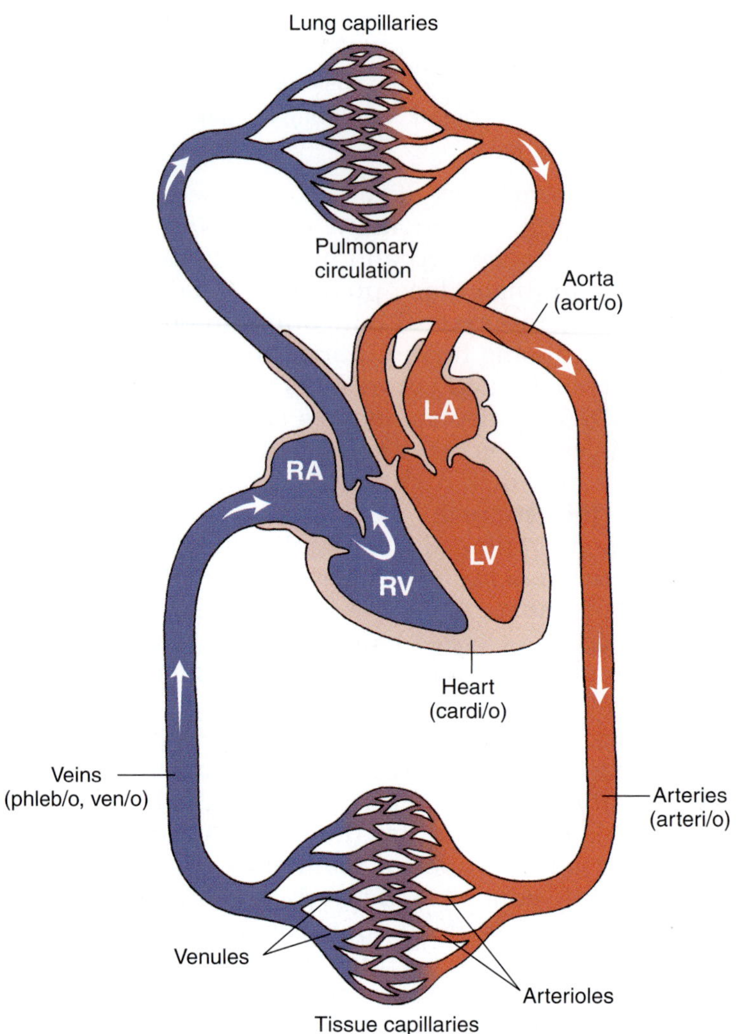

FIGURE 6-2 **The cardiovascular system**

the **bundle of His** located within the septum, and the **Purkinje fibers** distributed through the septum and throughout the ventricles. As the electrical impulse is transmitted throughout your ventricles, all ventricular muscle fibers contract in unison. This contraction occurs just slightly after the contraction of the atria, and the combination of the two results in one complete heartbeat. This entire process is repeated with each heartbeat.

The contraction and relaxation of the four heart chambers, known as the **cardiac cycle**, creates each heartbeat. Each cardiac cycle is quite rapid, taking an average of just 0.8 second. **Blood pressure**, created by the pumping of blood, is written as two numbers, one over the other: 120/80. The upper number, the **systolic pressure**, reflects the highest pressure exerted against artery walls during ventricular contraction, or **systole**. The lower number, the **diastolic pressure**, reflects the lowest pressure exerted against artery walls during ventricular relaxation, or **diastole**. Large arteries in the body that have a strong pulse and are easily palpated are known as **pulse points**. These points, sometimes called **pressure points**, may be compressed to slow bleeding in the case of hemorrhage (see Fig. 6-5).

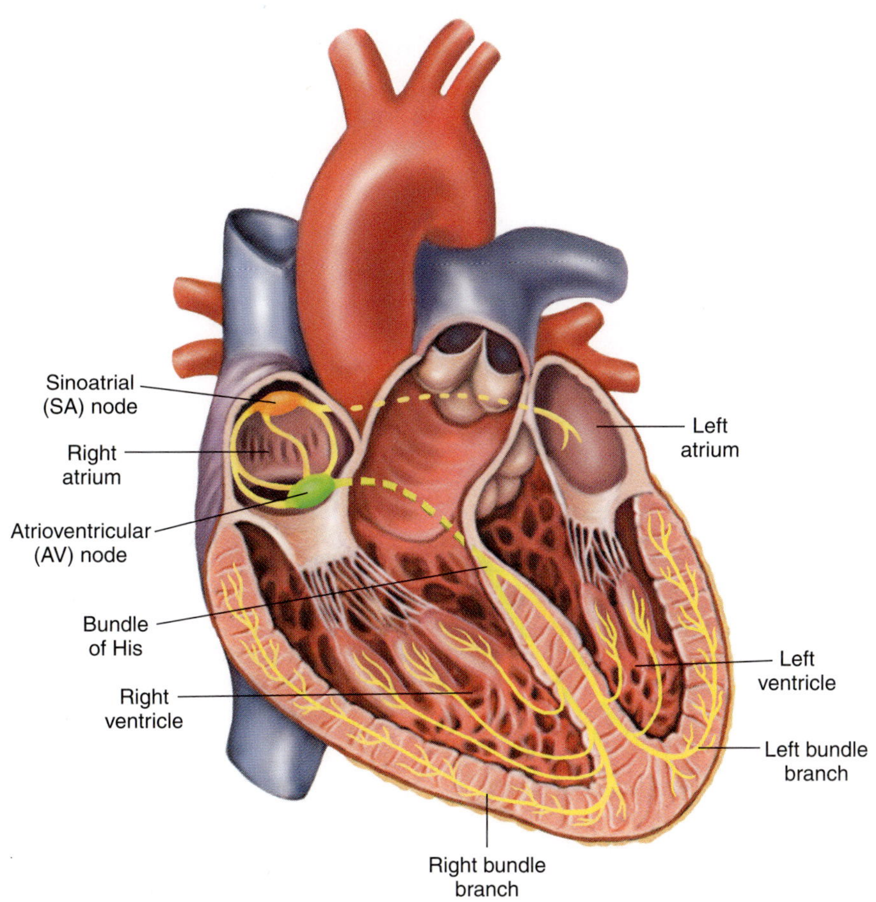

FIGURE 6-3 Electrical conduction system of the heart

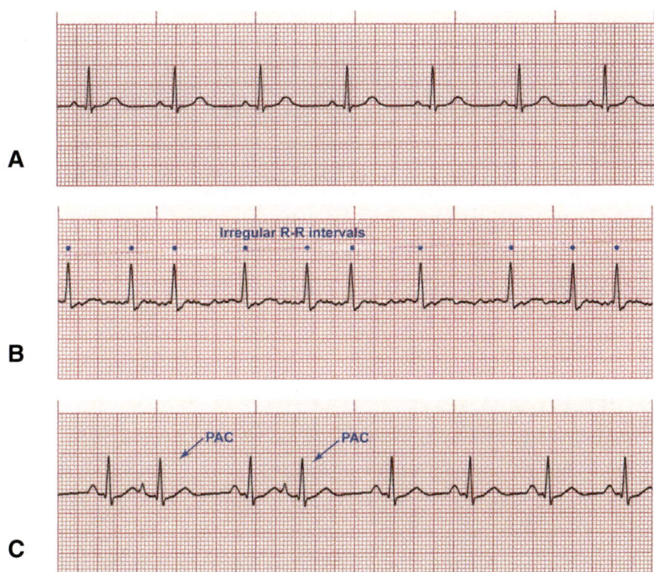

FIGURE 6-4 Cardiac rhythm (normal and abnormal rhythms): (A) Normal sinus rhythm (NSR); (B) Atrial fibrillation (AF, A-fib); (C) Sinus rhythm with premature atrial contractions (PACs)

(continued)

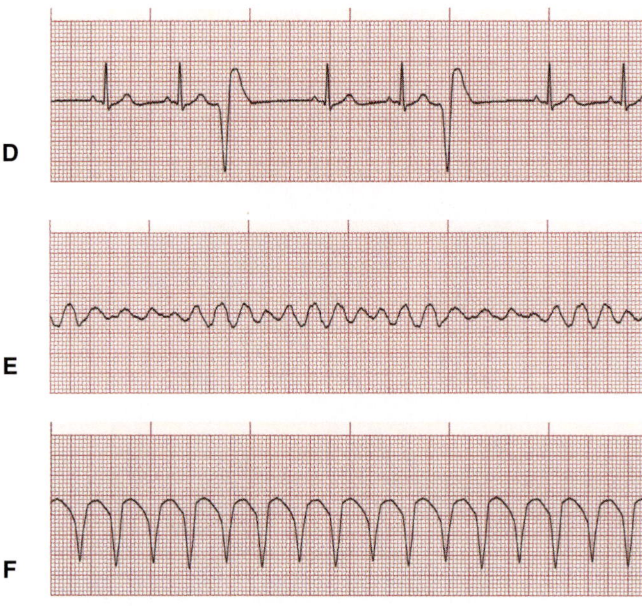

FIGURE 6-4—cont'd **(D) Sinus rhythm with premature ventricular contractions (PVCs); (E) Ventricular fibrillation (V-fib); (F) Ventricular tachycardia (VT, V-tach)** (From Eagle, S, et al.: *The Professional Medical Assistant.* F.A. Davis, Philadelphia, 2009, p. 465; with permission)

Flashpoint

Blood-pressure readings reflect the pressure exerted against the arterial walls during both phases of the cardiac cycle.

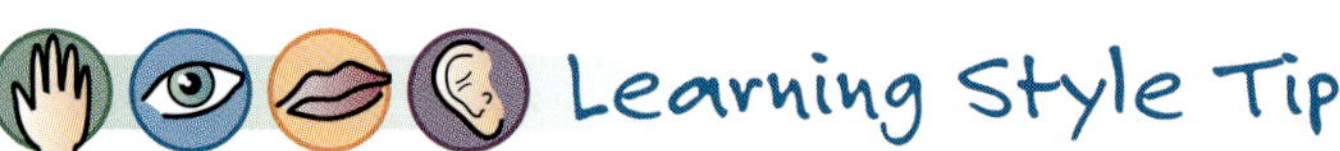

Learning Style Tip

If you can locate the resources in an on-campus lab or through a friend, use a stethoscope and blood-pressure cuff to practice taking blood-pressure readings on one another. Verbalize the readings as you obtain them and identify which is systolic and which is diastolic. Further define what these terms mean. Practice locating pulse points on one another as identified in Figure 6-19, and name each as you palpate (feel) it.

Combining Forms

Table 6-1 contains combining forms that pertain to the cardiovascular system, examples of terms that utilize the combining forms, and a pronunciation guide. Read aloud to yourself as you move from left to right across the table. Be sure to use the pronunciation guide so that you can learn to say the terms correctly.

STOP HERE.

Select the Combining Form Flash Cards for Chapter 6 and run through them at least three times before you continue.

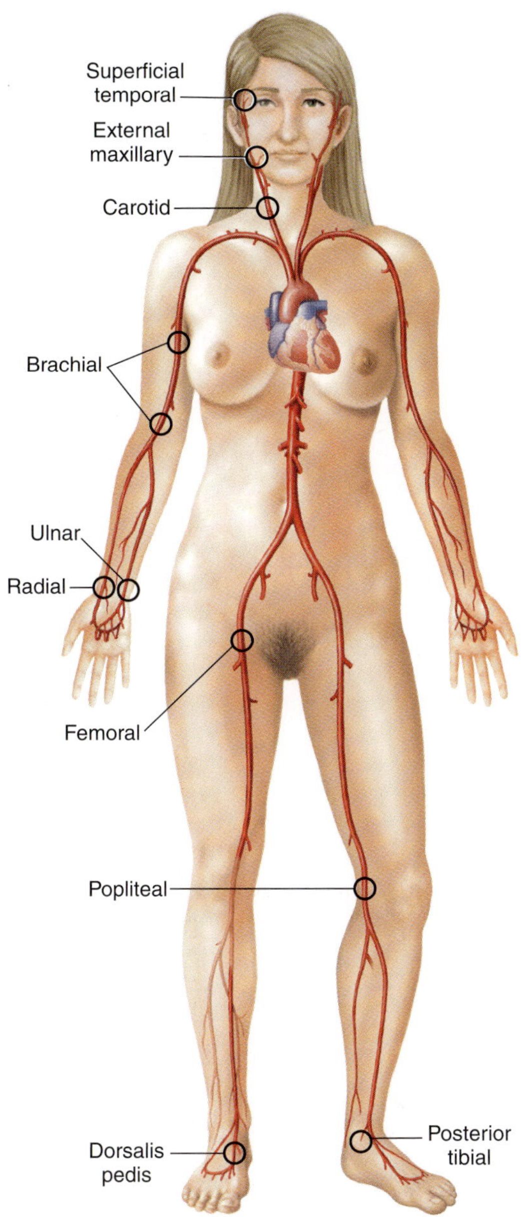

FIGURE 6-5 **Pulse points** (From Eagle, S, et al.: *The Professional Medical Assistant.* F.A. Davis, Philadelphia, 2009, p. 330; with permission)

TABLE 6-1

COMBINING FORMS

Combining Form	Meaning	Example (Pronunciation)	Meaning of New Term
angi/o	vessel	angioedema (ăn-jē-ō-ĕ-DĒ-mă)	swelling of a vessel
vas/o		vasorrhaphy (văs-OR-ă-fē)	suturing of a vessel
aort/o	aorta	aortostenosis (ā-or-tō-stĕ-NŌ-sĭs)	narrowing or stricture of the aorta

Continued

TABLE 6-1
COMBINING FORMS—cont'd

Combining Form	Meaning	Example (Pronunciation)	Meaning of New Term
arteri/o	artery	arteriosclerosis (ăr-tē-rē-ō-sklĕ-RŌ-sĭs)	abnormal condition of hardening of an artery
ather/o	thick, fatty	atheroma (ăth-ĕr-Ō-mă)	thick, fatty tumor
atri/o	atria	atrioventricular (ā-trē-ō-vĕn-TRĬK-ū-lăr)	pertaining to the atria and the ventricles
cardi/o	heart	tachycardia (tăk-ē-KĂR-dē-ă)	condition of a rapid heart
coron/o		coronary (KOR-ō-nă-rē)	pertaining to the heart
electr/o	electricity	electrocardiogram (ē-lĕk-trō-KĂR-dē-ō-grăm)	record of electricity of the heart
hem/o	blood	hemolytic (hē-mō-LĬT-ĭk)	pertaining to the destruction of blood
hemat/o		hematemesis (hĕm-ăt-ĔM-ĕ-sĭs)	vomiting of blood
phleb/o	vein	phleborrhexis (flĕb-ō-RĔK-sĭs)	rupture of a vein
ven/o		venostasis (vē-nō-STĀ-sĭs)	stopping of a vein
thromb/o	thrombus (clot)	thrombophlebitis (thrŏm-bō-flē-BĪ-tĭs)	inflammation of a vein with the presence of a clot
valv/o	valve	valvotomy (văl-VŎT-ō-mē)	cutting into or incision of a valve
valvul/o		valvuloplasty (VĂL-vū-lō-plăs-tē)	surgical repair of a valve
vascul/o	blood vessel	vasculogenesis (văs-kū-lō-JĔN-ĕ-sĭs)	creation of a blood vessel
ventricul/o	ventricle	ventriculostomy (vĕn-trĭk-ū-LŎS-tō-mē)	mouthlike opening into a ventricle

Practice Exercises

Fill in the Blanks

Fill in the blanks below using Table 6-1. Check Appendix G for the correct answers.

Exercise 1

1. mouthlike opening into a ventricle ____________________

2. swelling of a vessel ____________________

3. condition of a rapid heart ______________________________

4. cutting into or incision of a valve ______________________________

5. record of electricity of the heart ______________________________

6. abnormal condition of hardening of an artery ______________________________

7. rupture of a vein ______________________________

8. suturing of a vessel ______________________________

9. thick fatty tumor ______________________________

10. vomiting of blood ______________________________

11. surgical repair of a valve ______________________________

12. creation of a blood vessel ______________________________

13. narrowing or stricture of the aorta ______________________________

14. stopping of a vein ______________________________

15. pertaining to the atria and the ventricles ______________________________

16. pertaining to the destruction of blood ______________________________

17. inflammation of a vein with the presence of a clot ______________________________

18. pertaining to the heart ______________________________

19. **Fill in the blanks in Figure 6-6 with the appropriate anatomical terms and combining forms.**

20. **Fill in the blanks in Figure 6-7 with the appropriate anatomical terms and combining forms.**

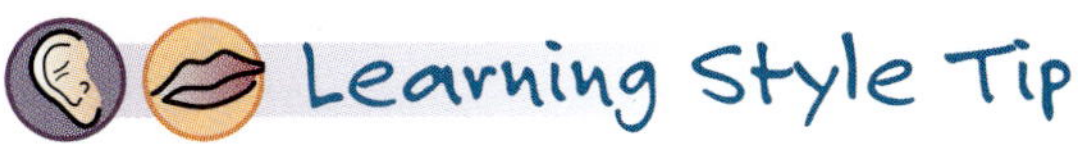

Play instrumental music (with no lyrics) when you study and sing the key terms, definitions, or phrases to the music.

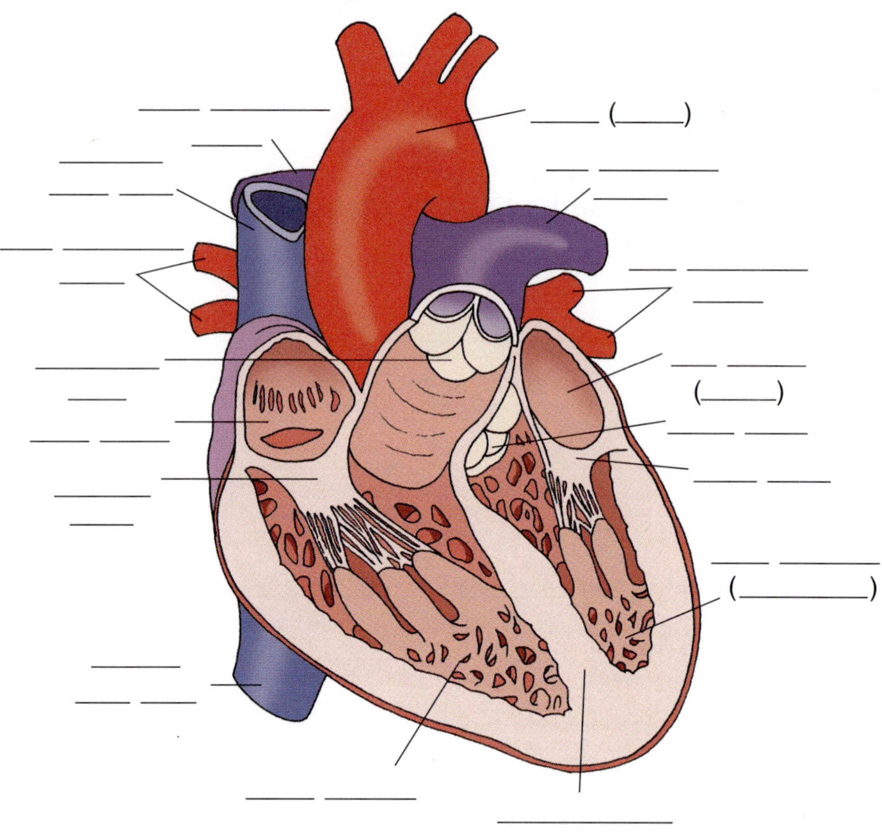

FIGURE 6-6 **The heart with blanks**

Abbreviations

Table 6-2 lists some of the most common abbreviations related to the cardiovascular system as well as others often used in medical documentation.

STOP HERE.
Select the Abbreviation Flash Cards for Chapter 6 and run through them at least three times before you continue.

Flashpoint
Heart disease is one of the most common causes of death among Americans.

Pathology Terms

Table 6-3 includes terms that relate to diseases or abnormalities of the cardiovascular system. Use the pronunciation guide and say the terms aloud as you read them. This will help you get in the habit of saying them properly.

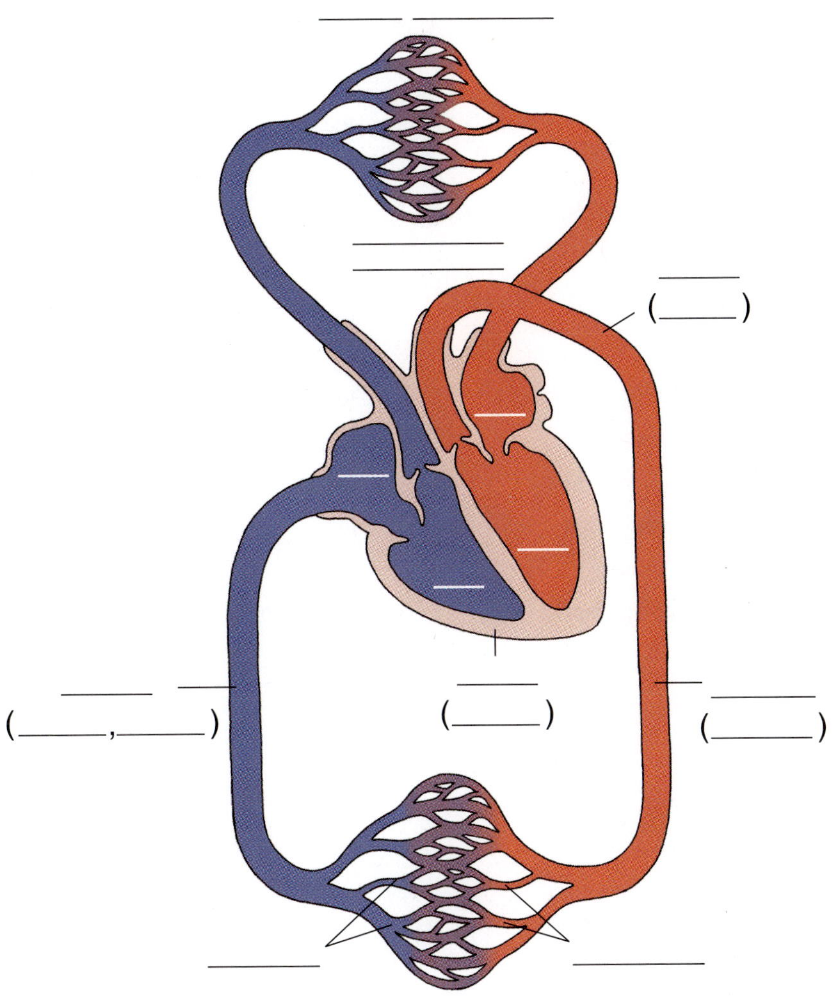

FIGURE 6-7 The cardiovascular system with blanks

TABLE 6-2
ABBREVIATIONS

Cardiovascular System			
AF, A-fib	atrial fibrillation	CCU	coronary care unit
ASHD	arteriosclerotic heart disease	CHF	congestive heart failure
AV, A-V	atrioventricular	CP	chest pain
BP	blood pressure	CPR	cardiopulmonary resuscitation
bpm	beats per minute	CV	cardiovascular
CABG	coronary artery bypass graft	DVT	deep vein thrombosis
CAD	coronary artery disease	ECG, EKG	electrocardiogram

Continued

TABLE 6-2
ABBREVIATIONS—cont'd

Cardiovascular System			
ECHO	echocardiogram	PAC	premature atrial contraction
HF	heart failure	PT	prothrombin time
HTN	hypertension (high blood pressure)	PTCA	percutaneous transluminal coronary angioplasty
ICU	intensive care unit	PTT	partial thromboplastin time
INR	international normalized ratio	PVC	premature ventricular contraction
LA	left atrium	RA	right atrium
LV	left ventricle	RBC	red blood cell
MI	myocardial infarction	ROM	range of motion
MR	mitral regurgitation	RV	right ventricle
MS	mitral stenosis	V-fib	ventricular fibrillation
MVP	mitral valve prolapse	VT, V-tach	ventricular tachycardia
P	pulse	VTE	venous thromboembolism
Dosing Schedules			
bid, b.i.d.	two times a day	q2h	every 2 hours
tid, t.i.d.	three times a day	qhs	each evening (hour of sleep)
qid, q.i.d.	four times a day	qam	each morning
qh	every hour		

STOP HERE.
Select the Pathology Term Flash Cards for Chapter 6 and run through them at least three times before you continue.

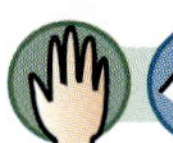
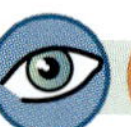
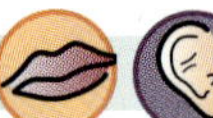

Learning Style Tip

Play charades or a Pictionary-type game with a study group or study buddy to act out or draw clues for each of the following procedures as your partners guess which one you are demonstrating. It is OK to be silly, laugh, and have fun. In fact, the more fun you have, the better you will remember the procedures.

TABLE 6-3
PATHOLOGY TERMS

Term	Definition
anemia (ă-NĒ-mē-ă)	group of disorders generally defined as a reduction in the mass of circulating red blood cells
aneurysm (ĂN-ū-rĭ-zum)	weakening and bulging of part of a vessel wall (see Fig. 6-8)

TABLE 6-3
PATHOLOGY TERMS—cont'd

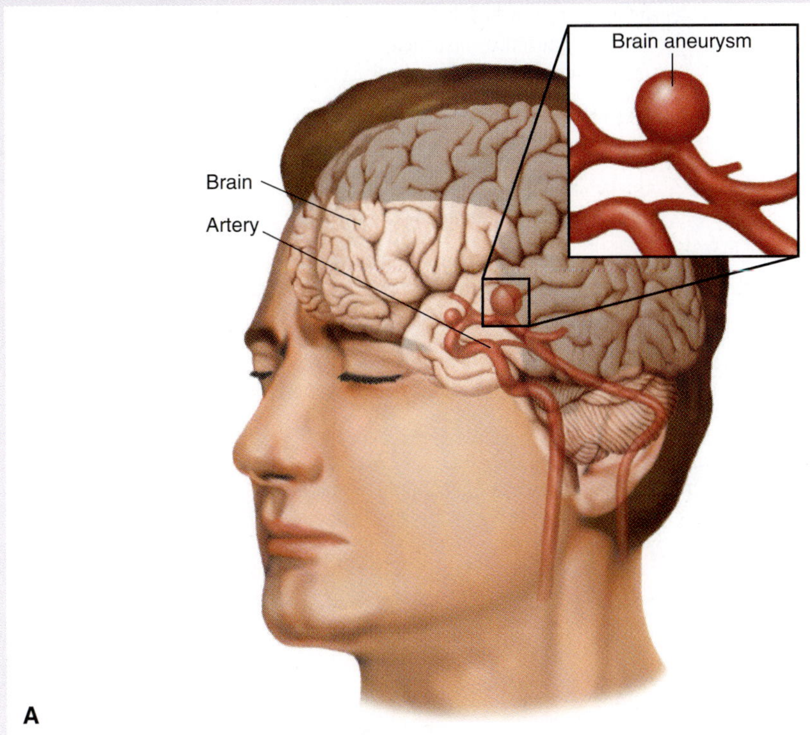

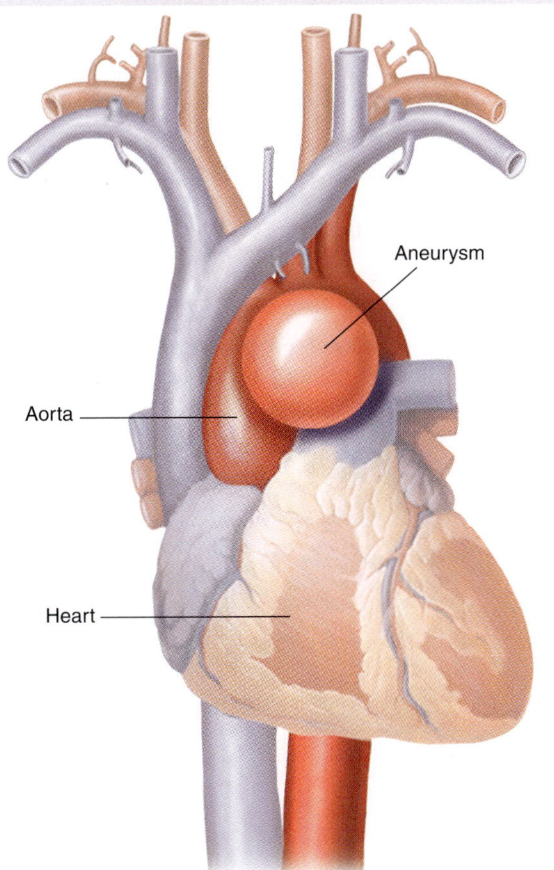

FIGURE 6-8 **Aneurysm** (From Eagle, S, et al.: *The Professional Medical Assistant.* F.A. Davis, Philadelphia, 2009, p. 476; with permission)

Continued

TABLE 6-3

PATHOLOGY TERMS—cont'd

angina (ăn-JĪ-nă)	heart pain or other discomfort felt in the chest, shoulders, arms, jaw, or neck, caused by insufficient blood and oxygen to the heart; usually a symptom of heart disease
arrhythmia (ă-RĬTH-mē-ă)	loss of heart rhythm (rhythmic irregularity)
arteriosclerosis (ăr-tē-rē-ō-sklĕ-RŌ-sĭs)	thickening, loss of elasticity, and loss of contractility of arterial walls; commonly called *hardening of the arteries*
atherosclerosis (ăth-ĕr-ō-sklĕ-RŌ-sĭs)	the most common form of arteriosclerosis, marked by deposits of cholesterol, lipids, and calcium on the walls of arteries, which may restrict blood flow
atrial fibrillation (AF, A-fib) (Ā-trē-ăl fĭ-brĭl-Ā-shŭn)	common irregular heart rhythm marked by uncontrolled atrial quivering and a rapid ventricular response (see Fig. 6-9)

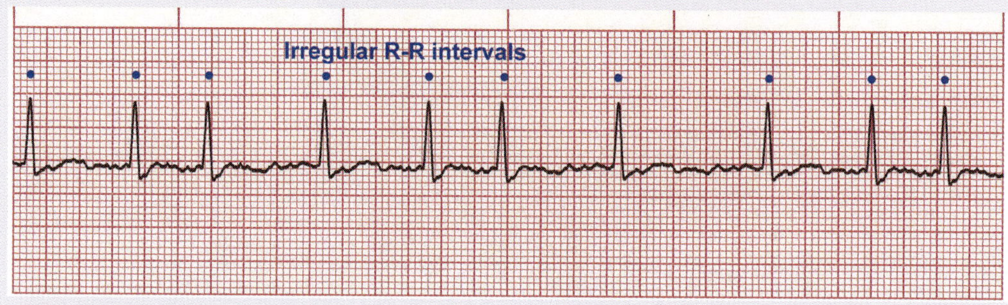

FIGURE 6-9 **Atrial fibrillation** (From Jones, S: *ECG Success*. F.A. Davis, Philadelphia, 2008, p. 32; with permission)

bruit (bruw-ē)	soft blowing sound caused by turbulent blood flow in a vessel
cardiac tamponade (KĂR-dē-ăk tăm-pŏn-ĀD)	serious condition in which the heart becomes compressed from an excessive collection of fluid or blood between the pericardial membrane and the heart
cardiomyopathy (kăr-dē-ō-mī-ŎP-ă-thē)	group of conditions in which the heart muscle has deteriorated and functions less effectively
congestive heart failure (CHF) (kŭn-JES-tĭv hărt FĀL-yĕr)	inability of the heart to pump enough blood to meet the needs of the body, resulting in lung congestion and dyspnea
cor pulmonale (kor pŭl-mă-NĂL-ē)	condition of right ventricular enlargement or dilation from increased right ventricular pressure; also called *pulmonary heart disease* or *right-sided heart failure*
coronary artery disease (CAD) (KOR-ō-nă-rē ĂR-tĕr-ē dĭ-ZĒZ)	narrowing of the lumen, or inner open space of a vessel, of heart arteries due to arteriosclerosis and atherosclerosis (see Fig. 6-10)

TABLE 6-3
PATHOLOGY TERMS—cont'd

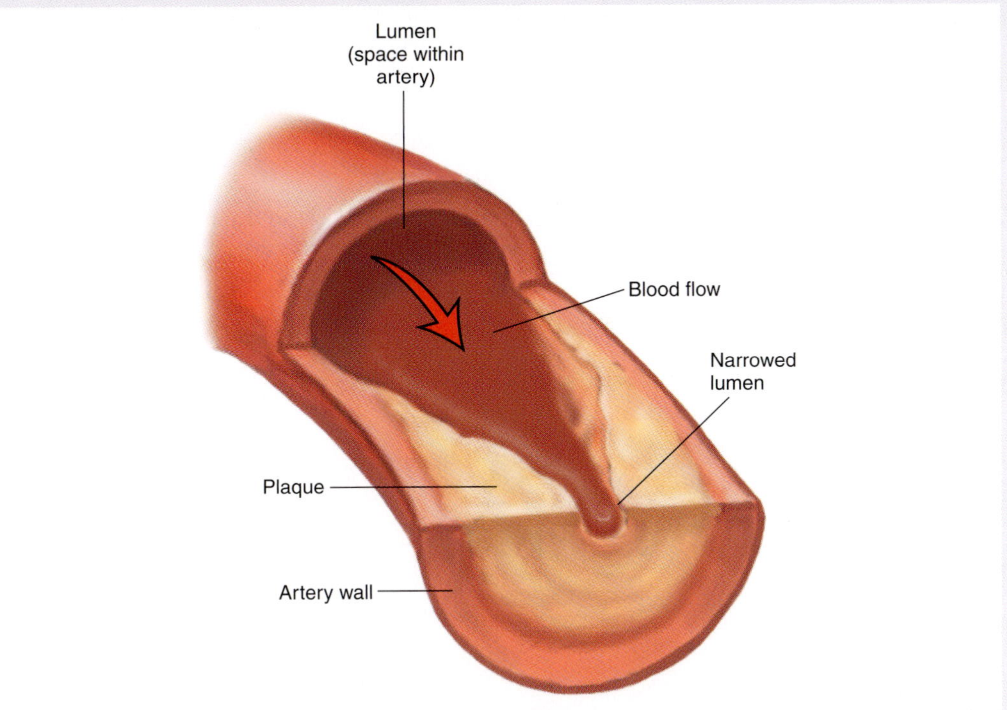

FIGURE 6-10 **Coronary artery disease** (From Eagle, S, et al.: *The Professional Medical Assistant.* F.A. Davis, Philadelphia, 2009, p. 473; with permission)

deep vein thrombosis (DVT) (dēp vān thrŏm-BŌ-sĭs)	development of a blood clot in a deep vein, usually in the legs; also known as *thrombophlebitis* (see Fig. 6-11)

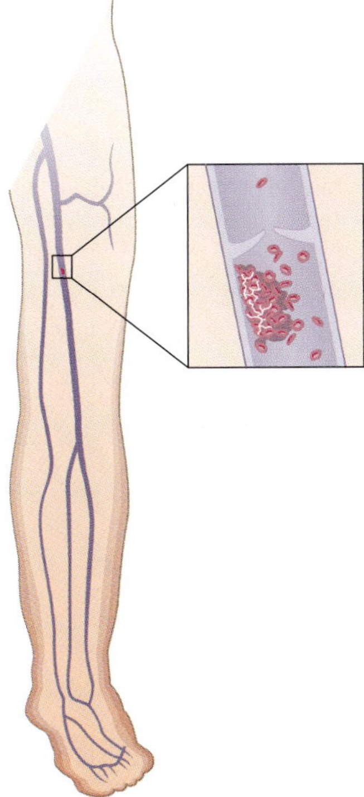

FIGURE 6-11 **Deep vein thrombosis**

Continued

TABLE 6-3

PATHOLOGY TERMS—cont'd

disseminated intravascular coagulation (DIC) (dĭ-SEM-ĭ-nāt-ĕd ĭn-tră-VĂS-kū-lăr kō-ăg-ū-LĀ-shŭn)	serious condition that arises as a complication of another disorder, in which widespread, unrestricted microvascular blood clotting occurs; primary symptom is hemorrhage
embolus (ĔM-bō-lŭs)	undissolved matter floating in blood or lymph fluid that may cause an occlusion and infarction
endocarditis (ĕn-dō-kăr-DĪ-tĭs)	infection of the inner lining of the heart that may cause vegetations to form within one or more heart chambers or valves (see Fig. 6-12)

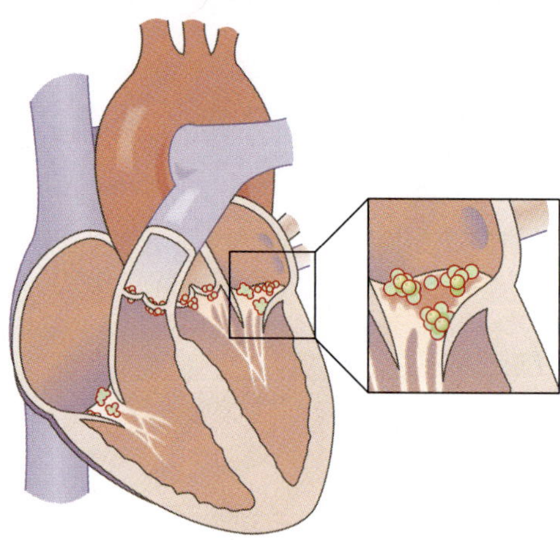

FIGURE 6-12 **Endocarditis**

fibrillation (fĭ-brĭl-Ā-shŭn)	quivering of heart muscle fibers instead of an effective heartbeat
hypertension (HTN) (hī-pĕr-TĔN-shŭn)	blood pressure that is consistently higher than 140 systolic, 90 diastolic, or both
ischemia (ĭs-KĒ-mē-ă)	temporary reduction in blood supply to a localized area of tissue
malignant hypertension (mă-LĬG-nănt hī-pĕr-TĔN-shŭn)	rare, life-threatening type of hypertension evidenced by optic-nerve (eye) edema and extremely high systolic and diastolic blood pressure
mitral regurgitation (MĪ-trăl rē-gŭr-jĭ-TĀ-shŭn)	condition in which the mitral valve does not close tightly, allowing blood to flow backward into the left atrium; also called *mitral insufficiency* or *mitral incompetence* (see Fig. 6-13)

TABLE 6-3
PATHOLOGY TERMS—cont'd

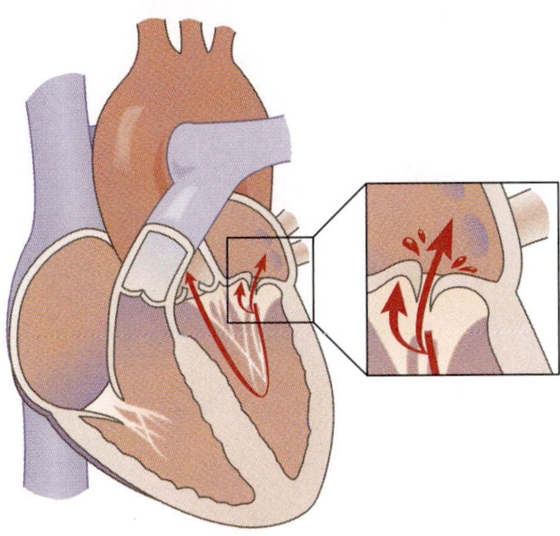

FIGURE 6-13 **Mitral regurgitation**

mitral stenosis (MĪ-trăl stĕ-NŌ-sĭs)	condition in which the mitral valve fails to open properly, thereby impeding normal blood flow and increasing pressure within the left atrium and lungs (see Fig. 6-14)

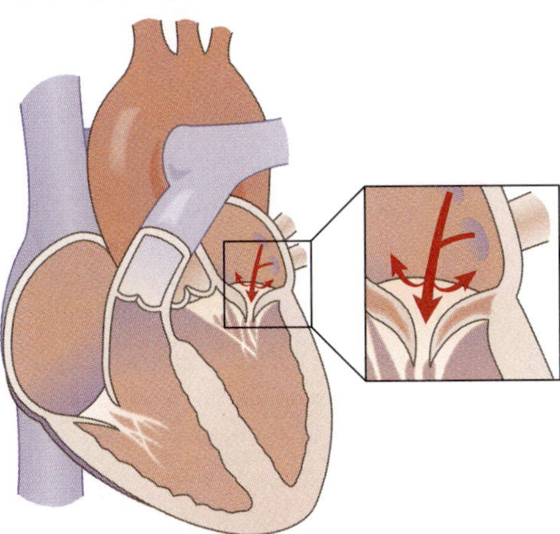

FIGURE 6-14 **Mitral stenosis**

murmur (MŬR-mŭr)	blowing or swishing sound in the heart, due to turbulent blood flow or backflow through a leaky valve
myocardial infarction (MI) (mī-ō-KĂR-dē-ăl ĭn-FĂRK-shŭn)	death of heart-muscle cells due to occlusion of a vessel; commonly called *heart attack* (see Fig. 6-15)

Continued

TABLE 6-3
PATHOLOGY TERMS—cont'd

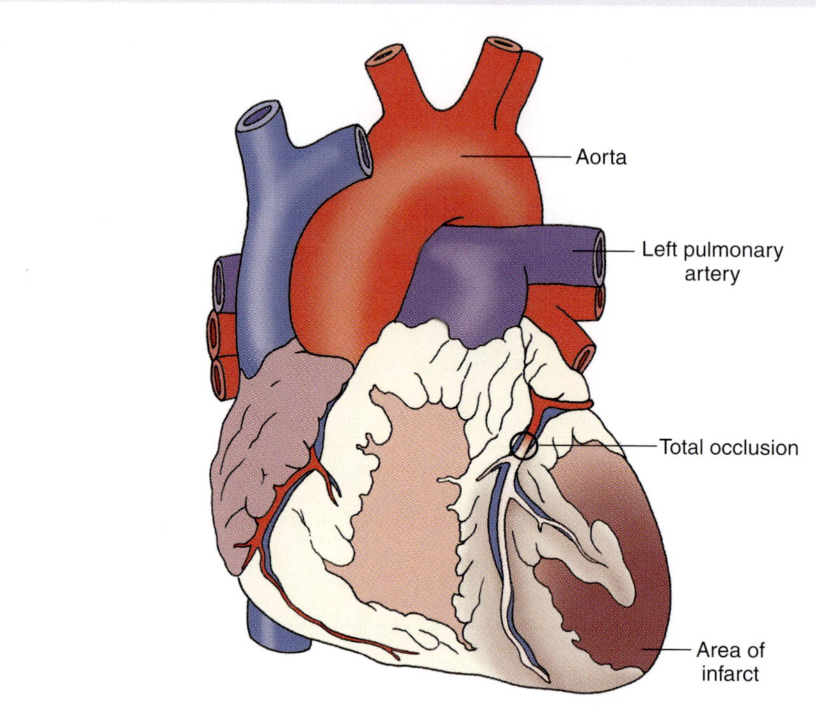

FIGURE 6-15 **Myocardial infarction**

myocarditis (mī-ō-kăr-DĪ-tĭs)	condition in which the middle layer of the heart wall becomes inflamed
pericarditis (pĕr-ĭ-kăr-DĪ-tĭs)	acute or chronic condition in which the fibrous membrane surrounding the heart becomes inflamed
peripheral artery disease (PAD) (pĕr-ĬF-ĕr-ăl ĂR-tĕr-ē dĭ-ZĒZ)	condition of partial or complete obstruction of the arteries of the arms or legs; similar to peripheral vascular disease (PVD), which includes both arteries and veins (see Fig. 6-16)

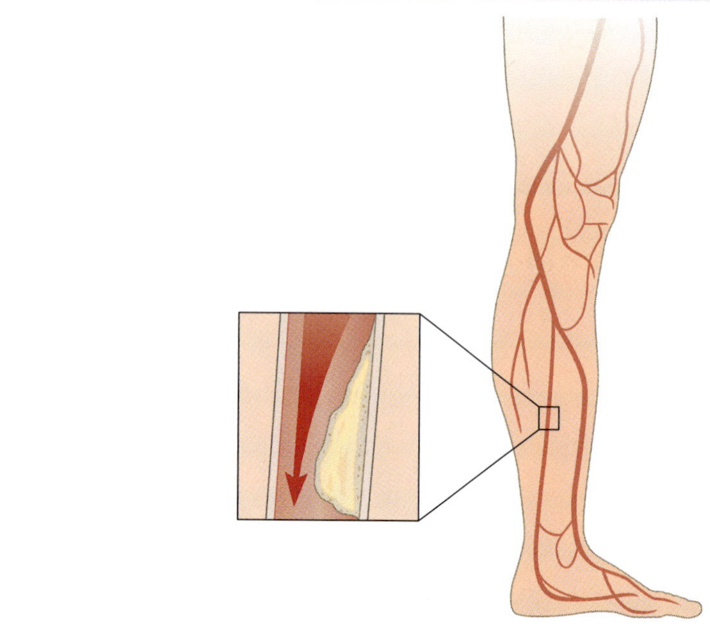

FIGURE 6-16 **Peripheral artery disease**

TABLE 6-3 PATHOLOGY TERMS—cont'd	
polycythemia vera (pŏl-ē-sī-THĒ-mē-ă VĔ-ră)	chronic disorder marked by increased number and mass of all bone marrow cells, especially RBCs, with increased blood viscosity and a tendency to develop blood clots
Raynaud disease (rĕ-NŌ dĭ-ZĒZ)	disorder that affects blood vessels in the fingers, toes, ears, and nose, marked by vessel constriction and reduced blood flow in response to triggers such as cold temperature (see Fig. 6-17)
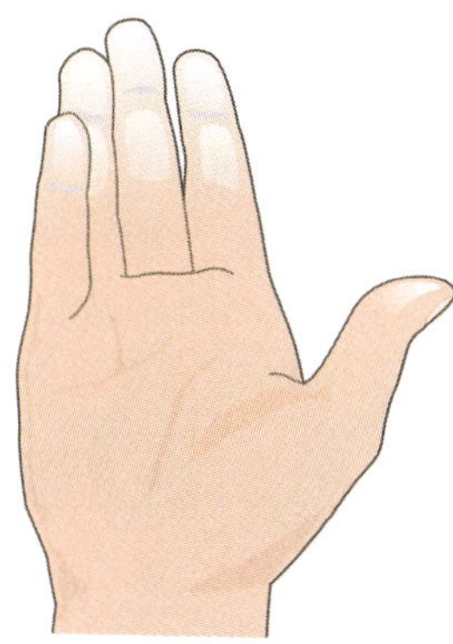 FIGURE 6-17 **Raynaud disease**	
rheumatic heart disease (roo-MĂT-ĭk hărt dĭ-ZĒZ)	complication of rheumatic fever in which inflammation and damage occur to parts of the heart, usually the valves
shock (shŏk)	syndrome of inadequate perfusion (circulation of blood, nutrients, and oxygen through tissues and organs) as a result of hypotension or low blood pressure
thromboangiitis obliterans (TAO) (thrŏm-bō-ăn-jē-Ī-tĭs ŏb-LĬT-ĕr-ănz)	type of vascular disease associated with tobacco use, marked by inflammation and clot formation within small vessels of the hands and feet, which may lead to gangrene and surgical amputation; sometimes called *Buerger disease*
varicose veins (VĂR-ĭ-kōs vānz)	bulging, distended veins due to incompetent valves, most commonly in the legs (see Fig. 6-18)

Continued

TABLE 6-3

PATHOLOGY TERMS—cont'd

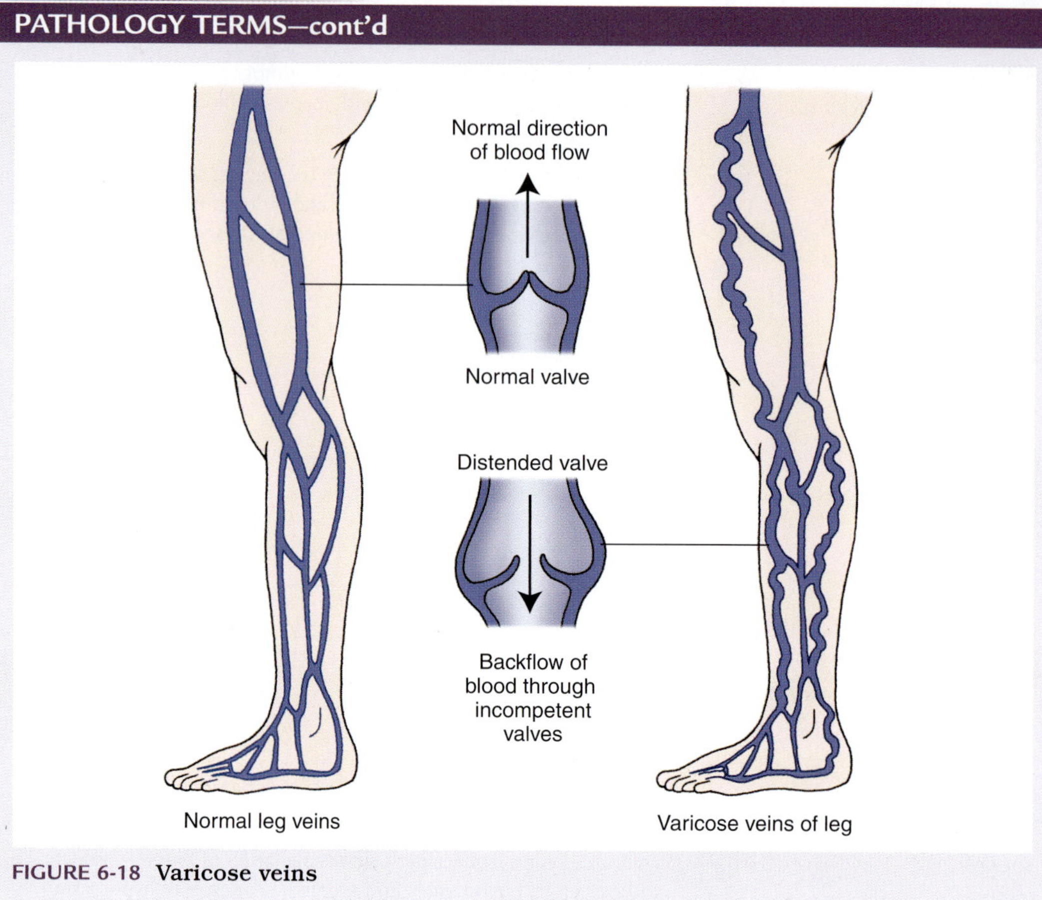

FIGURE 6-18 **Varicose veins**

Common Diagnostic Tests and Procedures

Angiography: Diagnostic or therapeutic radiography (radiological imaging) of the heart and blood vessels

Automated external defibrillator (AED): Small computer-driven defibrillator that analyzes the patient's rhythm, selects the appropriate energy level, charges the machine, and delivers a shock to the patient

Automatic implanted cardioverter defibrillator (AICD): Very small defibrillator, surgically implanted in patients with a high risk for sudden cardiac death, that automatically detects and treats life-threatening arrhythmias

Cardiac catheterization: Evaluation of the heart vessels and valves via the injection of dye that shows up under radiology (see Fig. 6-19)

Cardiopulmonary resuscitation (CPR): Emergency procedure that provides manual external cardiac compression and sometimes artificial respiration

Cardioversion: Restoration of normal sinus rhythm (NSR) by chemical or electrical means

Coronary artery bypass graft (CABG): Surgical creation of an alternate route for blood flow around an area of coronary arterial obstruction (see Fig. 6-20)

Defibrillation: Delivery of an electric shock with the goal of ending ventricular fibrillation and restoring normal sinus rhythm

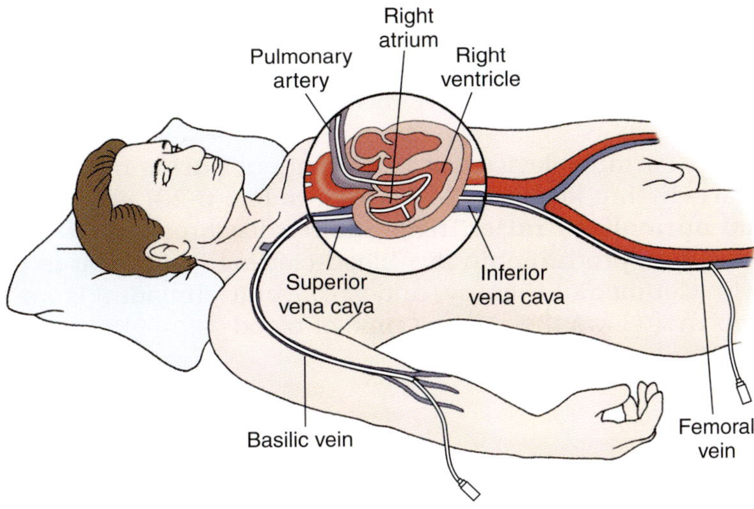

FIGURE 6-19 **Cardiac catheterization**

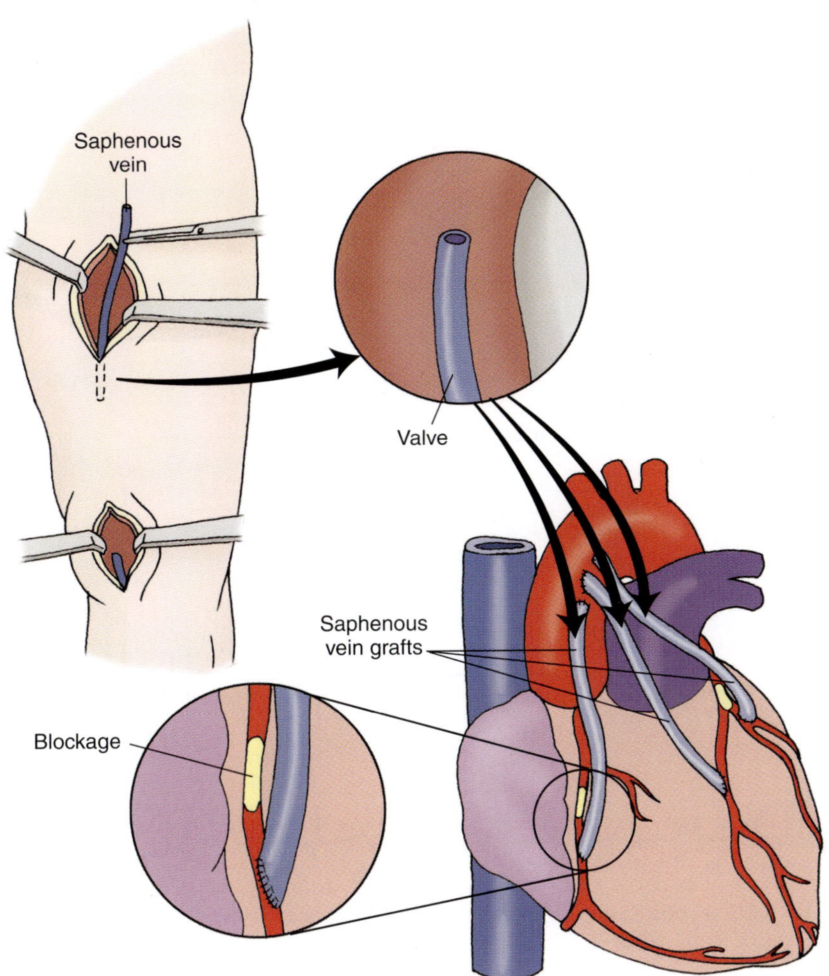

FIGURE 6-20 **Coronary artery bypass graft**

Electrocardiography (ECG, EKG): Creation and study of graphic records (electrocardiograms) of electric currents originating in the heart (see Fig. 6-21)

Event recorder: Portable monitoring device that transmits heart rhythms by telephone to a central laboratory, where dysrhythmias can be detected and analyzed (see Fig. 6-22)

Holter monitor: Portable device worn by a patient during normal activity that records heart rhythm for up to 24 hours (see Fig. 6-23)

International normalized ratio (INR): Standardized method of checking the prothrombin time (PT); prothrombin is a blood-clotting factor that is used to monitor warfarin (Coumadin) therapy, and warfarin (Coumadin) is an anticoagulant medication that slows the clotting time of blood

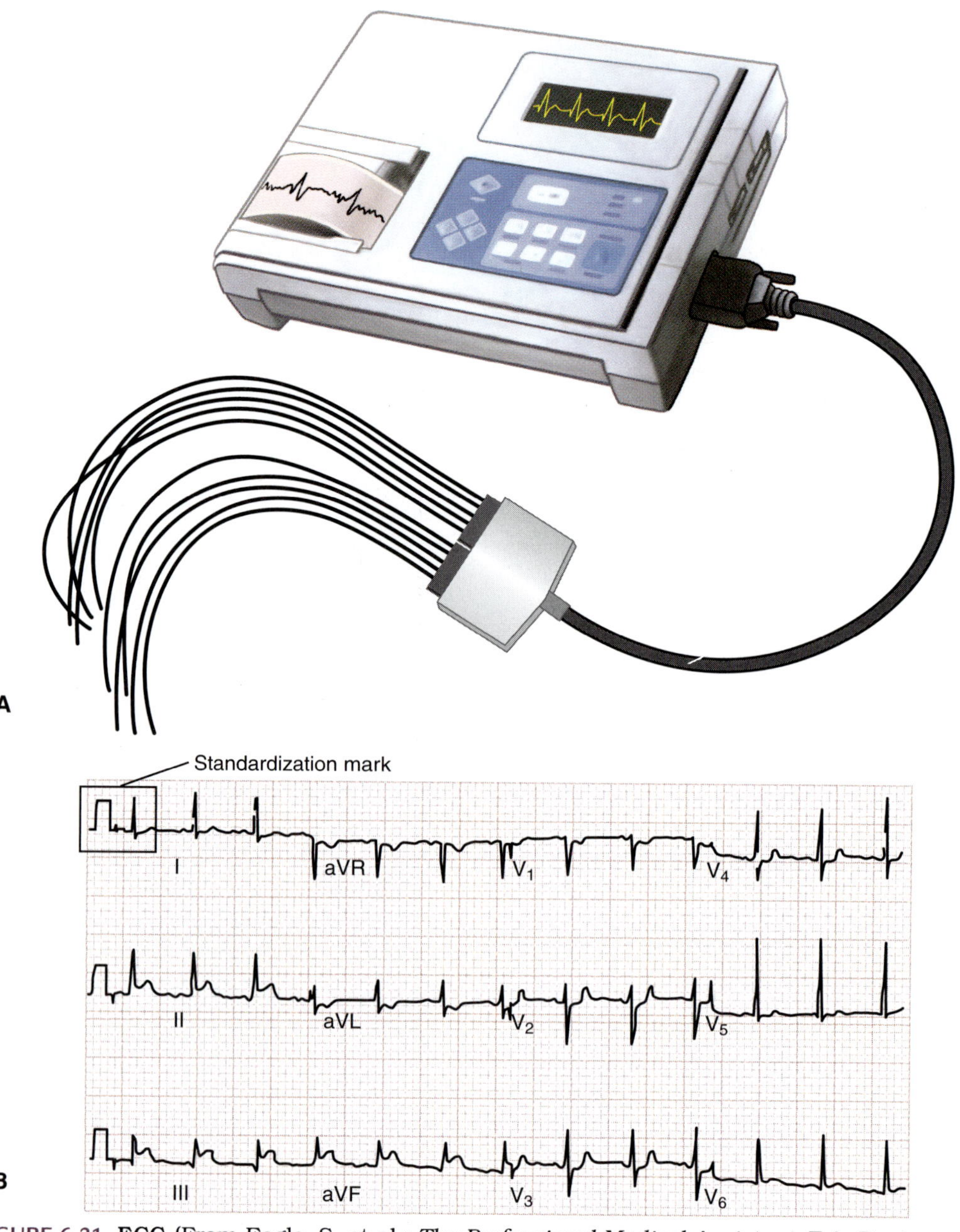

FIGURE 6-21 ECG (From Eagle, S, et al.: *The Professional Medical Assistant*. F.A. Davis, Philadelphia, 2009, pp. 482–483; with permission)

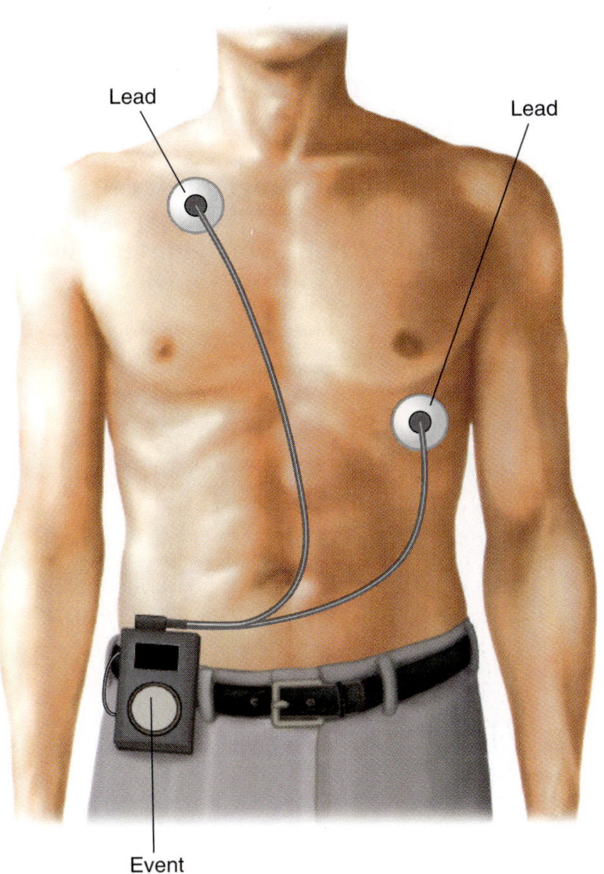

FIGURE 6-22 **Event recorder** (From Eagle, S, et al.: *The Professional Medical Assistant.* F.A. Davis, Philadelphia, 2009, p. 493; with permission)

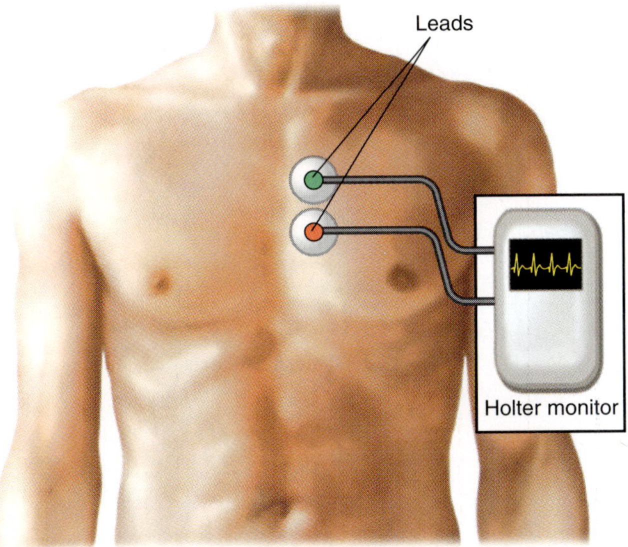

FIGURE 6-23 **Holter monitor** (From Eagle, S, et al.: *The Professional Medical Assistant.* F.A. Davis, Philadelphia, 2009, p. 493; with permission)

Pacemaker: Device that can trigger the mechanical contractions of the heart by emitting periodic electrical discharges

Partial thromboplastin time (PTT): Measure of blood-clotting time, used to monitor heparin therapy; heparin is an anticoagulant medication that slows the clotting time of blood

Percutaneous transluminal coronary angioplasty (PTCA): Method of treating a narrowed coronary artery via inflation and deflation of a balloon on a double-lumen catheter inserted through the right femoral artery (see Fig. 6-24)

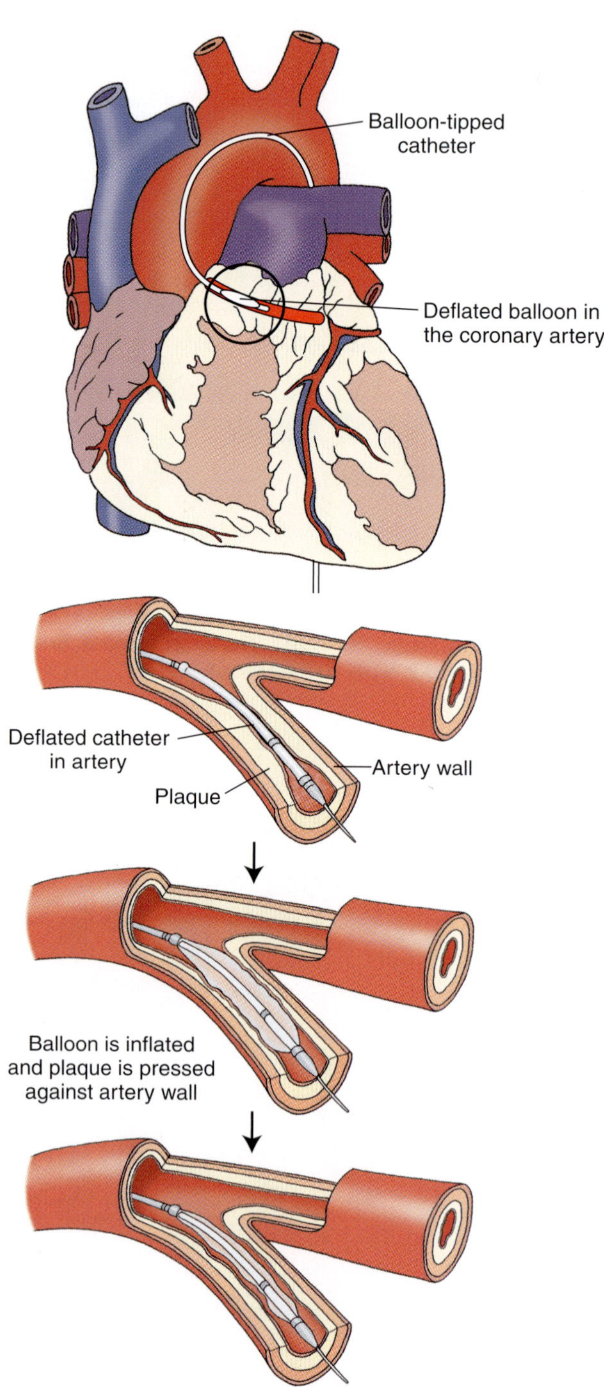

FIGURE 6-24 **Percutaneous transluminal coronary angioplasty**

Prothrombin time (PT): Procedure that measures the clotting time of blood; used to assess levels of anticoagulation in patients taking warfarin (Coumadin)

Stress test: Treadmill test that can show if the blood supply is reduced in the arteries that supply the heart

Transesophageal echocardiography (TEE): Study of the heart via a probe placed in the esophagus

Troponin: Protein released into the body by damaged heart muscle, considered the most accurate blood test to confirm the diagnosis of an MI

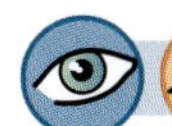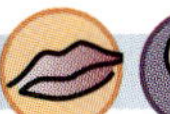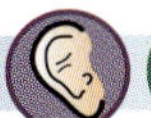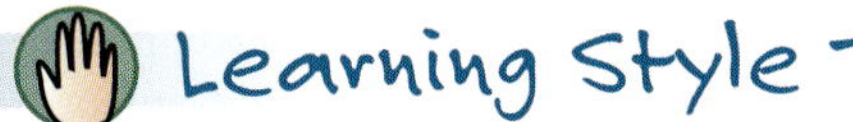

Don't skip the case studies. They are designed to engage your brain as well as your senses. To correctly answer the following questions you must reflect on what you just read and apply it. This type of application forces you to think about the terms in a meaningful (real-world) way. This greatly increases the chances that you will remember the material later. If you read and think aloud, thereby engaging your verbal and auditory senses, you will get even more out of this activity. Physically selecting and circling your answer engages your kinesthetic sense.

Case Study

Read the case study and answer the questions that follow. Most of the terms are included in this chapter. Refer to the glossaries (Appendixes B and D) or to your medical dictionary for the other terms.

Deep Vein Thrombosis

Arturo Espinoza is a 72-year-old retired cook with a history of ASHD and HTN. He also had an MI a year ago. He is 5′9″, weighs 220 lbs, and has been a pack-a-day smoker for 45 years. He recently noticed a deep, intense aching in his right lower leg but does not recall having injured it. Over the next few days, his right calf became tender and erythematous. In addition, his right lower leg, from the knee down, has become edematous.

After being evaluated by his family physician, Mr. Espinoza was diagnosed with deep vein thrombosis (DVT) and started on SubQ heparin injection therapy bid. After several days of heparin therapy, Coumadin was started as well. Both PTT and INR levels were monitored. Once Mr. Espinoza achieved a therapeutic level of his Coumadin, he was able to discontinue the heparin. Coumadin therapy is planned for the next 3 to 6 months, and he will return on a monthly basis for monitoring.

Venous thromboembolism (VTE) is a condition in which a thrombus, or blood clot, develops within a vein. When inflammation also develops, the condition is known as **deep vein thrombosis (DVT)** or **thrombophlebitis**. It can occur in any vein but is most common in the deep veins of the legs. Risk factors for DVT include venous stasis from immobility, obesity, increased blood coagulability, and vascular injury. People with an increased risk include the elderly, smokers, and women over 30 years old who use oral contraceptives.

In recent years, increased attention has been paid to the occurrence of DVT among airline passengers. Some have called it *economy-class syndrome* because of the prolonged sitting required of these passengers, which can cause venous stasis. Risk of this syndrome could be minimized if passengers were able to exercise their feet and legs every 1 to 2 hours by walking in the aisles or doing range-of-motion exercises while sitting. Remaining well hydrated and wearing support hose are also helpful. (**Note:** Support hose must have graduated compression and should **not** have a constricting band at the knee or anywhere else.)

Treatment of DVT may include rest, elevation of the extremity, and local heat application. Medications include nonsteroidal anti-inflammatory drugs (NSAIDs) and anticoagulant medication. A variety of anticoagulant medications are available; some of the most commonly used include heparin, Lovenox, and Fragmin. Heparin levels must be monitored by checking the PTT. This is not necessary with Lovenox. After several days, warfarin (Coumadin) therapy is started. Blood levels of this medication are monitored by checking the INR. These medications slow the patient's blood-clotting time, which prevents further clot formation while the body's natural mechanisms dissolve the present clot. A potential side effect of these medications is easy bruising and increased risk of bleeding. Therefore, patients are counseled to watch for signs of bleeding when, for example, passing bowel movements or brushing or flossing the teeth.

Case Study Questions

1. What known risk factor for DVT does Mr. Espinoza have?
- **a.** He is a Mexican-American
- **b.** He is a smoker
- **c.** He is a man
- **d.** He is a retired cook

2. Mr. Espinoza has a history of what disorder?
- **a.** Atherosclerotic heart disease
- **b.** Diabetes
- **c.** Epilepsy
- **d.** *Pneumocystis* pneumonia

3. By what route did Mr. Espinoza receive his heparin?
- **a.** By mouth
- **b.** Intramuscular injection
- **c.** Intradermal injection
- **d.** Subcutaneous injection

4. How often does Mr. Espinoza receive his heparin?
- **a.** Once each day
- **b.** Twice each day
- **c.** Three times each day
- **d.** Four times each day

5. What lab test was done to determine whether Mr. Espinoza's heparin dose was correct?
- **a.** PT
- **b.** PTT
- **c.** INR
- **d.** DVT

6. What lab test was done to determine whether Mr. Espinoza's Coumadin dose was correct?
- **a.** PT
- **b.** PTT
- **c.** INR
- **d.** DVT

7. Treatment of DVT includes which of the following measures?
   a. Application of cold therapy
   b. Vigorous exercise
   c. Nonsteroidal anti-inflammatory medication
   d. Topical application of creams or ointments

8. Why has *economy-class syndrome* become a recent popular name for DVT?
   a. Because flying in airplanes at high altitudes causes blood clot formation
   b. Because passengers who sit in economy class generally do not move about for the duration of the flight
   c. Because all airlines passengers are at high risk for blood-clot formation
   d. Because DVT happens only to airline passengers

9. People can reduce their risk for DVT formation by doing which of the following?
   a. Drinking less fluid
   b. Sitting and resting their legs whenever possible
   c. Taking oral contraceptives
   d. Losing excess body weight

Answers to Case Study Questions

1. b
2. a
3. d
4. b
5. b
6. c
7. c
8. b
9. d

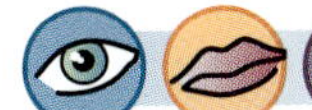
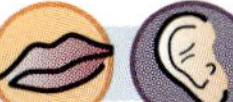

Learning Style Tip

Visit any of the following websites to read additional information about any cardiac topics that you find especially interesting. As always, if you read or verbalize key concepts aloud, thus engaging your verbal and auditory senses, you greatly increase the chance that you will understand and later remember what you read.

Websites

Please go to the F.A. Davis website at http://davisplus.fadavis.com/eagle/medterm to view resource websites for the cardiovascular system.

Practice Exercises

Deciphering Terms

Write the correct meaning of these medical terms. Check Appendix G for the correct answers.

Exercise 2

1. microcardia ______________________________
2. venule ______________________________
3. hemogram ______________________________
4. angiography ______________________________
5. aortoplasty ______________________________
6. arteriole ______________________________
7. atherocyte ______________________________
8. atriodynia ______________________________
9. electric ______________________________
10. hematuria ______________________________
11. valvular ______________________________
12. phlebitis ______________________________
13. venostasis ______________________________
14. vasculopathy ______________________________
15. thrombolysis ______________________________

Fill in the Blanks

Fill in the blanks below using Tables 6-2 and 6-3. Check Appendix G for the correct answers.

Exercise 3

1. Jim's heart no longer beats in a regular rhythm. Therefore, he has an ______________________.
2. When the physician listened to Martha's carotid arteries with a stethoscope, he heard a soft blowing sound caused by turbulent blood flow. This is also known as a ______________________.
3. Ismael has a heart condition that results in lung congestion and dyspnea. The medical term for this condition is ______________________ ______________________.

4. The abbreviation *qhs* stands for ______________________

______________________.

5. Victor was treated with an anticoagulant medication called heparin because of a blood clot in a deep vein of his legs. This condition is known as

______________________ ______________________ ______________________.

6. The abbreviation *q2h* stands for ______________________

______________________ ______________________.

7. The death of cardiac muscle cells due to occlusion of a vessel is known as a(n) ______________________ ______________________ and is abbreviated

______________________.

8. Cristobalina has bulging, distended veins in her legs. This condition is known as ______________________ ______________________.

9. The names of the two upper chambers of the heart are abbreviated

______________________ and ______________________.

10. The names of the two lower chambers of the heart are abbreviated

______________________ and ______________________.

11. After checking Jaemoon's BP, or ______________________

______________________, the physician diagnosed him with HTN, which stands for ______________________.

12. The physician ordered an EKG to record Jaemoon's heart rhythm. This stands for ______________________.

13. A medication is ordered qid. This means it should be taken

______________________ times a day.

14. The physician wants Oscar to weigh himself qam, which means

______________________ ______________________.

15. ______________________ ______________________ is a group of disorders generally defined as a reduction in the mass of circulating red blood cells.

16. Martha is suffering from ______________________, which is heart pain and usually a symptom of heart disease.

17. ______________________ is a group of conditions in which the heart muscle has deteriorated and functions less effectively.

18. Harold has vegetations growing on the inner lining of his heart. The doctor says this is probably caused by ______________________.

19. An acute or chronic condition in which the fibrous membrane surrounding the heart becomes inflamed is called ______________________.

Multiple Choice

Select the one best answer to the following multiple-choice questions. Check Appendix G for the correct answers.

Exercise 4

1. Which of the following disorders does **not** involve an interference in blood flow?
   a. Ischemia
   b. Myocardial infarction
   c. Mitral stenosis
   d. Arrhythmia

2. Which of the following does **not** involve the heart rhythm?
   a. V-tach
   b. PAC
   c. V-fib
   d. TIA

3. Which of the following abbreviations stands for the name of a chamber of the heart?
   a. BP
   b. EKG
   c. RA
   d. PCP

4. All of the following refer to a part of the heart **except**:
   a. RA
   b. RV
   c. MI
   d. LV

5. Which of the following may cause temporary strokelike symptoms?
   a. CHF
   b. TIA
   c. LA
   d. CPR

Word Building

*Using **only** the word parts in the lists provided, create medical terms with the indicated meanings. Check Appendix G for the correct answers.*

Exercise 5

Prefixes	Combining Forms	Suffixes
brady-	angi/o	-cele
micro-	aort/o	-cyte
tachy-	arteri/o	-gram
	ather/o	-graphy
	atri/o	-ia
	cardi/o	-ic
	coron/o	-logist
	electr/o	-megaly
	hemat/o	-metry
	phleb/o	-oid
	scler/o	-osis
	thromb/o	-pathy
	valvul/o	-plasty
	vascul/o	-rrhaphy
	ventricul/o	-rrhexis
		-sclerosis
		-tomy
		-version

1. record of a vessel ______________________________
2. pertaining to the aorta ______________________________
3. process of recording an artery ______________________________
4. abnormal condition of hardening of thick, fatty tissue
____
5. rupture of an artery ______________________________
6. condition of a slow heart ______________________________
7. enlargement of the heart ______________________________
8. condition of a rapid heart ______________________________
9. record of heart electricity ______________________________
10. specialist in the study of blood ______________________________
11. incision into a valve ______________________________
12. cutting into a vein ______________________________
13. inflammation of a blood vessel ______________________________
14. cell for clotting ______________________________

15. surgical repair of a vessel ______________________

16. hernia of a ventricle ______________________

17. measurement of the ventricle ______________________

18. condition of a small heart ______________________

19. rupturing of red blood cells ______________________

20. softening of the walls of the aorta ______________________

True or False

Decide whether the following statements are true or false. Check Appendix G for the correct answers.

Exercise 6

1. True False The abbreviation **PTT** stands for *platelets.*
2. True False A **murmur** is an abnormal blowing or swishing sound in the heart caused by turbulent blood flow or backflow through a leaky valve.
3. True False An **aneurysm** is a weakened area in the wall of a vessel.
4. True False The abbreviation **MI** stands for *muscle injury.*
5. True False The abbreviation **PTCA** stands for a type of food.
6. True False An **embolus** is a soft blowing sound caused by turbulent blood flow.
7. True False The abbreviation **CV** stands for *coronary vessel.*
8. True False **Ischemia** refers to a temporary reduction in blood supply to a localized area of tissue.
9. True False The abbreviation **ASHD** stands for *arteriosclerotic heart disease.*
10. True False **Fibrillation** refers to an abnormal quivering of heart muscle fibers instead of an effective heartbeat.

Deciphering Terms

Write the correct meaning of these medical terms. Check Appendix G for the correct answers.

Exercise 7

1. macrocardia ______________________________
2. ventriculoscopy ______________________________
3. vasotonic ______________________________
4. vasodilation ______________________________
5. vasodynia ______________________________
6. atriokinesis ______________________________
7. thrombolysis ______________________________
8. hematologist ______________________________
9. arteriorrhexis ______________________________
10. vasoconstriction ______________________________

Multiple Choice

Select the one best answer to the following multiple-choice questions. Check Appendix G for the correct answers.

Exercise 8

1. Which of the following terms is matched to the correct definition?
   a. Angi/o: thick, fatty
   b. Hem/o: heart
   c. Arteri/o: aorta
   d. Phleb/o: vein
2. Which of the following terms is matched to the correct definition?
   a. Atri/o: atria
   b. Vascul/o: valve
   c. Hem/o: thrombus
   d. Ventricul/o: blood vessel
3. All of the following terms are matched with the correct definition **except**:
   a. Aort/o: aorta
   b. Cardi/o: heart
   c. Hemat/o: blood
   d. Vas/o: vascular

4. Which of the following abbreviations represents a test or procedure?
   a. MR
   b. INR
   c. Bpm
   d. MVP

5. Which of the following abbreviations represents a dosing schedule?
   a. Bpm
   b. Bid
   c. PTT
   d. P

6. Which of the following abbreviations represents a type of heart disease?
   a. DVT
   b. ASHD
   c. PT
   d. PVC

7. All of the following terms are matched with the correct definition **except**:
   a. Anemia: reduction in the mass of circulating red blood cells
   b. Bruit: soft blowing sound caused by turbulent blood flow in a vessel
   c. Disseminated intravascular coagulation: serious condition in which widespread, microvascular blood clotting occurs while the patient has symptoms of hemorrhaging
   d. Raynaud disease: a chronic disorder marked by increased number and mass of all bone marrow cells, especially red blood cells (RBCs), with increased blood viscosity and a tendency to develop blood clots

8. All of the following terms are matched with the correct definition **except**:
   a. Aneurysm: weakening and bulging of part of a vessel wall
   b. Angina: heart pain or other discomfort felt in the chest
   c. Cardiomyopathy: condition in which the heart becomes compressed from an excessive collection of fluid or blood between the pericardial membrane and the heart
   d. Endocarditis: infection of the inner lining of the heart that may cause vegetations to form within one or more heart chambers or valves

9. All of the following terms are matched with the correct definition **except**:
   a. Embolus: undissolved matter floating in blood or lymph fluid
   b. Cor pulmonale: development of a blood clot in a deep vein, usually in the legs
   c. Arteriosclerosis: thickening, loss of elasticity, and loss of contractility of arterial walls; commonly called *hardening of the arteries*
   d. Ischemia: temporary reduction in blood supply to a localized area of tissue

10. Which of the following is a type of heart-rhythm abnormality?
    a. Cardiomyopathy
    b. Atrial fibrillation
    c. Murmur
    d. Thromboangiitis obliterans

11. Coronary artery disease includes which of the following components?
    a. Murmur and bruit
    b. Atherosclerosis and arteriosclerosis
    c. Heart failure and malignant hypertension
    d. Mitral regurgitation and mitral stenosis

12. Which of the following is related to incompetent valves?
    a. Hypertension
    b. Varicose veins
    c. Myocardial infarction
    d. Myocarditis

13. A surgeon performing a CABG will need to include which of the following?
    a. Angiorrhaphy
    b. Aortomalacia
    c. Valvuloplasty
    d. Hematemesis

14. Dr. Emily Shu is studying a piece of paper with the patient's heart-rhythm strip on it. The paper she is studying is an:
    a. Electrocardiography
    b. Electrocardiogram
    c. Electrocardiograph
    d. Electrocardiogravida

15. The process of dissolving or destroying a blood clot is called:
    a. Thrombocytosis
    b. Thrombosclerosis
    c. Thrombolytic
    d. Thrombolysis

16. A term that indicates the surgical puncture of a vein is:
    a. Ventoplasty
    b. Phlebocentesis
    c. Vasopexy
    d. Arteriotripsy

17. Which of the following terms means *bursting forth of blood?*
    a. Hemolysis
    b. Hemorrhage
    c. Hematoma
    d. Hematogenesis

18. An instrument used to cut the heart may be called a:
    a. Cardiotomy
    b. Cardiotome
    c. Cardiostomy
    d. Cardiectomy

19. As an aortic aneurysm develops, the following occurs:
    a. Aortomalacia
    b. Aortodilation
    c. Aortopexy
    d. Aortodesis

20. A test to examine heart vessels is:
    a. A CABG
    b. An angiography
    c. An arterioplasty
    d. A coronometry

LYMPHATIC-IMMUNE SYSTEM

7

Structure and Function

The lymphatic system includes an intricate network of vessels that collect excess tissue fluid, called **lymph**, and return it to the circulation. Lymph enters lymph capillaries and makes its way into larger lymphatic vessels (see Fig. 7-1). It is a clear, colorless, alkaline fluid made up mostly of water, along with some protein, salts, fats, white blood cells, and urea (a waste product of protein metabolism). Lymphatic vessels are found throughout the body alongside arteries, veins, and capillaries. While blood vessels rely on the pumping action of the heart, there is no pump for lymphatic vessels; instead, lymph flow is facilitated by the pumping action of skeletal muscles.

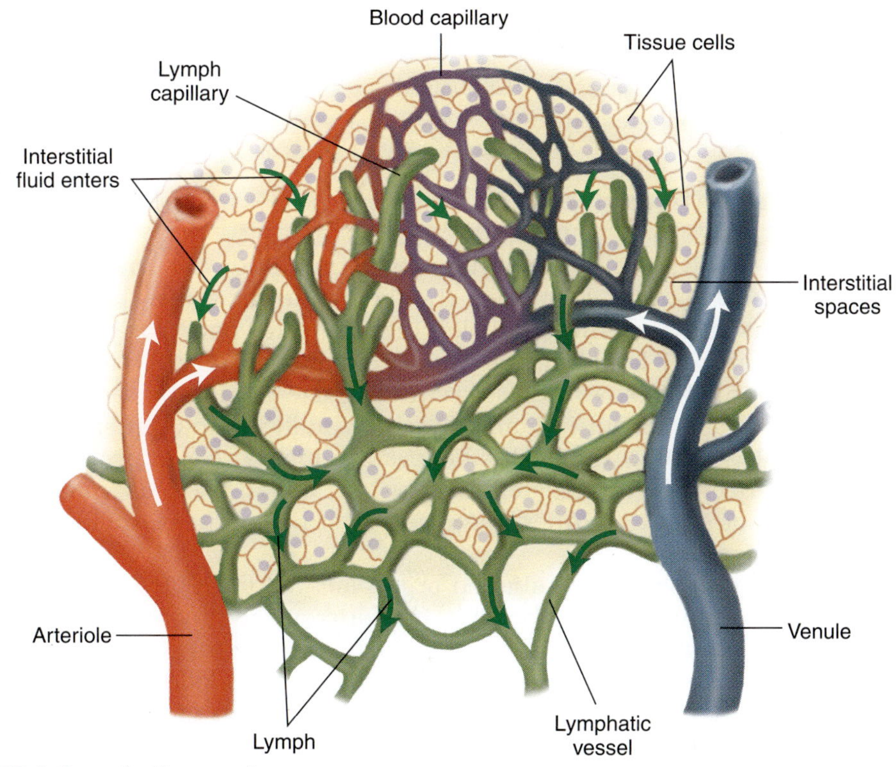

FIGURE 7-1 **Lymphatic vessels**

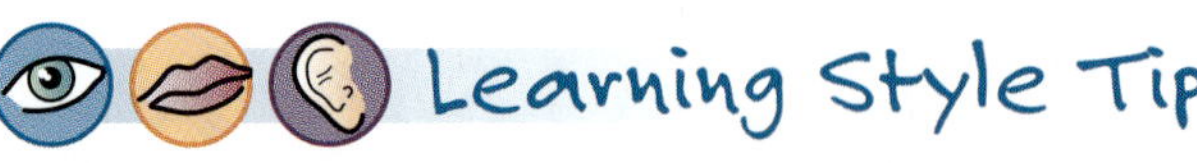

Read twice—slowly and aloud—any key sections of the text that you are struggling to grasp. This sometimes helps to slow your brain down so you can focus on each word and think about what it means before you continue.

Flashpoint
Lymph flow relies on the pumping action of skeletal muscles.

The lymphatic system includes **lymph nodes**, commonly called *glands*, which are rich in **phagocytes** (specialized white blood cells) and serve as filters to clean debris from lymph through the process of **phagocytosis**. In this process, white blood cells remove microorganisms, cell debris, and blood cells that are damaged, old, or abnormal by literally gobbling them up. Because of these functions, the lymphatic system is also considered part of the immune system. When infection and inflammation occur, the body is able to respond by increasing the production of phagocytes.

Lymphatic vessels are located throughout the body and are connected to the superior vena cava, which is where lymph enters the circulatory system and is combined with blood. Lymph nodes are distributed along lymphatic vessels with higher numbers in the neck, axillae (armpits), groin, and abdomen (see Fig. 7-2). There are two sets of lymph nodes in the throat commonly known as the **tonsils** and **adenoids**. These nodes may become tender and swollen when you have a cold or sore throat; this occurs when the lymph nodes, which have been working to filter lymph in that area, become overwhelmed and inflamed. An inflamed gland may be referred to as *lymphadenitis* or **lymphadenopathy**.

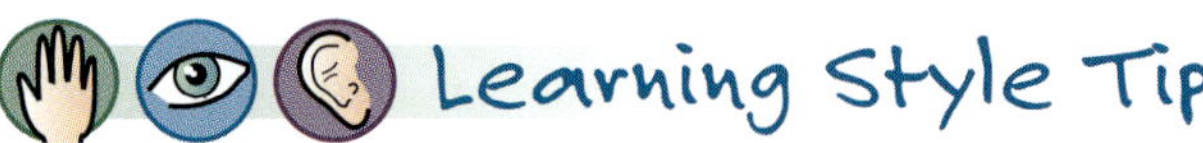

Move your body when you study. This helps even if what you are physically doing has nothing to do with what you are studying. While you flip through flash cards or read, try pacing around a room, going for a walk, running on a treadmill, pedaling on a stationary bicycle, or even working on an arts-and-crafts project. The movement helps keep you awake, keeps your brain engaged, and somehow helps you recall the information later. The same activities can also be done by auditory learners as you listen to taped lectures or audio terminology.

Flashpoint
The lymph nodes (glands) work like little filters, cleaning foreign matter from your lymph fluid.

The Thymus and the Spleen

Other structures involved in the lymphatic system include the thymus and the spleen. The **thymus gland** is located in the mediastinum above the heart. It consists of two fused lobes, and is divided into an outer part (cortex), mostly composed of immature T lymphocytes (a type of white blood cell), and an inner part (medulla). The thymus is most active during the prenatal period and early years of life. It grows until puberty and then gradually shrinks in size as we age. It plays a role in immunity and is believed to play a role in protecting our bodies against cancer. T lymphocytes, also known as *killer T cells*, mature in the thymus and then circulate to other immune-system structures, including the spleen and lymph nodes.

The **spleen** is a dark-red, oval-shaped organ located in the left upper quadrant of the abdomen, just under the ribs. It is surrounded by an outer capsule of connective tissue and is divided into compartments. During prenatal development, the spleen forms red blood cells (RBCs) and white blood cells (WBCs). After birth, RBCs are produced by the spleen only in cases of severe need; however, it continues creating WBCs as well as antibodies as part of its role in the immune system. It also acts as a type of storage container, generally holding a supply of 100 to 300 mL of blood as well as 30% of the body's total platelets.

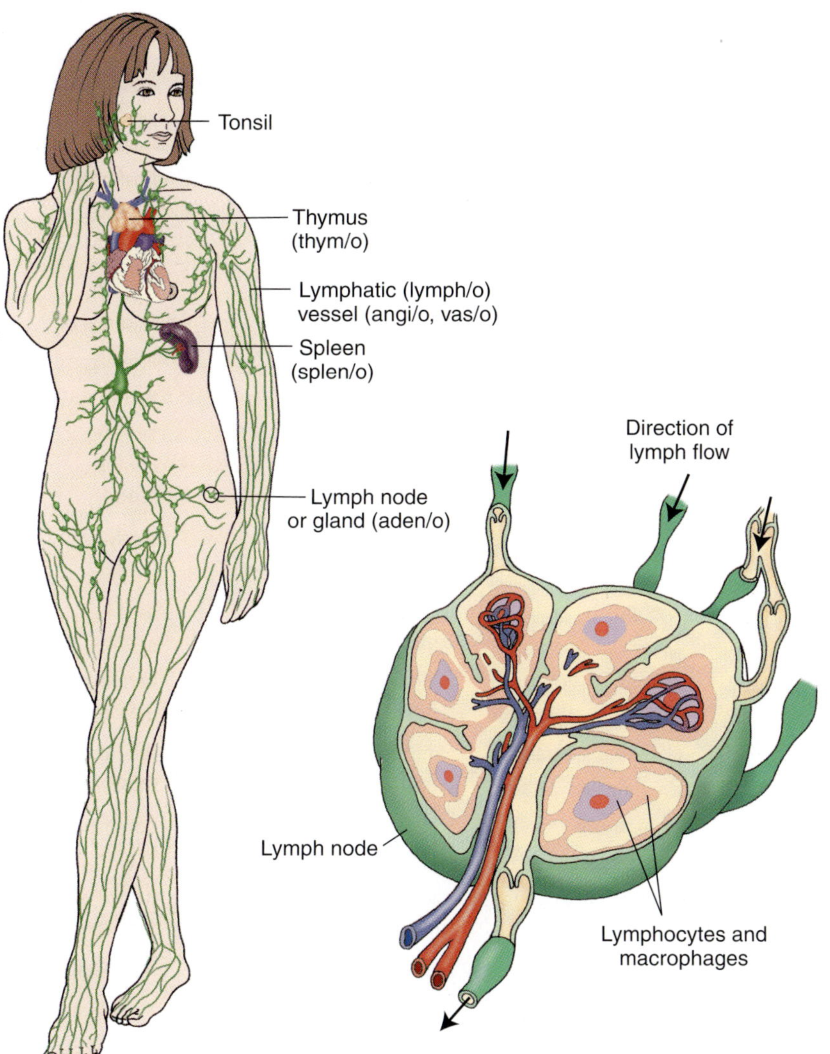

FIGURE 7-2 **Lymphatic system**

Platelets are important for blood clotting. In the event of hemorrhage, the spleen can return this extra blood and platelets to the circulation to help maintain blood pressure and help with blood clotting. Because of its location and rich blood supply, the spleen may be injured if you suffer a blow to the abdomen. This may require a splenectomy (surgical removal of the spleen) to stop any internal bleeding. Fortunately, most of us can survive without a spleen if we must. However, our immune system may be slightly weakened, leaving us more vulnerable to infection.

Flashpoint
The spleen is very vascular, and if it becomes injured, it may need to be removed to stop internal hemorrhaging.

Combining Forms

Table 7-1 contains combining forms that pertain to the lymphatic-immune system, examples of terms that utilize the combining forms, and a pronunciation guide. Read aloud to yourself as you move from left to right across the

TABLE 7-1
COMBINING FORMS

Combining Form	Meaning	Example (Pronunciation)	Meaning of New Term
aden/o	gland	adenoma (ăd-ĕ-NŌ-mă)	tumor of a gland
adenoid/o	adenoid	adenoidectomy (ăd-ĕ-noyd-ĔK-tō-mē)	excision or surgical removal of an adenoid
angi/o	vessel	angiasthenia (ăn-jē-ăs-THĒ-nē-ă)	absence of vessel strength
vas/o		vasorrhaphy (văs-OR-ă-fē)	suturing of a vessel
bacteri/o	bacteria	bacteriemia (băk-tĕr-Ē-mē-ă)	condition of bacteria in the blood
immun/o	immune	immunopathology (ĭm-ū-nō-pă-THŌL-ō-jē)	study of immune disease
lymph/o	lymph	lymphoma (lĭm-FŌ-mă)	lymph tumor
lymphaden/o	lymph gland	lymphadenocele (lĭm-FĂD-ĕ-nō-sēl)	hernia of a lymphatic vessel
lymphangi/o	lymphatic vessel	lymphangiectasis (lĭm-făn-jē-ĔK-tă-sĭs)	dilation of a lymphatic vessel
lymphocyt/o	lymph cell	lymphocytosis (lĭm-fō-sī-TŌ-sĭs)	abnormal condition of lymph cells
myel/o	bone marrow, spinal cord	myeloma (mī-ĕ-LŌ-mă)	tumor of the bone marrow
path/o	disease	pathophobia (păth-ō-FŌ-bē-ă)	fear of disease
ser/o	serum	serous (SĒR-ŭs)	pertaining to serum
splen/o	spleen	splenomegaly (splĕ-nō-MĔG-ă-lē)	enlargement of the spleen
thym/o	thymus	thymocyte (THĪ-mō-sīt)	thymus cell
tonsill/o	tonsil	tonsillitis (tŏn-sĭl-Ī-tĭs)	inflammation of the tonsil
tox/o	poison, toxin	toxoid (TŎKS-oyd)	resembling poison
toxic/o		toxicogenic (tŏks-ĭ-kō-JĔN-ĭk)	creating poison

table. Be sure to use the pronunciation guide so that you can learn to say the terms correctly.

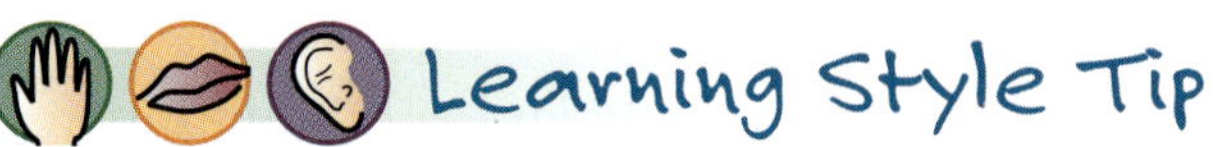

Using big motions, write each term in the air with your finger as you say it aloud and then state the definition.

STOP HERE.
Select the Combining Form Flash Cards for Chapter 7 and run through them at least three times before you continue.

Practice Exercises

Fill in the Blanks

Fill in the blanks below using Table 7-1. Check Appendix G for the correct answers.

Exercise 1

1. hernia of a lymphatic vessel ______________________________
2. absence of vessel strength ______________________________
3. creating poison ______________________________
4. enlargement of the spleen ______________________________
5. tumor of the bone marrow ______________________________
6. dilation of a lymph vessel ______________________________
7. abnormal condition of lymph cells ______________________________
8. inflammation of the tonsils ______________________________
9. pertaining to serum ______________________________
10. thymus cell ______________________________
11. tumor of a gland ______________________________
12. lymph tumor ______________________________
13. study of immune disease ______________________________
14. a condition of bacteria in the blood ______________________________
15. excision or surgical removal of an adenoid ______________________________
16. fear of disease ______________________________
17. suturing of a vessel ______________________________
18. resembling poison ______________________________

19. **Fill in the blanks in Figure 7-3 with the appropriate anatomical terms and combining forms.**

Abbreviations

Table 7-2 lists some of the most common abbreviations related to the lymphatic-immune system.

STOP HERE.
Select the Abbreviation Flash Cards for Chapter 7 and run through them at least three times before you continue.

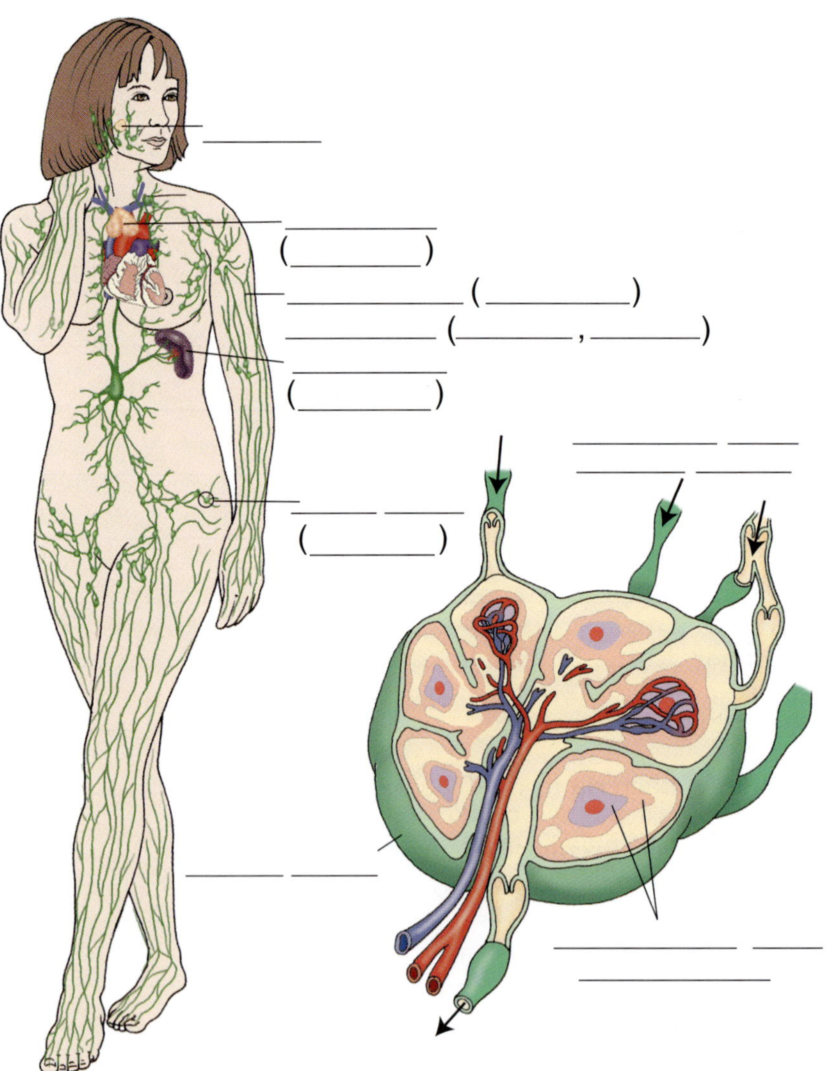

FIGURE 7-3 **Lymphatic vessels with blanks**

TABLE 7-2
ABBREVIATIONS

AB, Ab	antibody	GVHD	graft-versus-host disease
AG, Ag	antigen	HIV	human immunodeficiency virus
AIDS	acquired immunodeficiency syndrome	Ig	immunoglobulin
CA	cancer or carcinoma	KS	Kaposi sarcoma
EBV	Epstein-Barr virus	MET, met	metastasis, metastasize
EIA	enzyme immunosorbent assay	PCP	*Pneumocystis carinii* pneumonia, *Pneumocystis* pneumonia
ESR	erythrocyte sedimentation rate	SLE	systemic lupus erythematosus

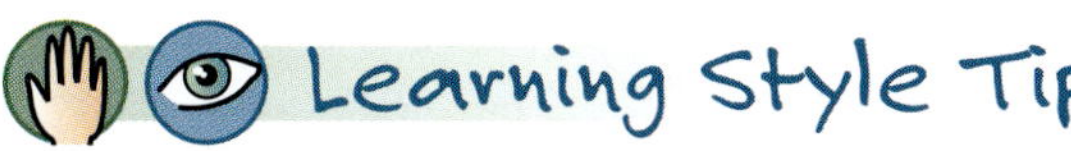

If you are highly kinesthetic, be sure to take notes in class even if the instructor does not require it. Embellish your notes with your own diagrams, illustrations, or flowcharts. Visual learners will get more out of this if you use colored pens or highlighters to jazz up your notes.

Pathology Terms

Table 7-3 includes terms that relate to diseases or abnormalities of the lymphatic-immune system. Use the pronunciation guide and say the terms aloud as you read them. This will help you get in the habit of saying them properly.

TABLE 7-3
PATHOLOGY TERMS

acquired immunodeficiency syndrome (AIDS) (ă-KWĪRD ĭm-ūn-ō-dē-FĬSH-ĕn-sē SĬN-drōm)	late-stage infection with the human immunodeficiency virus (HIV) which progressively weakens the immune system
anaphylaxis (ăn-ă-fĭ-LĂK-sĭs)	life-threatening systemic allergic reaction to a substance to which the body was previously sensitized
ankylosing spondylitis (AS) (ăng-kĭ-LŌ-sing spŏn-dĭl-Ī-tĭs)	inflammatory response that causes degenerative changes in the spinal vertebrae; sacroiliac joints; connective tissues such as tendons and ligaments in the hips, shoulders, knees, feet, and ribs; and tissues of the lungs, eyes, and heart valves (see Fig. 7-4)

Continued

TABLE 7-3

PATHOLOGY TERMS—cont'd

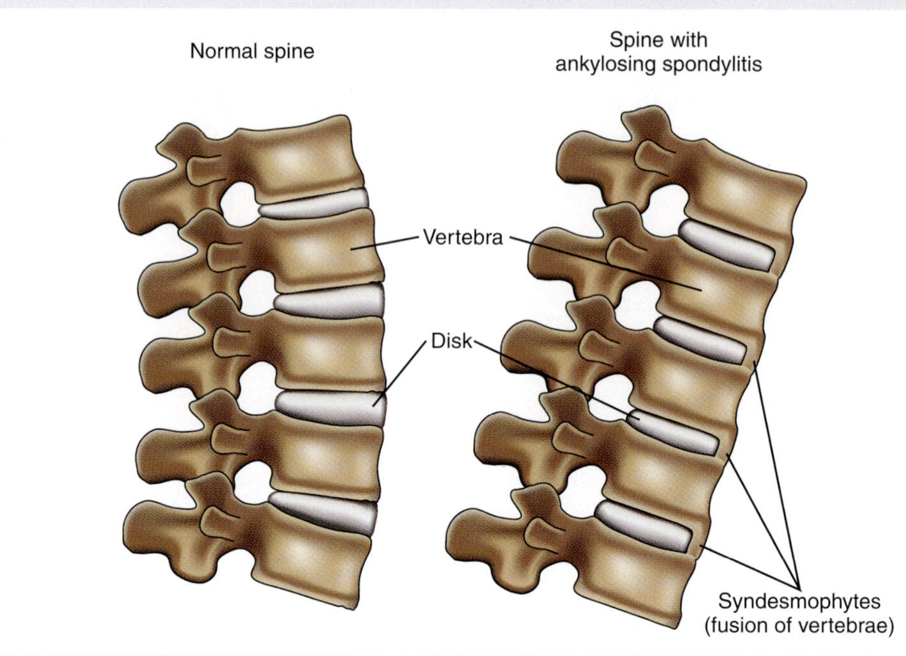

FIGURE 7-4 **Ankylosing spondylitis**

autoimmune hemolytic anemia (aw-tō-ĭm-MŪN hē-mō-LĬT-ĭk ă-NĒ-mē-ă)	group of disorders caused when the immune system misidentifies red blood cells (RBCs) as foreign and creates autoantibodies that attack them
chronic fatigue syndrome (CFS) (KRŎN-ĭk fă-TĒG SĬN-drōm)	complex chronic disorder marked by severe fatigue unrelieved by rest, often worsened by mental or physical activity; sometimes called *chronic fatigue and immune dysfunction syndrome (CFIDS)*
chronic mucocutaneous candidiasis (CMC) (KRŎN-ĭk mū-kō-kū-TĀ-nē-ŭs kăn-dĭ-DĪ-ă-sĭs	group of disorders in which persistent or recurrent *Candida* fungal infections develop on the skin, nails, or mucous membranes
Epstein-Barr virus (EBV) (ĔP-stēn-BĂR VĪ-rŭs)	acute infection which causes sore throat, fever, fatigue, and enlarged lymph nodes; also called *mononucleosis*
graft-versus-host disease (GVHD) (grăft VĔR-sŭz hōst dĭ-ZĒZ)	complication of bone-marrow transplantation in which lymphoid cells from donated tissue attack the recipient and cause damage to skin, liver, GI tract, and other tissues (see Fig. 7-5)

TABLE 7-3
PATHOLOGY TERMS—cont'd

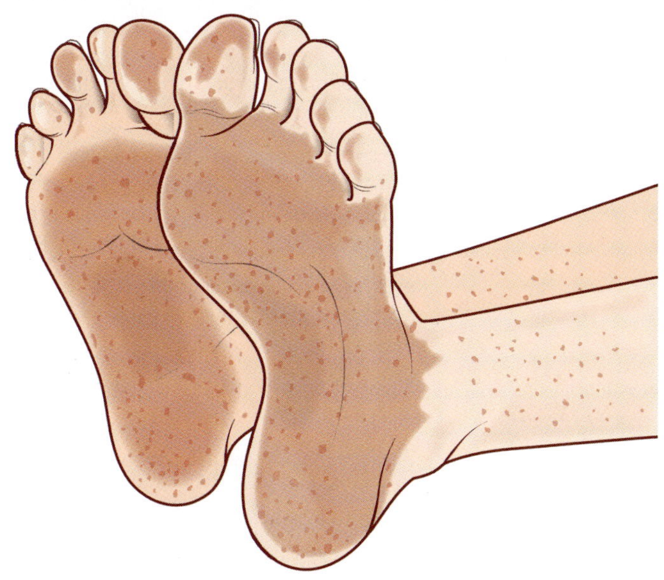

FIGURE 7-5 **Graft-versus-host disease**

Hodgkin disease (HŎJ-kĭn dĭ-ZĒZ)	type of lymphatic cancer; also called *lymphoma*
idiopathic thrombocytopenic purpura (ITP) (ĭd-ē-ō-PĂTH-ĭk thrŏm-bō-sī-tō-PĒ-nĭk PŬR-pū-ră)	disorder in which a deficiency of platelets results in abnormal blood clotting, marked by tiny purple bruises (purpura) that form under the skin (see Fig. 7-6)

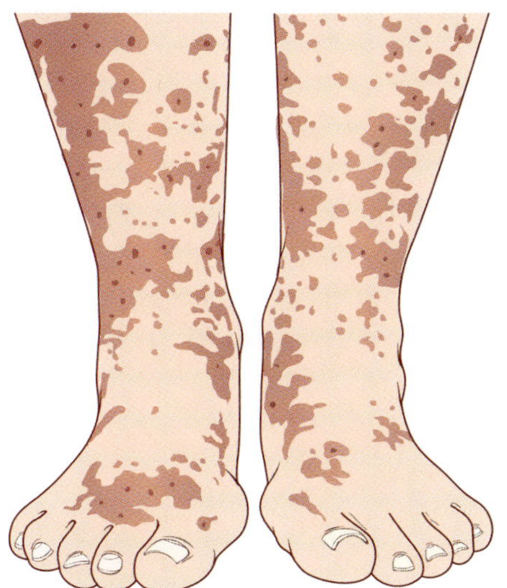

FIGURE 7-6 **Idiopathic thrombocytopenic purpura (ITP)**

Continued

TABLE 7-3

PATHOLOGY TERMS—cont'd	
lymphosarcoma (lĭm-fō-săr-KŌ-mă)	cancer of lymphatic tissue not related to Hodgkin disease
non-Hodgkin lymphom (nŏn-HŎJ-kĭn lĭm-FŌ-mă)	group of more than 30 types of malignancies of B and T lymphocytes
pernicious anemia (pĕr-NĬSH-ŭs ă-NĒ-mē-ă)	chronic form of megaloblastic anemia (producing many large, immature, dysfunctional RBCs), caused by a deficit in the absorption of vitamin B_{12}, that reduces the body's ability to produce sufficient numbers of healthy RBCs
phagocytosis (făg-ō-sī-TŌ-sĭs)	process in which specialized white blood cells (phagocytes) engulf and destroy microorganisms, foreign antigens, and cell debris
***Pneumocystis carinii* pneumonia** (nü-mə-SIS-təs kə-RĪ-nē nü-MŌ-nyə)	a type of pneumonia associated with AIDS
polymyositis (PM) (pŏl-ē-mī-ō-SĪ-tĭs)	disorder that causes the slow onset of muscle weakness and pain in the muscles of the trunk and progresses to affect muscles of the neck, shoulders, back, hip, and possibly hands and fingers
scleroderma (sklĕr-ă-DĔR-mă)	group of chronic autoimmune diseases that cause inflammatory and fibrotic changes to skin, muscles, joints, tendons, cartilage, and other connective tissues (see Fig. 7-7)

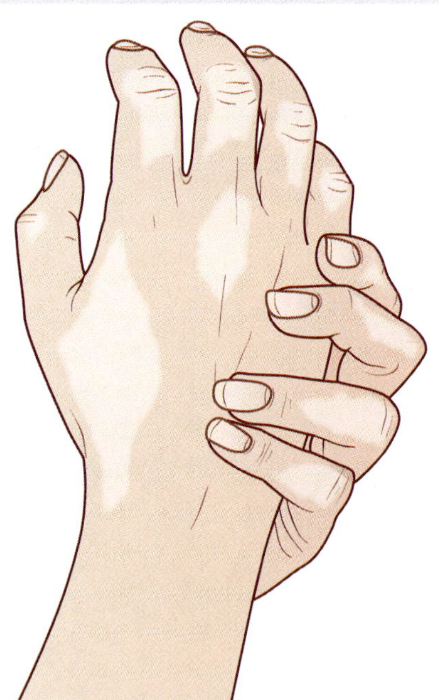

FIGURE 7-7 **Scleroderma**

Sjögren syndrome (SS) (SHŌ-grĕn SĬN-drōm)	autoimmune disorder that causes dysfunction of salivary glands in the mouth and lacrimal glands in the eyes, and affects other areas of the body

TABLE 7-3
PATHOLOGY TERMS—cont'd

systemic lupus erythematosus (SLE) (sĭs-TĔM-ĭk LOO-pŭs ĕr-ĭ-thē-mă-TŌ-sŭs)	chronic autoimmune disorder that causes inflammation and degeneration of various connective tissues and organs in the body, such as the skin, lungs, heart, joints, kidneys, blood, or nervous system (see Fig. 7-8)

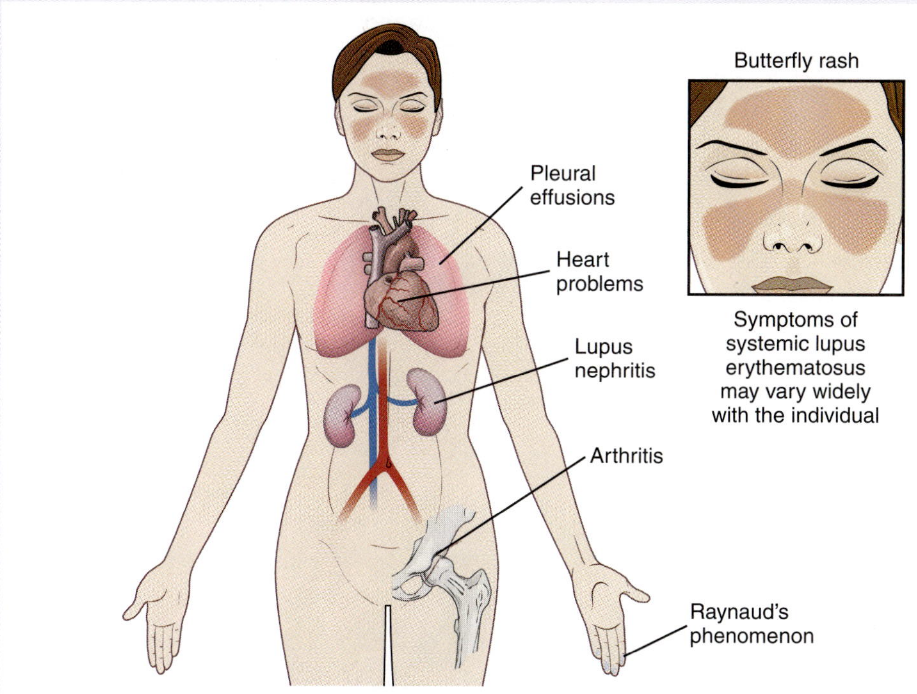

FIGURE 7-8 **Systemic lupus erythematosus**

transfusion incompatibility reaction (trănz-FŪ-zhŭn ĭn-kŏm-păt-ĭ-BĬL-ĭ-tē rē-ĂK-shŭn)	reaction of antibodies present in transfused blood to RBCs in the recipient's blood, or of antibodies in the recipient's blood to RBCs in the transfused blood
transplant rejection (TRĂNZ-plănt rē-JĔK-shŭn)	identification of transplanted tissue as foreign by the recipient's immune system, which responds by attacking the tissue

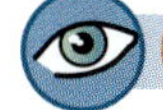 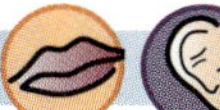

Learning Style Tip

Place sticky notes or tape flash cards around your house with the terms and definitions that you are learning. Recite the terms and definitions aloud each time you see the notes. Great locations to place the notes or cards include mirrors, cupboard doors, and the front of the refrigerator.

STOP HERE.
Select the Pathology Term Flash Cards for Chapter 7 and run through them at least three times before you continue.

Common Diagnostic Tests

Allergy Tests

Patch test: Test in which paper or gauze saturated with an allergen is applied to the skin beneath an occlusive dressing and the response is noted (see Fig. 7-9)

Scratch test: Test in which an allergen is placed on a scratched area of the skin and the response is noted (see Fig. 7-10)

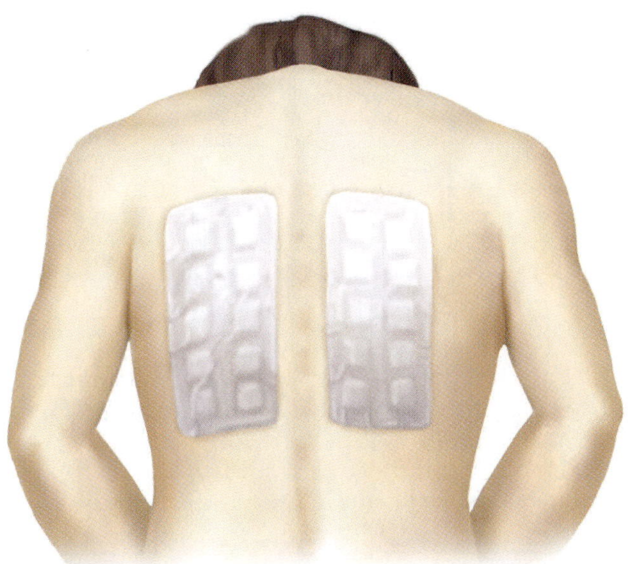

FIGURE 7-9 **Patch test** (From Eagle, S, et al.: *The Professional Medical Assistant.* F.A. Davis, Philadelphia, 2009, p. 430; with permission)

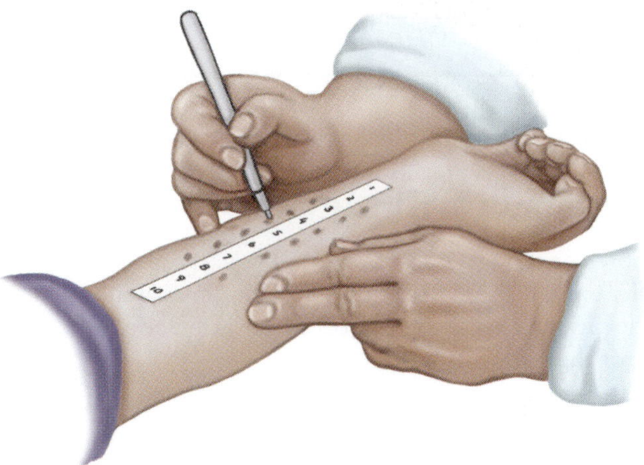

FIGURE 7-10 **Scratch test** (From Eagle, S, et al.: *The Professional Medical Assistant.* F.A. Davis, Philadelphia, 2009, p. 429; with permission)

Tests Used to Diagnose and Monitor HIV and AIDS

CD-4 lymphocyte count: Measurement of the number of specialized WBCs sometimes called *helper T cells*, used to identify whether a person's HIV infection is worsening

Enzyme immunosorbent assay (EIA): Rapid enzyme immunochemical method for identifying the presence of antigens, antibodies, or other substances in the blood, used as a primary diagnostic test for many infectious diseases including syphilis and HIV; formerly called *enzyme-linked immunosorbent assay (ELISA)*

Viral load: Measurement of the number of copies of the human immunodeficiency virus in the blood; used to monitor progression of HIV infection and AIDS

Flashpoint

As an individual's HIV worsens, his CD-4 count drops lower and his viral load climbs higher.

Other Tests

Erythrocyte sedimentation rate (ESR, sed rate): Test used in the diagnosis and monitoring of many diseases that cause acute or chronic inflammation; measures the rate at which RBCs settle in plasma or saline over a specific period of time

Monospot (heterophil): Quick test used to screen for the presence of the heterophil antibody that is present in individuals with Epstein-Barr virus infection

Case Study

Read the case study and answer the questions that follow. Most of the terms are included in this chapter. Refer to the glossaries (Appendixes B and D) or to your medical dictionary for the other terms.

Epstein-Barr Virus

Cindi is a 17-year-old high school student. She leads an active social life, gets good grades, and is a member of the track team. About 2 weeks ago she became ill with what she thought was the flu. Her symptoms included sore throat, enlarged and tender lymph nodes in her neck, inflamed tonsils, headache, fever, a brief maculopapular skin rash, and generalized muscle aches. She expected to feel better by now, but still has many of her symptoms. Therefore, her mother took her to their family physician for evaluation. He noted that Cindi's spleen is enlarged and that her blood reveals "leukocytosis with atypical lymphocytes and IgM antibodies." Based on these findings, the physician diagnosed Cindi with Epstein-Barr virus. He explained that there is no specific cure, but that treatment includes NSAIDs for fever, sore throat, and other discomfort. He also advised her to get plenty of rest and to refrain from vigorous physical activity or contact sports until she has recovered.

The **Epstein-Barr virus** is a member of the herpes virus group. It is most common in the United States in people between ages 15 and 25. Beyond that age, most people are immune to it. It is sometimes called the "kissing disease," because it is transmitted in saliva and infects epithelial cells of the oropharynx, nasopharynx, and salivary glands before spreading to the lymphatic system. It typically causes the symptoms that Cindi experienced, including splenic enlargement. Because splenic rupture could result in life-threatening internal hemorrhage, patients are cautioned to refrain from contact sports until they have fully recovered.

Case Study Questions

1. The illness that Cindi has is also sometimes called:
   a. Pernicious anemia
   b. Polymyositis
   c. Mononucleosis
   d. Sjögren syndrome
2. Cindi's symptoms include all of the following **except**:
   a. Pharyngitis
   b. Cervical lymphadenopathy
   c. Tonsillitis
   d. Jaundice
3. Upon examination, the physician noted that Cindi has:
   a. Splenomegaly
   b. Gastroenteritis
   c. Hepatoma
   d. Pharnygostenosis
4. Cindi's blood test revealed:
   a. An abnormal increase in her white blood cells
   b. Anemia
   c. Bacterial infection
   d. None of these
5. The Epstein-Barr virus is sometimes called the "kissing disease" because:
   a. It is only transmitted through kissing
   b. It is spread through oral secretions
   c. Teens should be discouraged from kissing
   d. None of these
6. A patient with Epstein-Barr virus should avoid which of these?
   a. Resting in bed
   b. Playing video games
   c. Playing football
   d. Watching movies
7. A complication patients must avoid is:
   a. Splenorrhexis
   b. Splenomegaly
   c. Splenitis
   d. Splenopathy

Answers to Case Study Questions

1. c
2. d
3. a
4. a
5. b
6. c
7. a

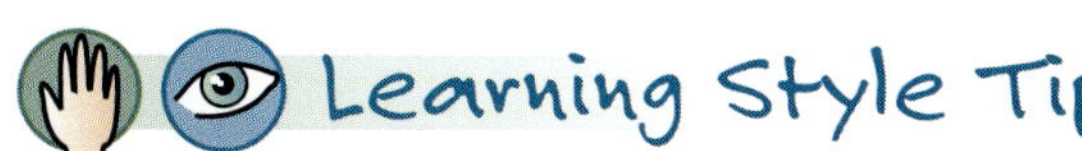

Use your computer to find clip art, photos, or graphics to paste into your class notes, homemade flash cards, or any other documents you create as you study.

Websites

Please go to the F.A. Davis website at http://davisplus.fadavis.com/eagle/medterm to view resource websites for the immune system.

Practice Exercises

Deciphering Terms

Write the correct meaning of these medical terms. Check Appendix G for the correct answers.

Exercise 2

1. pathologist ______________________
2. lymphangiogram ______________________
3. bacteriocidal ______________________
4. angiography ______________________
5. immunology ______________________
6. lymphocytic ______________________
7. toxemia ______________________
8. myelogenous ______________________
9. splenodynia ______________________
10. tonsillectomy ______________________
11. lymphadenopathy ______________________
12. vasorrhaphy ______________________
13. serology ______________________
14. thymotomy ______________________
15. vasalgia ______________________

Fill in the Blanks

Fill in the blanks below using Tables 7-2 and 7-3. Check Appendix G for the correct answers.

Exercise 3

1. An autoimmune disorder that causes dysfunction of salivary glands in the mouth and lacrimal glands in the eyes, and affects other areas of the body, is ____________ ____________.
2. ____________ is a life-threatening systemic allergic reaction.
3. Another name for mononucleosis is the ____________-____________ virus.
4. ____________ disease is a type of lymphatic cancer, also called *lymphoma.*
5. During ____________, specialized white blood cells engulf and destroy microorganisms, foreign antigens, and cell debris.
6. A group of chronic autoimmune diseases that cause inflammatory and fibrotic changes to skin, muscles, joints, tendons, cartilage, and other connective tissues is ____________.
7. ____________ ____________ is a group of more than 30 types of malignancies of B or T lymphocytes.
8. The abbreviation *SLE* stands for ____________ ____________ ____________.
9. The abbreviation *ESR* stands for ____________ ____________ ____________.
10. *Cancer* is often abbreviated as ____________.
11. The name of the virus that causes mononucleosis is abbreviated ____________.
12. Hodgkin disease is a type of ____________ ____________.
13. A complex chronic disorder marked by severe fatigue unrelieved by rest, often worsened by mental or physical activity, is ____________ ____________ syndrome.

14. The abbreviation for the test used to diagnose HIV is

_______________.

15. A type of pneumonia associated with AIDS is abbreviated

_______________.

16. The abbreviations for *antibody* are _______________ and

_______________.

17. The abbreviations for *antigen* are _______________ and

_______________.

18. Oscar has become very ill with AIDS, which stands for

_______________ _______________ _______________

_______________.

19. Oscar got AIDS after becoming infected with the _______________

_______________ virus.

20. Oscar has developed a serious respiratory complication of AIDS,

_______________ _______________ _______________.

Multiple Choice

Select the one best answer to the following multiple-choice questions. Check Appendix G for the correct answers.

Exercise 4

1. Which of the following terms means *creating disease?*
   - a. Pathogenic
   - b. Pathology
   - c. Pathologist
   - d. Pathogen

2. Which of the following is a type of cancer?
   - a. Hodgkin disease
   - b. CHF
   - c. DVT
   - d. TIA

3. A disorder that causes the slow onset of muscle weakness and pain in muscles of the trunk, and progresses to affect the muscles of the neck, shoulders, back, and hip is:
   a. Polymyositis
   b. Scleroderma
   c. Sjögren syndrome
   d. Systemic lupus erythematosus

4. Which of the following is responsible for causing acquired immunodeficiency syndrome?
   a. HIV
   b. RV
   c. CAD
   d. LV

5. Which of the following is related to a vitamin B deficit?
   a. Pernicious anemia
   b. Hodgkin disease
   c. Polymyositis
   d. Graft-versus-host disease

Word Building

*Using **only** the word parts in the lists provided, create medical terms with the indicated meanings. Check Appendix G for the correct answers.*

Exercise 5

Prefixes	Combining Forms	Suffixes
eu-	aden/o	-ar
peri-	angi/o	-genic
	adenoid/o	-gram
	bacteri/o	-ic
	immun/o	-logy
	lymph/o	-megaly
	myel/o	-oid
	path/o	-ous
	ser/o	-pathy
	splen/o	-plasty
	thym/o	-sclerosis
	tonsill/o	-tomy
	toxic/o	

1. record of a vessel ______________________________

2. study of bacteria ______________________________

3. creating immunity ______
4. pertaining to serum ______
5. study of poison ______
6. incision into the tonsil ______
7. study of disease ______
8. pertaining to around the tonsil ______
9. hardening of the thymus ______
10. produced by bone marrow ______
11. resembling lymph ______
12. enlarged spleen ______
13. surgical repair of a vessel ______
14. pertaining to a good thymus ______
15. disease of a gland ______

True or False

Decide whether the following statements are true or false. Check Appendix G for the correct answers.

Exercise 6

1. True False **Sjögren syndrome** is an autoimmune disorder.
2. True False **Lymphosarcoma** is a type of cancer of lymphatic tissue not related to Hodgkin disease.
3. True False The abbreviation **CA** stands for *carcinoma* or *cancer.*
4. True False **Hodgkin disease** occurs when the immune system misidentifies RBCs as foreign and creates autoantibodies that attack them.
5. True False The abbreviation **Ab** stands for *abnormal.*
6. True False **Phagocytosis** is a process in which specialized WBCs engulf and destroy microorganisms, foreign antigens, and cell debris.

7. True False **Rejection** occurs when a recipient's immune system identifies transplanted tissue as foreign and begins attacking it.

8. True False **Ankylosing spondylitis** affects vertebrae and connective tissue.

9. True False The abbreviation **EBV** refers to a test used to diagnose HIV infection.

10. True False **Ig** is the abbreviation for *antigen.*

Deciphering Terms

Write the correct meaning of these medical terms. Check Appendix G for the correct answers.

Exercise 7

1. adenolipoma ______________________________
2. adenoiditis ______________________________
3. angioedema ______________________________
4. vasoconstriction ______________________________
5. myeloma ______________________________
6. immunogen ______________________________
7. lymphadenectasis ______________________________
8. lymphorrhagia ______________________________
9. lymphangioma ______________________________
10. lymphocytopenia ______________________________

Multiple Choice

Select the one best answer to the following multiple-choice questions. Check Appendix G for the correct answers.

Exercise 8

1. Which of the following terms means *pertaining to bone-marrow cells?*
   - a. Lymphocytic
   - b. Myelogenous
   - c. Myelocytic
   - d. Lymphangiocyte

2. Which of the following terms means *tumor of a lymphatic vessel?*
    a. Lymphangioma
    b. Lymphadenoma
    c. Lymphadenopathy
    d. Angiomyoma
3. Which of the following terms means *abnormal condition of lymph cells?*
    a. Lymphogenesis
    b. Lymphocytosis
    c. Adenopathy
    d. Lymphokinesis
4. Which of the following terms means *hernia of the spinal cord and meninges?*
    a. Myeloma
    b. Myelomeningoma
    c. Myelomeningocele
    d. Myelomalacia
5. Which of the following terms is matched with the correct definition?
    a. Tox/o: disease
    b. Angi/o: vessel
    c. Path/o: poison
    d. Aden/o: adenoid
6. All of the following terms are matched with the correct definition **except**:
    a. Vas/o: vessel
    b. Ser/o: spleen
    c. Myel/o: bone marrow
    d. Lymphangi/o: lymphatic vessel
7. Which of the following has been called the kissing disease?
    a. EBV
    b. EIA
    c. ESR
    d. SLE

8. Which of the following abbreviations stands for the name of a test used to monitor disorders that cause inflammation in the body?

   a. EBV
   b. EIA
   c. ESR
   d. SLE

9. Which of the following abbreviations represents the name of a disorder that may affect transplant patients?

   a. AIDS
   b. KS
   c. PCP
   d. GVHD

10. Which of the following abbreviations is related to cancer?

    a. MET
    b. Ag
    c. EIA
    d. Ab

11. All of the following terms are matched with the correct definition **except**:

    a. Sjögren syndrome: autoimmune disorder that causes dysfunction of salivary and lacrimal glands
    b. Anaphylaxis: life-threatening systemic allergic reaction
    c. Ankylosing spondylitis: inflammatory response that causes degenerative changes in the spinal vertebrae, sacroiliac joints, and other connective tissues
    d. Chronic fatigue syndrome: acute infection that causes sore throat, fever, fatigue, and enlarged lymph nodes

12. All of the following terms are matched with the correct definition **except**:

    a. Chronic mucocutaneous candidiasis: group of disorders in which persistent or recurrent *Candida* fungal infections develop on the skin, nails, or mucous membranes
    b. Lymphosarcoma: cancer of lymphatic tissue not related to Hodgkin disease
    c. Pernicious anemia: group of disorders caused when the immune system misidentifies RBCs as foreign and creates autoantibodies that attack them
    d. Phagocytosis: process in which specialized white blood cells engulf and destroy microorganisms, foreign antigens, and cell debris

13. All of the following terms are matched with the correct definition **except**:

a. Graft-versus-host disease: complication of bone-marrow transplantation in which lymphoid cells from donated tissue attack the recipient and cause damage to the skin, liver, GI tract, and other tissues

b. Hodgkin disease: type of lymphatic cancer; also called *lymphoma*

c. Polymyositis: disorder that causes the slow onset of muscle weakness and pain in the trunk and progresses to affect the muscles of the neck, shoulders, back, and hip

d. Transplant rejection: reaction of antibodies present in transfused blood to RBCs in the recipient's blood, or of antibodies in the recipient's blood to RBCs in the transfused blood

14. A chronic autoimmune disorder that causes inflammation and degeneration of various connective tissues and organs in the body such as the skin, lungs, heart, joints, kidneys, blood, or nervous system is:

a. Acquired immunodeficiency syndrome

b. Systemic lupus erythematosus

c. Chronic fatigue syndrome

d. Idiopathic thrombocytopenic purpura

15. A disorder in which a deficiency of platelets results in abnormal blood clotting, marked by tiny purple bruises that form under the skin, is:

a. ITP

b. CFS

c. SS

d. SLE

16. A group of chronic autoimmune diseases that cause inflammatory and fibrotic changes to skin, muscles, joints, tendons, cartilage, and other connective tissues is:

a. Sjögren syndrome

b. Scleroderma

c. Systemic lupus erythematosus

d. Polymyositis

17. Which of the following terms means *skin (disease caused by a) poison?*

a. Toxicoderma

b. Dermopathy

c. Dermatomycosis

d. Toxicopathy

18. Which of the following terms means *suturing of the spleen?*
    a. Splenorrhexis
    b. Splenodesis
    c. Splenocentesis
    d. Splenorrhaphy

19. Which of the following terms means *condition of a good (healthy) thymus?*
    a. Dysthymic
    b. Euthymia
    c. Neothymia
    d. Endothymic

20. Which of the following terms means *study of serum?*
    a. Serologist
    b. Serous
    c. Serology
    d. Seroma

RESPIRATORY SYSTEM

8

Structure and Function

The most basic human need is the need to breathe. We take our first breaths as soon as we are born, and continue this vital function through the last moments of our lives. The complex and amazing structures of the respiratory system support this life-sustaining process.

When studying the respiratory system, we often divide it into the upper and lower airways. The **upper airway** consists of the **mouth, nose, sinuses,** and **pharynx.** The pharynx is further divided into the **nasopharynx** (back of the nose) and **oropharynx** (back of the mouth). The nose begins with the **nares** (nostrils) and extends back to the nasopharynx. The nasal passages are divided into right and left sides by the nasal septum. The hard palate divides the nasal cavity from the mouth, which sits beneath it. The sinus cavities are air-filled spaces named for the facial bones within which they are located. They include the maxillary, frontal, ethmoidal, and sphenoidal sinuses. Refer to Figure 8-1, which illustrates these structures, as we discuss the path that air takes into and out of the body.

Flashpoint

Structures of the upper airway filter, warm, and humidify air before it flows down to the lungs.

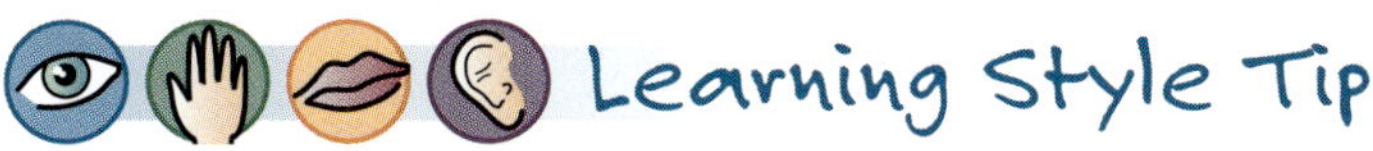

Learning Style Tip

Get permission to spend time in the biology laboratory and study the anatomical models, in this case the ones representing the respiratory system. Physically touch the various parts, naming them as you do, while you also name their associated combining forms.

As air moves through the upper airway, it is warmed, filtered, and humidified. Mucous membranes that line these structures contribute moisture to humidify the air. Cilia (tiny hairs) within the nasal cavity help filter the air by removing debris. The rich blood supply of all of these structures warms the air as it passes through. Sinus cavities serve to decrease the weight of the skull, provide resonance for the voice, and produce mucus, which helps eliminate microorganisms as it drains into the nasal cavities.

Air moves to the **lower airway** as it flows past the **epiglottis** and enters the **trachea**. The epiglottis acts as a doorway to the trachea and serves a vital protective function by opening to let in air and closing to keep out food and fluid. As air flows through the tracheal entrance, it passes through the **larynx**. This structure vibrates to create sound when we talk. Air then flows down the trachea and into the lower airways, which consist of the **bronchi** and **lungs**. The trachea is approximately 5 inches long and gets its shape and strength from numerous rings of cartilage. The bronchi split off into smaller bronchi and eventually into tiny **bronchioles**. The composition of the bronchi changes to less cartilage and more smooth muscle as they become smaller. The trachea

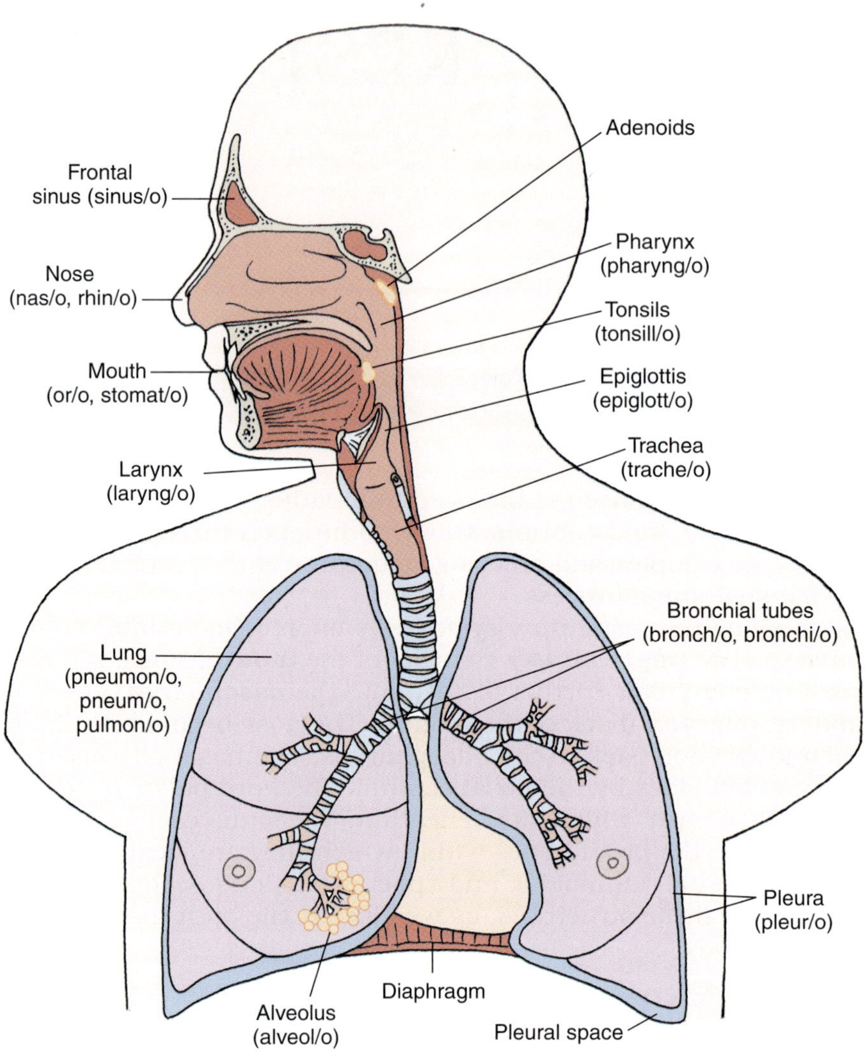

FIGURE 8-1 **Sinuses**

and bronchi have ciliated mucous-membrane linings, which further moisten air and secrete mucus to trap debris that has been inhaled. Cilia move in a wavelike fashion to propel debris upward. The trachea and bronchi are extremely sensitive, and the presence of foreign particles stimulates a powerful cough reflex that further helps to expel debris.

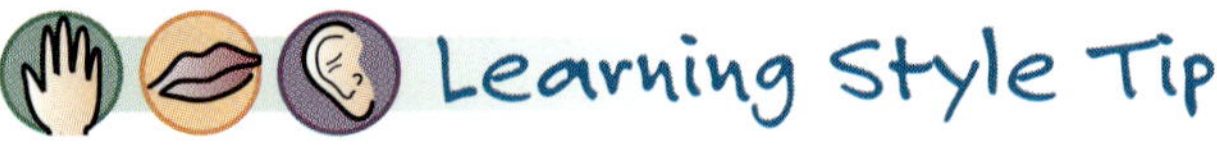

Use class breaks to get up and physically move. Walk briskly around the building or climb up and down several flights of stairs. As you do so, verbally repeat the definitions of two new terms. The physical activity will stimulate your circulation, wake you up, and energize you. You will return to class readier to learn—and as an added bonus, you will have just learned two new terms.

The Lungs

The lungs are divided into **lobes**; the right lung has three and the left lung has two. The lungs are covered with two thin membranes known as the **pleurae**. The term **intrapleural** means within the pleural space in general. The visceral pleura lies directly on the lungs, while the parietal pleura lines the inner wall of the thorax. The term **interpleural** refers to the specific area between the visceral pleura and the parietal pleura. A small amount of pleural fluid lies within the space between the two membranes. This space is sometimes referred to as a *potential* space, because there is nothing there other than this tiny amount of fluid. As we breathe in and out, our lungs expand and contract. The elastic quality that allows the lungs to do this is sometimes called *recoil*. As we breathe, the pleural fluid between the visceral and parietal pleurae acts as a sort of lubricant, which helps the process along as the lungs continually expand and contract.

As air continues on its journey into the lungs, it arrives at its final destination, the **alveoli**, which are microscopic-sized air sacs. We have approximately 300 million alveoli in each lung. They are covered with a delicate capillary bed (microscopic blood vessels) that provides a rich blood supply. The alveoli expand somewhat like tiny balloons during inspiration (also called inhalation) as air enters and fills them. They contract and partially deflate during expiration, as much of the air exits the lungs. Because the walls of the alveoli and the capillary beds are each just one cell thick, gases easily move back and forth across them. Excess carbon dioxide (CO_2) leaves the capillaries and moves into the air space within the alveoli, and is then exhaled. Oxygen (O_2) moves from the air space in the alveoli into the capillary blood, and is then distributed to various parts of the body via the circulatory system.

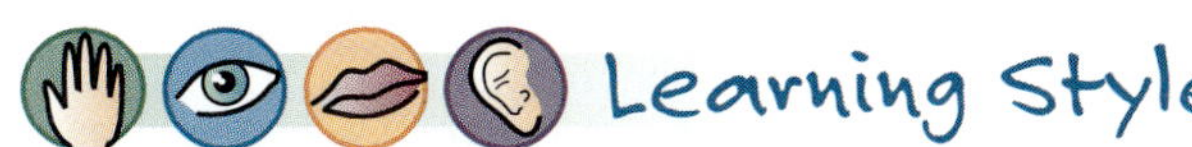

Take several deep, slow breaths. As you do so, visualize the path that oxygen is taking as it moves from your external environment into your respiratory system and finally into your bloodstream. Next, visualize the reverse path that carbon dioxide follows as it leaves your body. Now verbally describe both pathways to a real or imaginary partner.

Flashpoint

There are approximately 300 million alveoli in each lung!

We take oxygen into our lungs through the act of **inhalation**, or breathing in (also called inspiration), which is usually an unconscious act. However, we may exert conscious control to take extra-large breaths or even hold our breath for a short time. At some point, however, we feel an overwhelming urge to breathe, which is triggered by a buildup of CO_2. This buildup of CO_2 in the blood causes the blood to become more acidic. To be healthy, our blood must remain slightly alkaline—within the narrow range of 7.35 to 7.45 on the **pH scale**, which is a tool for measuring the acidity or alkalinity of a substance. As blood becomes more acidic, its pH level drops, triggering the urge to breathe. As we inhale, we bring fresh, oxygen-rich air into our lungs, where it can be absorbed into our blood. The act of **exhalation**, or breathing out (or expiration), allows our bodies to eliminate excess CO_2, thus restoring a normal blood pH level. Contrary to what most people think, the drive to breathe is not triggered by lower oxygen levels in the blood, but by the lowered pH level caused by CO_2 buildup.

Combining Forms

Table 8-1 contains combining forms that pertain to the respiratory system, examples of terms that utilize the combining forms, and a pronunciation guide. Read aloud to yourself as you move from left to right across the table. Be sure to use the pronunciation guide so that you can learn to say the terms correctly.

TABLE 8-1

COMBINING FORMS RELATED TO THE RESPIRATORY SYSTEM

Combining Form	Meaning	Example (Pronunciation)	Meaning of New Term
aer/o	air	aerophagia (ār-ō-FĀ-jē-ă)	eating or swallowing air
alveol/o	alveoli	alveolitis (ăl-vē-ŏ-LĪ-tĭs)	inflammation of the alveoli
anthrac/o	coal, coal dust	anthracosis (ăn-thră-KŌ-sĭs)	abnormal condition of coal (black lung)
bronch/o	bronchus	bronchitis (brŏng-KĪ-tĭs)	inflammation of the bronchus
bronchi/o		bronchiectasis (brŏng-kē-ĔK-tă-sĭs)	dilation or expansion of the bronchus
bronchiol/o	bronchiole	bronchiolitis (brŏng-kē-ō-LĪ-tĭs)	inflammation of the bronchiole
carcin/o	cancer	carcinoma (kăr-sĭ-NŌ-mă)	cancerous tumor
chondr/o	cartilage	chondroplasty (KŎN-drō-plăs-tē)	surgical repair of the cartilage
coni/o	dust	coniosis (kō-nē-Ō-sĭs)	abnormal condition caused by (inhalation of) dust
diaphragmat/o	diaphragm	diaphragmatocele (dī-ă-frăg-MĂT-ō-sēl)	hernia of the diaphragm
epiglott/o	epiglottis	epiglottal (ĕp-ĭ-GLŎT-ăl)	pertaining to the epiglottis
laryng/o	larynx	laryngitis (lăr-ĭn-JĪ-tĭs)	inflammation of the larynx
lob/o	lobe	lobectomy (lō-BĔK-tō-mē)	excision or surgical removal of a lobe
muc/o	mucus	mucoid (MŪ-koyd)	resembling mucus
nas/o	nose	nasogastric (nā-zō-GĂS-trĭk)	pertaining to the nose and stomach
rhin/o		rhinitis (rī-NĪ-tĭs)	inflammation of the nose
or/o	mouth, mouthlike opening	oral (Ō-răl)	pertaining to the mouth
stomat/o		stomatitis (stō-mă-TĪ-tĭs)	inflammation of the mouth
orth/o	straight	orthopnea (or-THŎP-nē-ă)	breathing in the straight position
ox/i	oxygen	oximeter (ŏk-SĬM-ĕ-tĕr)	measuring instrument for oxygen
ox/o		anoxia (ăn-ŎK-sē-ă)	condition of no oxygen
pharyng/o	pharynx	pharyngeal (făr-ĬN-jē-ăl)	pertaining to the pharynx

TABLE 8-1

COMBINING FORMS RELATED TO THE RESPIRATORY SYSTEM—cont'd

Combining Form	Meaning	Example (Pronunciation)	Meaning of New Term
phon/o	sound, voice	phonograph (FŌ-nō-grăf)	recording instrument for sound or voice
pleur/o	pleura	pleurodynia (ploo-rō-DĬN-ē-ă)	pain of the pleura
pneum/o	lung, air	pneumonia (nū-MŌ-nē-ă)	condition of the lung
pneumon/o		pneumonectomy (nū-mŏn-ĔK-tō-mē)	excision or surgical removal of the lung
pulmon/o	lung	pulmonary (PŬL-mō-nĕ-rē)	pertaining to the lung
sinus/o	sinus	sinusoid (SĪ-nŭs-oyd)	resembling a sinus
spir/o	breathing	spirometer (spī-RŎM-ĕt-ĕr)	measuring instrument for breathing
thorac/o	thorax	thoracentesis (thō-ră-sĕn-TĒ-sĭs)	surgical puncture of the thorax
tonsill/o	tonsil	tonsillitis (tŏn-sĭl-Ī-tĭs)	inflammation of the tonsil
trache/o	trachea	tracheotomy (trā-kē-ŎT-ō-mē)	cutting into or incision of the trachea

STOP HERE.
Select the Combining Form Flash Cards for Chapter 8 and run through them at least three times before you continue.

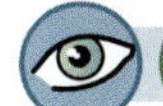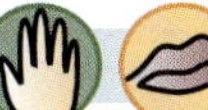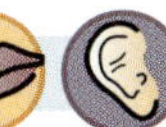

Learning Style Tip

Resist the temptation to skip over exercises like the following one. Completing them engages your visual and kinesthetic senses; verbalizing the terms as you read and write them also engages your verbal and auditory senses. Most importantly, these activities require you to read and review the new terms, which helps you learn and remember them.

Practice Exercises

Fill in the Blanks

Fill in the blanks below using Table 8-1. Check Appendix G for the correct answers.

Exercise 1

1. resembling mucus ______
2. inflammation of the tonsils ______
3. inflammation of the bronchus ______
4. dilation or expansion of the bronchus ______
5. pertaining to the epiglottis ______
6. eating or swallowing air ______
7. pertaining to the pharynx ______
8. surgical repair of the cartilage ______
9. breathing in the straight position ______
10. pertaining to the nose and stomach ______
11. cancerous tumor ______
12. pertaining to the mouth ______
13. condition of no oxygen ______
14. condition of the lung ______
15. inflammation of the nose ______
16. pain of the pleura ______
17. pertaining to the lung ______
18. resembling a sinus ______
19. surgical puncture of the thorax ______
20. excision or surgical removal of the lung ______
21. cutting into or incision of the trachea ______
22. inflammation of the larynx ______
23. inflammation of the mouth ______
24. abnormal condition caused by (inhalation of) dust ______
25. excision or surgical removal of a lobe ______
26. inflammation of the alveoli ______

27. abnormal condition of coal (black lung) ____________________

28. hernia of the diaphragm ____________________

29. inflammation of the bronchiole ____________________

30. measuring instrument for oxygen ____________________

31. recording instrument for sound or voice ____________________

32. measuring instrument for breathing ____________________

33. **Fill in the blanks in Figure 8-2 with the appropriate anatomical terms and combining forms.**

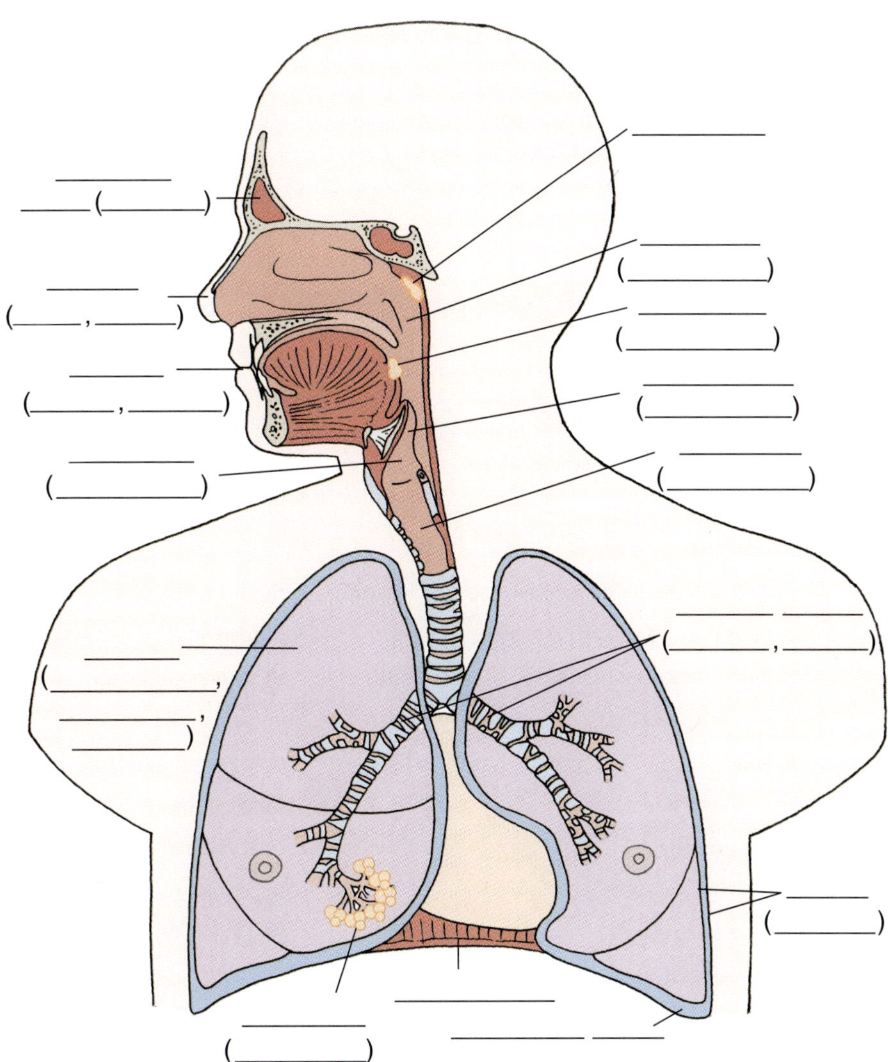

FIGURE 8-2 The respiratory system with blanks

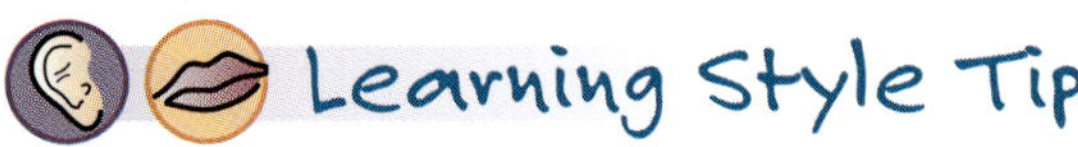

Most colleges have a free tutoring center on campus. Find yours and discover what types of services they offer. Working with a tutor will help you benefit from your auditory or verbal style. The tutor may also have additional study tips for you.

Abbreviations

Table 8-2 lists some of the most common abbreviations related to the respiratory system, as well as others often used in medical documentation.

STOP HERE.
Select the Abbreviation Flash Cards for Chapter 8 and run through them at least three times before you continue.

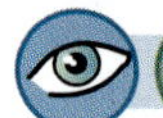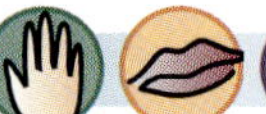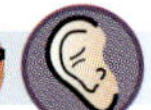

Learning Style Tip

Use your flash cards! They were created specifically to help you utilize your visual and kinesthetic styles. Verbal and auditory learners will benefit most by reading them aloud as you flip them over. Repetition is the key, so use them every day.

TABLE 8-2
ABBREVIATIONS

ABGs	arterial blood gases	PFT	pulmonary function test
AFB	acid-fast bacillus	pH	potential of hydrogen (measure of acidity or alkalinity)
ARDS	acute respiratory distress syndrome	PND	paroxysmal nocturnal dyspnea
CF	cystic fibrosis	PPD	purified protein derivative
CO_2	carbon dioxide	R	respiration
COPD	chronic obstructive pulmonary disease	RA	room air
CPAP	continuous positive airway pressure	SIDS	sudden infant death syndrome
CPR	cardiopulmonary resuscitation	SOB	short(ness) of breath
CPT	chest physiotherapy	stat	immediate(ly)
CXR	chest x-ray	T&A	tonsillectomy and adenoidectomy
DOE	dyspnea on exertion	TB	tuberculosis
MDI	metered dose inhaler	TV	tidal volume
O_2	oxygen	URI	upper respiratory infection
OSA	obstructive sleep apnea	VC	vital capacity
PE	pulmonary embolism		

Pathology Terms

Table 8-3 includes terms that relate to diseases or abnormalities of the respiratory system. Use the pronunciation guide and say the terms aloud as you read them. This will help you get in the habit of saying them properly.

TABLE 8-3
PATHOLOGY TERMS

acute bronchitis (ă-KŪT brŏng-KĪ-tĭs)	infection and inflammation of bronchial airways (see Fig. 8-3)

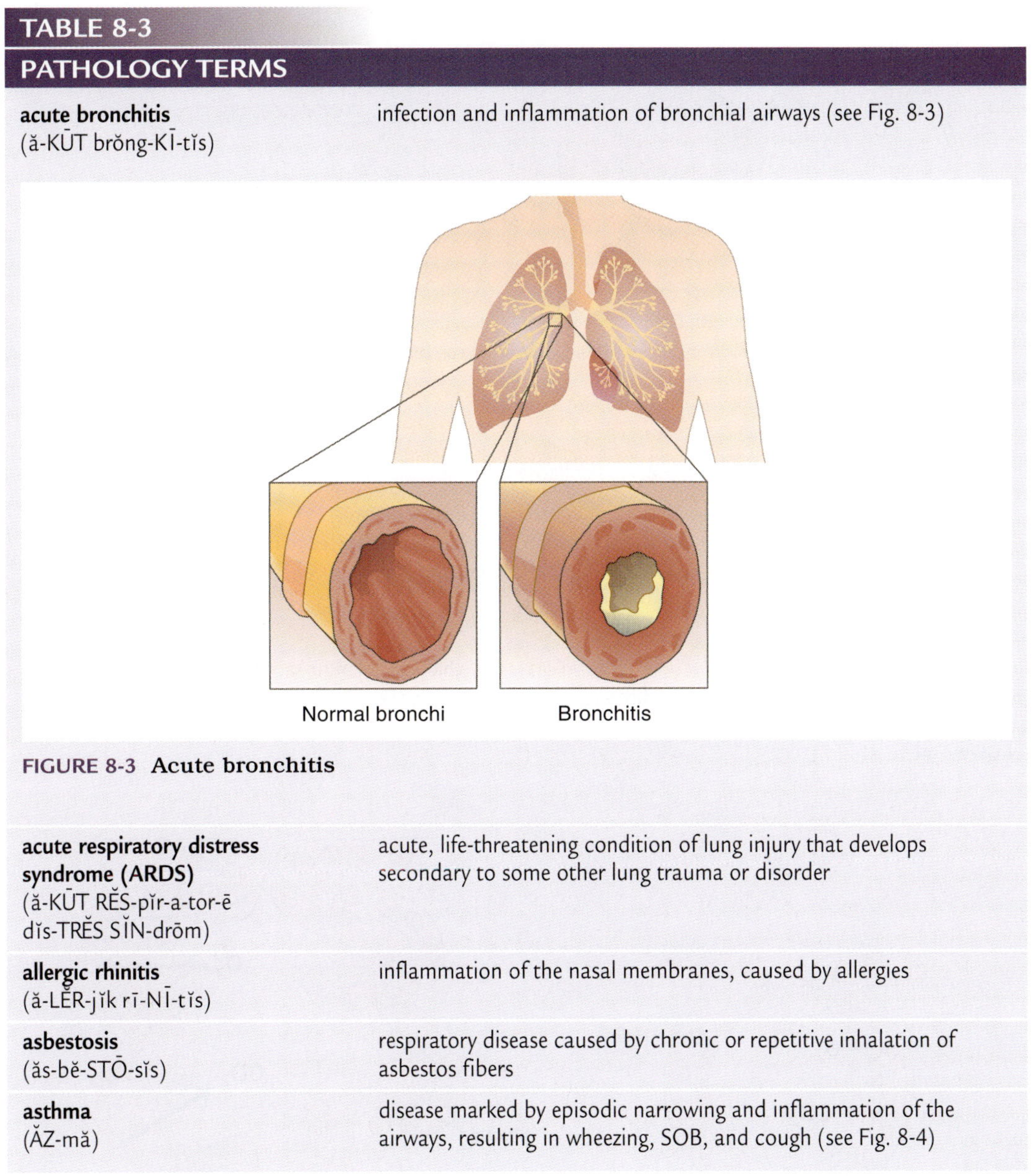

FIGURE 8-3 **Acute bronchitis**

acute respiratory distress syndrome (ARDS) (ă-KŪT RĔS-pĭr-a-tor-ē dĭs-TRĔS SĬN-drōm)	acute, life-threatening condition of lung injury that develops secondary to some other lung trauma or disorder
allergic rhinitis (ă-LĔR-jĭk rī-NĪ-tĭs)	inflammation of the nasal membranes, caused by allergies
asbestosis (ăs-bĕ-STŌ-sĭs)	respiratory disease caused by chronic or repetitive inhalation of asbestos fibers
asthma (ĂZ-mă)	disease marked by episodic narrowing and inflammation of the airways, resulting in wheezing, SOB, and cough (see Fig. 8-4)

Continued

TABLE 8-3
PATHOLOGY TERMS—cont'd

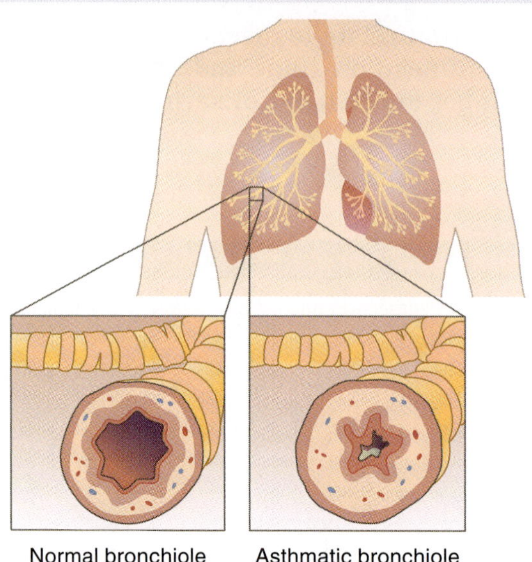

FIGURE 8-4 **Asthma**

atelectasis (ăt-ĕ-LĔK-tă-sĭs)	partial collapse of the alveoli and tiny airways of the lung
cardiopulmonary resuscitation (CPR) (KAR-dē-ō-pŭl-mō-nĕ-rē RĒ-su-sĭ-tā-shun)	a skill often taught in first-aid courses that helps restore a victim's breathing and circulation
chronic obstructive pulmonary disease (COPD) (KRŎN-ĭk ŏb-STRŬK-tĭv PŬL-mō-nĕ-rē dĭ-ZĒZ)	group of diseases in which alveolar air sacs are destroyed and chronic, severe SOB results (see Fig. 8-5)

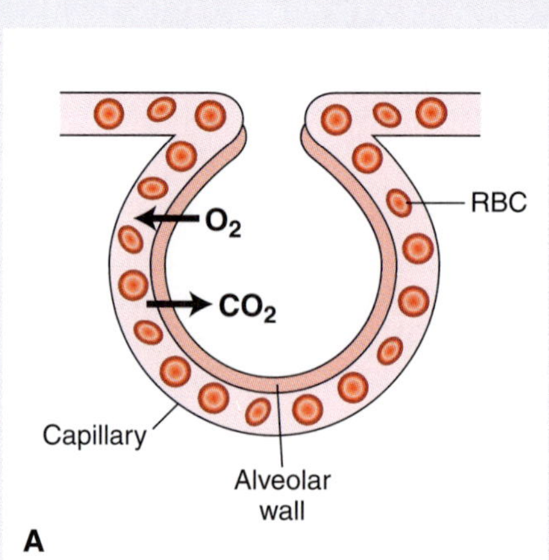

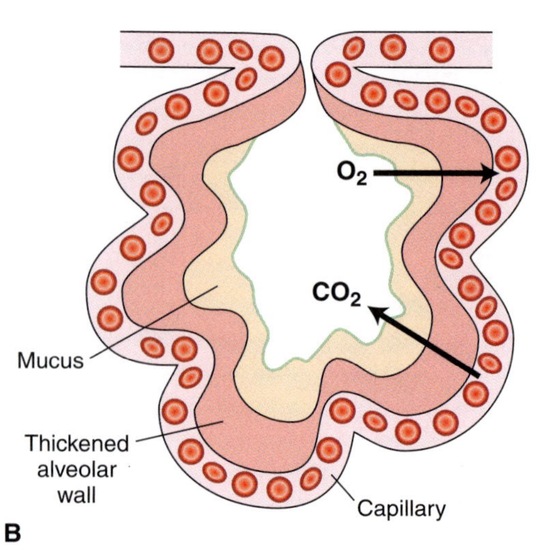

FIGURE 8-5 **Chronic obstructive pulmonary disease (COPD): (A) Normal alveoli, (B) Destructive changes of COPD**

TABLE 8-3 PATHOLOGY TERMS—cont'd	
coal worker's pneumoconiosis (CWP) (KŌL WER-kerz nū-mō-kō-nē-Ō-sĭs)	respiratory disease caused by chronic or repetitive inhalation of coal dust; often called *black lung* or *anthracosis*
coryza (kŏ-RĪ-ză)	acute inflammation of the nasal mucosa; the common cold
crackles (KRĂ-kuls)	abnormal crackly lung sound—like the sound of Rice Krispies—heard with a stethoscope, caused by air passing over retained secretions or by the sudden opening of collapsed airways
croup (croop)	acute viral disease, usually in children, marked by a barking, "seal-like" cough and respiratory distress
cystic fibrosis (CF) (SĬS-tĭk fī-BRŌ-sĭs)	fatal genetic disease that causes frequent respiratory infections, increased airway secretions, and COPD in children
deviated septum (DĒ-vē-ā-tĕd SĔP-tŭm)	condition in which the nasal septum is displaced to the side, causing the two nares (nasal passages) to be unequal (see Fig. 8-6)

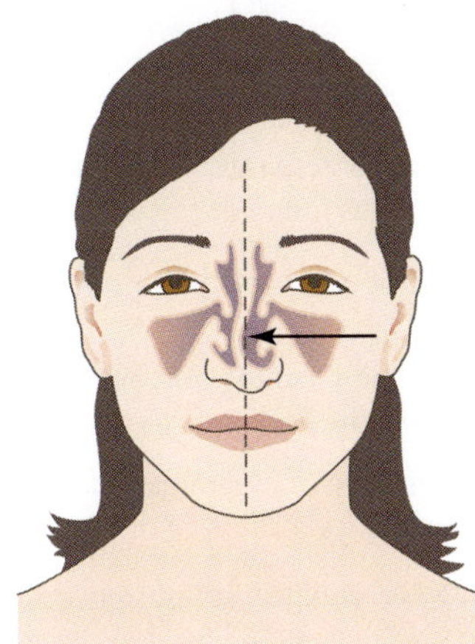

FIGURE 8-6 **Deviated septum**

emphysema (ĕm-fĭ-SĒ-mă)	disorder marked by abnormal increase in the size of air spaces distal to the terminal bronchiole and destruction of the alveolar walls, resulting in loss of normal elasticity and in progressive dyspnea
empyema (ĕm-pī-Ē-mă)	collection of infected fluid (pus) between the two pleural membranes that line the lungs
epistaxis (ĕp-ĭ-STĂK-sĭs)	episode of bleeding from the nose; commonly known as a *nosebleed*
hemoptysis (hē-MŎP-tĭ-sĭs)	coughing up blood from the respiratory tract
hemothorax (hē-mō-THŌ-răks)	condition in which blood or bloody fluid has collected within the intrapleural space, causing lung compression and respiratory distress (see Fig. 8-7)

Continued

TABLE 8-3
PATHOLOGY TERMS—cont'd

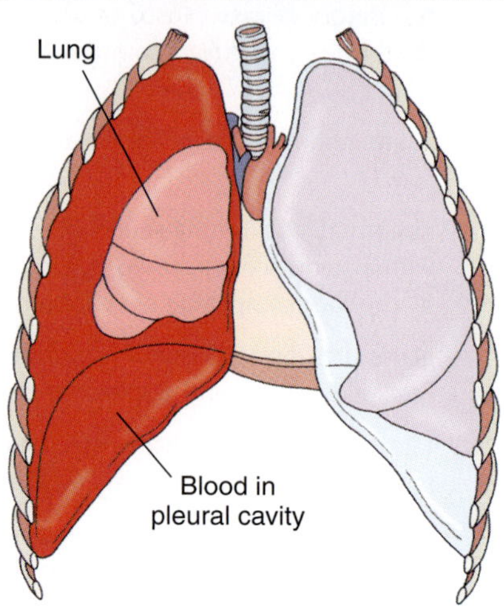

FIGURE 8-7 **Hemothorax**

histoplasmosis (hĭs-tō-plăz-MŌ-sĭs)	systemic respiratory disease caused by *Histoplasma capsulatum*, a fungus found in soil contaminated with bird droppings
hypercapnia (hī-pĕr-KĂP-nē-ă)	chronic retention of CO_2, causing symptoms of mental cloudiness and lethargy
influenza (ĭn-floo-ĔN-ză)	common, contagious, acute viral respiratory illness; commonly called the *flu*
laryngitis (lăr-ĭn-JĪ-tĭs)	condition of inflammation of the larynx, evidenced by a temporary hoarseness or loss of the voice
legionellosis (lē-jŭ-nĕ-LŌ-sĭs)	bacterial lung infection caused by the bacterium *Legionella pneumophila*
nasal polyps (NĀ-zul PŎL-ĭps)	rounded tissue growths on the nasal or sinal mucosa (see Fig. 8-8)

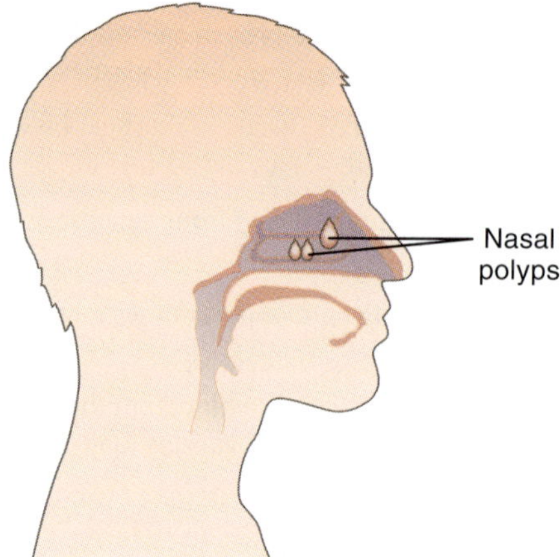

FIGURE 8-8 **Nasal polyps**

TABLE 8-3

PATHOLOGY TERMS—cont'd	
obstructive sleep apnea (OSA) (ŏb-STRŬK-tĭv slēp ăp-NĒ-ă)	dysfunctional breathing that occurs when the upper airway is intermittently blocked during sleep (see Fig. 8-9)

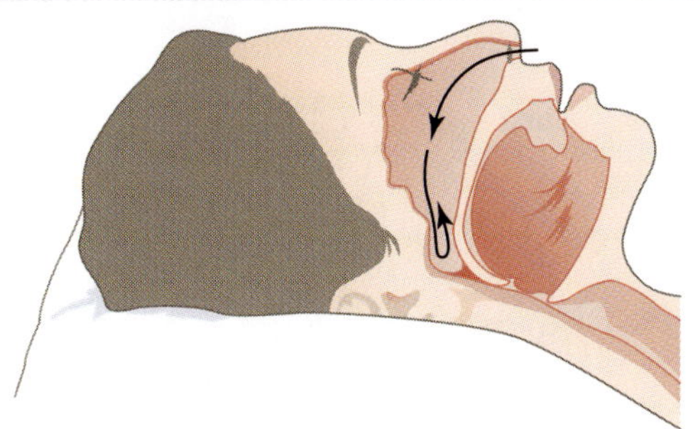

FIGURE 8-9 **Obstructive sleep apnea**

orthopnea (ōr-THŎP-nē-ă)	labored breathing that occurs when lying flat and improves when sitting up
pharyngitis (făr-ĭn-JĪ-tĭs)	inflammation of the pharynx; commonly called a *sore throat*
pleural effusion (PLOO-răl ĕ-FŪ-zhŭn)	excess collection of fluid in the intrapleural space
pleurisy (PLOO-rĭs-ē)	condition in which the pleurae become inflamed, causing sharp inspiratory chest pain; also called *pleuritis*
pneumoconiosis (nū-mō-kō-nē-Ō-sĭs)	any disease of the respiratory tract caused by chronic or repetitive inhalation of dust particles
pneumonia (nū-MŌ-nē-ă)	bacterial or viral infection of the lungs (see Fig. 8-10)

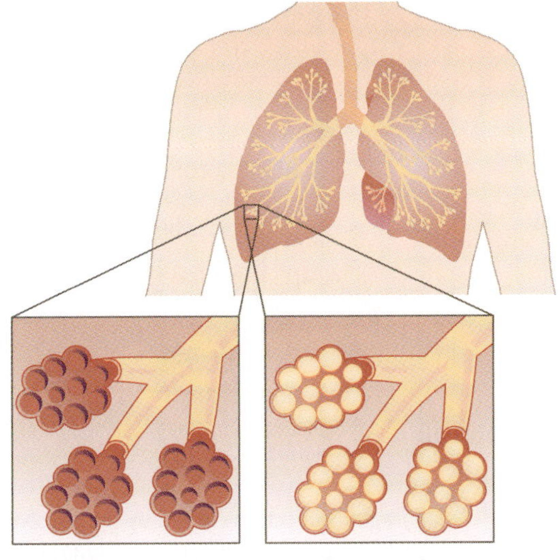

FIGURE 8-10 **Pneumonia**

Continued

TABLE 8-3

PATHOLOGY TERMS—cont'd

pneumothorax (nū-mō-THŌ-răks)	condition in which air collects in the intrapleural space; categorized as open, closed, spontaneous, or tension, and commonly called *collapsed lung* (see Fig. 8-11)

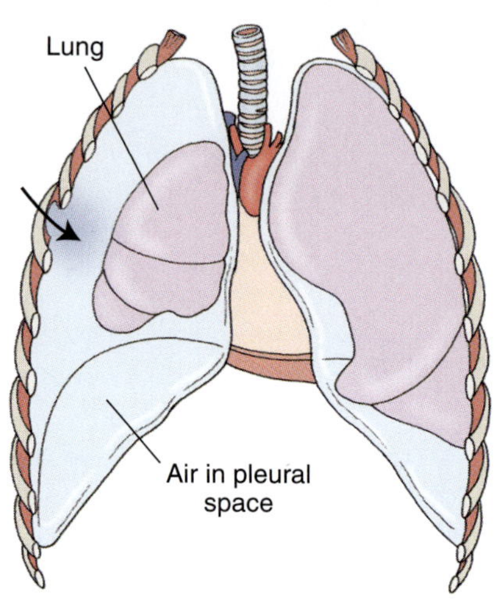

FIGURE 8-11 **Pneumothorax**

pulmonary embolism (PE) (PŬL-mō-nĕ-rē ĔM-bō-lĭ-zum)	sudden obstruction of a pulmonary blood vessel by debris, blood clots, or other matter (see Fig. 8-12)

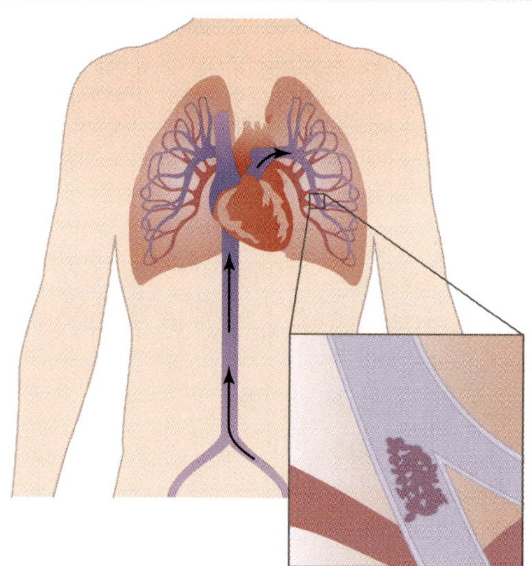

FIGURE 8-12 **Pulmonary embolism**

pulmonary tuberculosis (TB) (PŬL-mō-nĕ-rē tū-bĕr-kū-LŌ-sĭs)	contagious infection caused by the *Mycobacterium tuberculosis* organism, primarily affecting the lungs but sometimes also spreading to and affecting other organ systems
rhonchi (RŎNG-kī)	coarse, gurgling sound heard in the lungs with a stethoscope, caused by secretions in the air passages

TABLE 8-3
PATHOLOGY TERMS—cont'd

silicosis (sĭl-ĭ-KŌ-sĭs)	respiratory disease caused by chronic or repetitive inhalation of silica (quartz) dust
sinusitis (sī-nŭs-Ī-tĭs)	inflammation of the lining of the sinus cavities (see Fig. 8-13)

FIGURE 8-13 **Sinusitis**

stridor (STRĪ-dōr)	high-pitched upper-airway sound heard without a stethoscope, indicating airway obstruction; a medical emergency
upper respiratory infection (URI) (ŬP-ĕr RĔS-pĭr-a-tor-ē ĭn-FĔK-shŭn)	infection and inflammation of upper-airway structures, usually caused by a virus; often called the *common cold*
wheeze (hwēz)	somewhat musical sound heard in the lungs, usually with a stethoscope, caused by partial airway obstruction (such as with asthma)

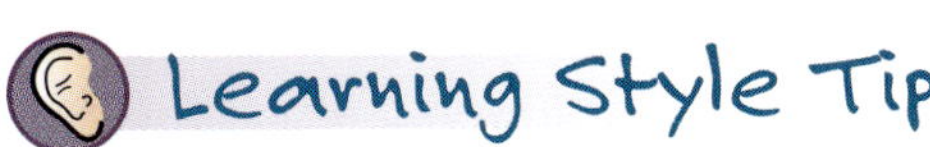

Ask the instructor to explain or describe terms you find confusing.

STOP HERE.
Select the Pathology Terms Flash Cards for Chapter 8 and run through them at least three times before you continue.

Common Diagnostic Tests and Procedures

Arterial blood gases (ABG): Measurement of O_2 and CO_2 levels and acid-base balance (pH balance) in arterial blood

Bronchoscopy: Visual examination of the airways of the lungs (see Fig. 8-14)

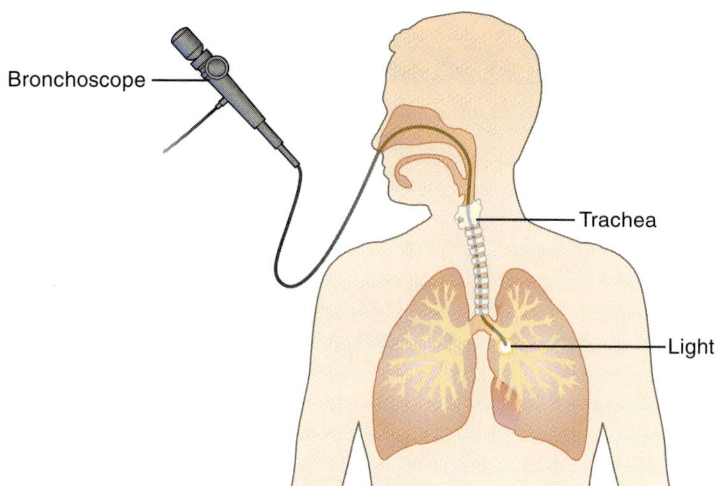

FIGURE 8-14 **Bronchoscopy**

Chest x-ray (CXR): Radiological picture of the lungs

Mantoux test: Intradermal injection of tuberculin purified protein derivative (PPD) just beneath the surface of the skin to identify whether the patient has been exposed to tuberculosis

Metered dose inhaler (MDI): Handheld device used to deliver medication to the patient's lower airways (see Figs. 8-15 and 8-16)

Nebulizer: Device that produces a fine spray or mist to deliver medication to a patient's deep airways (see Fig. 8-17)

Pleurodesis: Infusion of a sterile, irritating substance into the pleural space, causing the pleural linings to fuse to one another by developing scar tissue

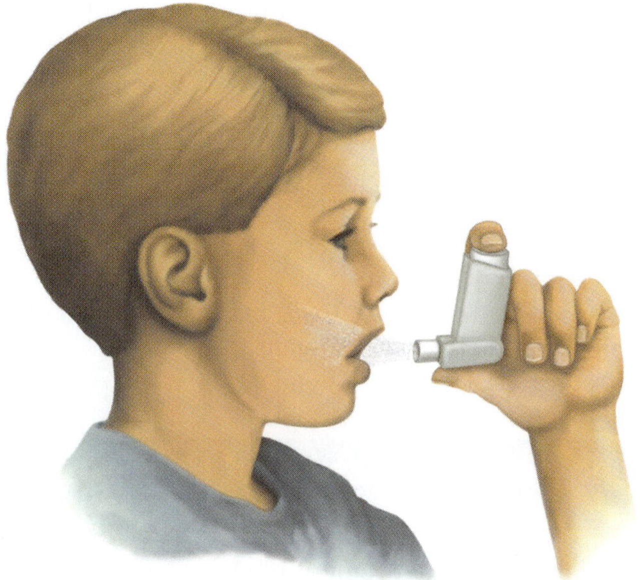

FIGURE 8-15 **Metered dose inhaler** (From Eagle, S, et al.: *The Professional Medical Assistant.* F.A. Davis, Philadelphia, 2009, p. 514; with permission)

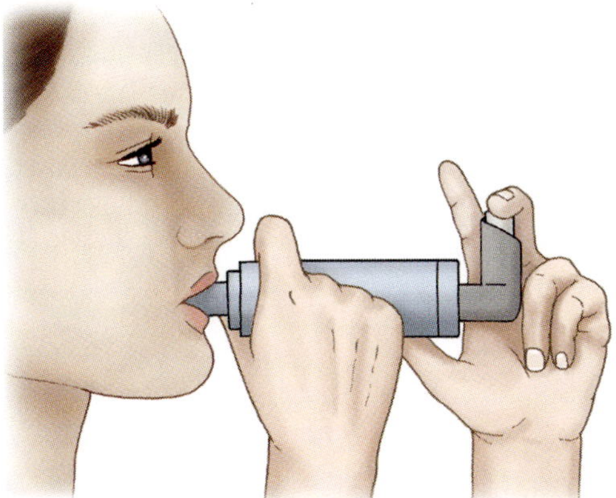

FIGURE 8-16 **Metered dose inhaler with spacer** (From Eagle, S, et al.: *The Professional Medical Assistant.* F.A. Davis, Philadelphia, 2009, p. 514; with permission)

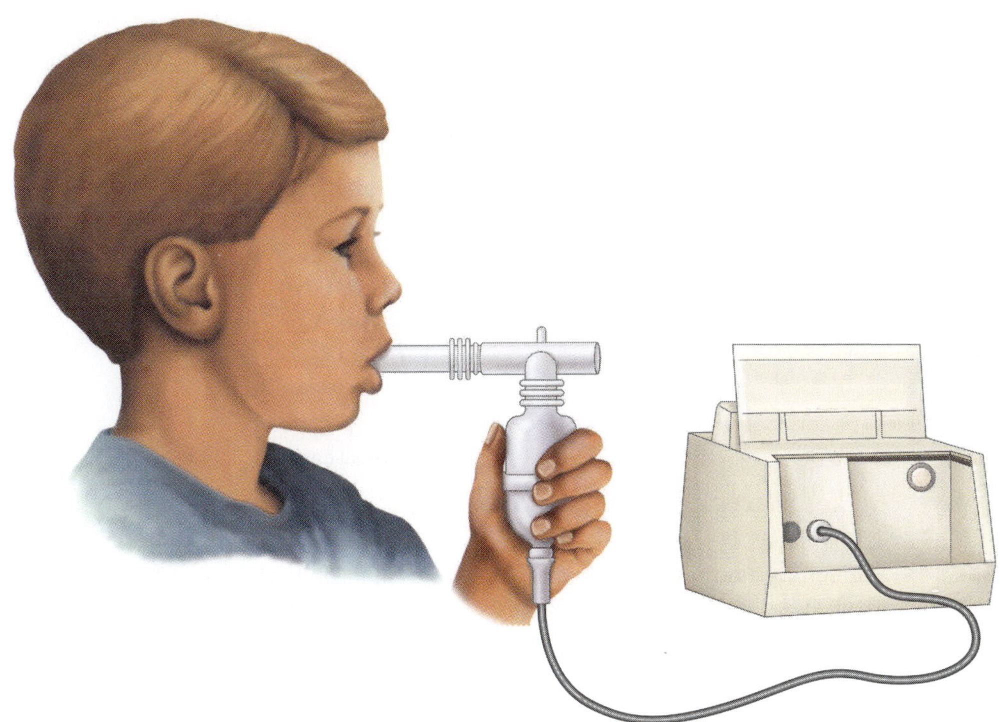

FIGURE 8-17 **Nebulizer** (From Eagle, S, et al.: *The Professional Medical Assistant.* F.A. Davis, Philadelphia, 2009, p. 514; with permission)

Postural drainage: Placement of the patient in various positions that facilitate drainage of secretions from the lungs, often done along with chest physiotherapy (CPT)

Pulmonary angiography: Radiographic examination of pulmonary circulation after injection of a contrast dye

Pulmonary function tests (PFTs): Group of tests that provide information regarding lung capacity; sometimes called *spirometry* (see Fig. 8-18)

Pulse oximetry: Indirect measurement of arterial-blood O_2 saturation level, also known as the Spo_2; the normal level in a person with healthy lungs is 97% to 99%

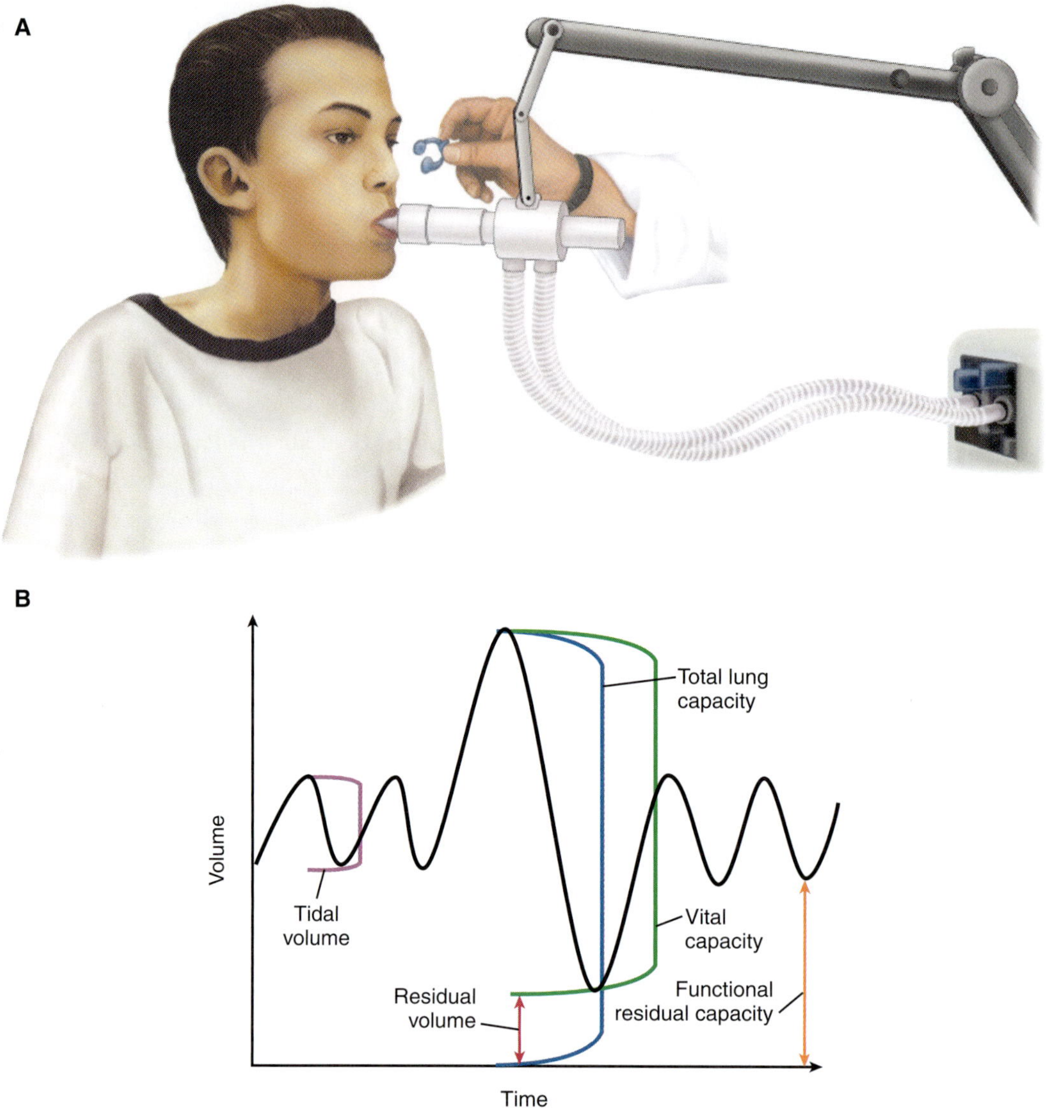

FIGURE 8-18 **Pulmonary function test** (From Eagle, S, et al.: *The Professional Medical Assistant.* F.A. Davis, Philadelphia, 2009, pp. 510–511; with permission)

Sputum analysis: Examination of mucus or fluid coughed up from the lungs

Thoracentesis: Surgical puncture of the chest wall to remove fluid from the interpleural space; also called *pleurocentesis* (see Fig. 8-19)

Vital capacity (VC): Measurement of the volume of air that can be exhaled after maximum inspiration

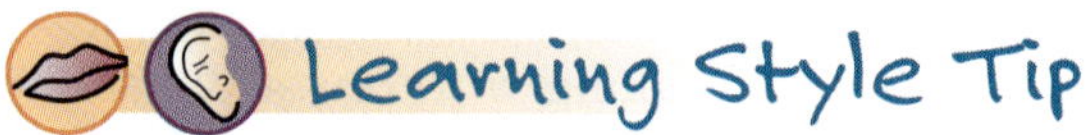

Sing content you need to remember, like these tests and procedures, to simple, easily remembered tunes such as "Happy Birthday to You" or nursery-school songs.

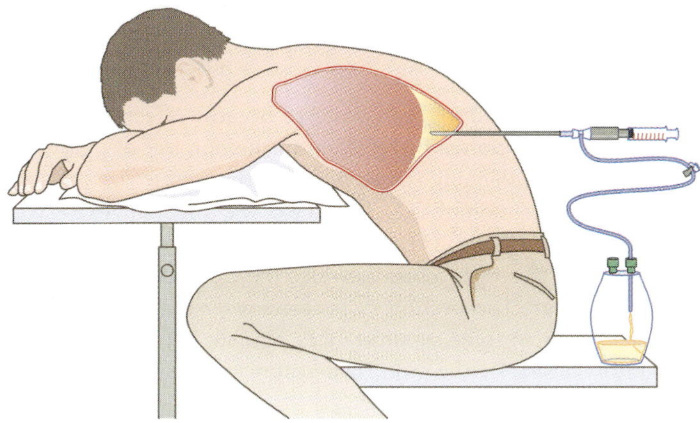

FIGURE 8-19 **Thoracentesis**

Case Study

Read the case study and answer the questions that follow. Most of the terms are included in this chapter. Refer to the glossaries (Appendixes B and D) or to your medical dictionary for the other terms.

Chronic Obstructive Pulmonary Disease (COPD)

Helga Freidericks is a 57-year-old woman who came to the urgent-care clinic today complaining of SOB. On admission, her respirations were labored, at a rate of 32 breaths per minute. Her Spo_2 was just 84%, and her VC was decreased. She appeared anxious and stated that she "[couldn't] get enough air." Her lungs had bilateral expiratory wheezes throughout, scattered rhonchi, and bibasilar crackles. She had a frequent cough, productive of thick green sputum.

Stat ABGs were drawn. She was put on O_2 at 2 liters per minute (lpm) per nasal cannula (NC) and given a nebulizer Tx. A sputum specimen was collected and sent for culture and sensitivity (C&S). She was given IV doses of a broad-spectrum antibiotic and a steroid drug. Upon review of her ABGs, it was determined that she was in a state of mild respiratory acidosis.

A short time later, Mrs. Freidericks's respiratory rate had decreased to 20 breaths per minute, her O_2 saturation was 91%, and she stated that she was breathing "much better." She was then transferred to the hospital for further monitoring and continued therapy.

COPD is a chronic disease with several different causes. The most common cause is smoking, because the lungs are subjected to chronic irritation by an inhaled substance 20 to 40 times each day for years on end. As a result, the lung tissue becomes inflamed. Under normal circumstances, body tissue is able to repair itself; however, in the case of smoking, chronic, repeated exposure to the irritants prevents healing and results in chronic inflammation. Over time, permanent damage occurs. The walls of the delicate alveoli lose their elasticity and become permanently distended, like balloons that have been inflated too many times. The walls of the alveoli also erode and thicken and, as a result, function less effectively. They begin to trap air rather than allowing it to escape during expiration. This decreases the amount of oxygen-rich air that can be inhaled in each breath.

As chronic air-trapping occurs, the chest changes dimension, becoming more barrel-like. The lungs also flatten on the bottom, robbing the diaphragm (an important respiratory muscle) of its effectiveness. Cilia in the airway normally move debris upward to be coughed out, but in COPD, cilia become clogged with tar and thus lose their effectiveness. As a result of these physical changes, the COPD patient may begin to experience some or all of the following symptoms:

Orthopnea: The need to remain upright in order to breathe effectively. Physicians often quantify the severity of orthopnea by referring to the number of pillows the patient must recline against while sleeping (three-pillow orthopnea).

Hypercapnia: The chronic retention of CO_2. In some cases, this changes the way the person's body determines when to breathe. The person may begin to function according to the "hypoxic drive," and feel the urge to breathe when the O_2 level gets too low instead of when the CO_2 level gets too high. This becomes a problem when the person requires supplemental O_2. Too much O_2 can, in some circumstances, actually knock out the urge to breathe, leading to respiratory arrest. Furthermore, hypercapnia can lead to symptoms of mental cloudiness and lethargy.

Chronic hypoxia: A chronic lack of oxygen. As gas exchange becomes less effective, breathing becomes more and more difficult. Eventually the person becomes dependent on oxygen. Yet in the last stages of the disease, supplemental O_2 is of little help. The person feels chronically short of breath and becomes severely dyspneic with the slightest exertion.

Case Study Questions

1. Upon admission, Mrs. Freidericks was:
- **a.** Having chest pain
- **b.** Very short of breath
- **c.** Breathing very slowly
- **d.** Unconscious

2. Mrs. Freidericks had:
- **a.** An increased ability to breathe in
- **b.** A decreased ability to breathe in
- **c.** An increased ability to breathe out
- **d.** A decreased ability to breathe out

3. Mrs. Freidericks's oxygen saturation level was:
- **a.** Checked by pulse oximetry
- **b.** At a normal level
- **c.** Not known
- **d.** Higher than normal

4. When listening to Mrs. Freidericks's lungs, the physician heard:
- **a.** Normal sounds of air movement
- **b.** A somewhat musical sound caused by partial airway obstruction
- **c.** A high-pitched upper airway sound that indicates airway obstruction
- **d.** A barking, "seal-like" cough

5. Which of the following statements is true?
- **a.** Mrs. Freidericks normally slept lying down
- **b.** It is always safe to give high levels of oxygen to people with COPD
- **c.** Supplemental O_2 effectively relieves dyspnea in the final stages of COPD
- **d.** Mrs. Freidericks's chest cavity had most likely become more barrel-like in shape

6. Which of the following statements is correct?
   a. Cilia continue to work effectively in people with late-stage COPD
   b. The only cause of COPD is smoking
   c. People with COPD tend to develop chronic O_2 retention
   d. Arterial blood was immediately drawn to analyze the levels of O_2, CO_2, and pH
7. In a person with healthy lungs, the drive to breathe is stimulated by:
   a. Low levels of oxygen
   b. A drop in blood pH caused by high levels of CO_2
   c. A feeling of emptiness in the lungs
   d. A neurological message sent from the brain to the lungs

Answers to Case Study Questions

1. b
2. d
3. a
4. b
5. d
6. d
7. b

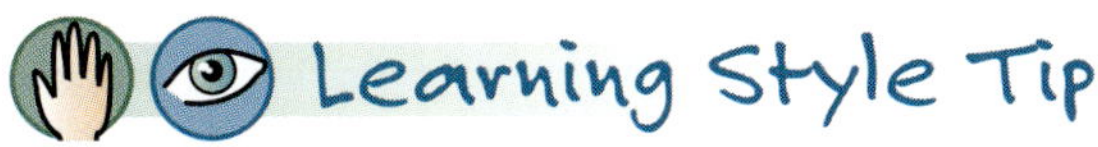

Take a few minutes to visit at least one of the websites listed below. Locate information about one of the pathologic conditions mentioned in this chapter and read the description and definition.

Flashpoint
Sadly, COPD is a very common disorder in the United States.

Websites

Please go to the F.A. Davis website at http://davisplus.fadavis.com/eagle/medterm to view resource websites for the respiratory system.

Practice Exercises

Deciphering Terms

Write the correct meaning of these medical terms. Check Appendix G for the correct answers.

Exercise 2

1. laryngeal ____________________
2. pleuralgia ____________________
3. pneumatic ____________________

4. pneumonia ________________

5. pulmonary ________________

6. sinusotomy ________________

7. thoracentesis ________________

8. tonsillectomy ________________

9. dyspnea ________________

10. hemothorax ________________

11. pneumothorax ________________

12. eupnea ________________

13. orthopnea ________________

14. rhinitis ________________

15. tracheostomy ________________

Fill in the Blanks

Fill in the blanks below using Tables 8-2 and 8-3. Check Appendix G for the correct answers.

Exercise 3

1. The combining form that means *coal* or *coal dust* is ________________.

2. A group of diseases in which the alveoli are destroyed, resulting in chronic SOB, is ________________ ________________ ________________ ________________.

3. The name of the disease in the previous question is abbreviated ________________.

4. To determine whether he has been exposed to tuberculosis, Victor has a skin test done and is injected with ________________ ________________ ________________.

5. Julio has ________________, which causes him to experience SOB and wheezing in response to various triggers.

6. A medical term for the common cold is ________________.

7. A collection of air in the intrapleural space is known as

_______________________.

8. Edelia is allergic to bees. If she gets stung, she has a severe reaction known as anaphylaxis, and has great difficulty breathing. In addition to sounding wheezy, she develops a high-pitched upper-airway sound caused by obstruction of her airways. This is known as _______________________.

9. When a physician gives a _______________________ order, the expectation is that the order will be carried out immediately.

10. Sophie has a cold. This might also be called an _______________________

_______________________ _______________________.

11. The abbreviation for the name of the condition referred to in the previous question is _______________________.

12. Acute inflammation of the nasal mucosa is known as

_______________________.

13. A skill often taught in first-aid courses that helps restore a victim's breathing and circulation is known as _______________________

_______________________.

14. The name of the procedure referred to in the previous question is abbreviated _______________________.

15. Miguel was treated in the urgent-care clinic for epistaxis. This is more commonly known as a _______________________.

16. A fungus found in soil contaminated with bird droppings can cause a systemic respiratory disease known as _______________________.

17. Albert has temporarily lost his voice because his larynx is inflamed. He has

_______________________.

18. Vaishali has suffered from a partial collapse of the alveoli and tiny airways in her lungs. She has _______________________.

19. Vita is currently suffering from chronic retention of CO_2 and has symptoms of mental cloudiness and lethargy. She has _______________________.

20. Missy has had a T&A. Therefore she has had her _______________________ and _______________________ removed.

Multiple Choice

Select the one best answer to the following multiple-choice questions. Check Appendix G for the correct answers.

Exercise 4

1. A coarse, gurgling sound heard with a stethoscope in the lungs, caused by secretions in the air passages, is known as:
   a. Crackles
   b. Stridor
   c. Rhonchi
   d. Wheezes

2. Which of the following tests provides an indirect measure of the level of arterial-blood oxygen saturation?
   a. Pulse oximetry
   b. Arterial blood gases
   c. Vital capacity
   d. Sputum analysis

3. Which of the following terms indicates a condition of low oxygen?
   a. Apnea
   b. Hypoxia
   c. Dyspnea
   d. Eupnea

4. Which of the following terms means *mouthlike opening in the trachea?*
   a. Tracheotomy
   b. Tracheotome
   c. Tracheostomy
   d. Tracheoscopy

5. Mrs. Yachinich sleeps propped up on three pillows so she can breathe better. Which of the following terms best describes this condition?
   a. Orthopnea
   b. Aerophagia
   c. Pneumonplegia
   d. Aerophobia

Word Building

*Using **only** the word parts in the lists provided, create medical terms with the indicated meanings. Check Appendix G for the correct answers.*

Exercise 5

Prefixes	**Combining Forms**	**Suffixes**
dys-	aer/o	-al
eu-	bronch/o	-ary
peri-	carcin/o	-dynia
tachy-	chondr/o	-gen
	cutane/o	-genesis
	epiglott/o	-genic
	laryng/o	-ic
	muc/o	-itis
	myc/o	-malacia
	nas/o	-oid
	pharyng/o	-oma
	pleur/o	-osis
	pneum/o	-ous
	pulmon/o	-pathy
	sinus/o	-pexy
	thorac/o	-pnea
	tonsill/o	-scopy
	trache/o	-stomy
		-tomy

1. pertaining to the bronchus and lung ______________
2. tumor of cartilage ______________
3. creation of air ______________
4. pertaining to mucus and skin ______________
5. visual examination of the trachea and bronchus ______________
6. disease of the tonsil ______________
7. softening of the trachea ______________
8. inflammation of the epiglottis ______________
9. pertaining to bad, painful, or difficult breathing ______________
10. good or normal breathing ______________
11. cutting into or incision of the thorax ______________
12. fungal infection of the pharynx ______________

13. pain of the pleura ________________

14. surgical fixation of the lung ________________

15. pertaining to the lung ________________

16. resembling the sinus ________________

17. mouthlike opening in the trachea ________________

18. pertaining to causing cancer ________________

19. rapid breathing ________________

20. visual examination of the larynx ________________

True or False

Decide whether the following statements are true or false. Check Appendix G for the correct answers.

Exercise 6

1. True False A collection of air in the intrapleural space is known as **hemothorax**.

2. True False The abbreviation **PND** stands for *pulmonary neoplastic disease.*

3. True False A collection of pus in the pleural cavity is known as **empyema**.

4. True False The abbreviation **ARDS** stands for *adult research drug study.*

5. True False A nosebleed is known as **epistaxis**.

6. True False The abbreviation **ABG** stands for *arterial blood gases.*

7. True False Another name for the common cold is **croup**.

8. True False The abbreviation **VC** stands for *very critical.*

9. True False A collection of fluid in the intrapleural space is known as **pleural effusion**.

10. True False An abnormal "Rice Krispies" sound heard in the lungs with a stethoscope is known as **crackles**.

Deciphering Terms

Write the correct meaning of these medical terms. Check Appendix G for the correct answers.

Exercise 7

1. aerophagia ______________________________
2. alveolar ______________________________
3. pharyngeal ______________________________
4. spirogram ______________________________
5. nasal ______________________________
6. anthracoid ______________________________
7. mucolysis ______________________________
8. phonophobia ______________________________
9. carcinoma ______________________________
10. oxygenic ______________________________

Multiple Choice

Select the one best answer to each of the following multiple-choice questions. Check Appendix G for the correct answers.

Exercise 8

1. Which of the following terms is matched with the correct definition?
   a. Coni/o: dust
   b. Chondr/o: cancer
   c. Phon/o: pharynx
   d. Spir/o: sinus
2. All of the following terms are matched with the correct definition **except**:
   a. Chondr/o: cartilage
   b. Rhin/o: nose
   c. Stomat/o: mouth
   d. Pleur/o: lung

3. Which of the following is related to coryza?
   a. CWP
   b. URI
   c. AFB
   d. ARDS

4. Which of the following indicates a surgical procedure?
   a. T&A
   b. PPD
   c. PND
   d. MDI

5. All of the following terms refer to abnormal breathing sounds **except**:
   a. Crackles
   b. Stridor
   c. Orthopnea
   d. Wheeze

6. Which of the following terms indicates the surgical removal of a portion of a lung?
   a. Pneumothorax
   b. Pleurocentesis
   c. Pneumotomy
   d. Lobectomy

7. If the surgeon places a drainage tube through the patient's chest cavity, it may be described as:
   a. Pneumatic
   b. Transthoracic
   c. Intrapleural
   d. Lobar

8. What word describes the normal location of pleural fluid?
   a. Interpleural
   b. Endotracheal
   c. Contralateral
   d. Circumoral

9. A patient who is breathing normally may be described as demonstrating:
   a. Hyperpnea
   b. Eupnea
   c. Dyspnea
   d. Tachypnea

10. An artificial opening in the neck which helps a person breathe is:
   a. A tracheostomy
   b. A tracheotomy
   c. A tracheotome
   d. None of these

11. Which of the following indicates a sense of urgency?
   a. CPAP
   b. CXR
   c. Stat
   d. R

12. Which of the following conditions involves infection?
   a. Hemothorax
   b. Empyema
   c. Epistaxis
   d. Hemoptysis

13. Which of the following involves abnormal tissue growths?
   a. Nasal polyps
   b. Histoplasmosis
   c. Pneumoconiosis
   d. Silicosis

14. Which of the following conditions involves birds?
   a. Histoplasmosis
   b. Asbestosis
   c. Coryza
   d. Legionellosis

15. Which of the following might cause a person to belch more frequently?

   a. Bronchitis
   b. Aerophagia
   c. Coniosis
   d. Dysphonia

16. Which of the following conditions is most likely to block a patient's airway?

   a. Pneumonitis
   b. Anthracosis
   c. Epiglottedema
   d. Thoracentesis

17. All of the following involve the collection of a substance within the intrapleural space **except**:

   a. Hemothorax
   b. Pneumothorax
   c. Empyema
   d. Emphysema

18. Which of the following tests is most useful when the physician needs to evaluate circulation within the patient's lungs?

   a. Spirometry
   b. Pulmonary angiography
   c. Vital capacity
   d. Thoracentesis

19. Which of the following is done to cause the two membranes covering the lungs to adhere to one another?

   a. Oximetry
   b. Pleurodesis
   c. Angiography
   d. Sputum analysis

20. Which of the following is most useful in measuring the patient's lung capacity?

   a. Pulmonary function tests
   b. Mantoux test
   c. Postural drainage
   d. Sputum analysis

DIGESTIVE SYSTEM

9

Structure and Function

The digestive system is also known as the **gastrointestinal (GI) system**. It includes all the structures of the alimentary canal, from the mouth to the anus, and the **accessory organs**. The digestive system has two key functions: **digestion** and **excretion**. The organs of the GI system break down food into usable nutrients and then eliminate bulk waste in the form of feces.

We will discuss the parts of the GI system in the same order in which food passes through it. As we do this, please refer to Figure 9-1 to see the various parts of the GI system.

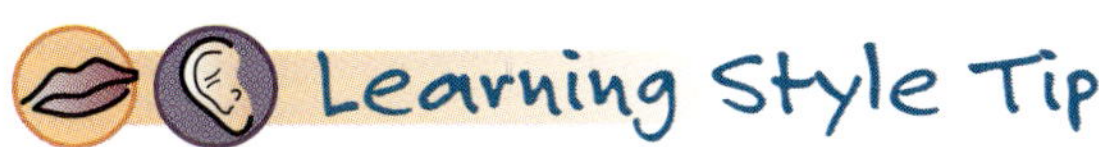

"Teach" your study buddy or a friend about the GI tract. Beginning with the mouth and working all the way to the anus, list each anatomical part and its associated combining form. Then briefly describe its function.

The first or most proximal part of the digestive system is the mouth, also known as the **oral** or **buccal cavity**. When we take a bite of food (**ingestion**) and begin chewing it, our tongue and teeth aid in the process of **mechanical digestion** as food is broken down into smaller and smaller parts. It is mixed and moistened with **saliva**, which is secreted from three different **salivary glands**. Saliva also contains ptyalin, a chemical that starts to break down starches. The tongue helps to form chewed food into a **bolus**, which is a rounded mass ready to be swallowed. The tongue also allows us to taste food, which can make eating an enjoyable process. Specific areas on the tongue identify sweet, salty, sour, and bitter flavors (see Fig. 9-2).

The **uvula** is a small, finger-shaped portion of soft tissue that hangs from the upper back of the mouth. It prevents food from entering the nasal cavity as we eat. At the back of the mouth is the **pharynx**, which is shaped something like a funnel. The pharynx extends down to the esophagus, which is a long, tubelike structure that passes through the diaphragm and connects to the stomach. At the top of the esophagus is a small flap of cartilage covered with epithelial tissue; it is called the **epiglottis**. It acts to cover the trachea when we swallow, to keep food from entering the respiratory tract. Muscles in the esophageal wall contract intermittently and involuntarily, causing **peristalsis**, which moves the food bolus downward into the stomach. At the lower end of the esophagus is a muscular opening called the **lower esophageal sphincter (LES)**, also called the **cardiac sphincter** because of its location near the heart. The LES acts as a doorway between the esophagus and the stomach, and prevents backflow of gastric secretions.

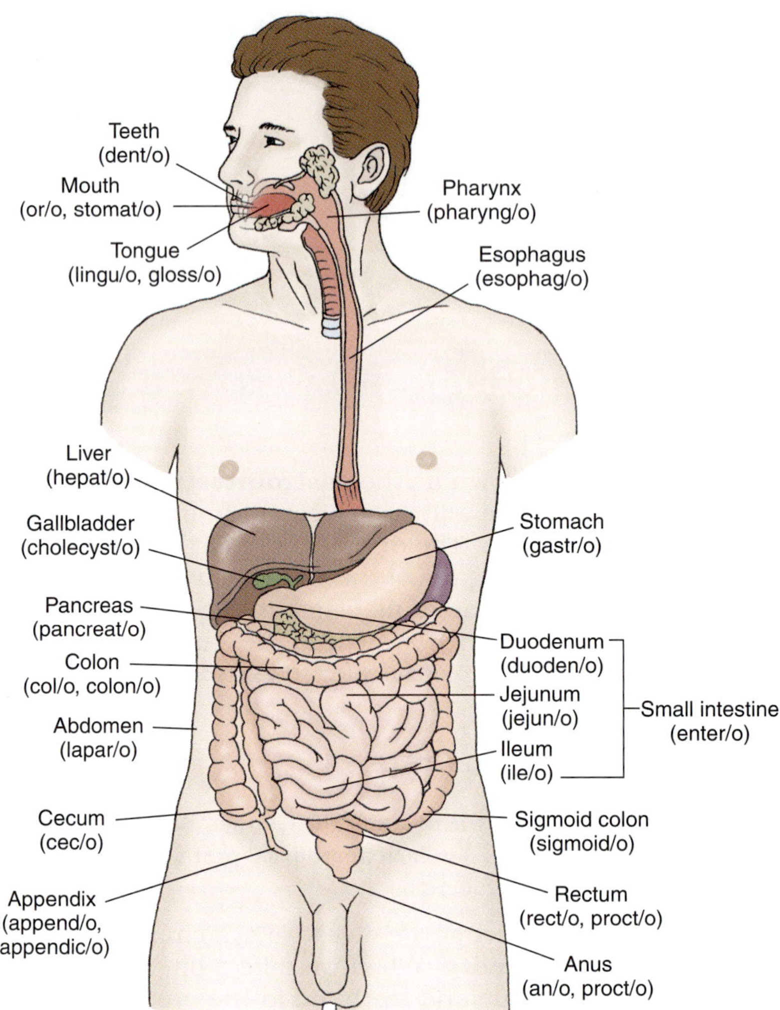

FIGURE 9-1 **The gastrointestinal system**

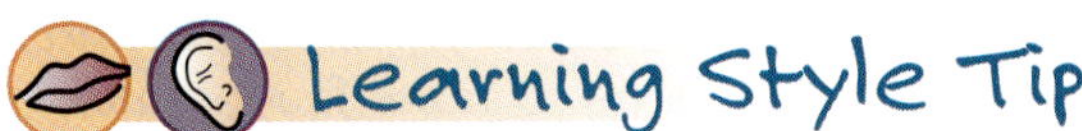

Orally summarize the content and key points after reading each paragraph in this chapter before moving on to the next one.

Flashpoint

Peristalsis is the rhythmic muscular contractions that propel food along the GI tract.

The abdominal cavity holds the stomach, small intestine, large intestine, rectum, and anus. This cavity is lined with a membrane called the **peritoneum**. The inside of the stomach is lined with folds called rugae that allow the stomach to expand when we eat a large amount of food. The stomach is composed of three major areas: the **fundus** (upper portion), **body** (middle portion), and **pylorus** (lower portion). The fundus and body of the stomach are mostly holding areas for food; the majority of activity occurs in the pylorus. Gastric secretions—which are very acidic, with an average pH of 1.7—act on food to continue breaking it down and preparing it for **absorption** within the intestines. At this point the food is now referred to as **chyme**, a more liquid material made up of chewed food, saliva, and digestive juices. The **pyloric sphincter** lies between the pylorus and the small intestine. It acts as the stomach's exit way and releases chyme into the small intestine a little at a time.

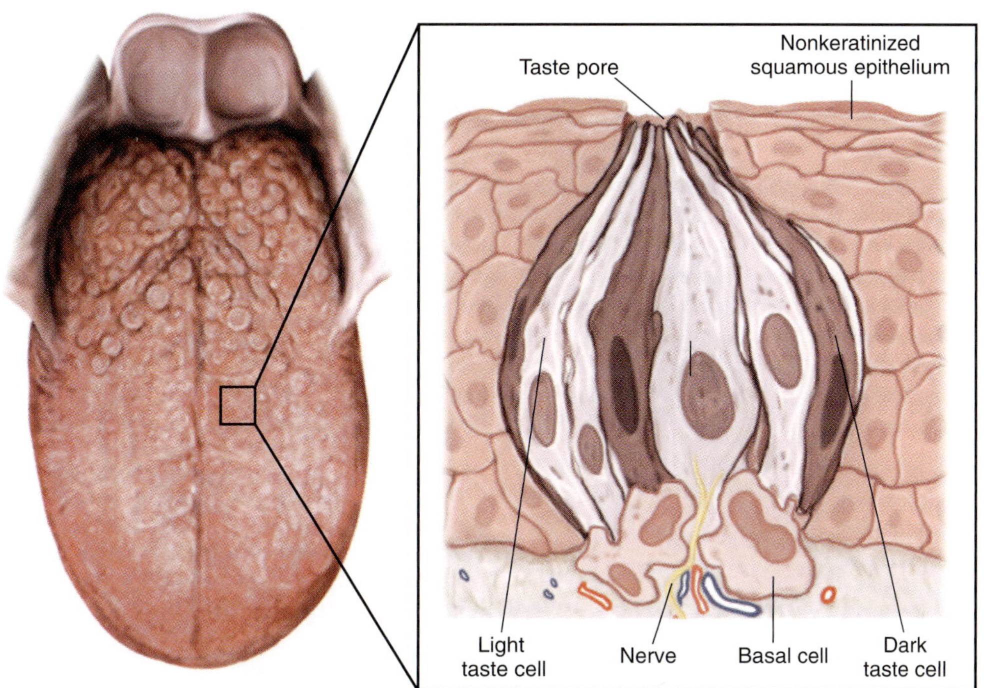

FIGURE 9-2 **The tongue with structure of a taste bud and taste cells** (From Eagle, S, et al.: *The Professional Medical Assistant.* F.A. Davis, Philadelphia, 2009, p. 540; with permission)

The real digestive action occurs within the small intestine. It is small only in the sense that it is relatively narrow; however, it is really quite long, around 20 feet in the average adult. Peristalsis continues to move the contents through the three parts of the small intestine: the **duodenum** (upper portion), **jejunum** (middle portion), and **ileum** (end portion). Here the majority of digestion is completed and most nutrients are absorbed.

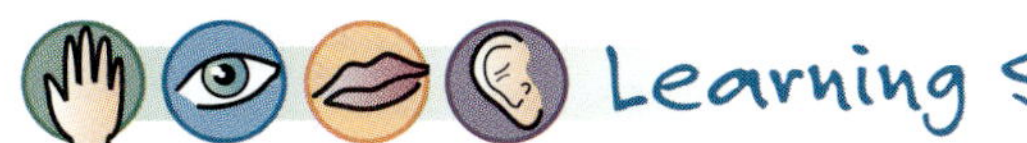

Learning Style Tip

Use inexpensive watercolor paints or colorful markers and sheets of paper to draw the GI system. Label anatomical parts and include the associated combining forms. Speak aloud as you do this.

> **Flashpoint**
> It's easy to remember the correct order of the three parts of the small intestine. Just think of the phrase "**D**on't **j**uggle **i**ce."

The small intestine is lined with **villi**, which are tiny, fingerlike structures surrounded by capillaries and lymphatic vessels. Villi increase the surface area of the small intestine, allowing greater absorption of water and nutrients into the blood (see Fig. 9-3). All other products of digestion pass from the small intestine to the large intestine through the **ileocecal valve**. The first part of the large intestine is the cecum. A small tubelike structure called the **appendix** hangs from the cecum in the right lower quadrant (RLQ) of the abdomen. For years, the appendix was thought to serve no useful function. More recently, however, some experts have suggested that it may serve as a storage facility for normal bacteria, which may serve to repopulate the GI tract in the event that normal bacteria are eliminated (as can happen with certain GI disorders). Unfortunately, the appendix occasionally becomes clogged with intestinal matter and then becomes inflamed and infected. This condition is known as ***appendicitis***. When this occurs, the appendix must be surgically removed by a procedure known as an **appendectomy**.

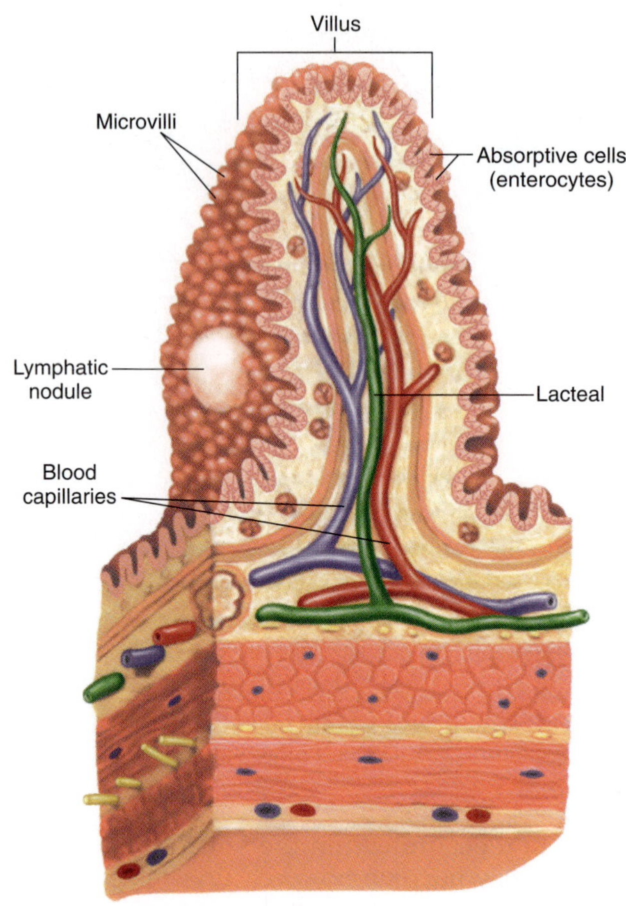

FIGURE 9-3 **Villi of the small intestine** (From Eagle, S, et al.: *The Professional Medical Assistant.* F.A. Davis, Philadelphia, 2009, p. 540; with permission)

The portion of the colon that progresses upward from the cecum is known as the **ascending colon**. It takes a 90-degree turn as it nears the top of the abdomen, beneath the liver, and becomes the **transverse colon** as it passes horizontally across the uppermost part of the abdomen. It again takes a 90-degree turn, beneath the spleen, and heads down along the left side of the abdomen. This portion is known as the **descending colon**. The key function of the colon is absorption of water as the remaining waste products become less liquid and more solid. The colon then takes a gentle turn inward and becomes the **sigmoid colon**, which descends into the **rectum** and finally the **anus**. It is here that intestinal contents, now a waste product known as **feces**, are excreted in the process of **defecation**.

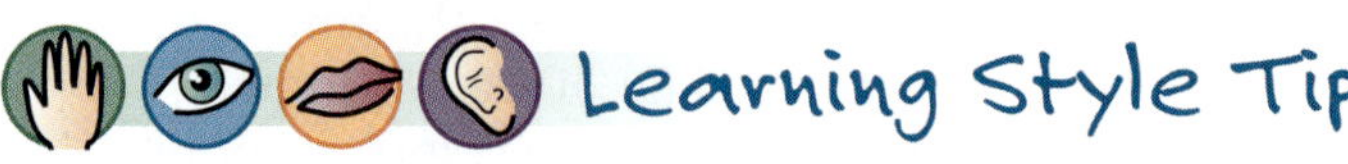

Trace the GI system in Figure 9-1 with the tip of your finger as you recite the associated combining forms that go with each anatomical part.

Flashpoint
The liver, gallbladder, and pancreas are considered *accessory organs* of the digestive system because they assist with its many functions.

Accessory Organs

There are several accessory organs that contribute to the process of digestion. These include the liver, gallbladder, and pancreas.

The **liver**, located in the upper right and center of the abdominal cavity, is the largest glandular organ of the body. Its many functions include digestion, absorption, storage, and excretion.

The **gallbladder** is a sac, 3 to 4 inches long, on the inner surface of the liver. It is connected to the common bile duct, which also connects to the duodenum. The gallbladder acts as a storage pouch for bile. When we eat fatty food, the gallbladder responds by secreting bile into the duodenum through the common bile duct to break down those fats for digestion and absorption.

The **pancreas** is a long, somewhat flat organ that lies just behind and beneath the stomach. Within the pancreas are specialized cells called the **islets of Langerhans**. The two types include alpha and beta cells. The pancreas is connected to the hepatic duct via the pancreatic duct at the duodenum. The pancreas secretes several substances into the duodenum through the pancreatic duct and directly into the bloodstream through capillaries of the islets of Langerhans. One of these substances is sodium bicarbonate, which acts to neutralize stomach acid. Others include the pancreatic enzymes trypsin, which breaks down proteins; lipase, which breaks down fats; and amylase, which breaks down carbohydrates.

The cells of the islets of Langerhans also secrete the hormones insulin and glucagon, which work together to regulate blood glucose levels. **Insulin** is secreted by beta cells in response to rising blood glucose levels after we eat. It binds to glucose molecules in the blood, which then allows them to diffuse into the tissues and enter cells to provide energy. **Glucagon** is secreted by alpha cells in response to dropping blood glucose levels. It stimulates the liver to release a storage form of glucose called **glycogen**. The liver then converts the glycogen into glucose for energy.

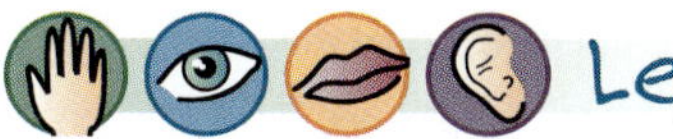

Learning Style Tip

On a whiteboard, poster board, or even your notepaper, create a flowchart with boxes, circles, and arrows that illustrates the following:

- the production of insulin and glucagon by the pancreas and their effects on the liver
- the liver's response (glycogen release)
- the effect these substances have on the blood and body cells

When your flowchart is complete, verbally explain it to your study buddy.

Flashpoint

To remember which comes first, glucagon or glycogen, remember this rhyme: "Glucagon acts upon." Glucagon acts upon the liver to convert glycogen to glucose.

Combining Forms

Table 9-1 contains combining forms that pertain to the digestive system, examples of medical terms that utilize the combining forms, and a pronunciation guide. Read aloud to yourself as you move from left to right across the table. Be sure to use the pronunciation guide so you can learn to say the terms correctly.

STOP HERE.

Select the Combining Form Flash Cards for Chapter 9 and run through them at least three times before you continue.

TABLE 9-1

COMBINING FORMS

Combining Form	Meaning	Example (Pronunciation)	Meaning of New Term
an/o	anus	anal (Ā-năl)	pertaining to the anus
append/o	appendix	appendectomy (ăp-ĕn-DĔK-tŏ-mē)	excision or surgical removal of the appendix
appendic/o		appendicitis (ă-pĕn-dĭ-SĪ-tĭs)	inflammation of the appendix
bil/i	bile	biliary (BĬL-ē-ăr-ē)	pertaining to bile
bucc/o	cheek	buccogingival (bŭk-kō-JĬN-jĭ-văl)	pertaining to the cheek and gums
cec/o	cecum	cecectomy (sē-SĔK-tō-mē)	excision or surgical removal of the cecum
cheil/o	lip	cheiloplasty (KĪ-lō-plăs-tē)	surgical repair of the lip
labi/o		labiodental (lā-bē-ō-DĔN-tăl)	pertaining to the lips and teeth
chol/e	bile, gall	cholecystitis (kō-lē-sis-TĪ-tus)	inflammation of the gallbladder
cholangi/o	bile duct	cholangiography (kō-lăn-jē-ŎG-ră-fē)	process of recording a bile duct
cholecyst/o	gallbladder	cholecystectomy (kō-lē-sĭs-TĔK-tŏ-mē)	excision or surgical removal of the gallbladder
choledoch/o	common bile duct	choledocholith (kō-LĔD-ŏ-kō-lĭth)	stone of the common bile duct
col/o	colon	colectomy (kō-LĔK-tŏ-mē)	excision or surgical removal of the colon
colon/o		colonoscopy (kō-lŏn-ŎS-kō-pē)	visual examination of the colon
dent/o	teeth	dental (DĔN-tăl)	pertaining to the teeth
odont/o		odontodynia (ō-dŏn-tō-DĬN-ē-ă)	pain of the teeth
duoden/o	duodenum	duodenoscopy (dū-ŏd-ĕ-NŎS-kō-pē)	visual examination of the duodenum
enter/o	small intestine	enteritis (ĕn-tĕr-Ī-tĭs)	inflammation of the small intestine
esophag/o	esophagus	esophagostenosis (ē-sŏf-ă-gō-stĕn-Ō-sĭs)	narrowing or stricture of the esophagus
gastr/o	stomach	gastralgia (găs-TRĂL-jē-ă)	pain of the stomach
gingiv/o	gums	gingivoglossitis (jĭn-jĭ-vō-glŏs-SĪ-tĭs)	inflammation of the gums and tongue

TABLE 9-1

COMBINING FORMS—cont'd

Combining Form	Meaning	Example (Pronunciation)	Meaning of New Term
gloss/o	tongue	glossokinesthetic (glŏs-ō-kĭn-ĕs-THĔT-ĭk)	pertaining to tongue movement
lingu/o		sublingual (sŭb-LĬNG-gwăl)	pertaining to beneath the tongue
hepat/o	liver	hepatitis (hĕp-ă-TĪ-tĭs)	inflammation of the liver
ile/o	ileum	ileotomy (ĭl-ē-ŎT-ō-mē)	cutting into or incision of the ileum
jejun/o	jejunum	jejunostomy (jē-jū-NŎS-tō-mē)	mouthlike opening into the jejunum
lapar/o	abdomen, abdominal wall	laparoscope (LĂP-ă-rō-skōp)	instrument used to view inside the abdominal cavity
or/o	mouth	oral (ŌR-ăl)	pertaining to the mouth
pancreat/o	pancreas	pancreatitis (păn-krē-ă-TĪ-tĭs)	inflammation of the pancreas
pept/o	digestion	peptic (PĔP-tĭk)	pertaining to digestion
phag/o	eating, swallowing	phagocyte (FĂG-ō-sīt)	eating cell (specialized type of WBC)
pharyng/o	pharynx	pharyngeal (făr-ĬN-jē-ăl)	pertaining to the pharynx
proct/o	rectum, anus	proctoscopy (prŏk-TŎS-kō-pē)	visual examination of the rectum and/or anus
pylor/o	pylorus	pylorostenosis (pī-lōr-ō-stĕn-Ō-sĭs)	narrowing or stricture of the pylorus
rect/o	rectum	rectal (RĔK-tăl)	pertaining to the rectum
sial/o	saliva, salivary gland	sialolithiasis (sī-ă-lō-lĭ-THĪ-ă-sĭs)	pathological condition of a salivary-gland stone
sigmoid/o	sigmoid colon	sigmoidoscope (sĭg-MOY-dō-skōp)	viewing instrument for the sigmoid colon
steat/o	fat	steatorrhea (stē-ă-tō-RĒ-ă)	flow or discharge of fat (fatty stool)
stomat/o	mouth, mouthlike opening	stomatitis (stō-mă-TĪ-tĭs)	inflammation of the mouth

Practice Exercises

Fill in the Blanks

Fill in the blanks below using Table 9-1. Check Appendix G for the correct answers.

Exercise 1

1. pertaining to the rectum ______
2. instrument used to view inside the abdominal cavity ______
3. pertaining to the mouth ______
4. pertaining to the pharynx ______
5. pertaining to the anus ______
6. narrowing or stricture of the esophagus ______
7. excision or surgical removal of the gallbladder ______
8. inflammation of the small intestine ______
9. mouthlike opening into the jejunum ______
10. visual examination of the colon ______
11. pertaining to beneath the tongue ______
12. visual examination of the duodenum ______
13. cutting into or incision of the ileum ______
14. inflammation of the mouth ______
15. pain of the stomach ______
16. inflammation of the liver ______
17. excision or surgical removal of the appendix ______
18. inflammation of the appendix ______
19. visual examination of the rectum and anus ______
20. excision or surgical removal of the colon ______

21. pertaining to the teeth ______________________________

22. spasm of the tongue ______________________________

23. inflammation of the pancreas ______________________________

24. viewing instrument for the sigmoid colon ______________________________

25. flow or discharge of fat (fatty stool) ______________________________

26. pertaining to bile ______________________________

27. pertaining to the cheeks and gums ______________________________

28. stone of the common bile duct ______________________________

29. pathological condition of a salivary-gland stone ______________________________

30. excision or surgical removal of the cecum ______________________________

31. process of recording a bile duct ______________________________

32. surgical repair of the lip ______________________________

33. pain of the teeth ______________________________

34. pertaining to the lips and teeth ______________________________

35. inflammation of the gums and tongue ______________________________

36. pertaining to tongue movement ______________________________

37. inflammation of the gallbladder ______________________________

38. pertaining to digestion ______________________________

39. eating cell (specialized type of WBC) ______________________________

40. narrowing or stricture of the pylorus ______________________________

41. **Fill in the blanks in Figure 9-4 with the appropriate anatomical terms and combining forms.**

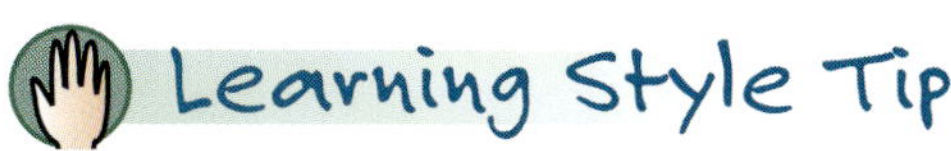

Take short (5-to-10-minute) but frequent (every 30 to 60 minutes) study breaks and move your body. Exercise wakes you up, helps you feel better, and increases your ability to learn.

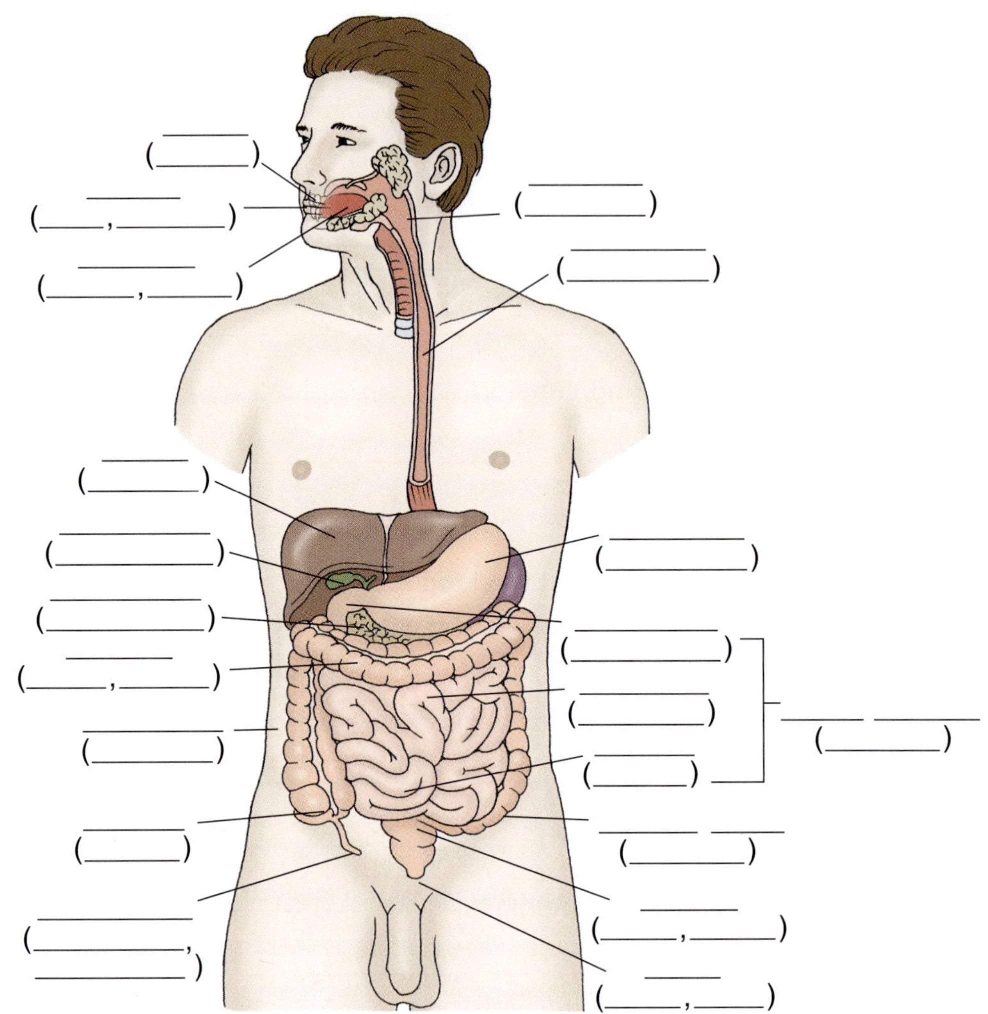

FIGURE 9-4 **Gastrointestinal system with blanks**

Abbreviations

Table 9-2 lists some of the most common abbreviations related to the GI system, as well as others often used in medical documentation.

Flashpoint

The abbreviations *NG, PO,* and *PR* are often used to indicate a specific route for medication administration.

STOP HERE.

Select the Abbreviation Flash Cards for Chapter 9 and run through them at least three times before you continue.

TABLE 9-2
ABBREVIATIONS

Abd	abdomen	IBS	irritable bowel syndrome
BM	bowel movement	LFT	liver function test
BR	bedrest	N&V	nausea and vomiting
BRP	bathroom privileges	NG	nasogastric
c̄	with	NPO	nothing by mouth
CA	cancer	PO	by mouth
c/o	complain(ed/ing/s/t) of	PR	per rectum
Dx	diagnosis	PUD	peptic ulcer disease
EGD	esophagogastroduodenoscopy	q	every
ERCP	endoscopic retrograde cholangiopancreatography	qd	every day
GERD	gastroesophageal reflux disease	s̄	without
GI	gastrointestinal	SBO	small bowel obstruction
h, hr	hour	UGI	upper GI x-ray
IBD	inflammatory bowel disease	VS	vital signs

Pathology Terms

Table 9-3 includes terms that relate to diseases or abnormalities of the digestive system. Use the pronunciation guide and say the terms out loud as you read them. This will help you get in the habit of saying the terms properly.

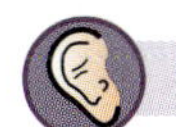

Learning Style Tip

Record your instructor's lectures, with his or her permission, and then play them back when you study. This allows you to hear information again later, as often as you wish. This technique will be especially helpful when your instructor discusses pathology terms and medical procedures.

STOP HERE.
Select the Pathology Terms Flash Cards for Chapter 9 and run through them at least three times before you continue.

TABLE 9-3
PATHOLOGY TERMS

achalasia (ăk-ă-LĀ-zē-ă)	dilation and expansion of the lower esophagus, due to pressure from food accumulation (see Fig. 9-5)

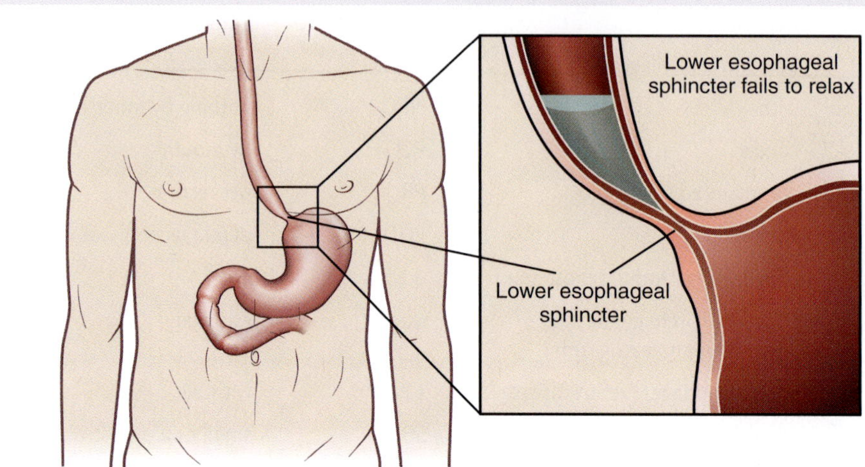

FIGURE 9-5 Achalasia

anorexia nervosa (ăn-ō-RĔK-sē-ă nĕr-VŌ-să)	physical and psychiatric disorder that involves a combination of an intense fear of weight gain, distorted body image, and self-imposed starvation (see Fig. 9-6)

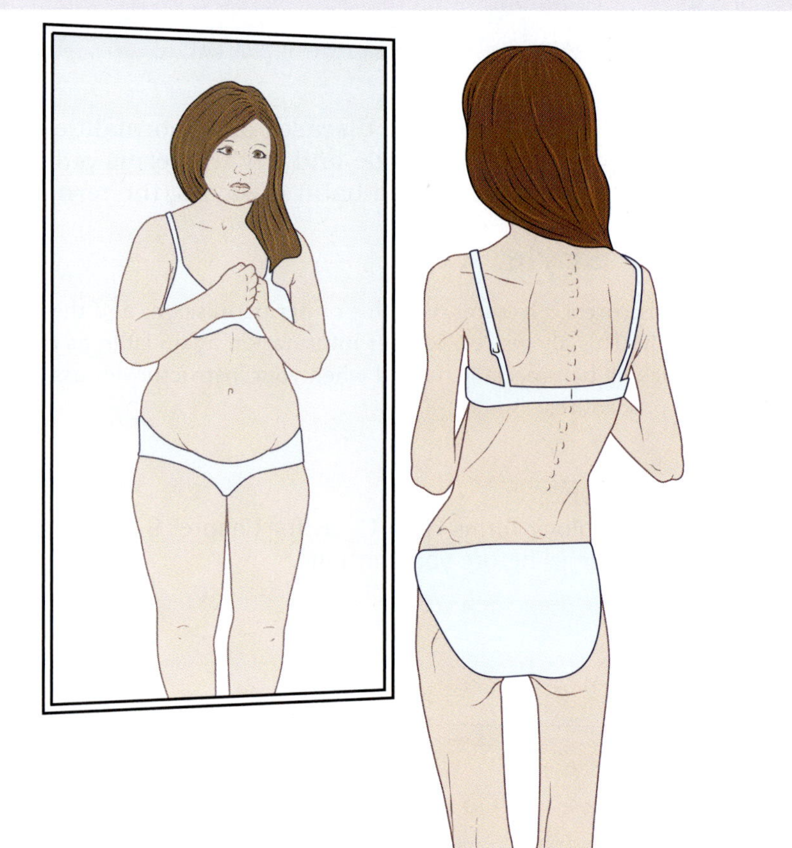

FIGURE 9-6 Anorexia

TABLE 9-3
PATHOLOGY TERMS—cont'd

Term	Definition
appendicitis (ă-pĕn-dĭ-SĪ-tĭs)	inflammation of the appendix (see Fig. 9-7)

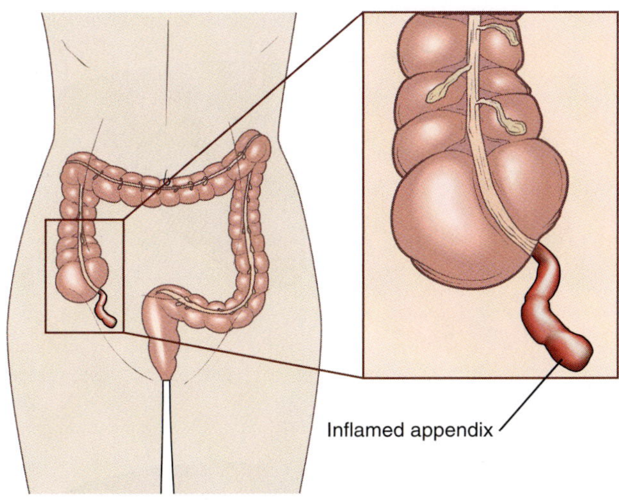

FIGURE 9-7 **Appendicitis**

Term	Definition
ascites (ă-SĪ-tēz)	accumulation of serous fluid in the peritoneal (abdominal) cavity
bowel obstruction (BOW-ĕl ŏb-STRŬK-shŭn)	partial or complete blockage of the small or large intestine; common causes include volvulus, intussusception, tumors, and adhesions (scar tissue)
bulimia nervosa (bū-LĒ-mē-ă nĕr-VŌ-să)	physical and psychiatric disorder that involves a combination of obsessively eating huge quantities of food with purging behaviors
***Campylobacter* infection** (kăm-pĭ-lō-BĂK-tĕr ĭn-FĔK-shŭn)	infection with *Campylobacter* organisms via contaminated food or water, resulting in intestinal illness
celiac disease (SĒ-lē-ăk dĭ-ZĒZ)	disorder in which the lining of the small intestine is damaged due to dietary factors, resulting in impaired nutrient absorption
cholecystitis (kō-lē-sĭs-TĪ-tĭs)	inflammation of the gallbladder, usually secondary to the presence of gallstones
cholelithiasis (kō-lă-lĭ-THĪ-ăs-ĭs)	condition in which gallstones are present in the gallbladder, liver, or biliary ducts (see Fig. 9-8)

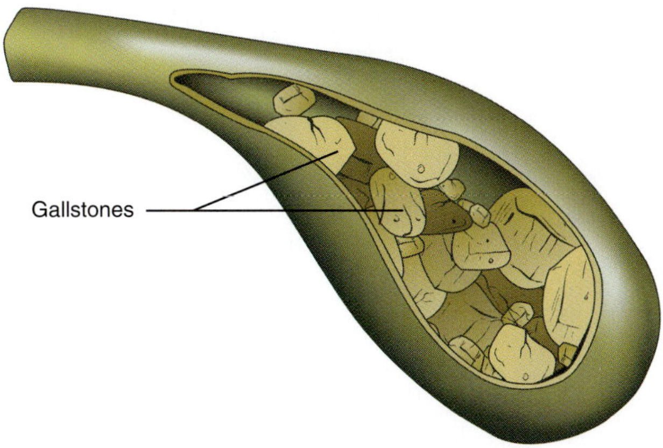

FIGURE 9-8 **Cholelithiasis**

Continued

TABLE 9-3
PATHOLOGY TERMS—cont'd

cirrhosis (sĭ-RŌ-sĭs)	chronic liver disease characterized by scarring and loss of normal structure (see Fig. 9-9)

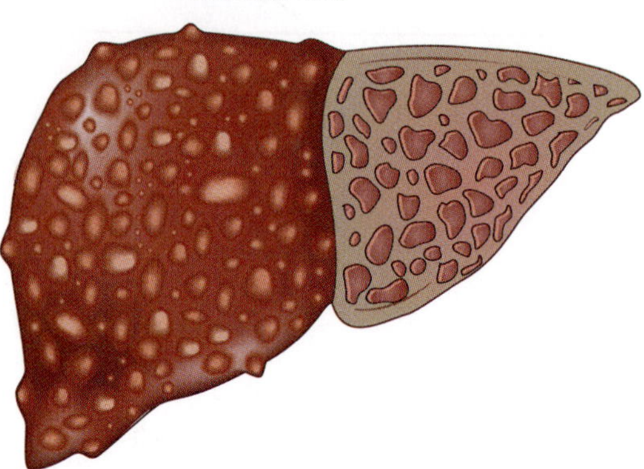

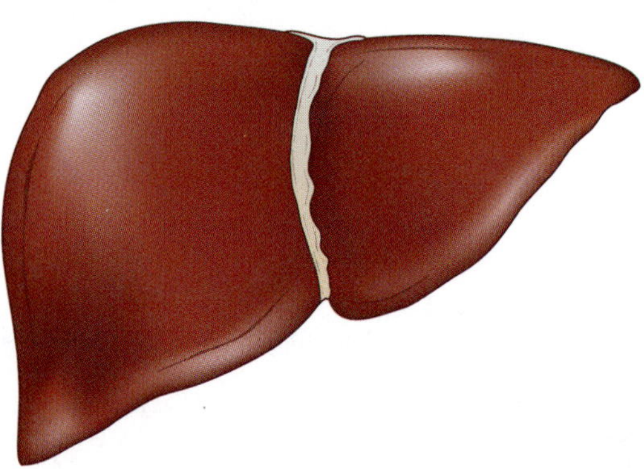

FIGURE 9-9 **Cirrhosis**

Crohn disease (krōn dĭ-ZĒZ)	disorder involving inflammation and edema deep into the layers of the lining of any part of the GI tract
diverticulitis (dī-vĕr-tĭk-ū-LĪ-tĭs)	inflammation of one or more diverticula (tiny pouches in the intestinal wall) (see Fig. 9-10)

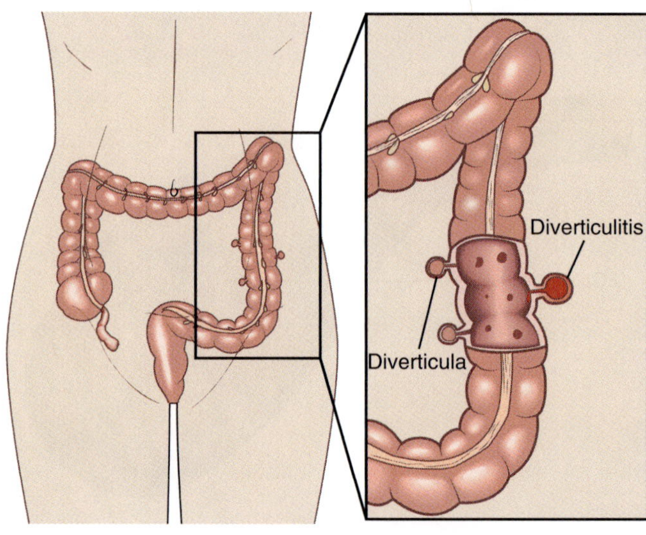

FIGURE 9-10 **Diverticulitis**

TABLE 9-3
PATHOLOGY TERMS—cont'd

diverticulosis (dī-vĕr-tĭk-ū-LŌ-sĭs)	condition in which diverticula form in the intestinal wall due to increased pressure (see Fig. 9-11)

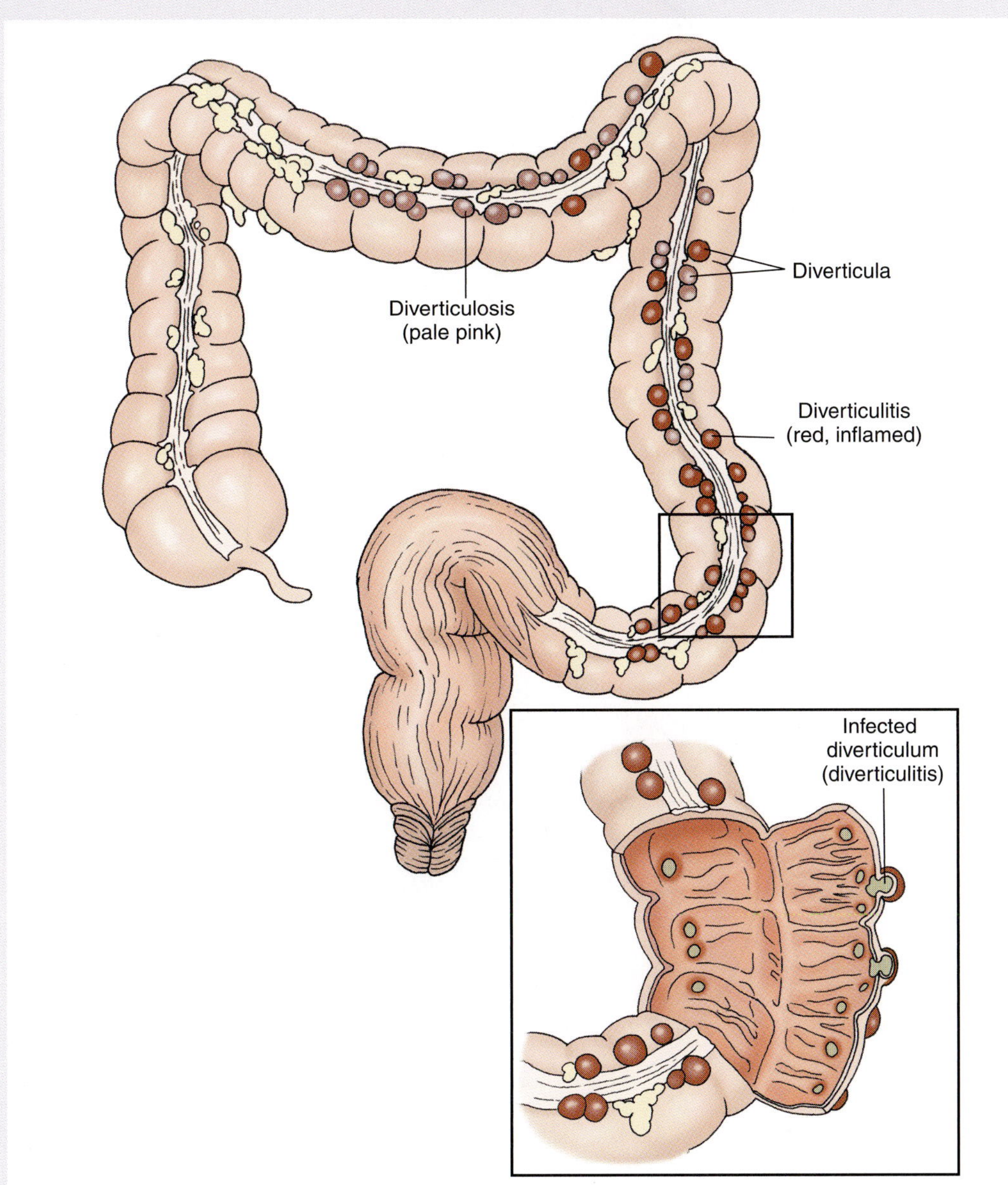

FIGURE 9-11 **Diverticulosis**

***E. coli* O157:H7 infection** (ē KŌ-lī ĭn-FĔK-shŭn)	dangerous strain of *Escherichia coli* that produces toxins that can severely damage the intestinal lining, resulting in bloody diarrhea
emesis (ĔM-ĕ-sĭs)	vomiting
esophageal varices (ē-sŏf-ă-JĒ-ăl VĂR-ĭ-sēz)	varicose veins of the distal end of the esophagus (see Fig. 9-12)

Continued

TABLE 9-3

PATHOLOGY TERMS—cont'd

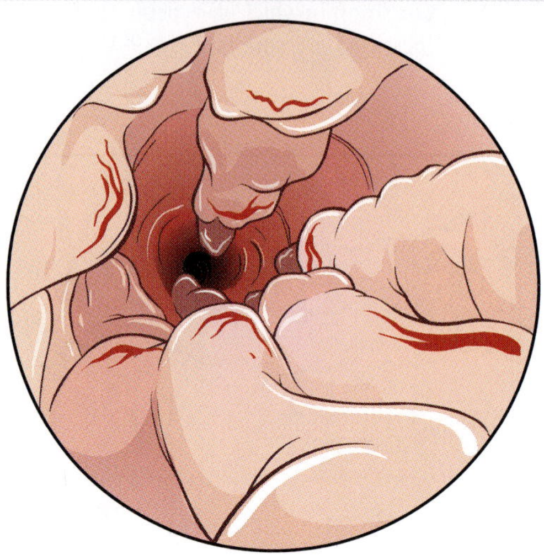

FIGURE 9-12 **Esophageal varices**

esophagitis (ē-sŏf-ă-JĪ-tĭs)	inflammation of the lower esophageal lining (see Fig. 9-13)

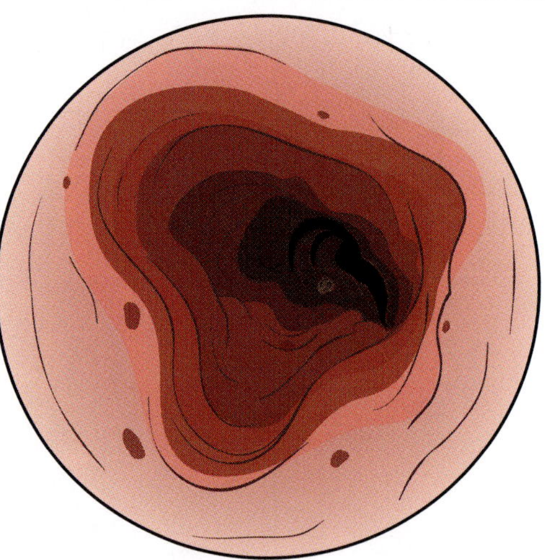

FIGURE 9-13 **Esophagitis**

food poisoning (fūd POY-zun-ing)	common term for a number of illnesses caused by eating food contaminated with bacterial or toxic organisms; sometimes called *dysentery*
gastritis (găs-TRĪ-tĭs)	inflammation of the stomach's mucosal lining (see Fig. 9-14)

TABLE 9-3
PATHOLOGY TERMS—cont'd

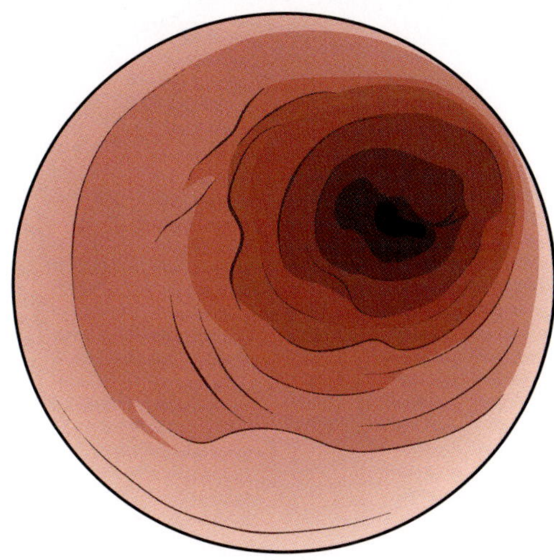

FIGURE 9-14 **Gastritis**

gastroenteritis (găs-trō-ĕn-tĕr-Ī-tĭs)	inflammation of the stomach and intestines; often referred to as the *stomach flu* (although influenza is not the cause)
gastroesophageal reflux disease (GERD) (găs-trō-ĕ-sŏf-ă-JĒ-ăl RĒ-flŭks dĭ-ZĒZ)	backflow of acidic gastric contents into the esophagus, causing esophagitis (see Fig. 9-15)

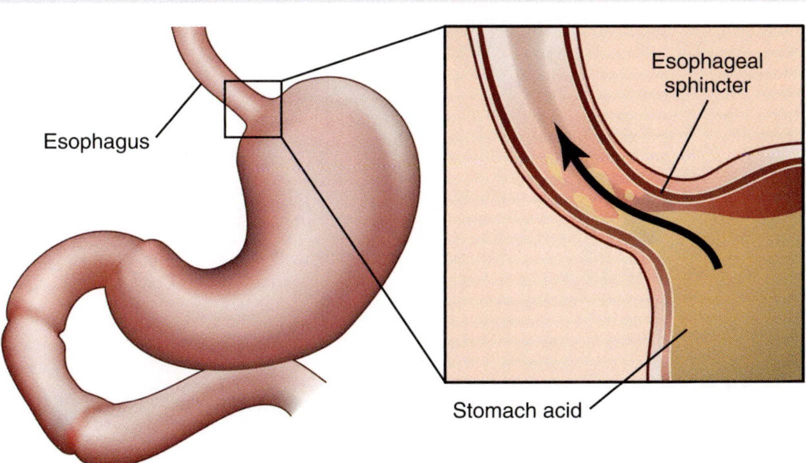

FIGURE 9-15 **Gastroesophageal reflux disease**

hemorrhoids (HĔM-ō-roydz)	internal or external varicose veins of the anal area (see Fig. 9-16)

Continued

TABLE 9-3
PATHOLOGY TERMS—cont'd

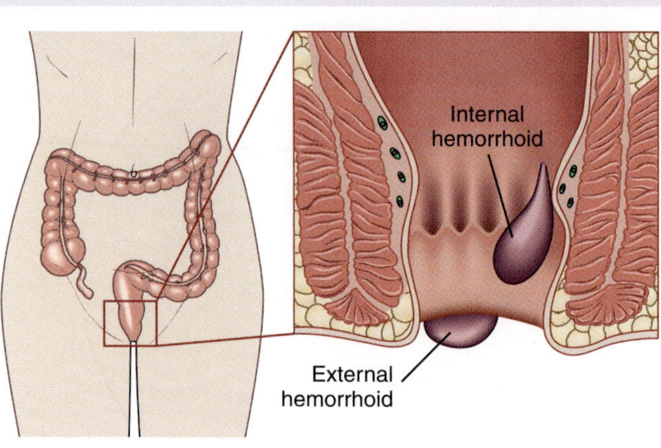

FIGURE 9-16 **Hemorrhoids**

hepatitis (hĕp-ă-TĪ-tĭs)	chronic inflammation of the liver, caused by one of several viruses (types A, B, C, D, or E)
hernia (HĔR-nē-ă)	protrusion of a structure through the wall that normally contains it (see Fig. 9-17)

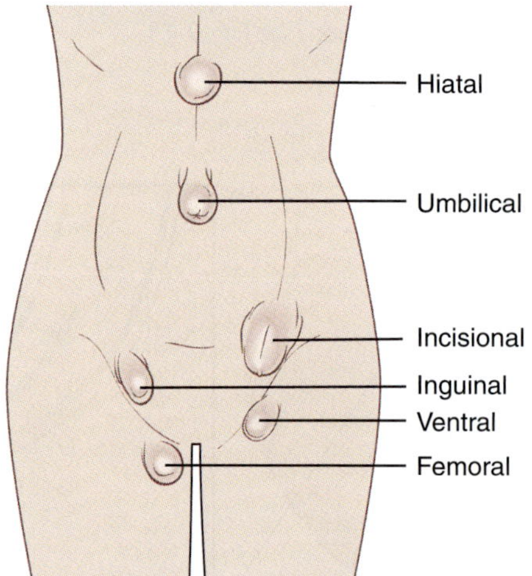

FIGURE 9-17 **Abdominal hernia**

hiatal hernia (hī-Ā-tăl HĔR-nē-ă)	protrusion of a portion of the stomach through the diaphragm into the chest cavity; also called *hiatus hernia* (see Fig. 9-18)

TABLE 9-3
PATHOLOGY TERMS—cont'd

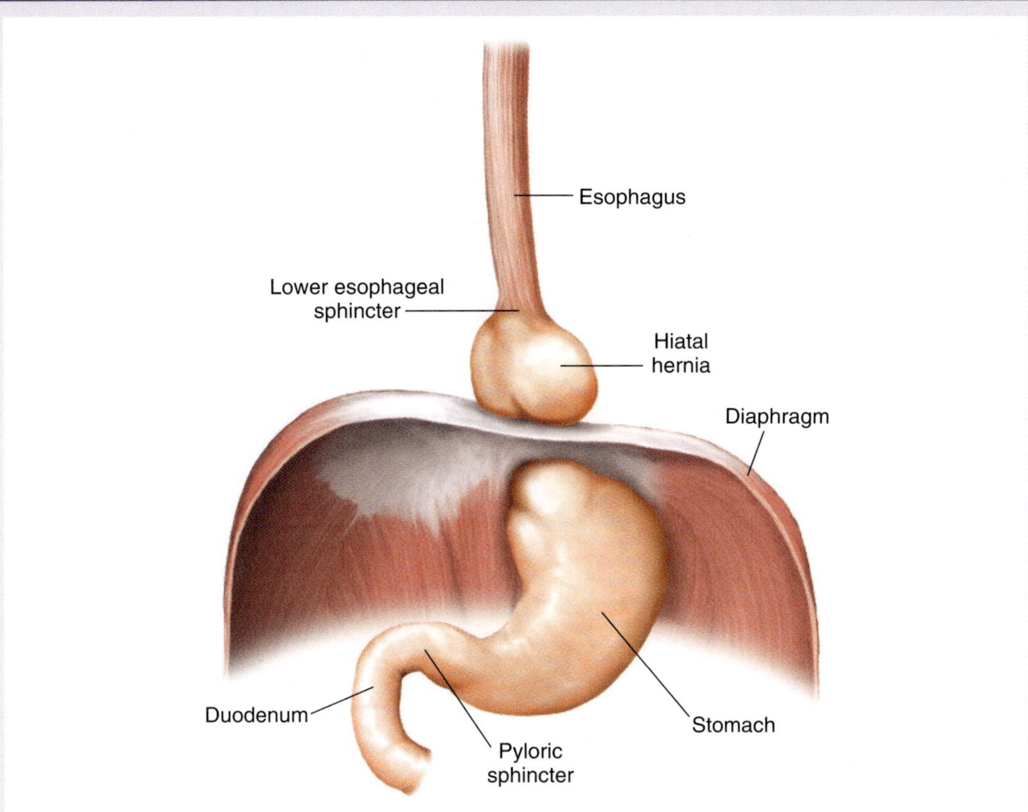

FIGURE 9-18 **Hiatal hernia** (From Eagle, S, et al.: *The Professional Medical Assistant.* F.A. Davis, Philadelphia, 2009, p. 545; with permission)

intussusception (ĭn-tŭ-sŭ-SĔP-shŭn)	slipping or telescoping of a portion of the bowel into itself (see Fig. 9-19)

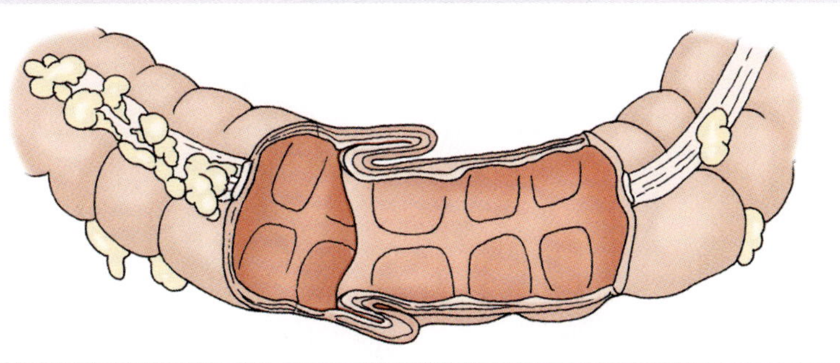

FIGURE 9-19 **Intussusception**

Continued

TABLE 9-3

PATHOLOGY TERMS—cont'd	
irritable bowel syndrome (ĬR-ĭt-ă-bul BOW-ĕl SĬN-drōm)	chronic condition characterized by alternating episodes of constipation and diarrhea
jaundice (JAWN-dĭs)	condition marked by yellow staining of body tissues and fluids as a result of excessive levels of bilirubin in the blood
malabsorption syndrome (măl-ăb-SŌRP-shŭn SĬN-drōm)	inadequate absorption of nutrients from the intestinal tract, especially the small intestine
malnutrition (măl-nū-TRĬ-shŭn)	nutritional deficiency due to inadequate intake or absorption of protein, vitamins, minerals, or other vital nutrients
oral herpes (OR-ăl HĔR-pēz)	vesicular eruption in or on the mouth caused by herpesvirus; also called *herpes labialis* or *cold sore* (see Fig. 9-20) 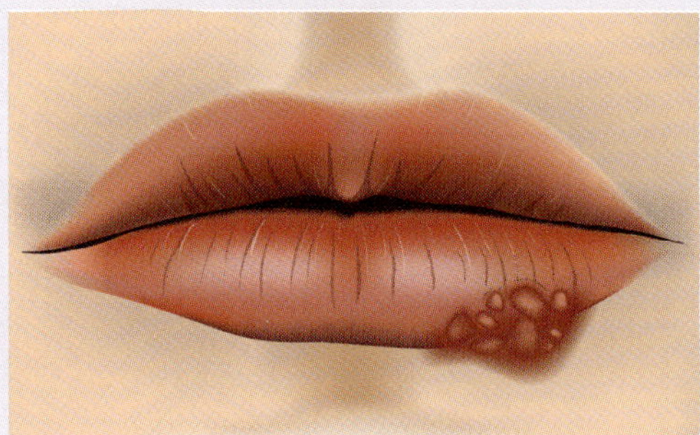 FIGURE 9-20 **Oral herpes lesion**
oral thrush (OR-ăl thrŭsh)	infection of the skin or mucous membrane with any species of candida, but mainly *Candida albicans;* also called *candidiasis* (see Fig. 9-21) 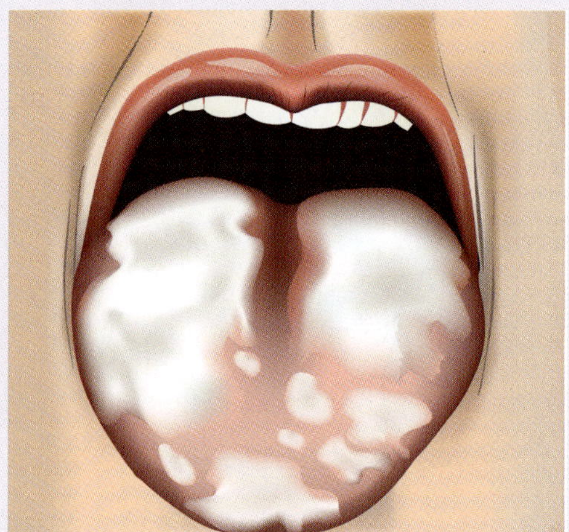 FIGURE 9-21 **Oral thrush**
pancreatitis (păn-krē-ă-TĪ-tĭs)	acute or chronic inflammation of the pancreas
peptic ulcer (PĔP-tĭk ŬL-sĕr)	inflamed lesion in the gastric or duodenal lining (see Fig. 9-22)

TABLE 9-3
PATHOLOGY TERMS—cont'd

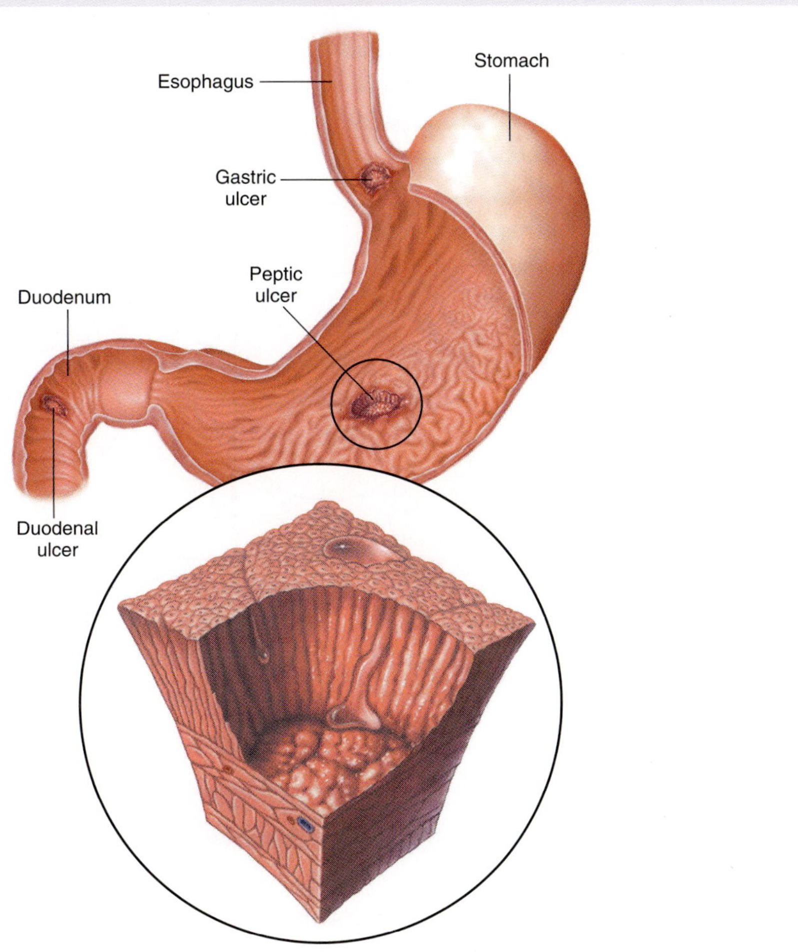

FIGURE 9-22 **Peptic ulcer** (From Eagle, S, et al.: *The Professional Medical Assistant.* F.A. Davis, Philadelphia, 2009, p. 547; with permission)

peritonitis (pĕr-ĭ-tō-NĪ-tĭs)	inflammation of the organs and structures within the peritoneal cavity
pseudomembranous enterocolitis (soo-dō-MĔM-brān-ŭs ĕn-tĕr-ō-kō-LĪ-tĭs)	inflammatory condition of both small and large bowels that results in severe watery diarrhea; also commonly called *C. diff. colitis*
salmonellosis (săl-mō-nĕ-LŌ-sĭs)	intestinal infection caused by various types of salmonella organisms
short bowel syndrome (shōrt BOW-ĕl SĬN-drōm)	malabsorption and malnutrition disorder created by the loss of a significant portion of functioning bowel
small bowel obstruction (SBO) (smăl BOW-ĕl ŏb-STRŬK-shŭn)	blockage of normal passage of intestinal contents
ulcerative colitis (ŬL-sĕr-ā-tĭv kō-LĪ-tĭs)	chronic inflammatory disease of the lining of the colon and rectum marked by up to 20 liquid, bloody stools per day
volvulus (VŎL-vū-lŭs)	twisting of the bowel upon itself, causing obstruction (see Fig. 9-23)

Continued

TABLE 9-3
PATHOLOGY TERMS—cont'd

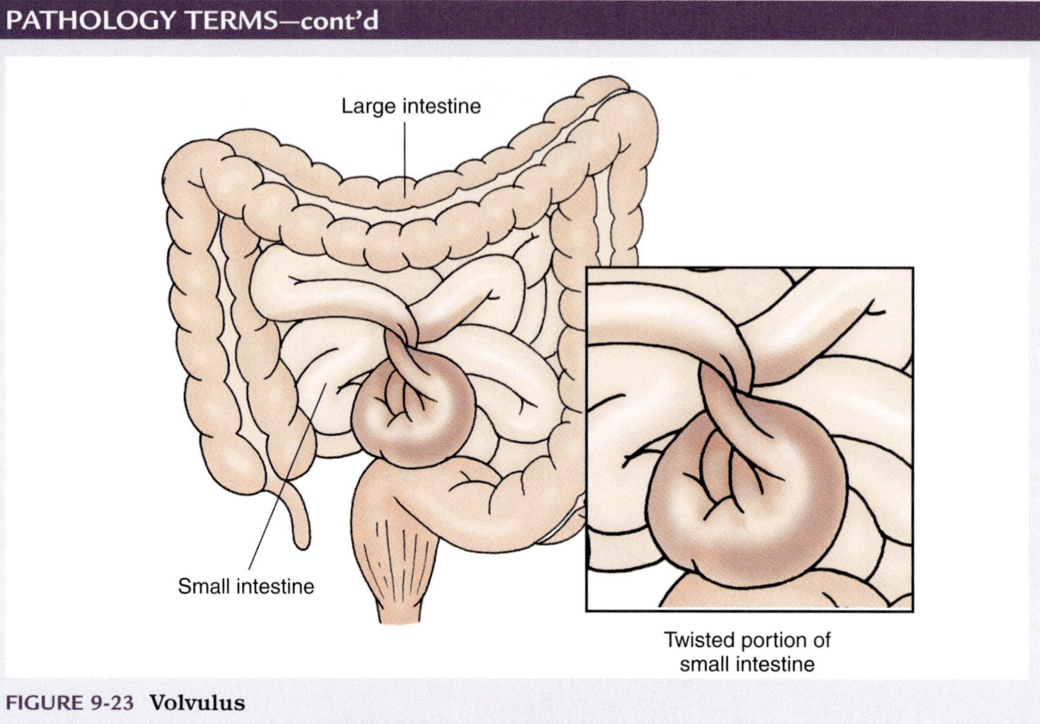

FIGURE 9-23 **Volvulus**

Common Diagnostic Tests and Procedures

Barium enema: Enema containing a substance that shows up clearly under x-ray and fluoroscopic examination

Barium swallow: X-ray examination of the esophagus after the patient has swallowed a liquid that contains barium

Computed tomography (CT) scan: Computerized collection and translation of multiple x-rays into a 3-dimensional picture, creating a more detailed and accurate image than traditional x-rays (see Fig. 9-24)

Endoscopic retrograde cholangiopancreatography (ERCP): Radiographic examination through a fiberoptic endoscope of vessels that connect the liver, gallbladder, and pancreas to the duodenum after a radiopaque material has been injected

Fecal occult blood test (Hemoccult): Test of fecal specimen for presence of hidden blood

Gastroccult: Test of gastric contents for pH level and presence of blood

***Helicobacter pylori* test:** Test that detects the presence of antibodies to *Helicobacter pylori*, the most common cause of gastric ulcers

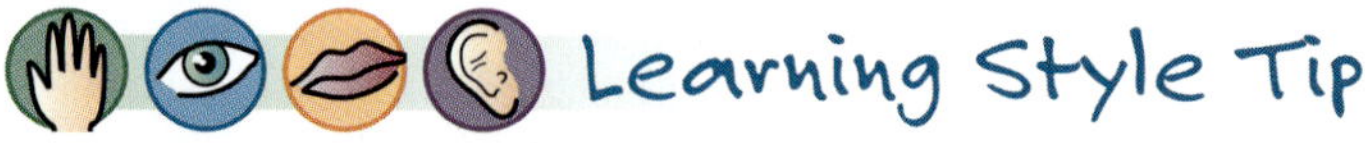

Visit a medical clinic to obtain patient-education pamphlets about some (or all) of these diagnostic tests and procedures; then read them aloud.

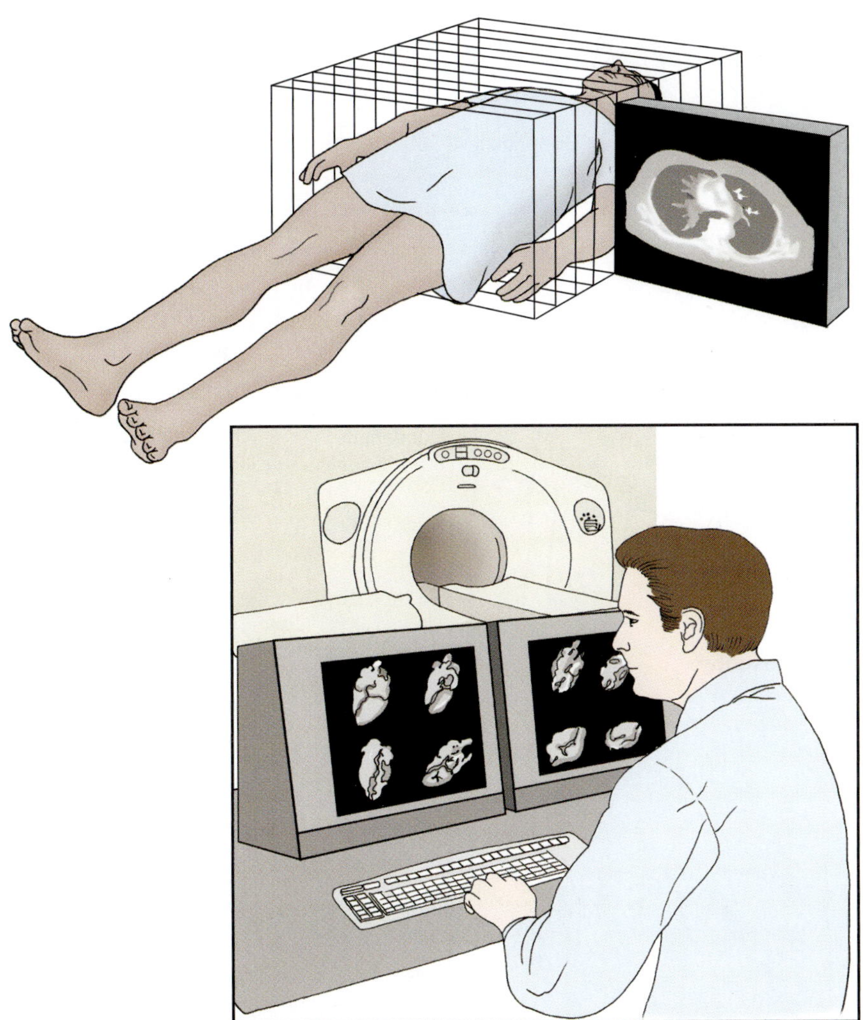

FIGURE 9-24 **Computed tomography scan**

Laparoscopy: Exploration of abdominal contents with a laparoscope

Liver function tests (LFTs): Tests, including aspartate aminotransferase (AST) and alanine aminotransferase (ALT), that determine the liver's ability to perform its many complex functions

Lower endoscopy: Visual examination of the GI tract from rectum to cecum; variations include the colonoscopy, sigmoidoscopy, and proctoscopy (see Fig. 9-25)

Lower GI x-ray: X-ray of the large intestine after rectal instillation of barium sulfate

Stool culture: Examination of a fecal specimen for abnormal bacteria and other microorganisms

Ultrasound: Test in which ultrahigh-frequency sound waves are used to outline the shapes of various body structures

Upper endoscopy: Visual examination of the GI tract, from esophagus to duodenum (see Fig. 9-26)

Upper GI x-ray (UGI): X-ray that involves the use of a contrast medium to help visualize abdominal organs, including the stomach and esophagus

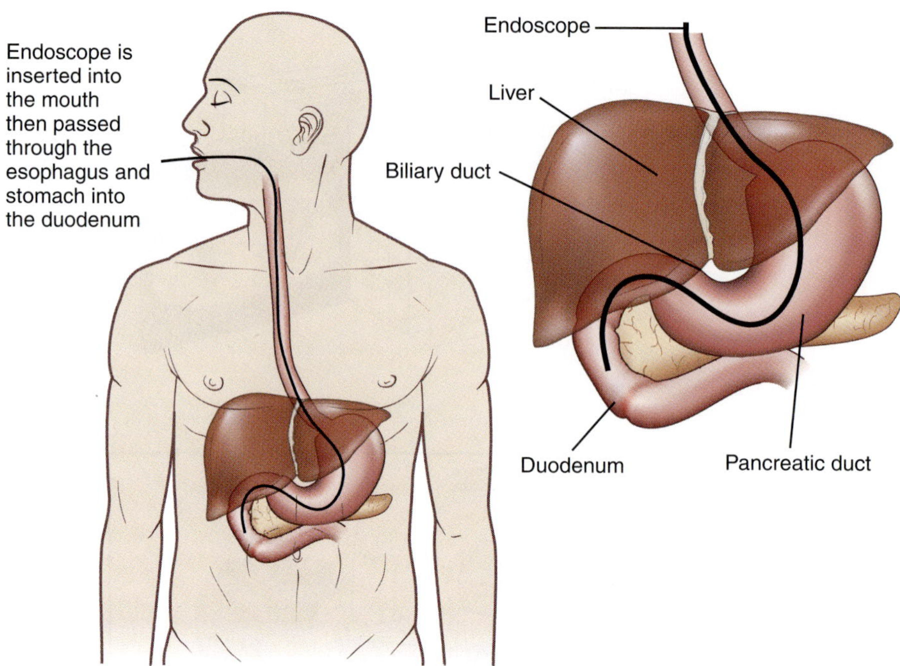

FIGURE 9-25 **Lower endoscopy**

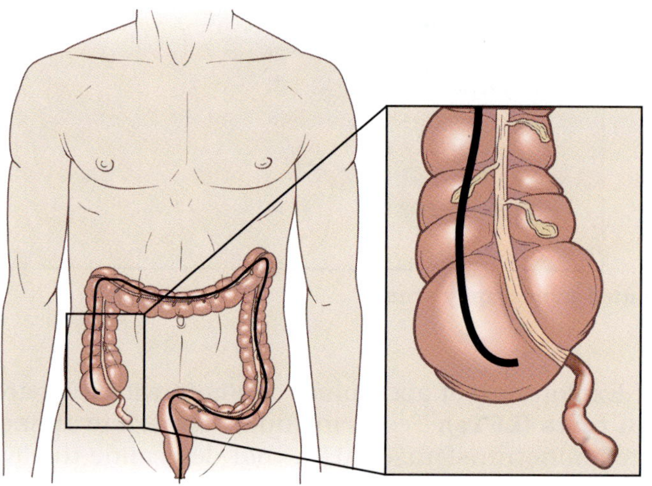

FIGURE 9-26 **Upper endoscopy**

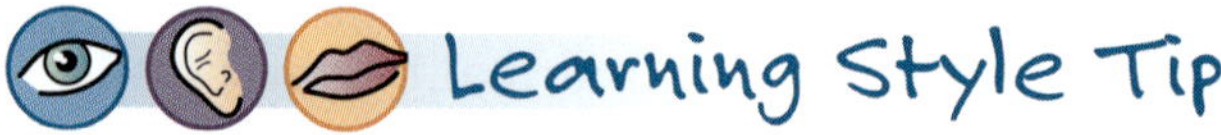

Be sure to complete the following case study. If you are an auditory or verbal learner, make sure you read it aloud. Then answer the questions that follow. This forces you to think about the information and greatly increases the chances that you will remember it later.

CASE STUDY

Read the case study and answer the questions that follow. Most of the terms are included in this chapter. Refer to the glossaries (Appendixes B and D) or to your medical dictionary for the other terms.

Ulcerative Colitis

Cynthia Summers is a 34-year-old married woman with two small children. She was seen by a physician at Valley Clinic this morning for an exacerbation of her ulcerative colitis. Her chief complaints were three to five episodes of bloody diarrhea per day, cramping abdominal pain, and fatigue. Mrs. Summers is thin and pale. She appears anxious and is reluctant to go to the hospital, stating that she needs to go home to take care of her family.

The physician prescribed prednisone and gave her the following dietary recommendations: Eat high-calorie foods, avoid strong spices and caffeine, and drink plenty of fluids. She is to return in 3 days for a follow-up visit, or sooner if her condition worsens. If her condition cannot be controlled with medications and dietary changes, hospitalization and possibly surgery will be considered.

Ulcerative colitis is characterized by chronic inflammation of the large intestine, primarily the rectum and sigmoid colon. Onset is usually in a patient's early 20s. Lesions form in the mucosal layer, causing very tiny hemorrhages that may, in time, develop abscesses. The lesions may become necrotic and may ulcerate. The primary symptom of ulcerative colitis is bloody diarrhea accompanied by cramping abdominal pain. Episodes of diarrhea may vary from once or twice a day to as many as 30 to 40 times a day in very severe cases. As a result, anorexia, anemia, and fatigue are common. The disease usually has periods of exacerbation and remissions. Treatment includes steroid medication such as prednisone, which has a powerful anti-inflammatory effect, and dietary modifications. Severe cases may require partial or complete colectomy. People with ulcerative colitis are at increased risk for developing colon cancer.

Case Study Questions

1. Ulcerative colitis usually affects which part of the intestine?
- **a.** Ileum
- **b.** Jejunum
- **c.** Proximal colon
- **d.** Distal colon

2. The medication the physician prescribed should help Mrs. Summers because:
- **a.** It is an analgesic, which reduces pain
- **b.** It is an antibiotic, which promotes healing
- **c.** It will reduce inflammation in her colon
- **d.** It reduces pain by reducing acids in the intestine

3. The age of onset of ulcerative colitis is usually:
- **a.** Childhood
- **b.** The early 20s
- **c.** The 40s
- **d.** After 60

4. Lesions may become abscessed, which means that they:
- **a.** Become infected
- **b.** Bleed
- **c.** Swell
- **d.** Contain dead tissue

5. The lesions may eventually become necrotic, which means that they:
   a. Heal
   b. Contain dead tissue
   c. Swell
   d. Bleed
6. In severe cases of ulcerative colitis, the patient experiences:
   a. Weight gain
   b. Constipation
   c. Frequent nausea
   d. Loss of appetite
7. Ulcerative colitis is characterized by:
   a. Periods of improvement alternating with periods of worsening
   b. Sudden, acute onset, short duration, and total healing
   c. Gradual onset, lengthy illness, and eventual complete healing
   d. Gradual onset, chronic disability, and eventual death

Answers to Case Study Questions

1. d
2. c
3. b
4. a
5. b
6. d
7. a

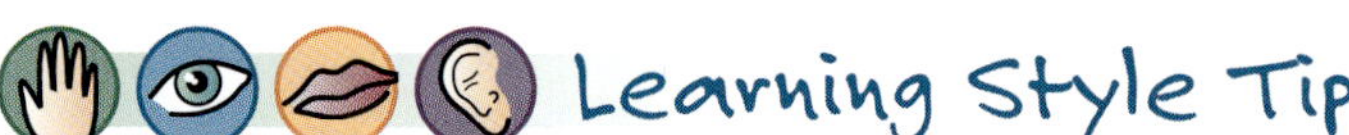

Learning Style Tip

Look up terms, diseases, or procedures on some of the following websites. They have great information! Remember to read aloud if you are an auditory or verbal learner.

Websites

Please go to the F.A. Davis website at http://davisplus.fadavis.com/eagle/medterm to view resource websites for the gastrointestinal system.

Practice Exercises

Deciphering Terms

Write the correct meaning of these medical terms. Check Appendix G for the correct answers.

Exercise 2

1. cholecystectomy ______________________________
2. enteritis ______________________________

3. proctoscopy ____________________

4. gastroscope ____________________

5. laparoscopy ____________________

6. jejunoplasty ____________________

7. pancreatolith ____________________

8. sublingual ____________________

9. pharyngitis ____________________

10. gastroenterologist ____________________

11. microgastric ____________________

12. dyskinesia ____________________

13. diarrhea ____________________

14. gastroparesis ____________________

15. dysphoria ____________________

Fill in the Blanks

Fill in the blanks below using Tables 9-2 and 9-3. Check Appendix G for the correct answers.

Exercise 3

1. ____________________ is the accumulation of serous fluid in the peritoneal cavity.

2. A condition in which tiny pouches form in the intestinal wall is ____________________.

3. When the condition in the previous question includes inflammation, it is known as ____________________.

4. The abbreviation *ERCP* stands for ____________________ ____________________ ____________________.

5. Another term for *vomiting* is ____________________.

6. The abbreviation ____________________ means *with.*

7. A chronic disease of the colon marked by inflammation and frequent bloody diarrhea is ____________________ ____________________.

8. *Abdomen* may be abbreviated as ______________________.

9. The abbreviation *UGI* stands for ______________________

______________________.

10. The abbreviation *SBO* stands for ______________________

______________________ ______________________.

11. If a patient is not to eat or drink anything, the physician may write this order: ______________________.

12. If a medication is to be taken orally, the order will be

______________________.

13. A suppository medication that is given rectally may be ordered

______________________.

14. If vital signs are to be taken once every hour, the physician may write the following order: ______________________ ______________________.

15. If a patient is to be weighed every day, the physician may write the following order: "weigh ______________________".

16. When a portion of the bowel slips inside of itself, it is called

______________________.

17. Excessive levels of bilirubin in the blood may result in a yellow staining of body tissues, known as ______________________.

18. ______________________ is the abbreviation for *cancer.*

19. To order bedrest with bathroom privileges, a physician might write

"______________________ ______________________

______________________."

20. The physician dictates that the patient "c/o N&V." This means that the patient ______________________ ______________________

______________________ ______________________ ______________________.

Multiple Choice

Select the one best answer to the following multiple-choice questions. Check Appendix G for the correct answers.

Exercise 4

1. Mr. Green is a 63-year-old man with heartburn (GERD). When it flares up, he experiences:
   a. Gastromegaly
   b. Esophagoplegia
   c. Esophagodynia
   d. Gastromalacia

2. Mr. Smith, a 36-year-old man, has come to the clinic complaining of symptoms that are consistent with heartburn (GERD). Which of the following will accurately diagnose this condition?
   a. Laparoscopy
   b. Upper endoscopy
   c. Esophagectomy
   d. Enteropathy

3. Ms. Diaz is a 47-year-old woman with a bowel obstruction caused by a portion of her bowel twisting upon itself. This condition is known as:
   a. Intussusception
   b. Ulcerative colitis
   c. Volvulus
   d. Cirrhosis

4. Which of the following terms is **not** related to a part of the small intestine?
   a. Duoden/o
   b. Jujen/o
   c. Colon/o
   d. Ile/o

5. To obtain multiple three-dimensional images of a body structure, the physician will order:
   a. A barium swallow
   b. A CT scan
   c. An ERCP
   d. A UGI

Word Building

*Using **only** the word parts in the lists provided, create medical terms with the indicated meanings. Check Appendix G for the correct answers.*

Exercise 5

Prefixes	Combining Forms	Suffixes
circum-	an/o	-al
hyper-	append/o	-ectomy
hypo-	appendic/o	-emesis
peri-	chol/e	-ic
	cholecyst/o	-itis
	colon/o	-lith
	dent/o	-megaly
	esophag/o	-oma
	gastr/o	-pathy
	hepat/o	-scopy
	ile/o	-stomy
	jejun/o	-tomy
	or/o	

1. disease of the liver ______________________
2. inflammation of the esophagus ______________________
3. visual examination of the esophagus and stomach ______________________
4. pertaining to around the mouth ______________________
5. excision or surgical removal of the gallbladder ______________________
6. enlargement of the stomach ______________________
7. pertaining to excessive colon ______________________
8. pertaining to near the anus ______________________
9. instrument used in examining the pharynx ______________________
10. tumor of the liver ______________________
11. inflammation of the appendix ______________________
12. excision or surgical removal of the appendix ______________________
13. cutting into or incision of the ileum ______________________
14. excessive vomiting ______________________
15. pertaining to the teeth ______________________
16. inflammation of the gallbladder ______________________
17. pertaining to below or beneath the stomach ______________________
18. visual examination of the colon ______________________

19. bile stone ______________________________

20. disease of the colon ______________________________

True or False

Decide whether the following statements are true or false. Check Appendix G for the correct answers.

Exercise 6

1. True False The abbreviation **s̄** means *with.*
2. True False The abbreviation **q** stands for *every.*
3. True False **Crohn disease** is a chronic inflammatory disease of the lining of the colon, marked by up to 20 liquid, bloody stools per day.
4. True False The abbreviation **LFT** stands for *liver function test.*
5. True False **Irritable bowel syndrome** is a chronic condition characterized by alternating episodes of constipation and diarrhea.
6. True False The abbreviation **PUD** stands for *peptic ulcer disease.*
7. True False An **EGD** is a procedure that involves examination of the liver.
8. True False The abbreviation **BM** stands for *basal metabolic rate.*
9. True False An accumulation of fluid in the peritoneal cavity is known as **cirrhosis**.
10. True False The abbreviation **GI** stands for *gastrointestinal.*

Deciphering Terms

Write the correct meaning of these medical terms. Check Appendix G for the correct answers.

Exercise 7

1. atrophy ______________________________
2. gingivostomatitis ______________________________
3. proctology ______________________________
4. glossospasm ______________________________

5. lithotripsy ______________________________

6. phagophobia ______________________________

7. dyspepsia ______________________________

8. labionasal ______________________________

9. oralgia ______________________________

10. cecectomy ______________________________

Multiple Choice

Select the one best answer to the following multiple-choice questions. Check Appendix G for the correct answers.

Exercise 8

1. Mr. Washington, a 27-year-old man, has a sore throat caused by inflammation. Which of the following is the correct medical term for this condition?

   a. Pharyngitis

   b. Pharyngostenosis

   c. Colitis

   d. Stomatitis

2. Which of the following terms means *bad, difficult, or painful swallowing?*

   a. Dyspepsia

   b. Dysphagia

   c. Dysphasia

   d. Dyspnea

3. Which of the following tests most accurately detects the cause of gastric ulcers?

   a. Gastroccult

   b. *H. pylori* test

   c. Laparoscopy

   d. Ultrasound

4. To detect gastrointestinal bleeding, the physician may order which of the following?

   a. Barium enema

   b. Lower endoscopy

   c. Stool culture

   d. Fecal occult blood test

5. Which of the following abbreviations refers to measurement of the patient's pulse, respiratory rate, blood pressure, and temperature?
   a. VS
   b. N&V
   c. CA
   d. LFT

6. Which of the following abbreviations involves the pancreas?
   a. GERD
   b. BRP
   c. ERCP
   d. EGD

7. Which of the following abbreviations refers to a procedure?
   a. IBS
   b. IBD
   c. PUD
   d. UGI

8. Which of the following indicates a route of medication administration?
   a. PO
   b. C/o
   c. GI
   d. Q

9. Which of the following disorders involves dilation and expansion of the lower esophagus due to pressure from food accumulation?
   a. Cholelithiasis
   b. Achalasia
   c. Esophageal varices
   d. Ascites

10. The definition of *pseudomembranous enterocolitis* is:
    a. Accumulation of serous fluid in the peritoneal (abdominal) cavity
    b. Inflammatory condition of both small and large bowels that results in severe watery diarrhea
    c. Disorder of inflammation and edema deep into the layers of the lining of any part of the GI tract
    d. Chronic condition characterized by alternating episodes of constipation and diarrhea

11. Which of the following is **not** a common cause of bowel obstruction?
    a. Volvulus
    b. Intussusception
    c. Adhesions
    d. Hernia

12. All of the following disorders involve the large intestine **except**:
    a. Celiac disease
    b. Pseudomembranosus enterocolitis
    c. Ulcerative colitis
    d. Diverticulosis

13. The term *enterobiliary* means:
    a. Abnormal condition of the cheek and esophagus
    b. Pertaining to the small intestine and bile
    c. Disease of the bowel
    d. Within the small intestine

14. The term *gingivostomatitis* means:
    a. Inflammation of the tongue and mouth
    b. Inflammation of the teeth and gums
    c. Inflammation of the gums and mouth
    d. Inflammation of the cheek and throat

15. The term *glossolabial* means:
    a. Pertaining to the gums and teeth
    b. Pertaining to the gallbladder and liver
    c. Pertaining to the cheek and tongue
    d. Pertaining to the tongue and lips

16. Which of the following terms means *inflammation of the salivary gland?*
    a. Steatitis
    b. Sialadenitis
    c. Stomatitis
    d. Lymphadenitis

17. Which of the following terms means *enlargement of the liver and spleen?*

   a. Hepatosplenomegaly
   b. Linguostomatomalacia
   c. Macrosplenism
   d. Microlipolysis

18. Which of the following terms means *suturing of the rectum?*

   a. Proctorrhaphy
   b. Rectostenosis
   c. Anoptosis
   d. Sigmoidosurgery

19. Which of the following terms means *cutting instrument for the pharynx?*

   a. Pharyngoscopy
   b. Pharyngoscope
   c. Pharyngotome
   d. Pharyngotomy

20. Which of the following terms means *cutting into or incision of the abdomen and spleen?*

   a. Pylorosplenotome
   b. Laparosplenotomy
   c. Splenomalacia
   d. Hepatopexy

10 URINARY SYSTEM

Structure and Function

The urinary system consists of the kidneys, ureters, bladder, and urethra. Each structure is uniquely designed and suited to its purpose. The urinary system's main functions are to filter and excrete waste products from the body, help regulate blood pressure, and maintain an optimal level of fluid and electrolytes within the body (see Fig. 10-1).

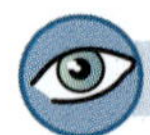
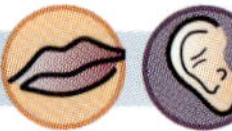

Learning Style Tip

Study Figure 10-1 carefully. Now close your eyes and visualize the urinary system. Note each structure in the order of urine creation and flow. As you do so, visualize it, name it aloud, and name the associated combining forms.

The key organs of the urinary system are the **kidneys**, which are located in the back of the abdominal cavity in the **retroperitoneal space**, to either side of the vertebral column. The right kidney is slightly lower than the left. Each one is surrounded by a renal capsule, made up of connective tissue and a thick layer of fat. This provides protection by acting as a cushion and a shock absorber. The renal artery, vein, nerves, and ureter exit the kidneys on the medial (inner) side. Both kidneys are highly vascular organs made up of an outer cortex and an inner medulla. In fact, over 20% of the blood pumped by the heart each minute passes through the kidneys. The vascular nature of the kidneys lends itself to their function, which is to filter blood for the elimination of wastes and excess fluid, and to regulate electrolytes. Major electrolytes include sodium (Na), potassium (K), magnesium (Mg) and calcium (Ca).

> **Flashpoint**
> There are approximately one million nephrons in each kidney!

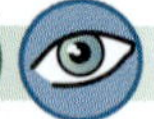

Learning Style Tip

Give yourself permission to write in your book. Use colorful markers to highlight terms and definitions. Add your own notes, diagrams, or flowcharts.

Located primarily within the outer cortex of the kidneys are the **nephrons** (see Fig. 10-2). There are more than one million nephrons in each kidney. Each one is a complex microscopic structure composed of an arteriole, venule, Bowman capsule, glomerulus (capillary cluster within the Bowman capsule), proximal tubule, loop of Henle, distal tubule, and capillary bed. The nephron has long been called the functional unit of the kidney, because it is where most of the action takes place. To begin the filtration process, blood passes from a tiny arteriole into the glomerulus. The walls of the glomerulus and Bowman capsule are designed to permit filtration of water, electrolytes, urea, and other

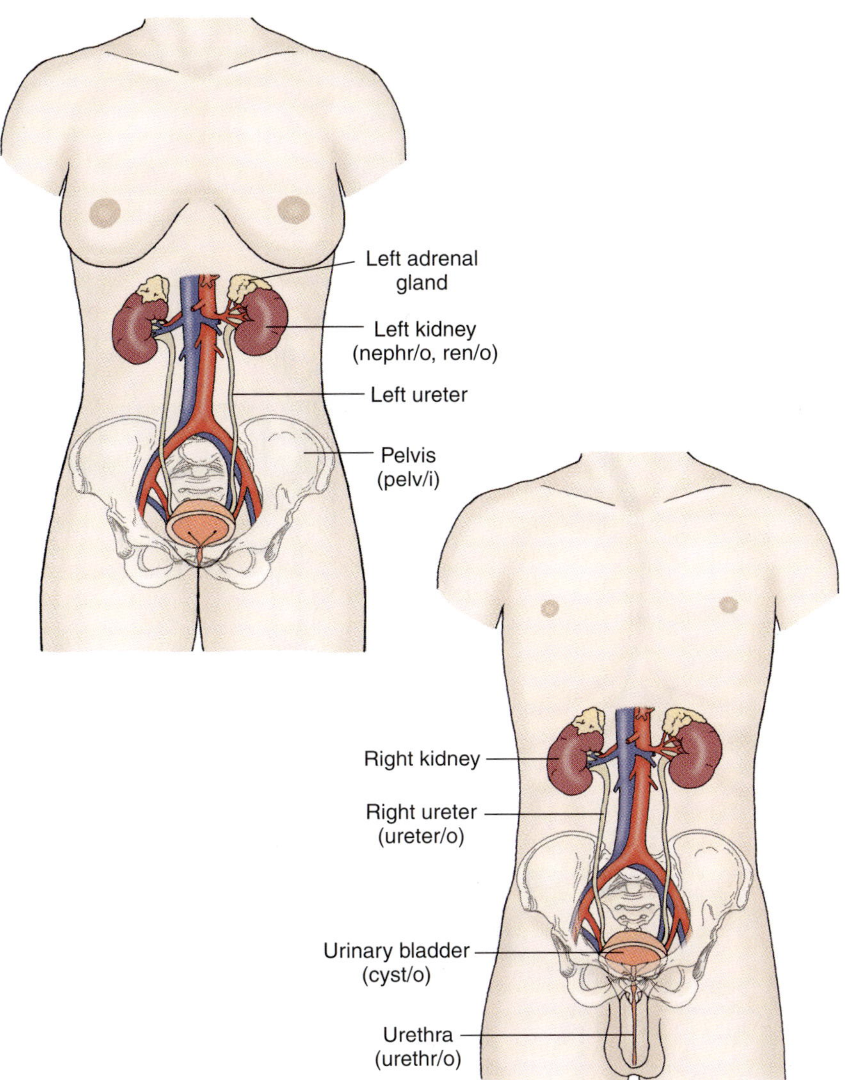

FIGURE 10-1 **The urinary system**

small molecules. A large amount of this fluid (approximately 180 liters), called **filtrate**, is created each day. However, as it moves on through the proximal tubule, loop of Henle, and distal tubule, nearly all of the water and useful solutes (99%) are reabsorbed, and additional wastes are excreted. After the kidneys make final adjustments in the composition of the fluid, it is called *urine.* The kidneys produce and excrete an average of 1 to 2 liters of urine each day.

Within the kidney's medulla, the innermost part of the kidney, are several oval-shaped renal pyramids, which point inward. Cupping each one is a calyx. The area where all of the calyces join is called the **renal pelvis**. As the renal pelvis narrows, it joins the uppermost part of the **ureter**. When urine is formed, it drains into the calyces, which funnel the urine inward through the renal pelvis and into the ureter, which in turn drains urine from the kidney downward to the **urinary bladder**.

In addition to filtering fluid and wastes from the body, the kidneys play active roles in maintaining blood pressure and blood pH (acidity or alkalinity). They

Flashpoint

The kidneys create 1 to 2 liters of urine each day. That is about 1 to 2 quarts.

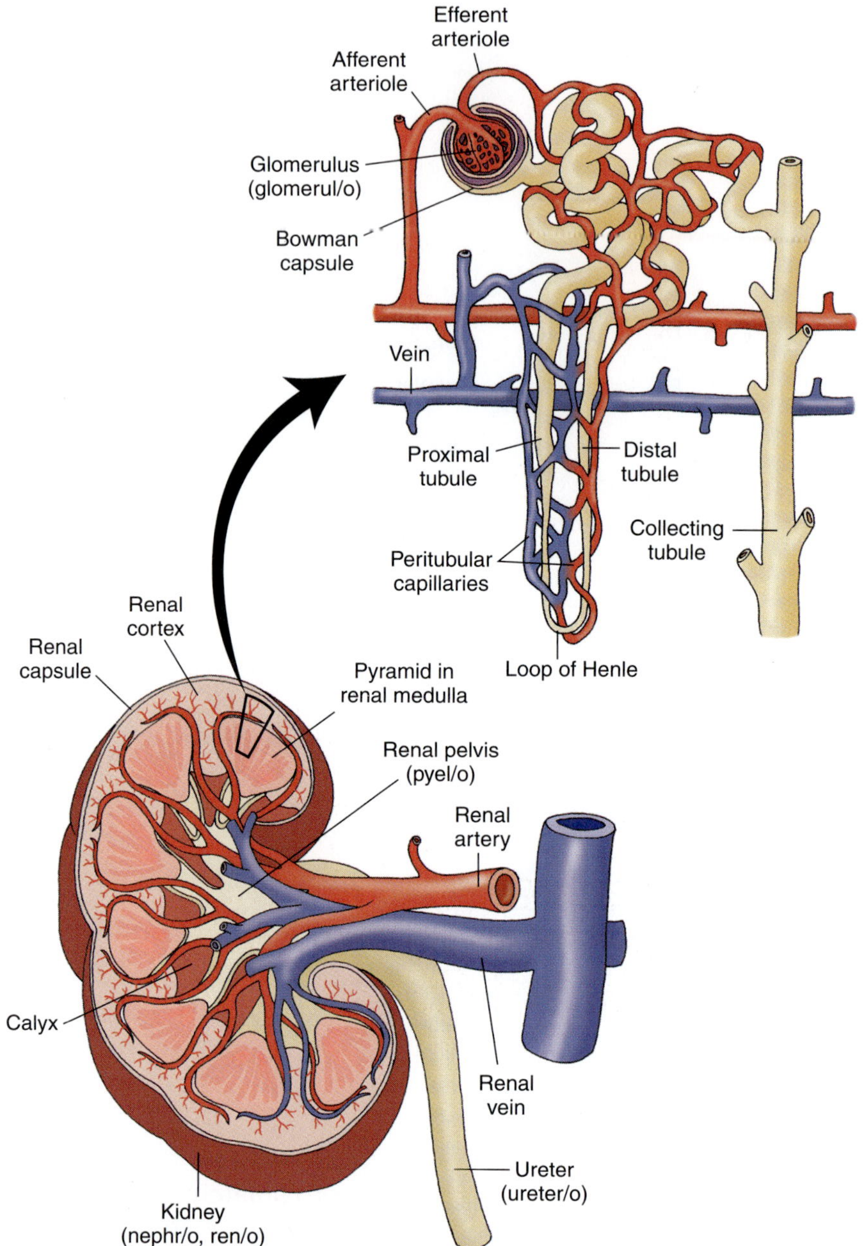

FIGURE 10-2 **The kidney and the nephron**

help regulate blood pressure by retaining or excreting more fluid and electrolytes (especially sodium). They help maintain a healthy acid-base balance by retaining or excreting buffers and acids as needed. Acid-base level is measured according to the **pH scale**, which ranges from 0 to 14 (see Fig. 10-3). The pH level of human blood must remain slightly alkaline, within the very narrow range of 7.35 to 7.45. Even minor fluctuations in this balance will result in illness or even death.

Flashpoint

The kidneys play an important role in maintaining the body's acid-base balance.

The ureters are long, narrow tubes that drain urine from the renal pelvis to the urinary bladder. The bladder is a flexible, muscular container for urine; its lining is uniquely designed to stretch to accommodate varying amounts of fluid. Urine accumulates here until the volume reaches a level that stimulates stretch

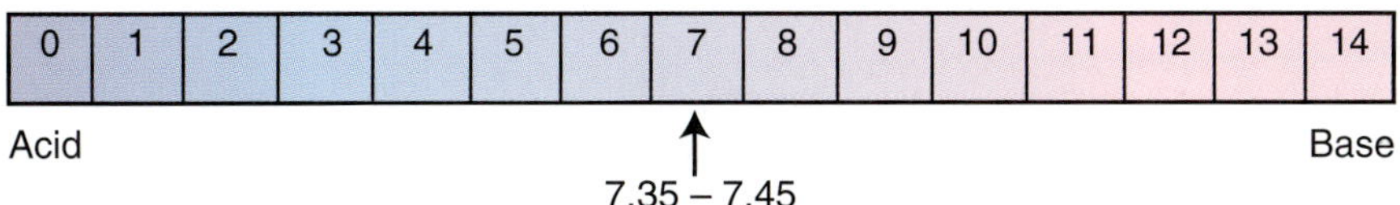

FIGURE 10-3 **pH scale**

receptors and initiates the **micturition reflex**, which is the urge to urinate. We may temporarily ignore this urge; however, eventually, the increased urine volume stimulates the stretch receptors again, and our urge to urinate will be even stronger. At the base of the bladder is the exit into the urethra, a tube that varies in length depending on the patient's sex. The male urethra is approximately 20 cm (just under 8 inches) long and the female urethra is approximately 4 cm (just over $1\frac{1}{2}$ inches) long. The urethra functions as a passageway for final urine elimination and emptying of the bladder.

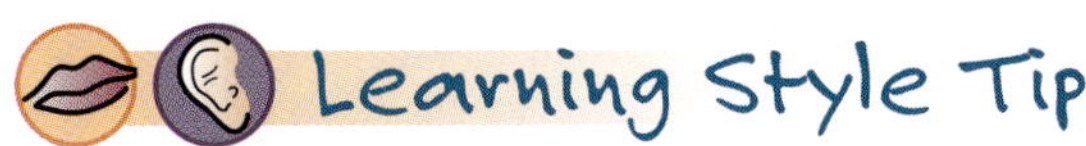

Collaborate with your study buddy to create sales pitches for terms (definitions included) that you might (theoretically) sell on TV or the Internet. The sillier your sales pitches, the more likely you will remember them later, so have fun with this.

Occasionally, a person may experience kidney failure, also known as ***renal failure***. A common cause is the destructive effects of poorly controlled **diabetes**. This is a disorder in which the pancreas does not produce enough insulin, or the body is resistant to the insulin that is produced. This results in abnormal metabolism of **glucose** (sugar) and fat. (This disorder is discussed more thoroughly in Chapter 12, Endocrine System.)

In some cases, when a person experiences renal failure, he or she is able to receive a kidney **transplant**. You may have heard of situations in which one person donates a kidney to another person. This illustrates two important points: One is that most people can live a long and normal life with only one healthy kidney; the other is that it is very difficult to lead a long and normal life without any kidneys at all.

If the person is not able to receive a transplant, he or she may live for months or even years by having regular **hemodialysis**. This is a process in which the blood is filtered through a special membrane in a dialysis machine to remove excess fluid and wastes (see Fig. 10-4). Another type of dialysis, in which the patient is not hooked up to a machine, is **peritoneal** dialysis. In this case, the patient's own peritoneal membrane (in the abdominal cavity) is used as a filter (see Fig. 10-5).

Combining Forms

Table 10-1 contains combining forms that pertain to the urinary system, examples of terms that utilize the combining forms, and a pronunciation guide. Read aloud to yourself as you move from left to right across the table. Be sure to use the pronunciation guide so that you can learn to say the terms correctly.

Flashpoint

Many of the combining forms in Table 10-1 are paired with the commonly used suffix *-uria* to describe abnormalities of urine.

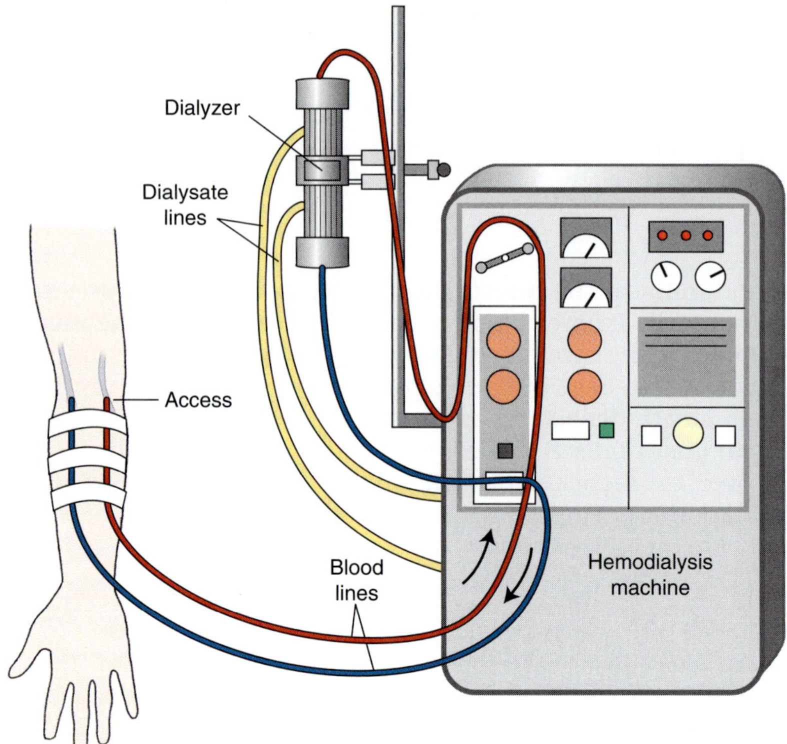

FIGURE 10-4 **Hemodialysis**

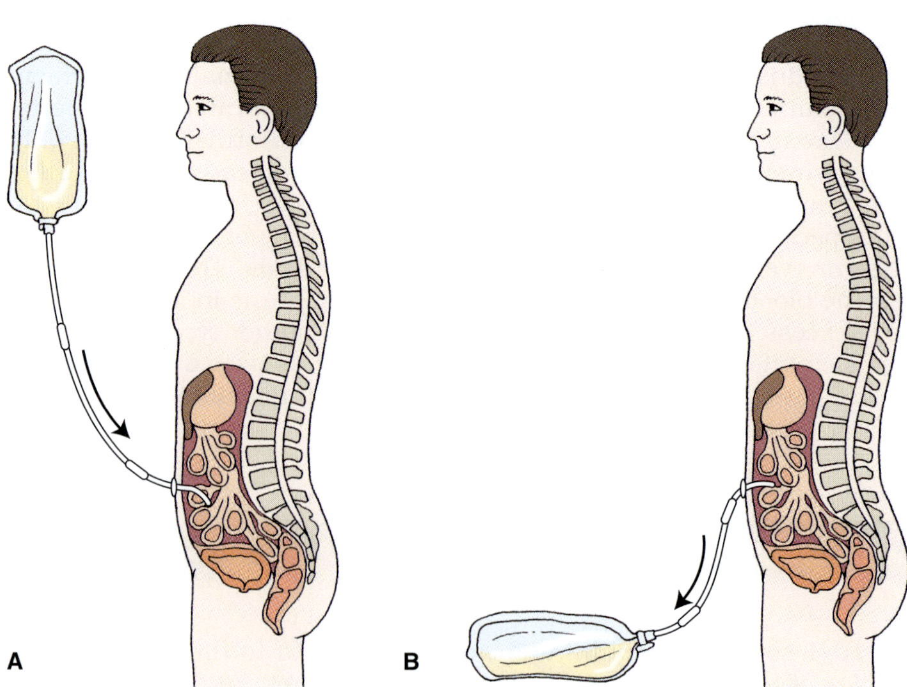

FIGURE 10-5 **Peritoneal dialysis**

TABLE 10-1
COMBINING FORMS

Combining Form	Meaning	Example (Pronunciation)	Meaning of New Term
azot/o	nitrogenous compounds	azoturia (ăz-ō-TŪ-rē-ă)	nitrogenous compounds in the urine
bacteri/o	bacteria	bacteriuria (BĂK-tē-rē-ū-rē-ă)	bacteria in the urine
cyst/o	bladder	cystoscopy (sĭs-TŎS-kō-pē)	visual examination of the bladder
vesic/o		vesicocele (VĔS-ĭ-kō-sēl)	hernia of the bladder
		vesicoscopy (VĔS-ĭ-kō-skō-pē)	visual examination of the bladder
glomerul/o	glomerulus	glomerulopathy (glō-mĕr-ū-LŎP-ă-thē)	disease of the glomerulus
gluc/o	glucose, sugar, sweet	glucogenesis (gloo-kō-JĔN-ĕ-sĭs)	creation of glucose
glucos/o		glucosuria (gloo-kō-SŪR-ē-ă)	sugar in the urine
glyc/o		glycemia (glī-SĒ-mē-ă)	sugar in the blood
glycos/o		glycosuria (glī-kō-SŪ-rē-ă)	sugar in the urine
keton/o	ketone bodies (acids and acetones)	ketonuria (kē-tō-NŪ-rē-ă)	ketone bodies in the urine
lith/o	stone	nephrolithiasis (nĕf-rō-lĭth-Ī-ă-sĭs)	pathological condition of kidney stones
meat/o	meatus, opening	meatotome (mē-ĂT-ŏ-tōm)	cutting (enlarging) instrument for a meatus
nephr/o	kidney	nephrologist (nĕ-FRŎL-ō-jĭst)	specialist in the study of the kidneys
ren/o		renal (RĒ-năl)	pertaining to the kidneys
noct/o	night	nocturia (nŏk-TŪ-rē-ă)	urination at night
olig/o	deficiency	oliguria (ōl-ĭ-GŪR-ē-ă)	deficiency of urine
peritone/o	peritoneum	peritoneal (pĕr-ĭ-tō-NĒ-ăl)	pertaining to the peritoneum
py/o	pus	pyuria (pī-ŪR-ē-ă)	pus in the urine
pyel/o	renal pelvis	pyelonephritis (pī-ĕ-lō-nĕ-FRĪ-tĭs)	inflammation of the renal pelvis and kidney
pelv/i	pelvis	pelvic	pertaining to the pelvis

Continued

TABLE 10-1
COMBINING FORMS—cont'd

Combining Form	Meaning	Example (Pronunciation)	Meaning of New Term
ur/o	urine	urology (ū-RŎL-ō-jē)	study of disorders of the urinary tract
urin/o		urinometer (ū-rĭ-NŎM-ĕ-tĕr)	measuring instrument for urine
ureter/o	ureter	ureterostenosis (ū-rē-tĕr-ō-stĕ-NŌ-sĭs)	narrowing or stricture of the ureter
urethr/o	urethra	urethropexy (ū-RĒ-thrō-pĕk-sē)	surgical fixation of the urethra

STOP HERE.
Select the Combining Form Flash Cards for Chapter 10 and run through them at least three times before you continue.

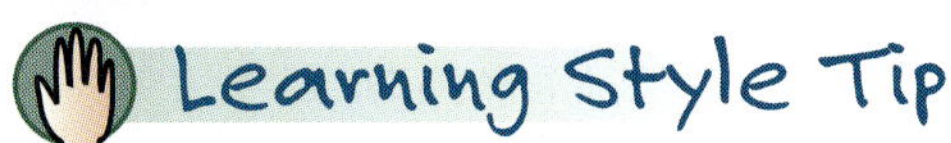

You will get more out of class if you remain awake and alert. Therefore, if you sometimes find yourself feeling sleepy, ask permission (before class) to stand up occasionally. To avoid disrupting others, you may elect to sit near the back of the room or on an aisle.

Practice Exercises

Fill in the Blanks

Fill in the blanks below using Table 10-1. Check Appendix G for the correct answers.

Exercise 1

1. pertaining to the peritoneum ______________________
2. urination at night ______________________
3. hernia of the bladder ______________________
4. sugar in the blood ______________________
5. surgical fixation of the urethra ______________________
6. inflammation of the renal pelvis and kidney ______________________
7. disease of the glomerulus ______________________
8. visual examination of the bladder ______________________

9. nitrogenous compounds in the urine ______________________________

10. specialist in the study of the kidneys ______________________________

11. narrowing or stricture of the ureter ______________________________

12. study of disorders of the urinary tract ______________________________

13. measuring instrument for urine ______________________________

14. sugar in the urine ______________________________

15. ketone bodies in the urine ______________________________

16. abnormal condition of kidney stones ______________________________

17. deficiency of urine ______________________________

18. pus in the urine ______________________________

19. pertaining to the kidneys ______________________________

20. cutting (enlarging) instrument for a meatus ______________________________

21. creation of glucose ______________________________

22. bacteria in the urine ______________________________

23. **Fill in the blanks in Figure 10-6 with the appropriate anatomical terms and combining forms.**

24. **Fill in the blanks in Figure 10-7 with the appropriate anatomical terms and combining forms.**

Abbreviations

Table 10-2 lists some of the most common abbreviations related to the urinary system, as well as others often used in medical documentation.

STOP HERE.
Select the Abbreviations Flash Cards for Chapter 10 and run through them at least three times before you continue.

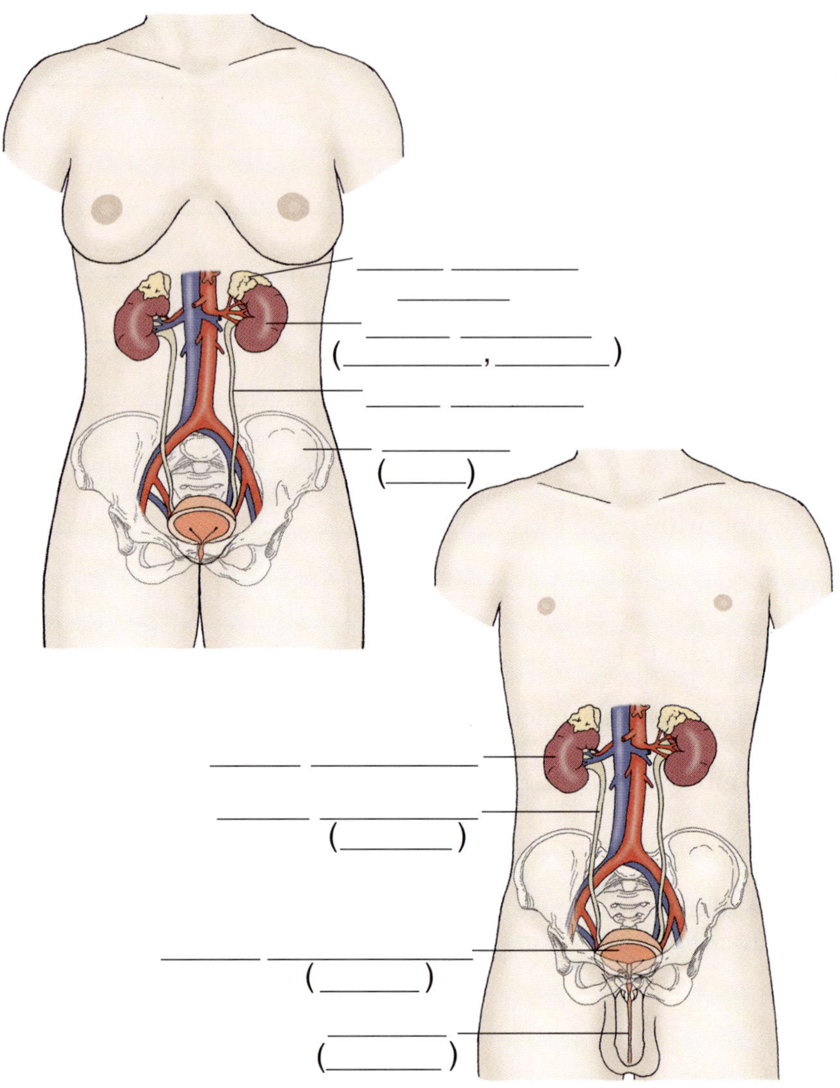

FIGURE 10-6 **Urinary system with blanks**

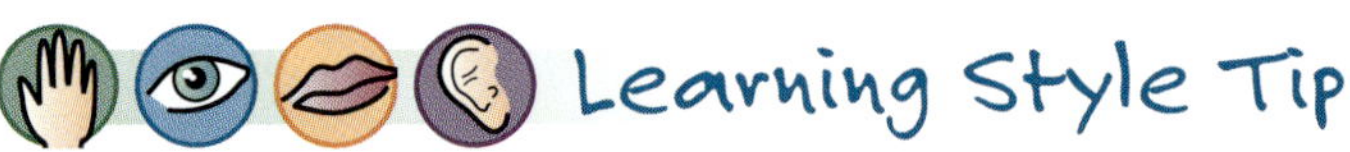

Learning Style Tip

Choose several of the pathology terms that you are especially interested in learning about. Use a computer to create a colorful, visually interesting one-page flyer about each of the selected disorders. Keep text to a minimum; instead use photos or illustrations from the Internet, symbols, and diagrams. Share your flyers with your study buddy and verbally "teach" her about the disorders you researched.

Flashpoint

A TURP is a procedure performed to relieve the symptoms caused by an enlarged prostate (BPH). Remember this relationship by connecting the two abbreviations in the following manner:

B
TURP
H

Pathology Terms

Table 10-3 includes terms that relate to diseases or abnormalities of the urinary system. Use the pronunciation guide and say the terms aloud as you read them. This will help you get in the habit of saying them properly.

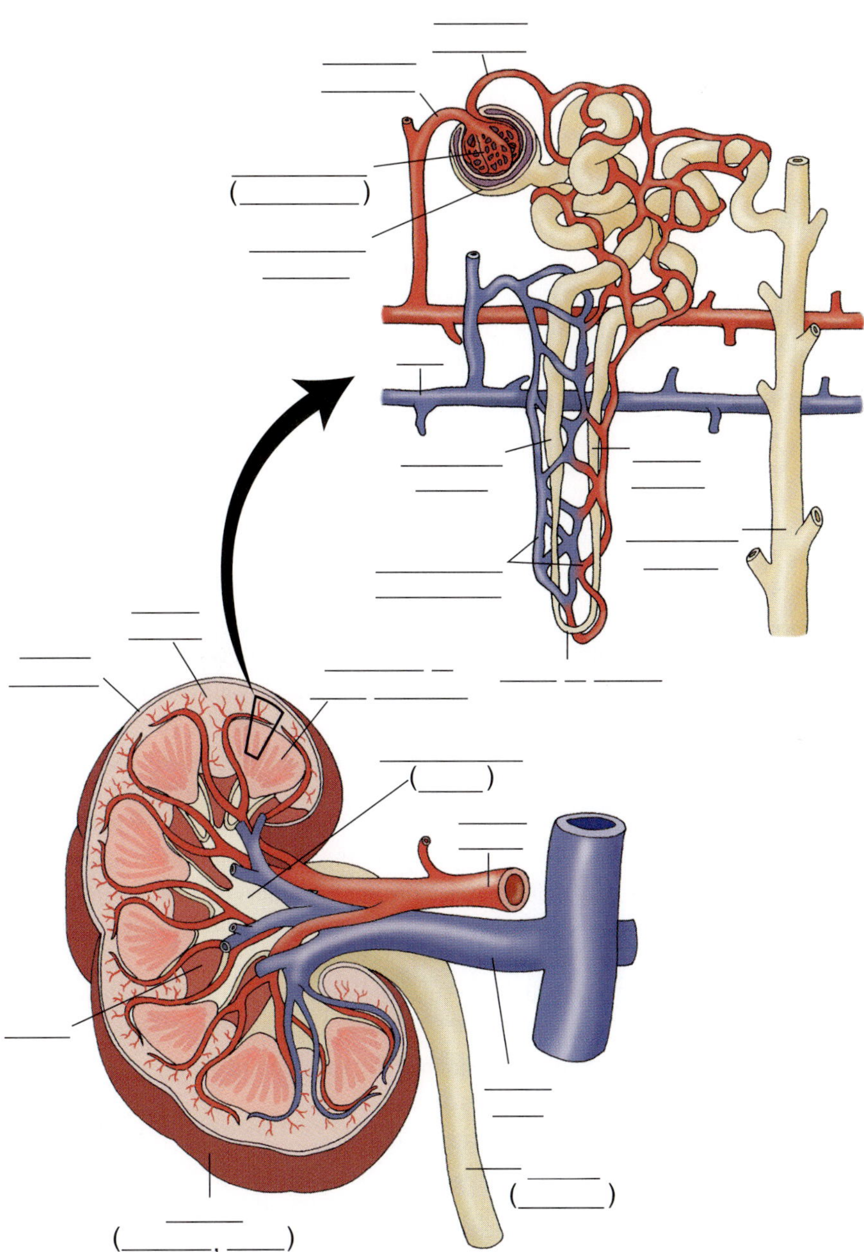

FIGURE 10-7 **Kidney and nephron with blanks**

TABLE 10-2 ABBREVIATIONS			
AGN	acute glomerulonephritis	BUN	blood urea nitrogen
ARF	acute renal failure	C&S	culture and sensitivity
ATN	acute tubular necrosis	Cath	catheterization, catheter
BNO	bladder neck obstruction	CRF	chronic renal failure
BPH	benign prostatic hypertrophy (benign prostatic hyperplasia)	Cysto	cystoscopy

Continued

TABLE 10-2
ABBREVIATIONS—cont'd

ESRD	end-stage renal disease	SG, sp. gr.	specific gravity
HD	hemodialysis	TURP	transurethral resection of the prostate
H_2O	water	UA	urinalysis
I&O	intake and output	UC	urine culture
IVP	intravenous pyelogram	UTI	urinary tract infection
KUB	kidney, ureter, and bladder	VCUG	voiding cystourethrography
PKD	polycystic kidney disease	VUR	vesicoureteral reflux
RP	retrograde pyelogram		

TABLE 10-3
PATHOLOGY TERMS

acute glomerulonephritis (ă-KYŪT glō-mĕr-ū-lō-nĕ-FRĪ-tĭs)	type of nephritis (kidney infection) in which the glomeruli are the key structures affected; also called *acute nephritic syndrome*
bacterial cystitis (bak-TIR-ē-ul sĭs-TĪ-tĭs)	inflammation of the bladder caused by bacterial infection, commonly coexisting with bacterial urethritis, both of which together constitute a urinary tract infection (UTI), sometimes referred to as a *bladder infection*
chronic glomerulonephritis (KRĂN-ik glō-mĕr-ū-lō-nĕ-FRĪ-tĭs)	condition in which the glomeruli suffer gradual, progressive, destructive changes, with resulting loss of kidney function; also called *chronic nephritis*
diabetic nephropathy (dī-ă-BĔT-ĭk nĕ-FRŎP-ă-thē)	kidney disease associated with diabetes that results in inflammation, degeneration, and sclerosis of the kidneys
diuresis (dī-ū-RĒ-sĭs)	abnormal secretion of large amounts of urine
end-stage renal disease (ESRD) (END-stāj RĒ-năl dĭ-ZĒZ)	final phase of kidney disease
enuresis (ĕn-ū-RĒ-sĭs)	involuntary urination during sleep; also called *bedwetting*
frequency (FRĒ-kwun-sē)	need to urinate more often than normal
glucosuria, glycosuria (gloo-kō-SŪ-rē-ă, glī-kō-SŪ-rē-ă)	sugar in the urine
hydronephrosis (hī-drō-nĕf-RŌ-sĭs)	condition in which the renal pelvis and calyces become distended and dilated and begin to atrophy due to urine outflow obstruction (see Fig. 10-8)

TABLE 10-3
PATHOLOGY TERMS—cont'd

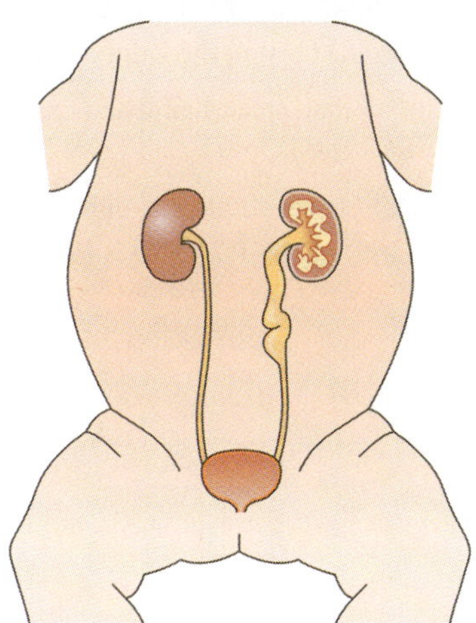

FIGURE 10-8 **Hydronephrosis**

interstitial cystitis (ĭn-tĕr-STĬSH-ăl sĭs-TĪ-tĭs)	chronic inflammatory condition of the bladder lining not caused by infection or other identified pathology
interstitial nephritis (ĭn-tĕr-STĬSH-ăl nĕf-RĪ-tĭs)	pathological changes in renal tissue that destroy nephrons and impair kidney function
nephrotic syndrome (nĕ-FRŎT-ĭk SĬN-drōm)	uncommon disorder marked by massive proteinuria, edema, hypoalbuminemia (low blood albumin), hyperlipidemia (high blood lipids), and hypercoagulability (high tendency to form blood clots)
neurogenic bladder (nū-rō-JĔN-ĭk BLĂD-ĕr)	bladder dysfunction (retention, incontinence, or altered capacity) due to disease or injury of the central nervous system or certain peripheral nerves
phimosis (fī-MŌ-sĭs)	narrowing or stricture of the foreskin opening of the penis (see Fig. 10-9)

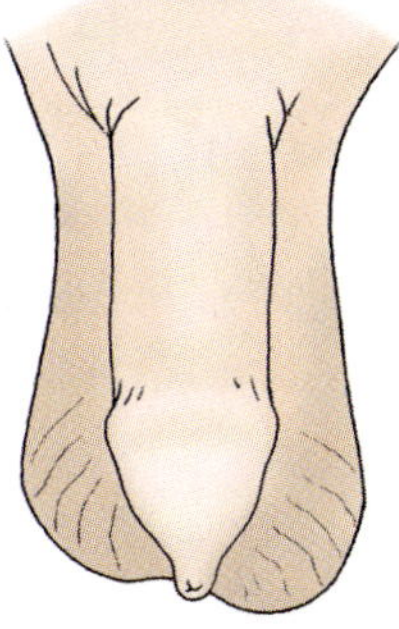

FIGURE 10-9 **Phimosis**

Continued

TABLE 10-3

PATHOLOGY TERMS—cont'd

polycystic kidney disease (PKD) (pŏl-ē-SĬS-tĭk KĬD-nē dĭ-ZĒZ)	group of hereditary, progressive disorders in which cysts (small sacs of fluid) form in the kidneys, eventually destroying them
pyelonephritis (pī-ĕ-lō-nĕ-FRĪ-tĭs)	inflammation and infection caused by bacterial growth in the renal pelvis and kidney
renal calculus (RĒ-năl KĂL-kū-lŭs)	small stone, composed of mineral salts, that may obstruct portions of the kidneys or a ureter; also called *kidney stone* (see Fig. 10-10)

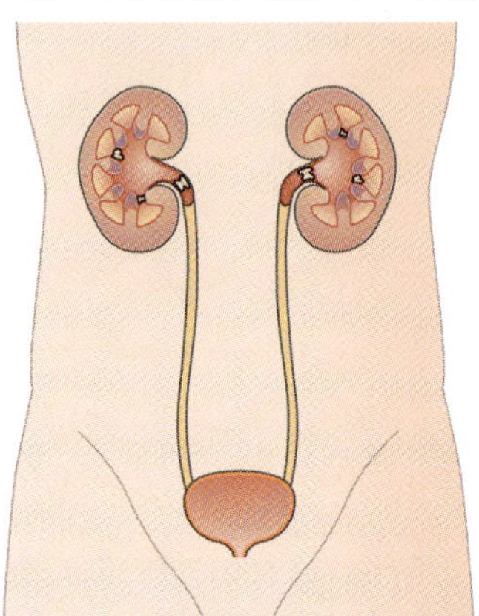

FIGURE 10-10 **Renal calculus**

renal colic (RĒ-năl KĂL-ik)	severe, intermittent pain caused by spasms of the ureter
renal failure (RĒ-năl FĀL-yĕr)	acute or chronic failure of the kidneys to effectively eliminate fluids or wastes from the body
stress incontinence (strĕs ĭn-KŎNT-ĭn-ĕns)	involuntary urine leakage upon physical stress, such as a cough or sneeze (see Fig. 10-11)

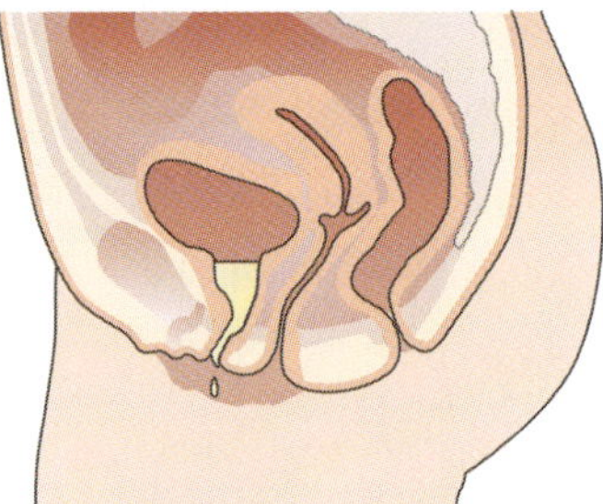

FIGURE 10-11 **Stress incontinence**

tubular necrosis (TŪ-bū-lăr nĕ-KRŌ-sĭs)	renal failure caused by acute injury to the renal tubules
uremia (ū-RĒ-mē-ă)	increased level of urea or other wastes in the blood

TABLE 10-3

PATHOLOGY TERMS—cont'd

urgency (UR-jən-sē)	need to urinate immediately
urinary retention (Ū-rĭ-nār-ē rĭ-TĔN-shŭn)	inability to urinate
urinary tract infection (UTI) (Ū-rĭ-nār-ē trăkt ĭn-FĔK-shŭn	inflammation and infection caused by bacterial growth in the urinary tract, usually the bladder
vesicoureteral reflux (VUR) (ves-i-kō-yū-RĒT-ə-rəl RĒ-fluks)	abnormal flow of urine from the bladder back into the ureter
Wilms tumor (vĭlmz TŪ-mor)	rapidly growing type of kidney cancer that most commonly affects children; also known as *nephroblastoma*

STOP HERE.
Select the Pathology Terms Flash Cards for Chapter 10 and run through them at least three times before you continue.

Common Diagnostic Tests and Procedures

Flashpoint

Remember the differences in the meanings of the following terms by using the associations shown below:

Diuresis happens in the **d**aytime (usually) in response to **d**rugs
Enuresis occurs **"en"** (in) bed while you sleep
Nocturia **n**udges you from bed (wakes you) at **n**ight

24-hour urine specimen: Total urine excreted over 24 hours, collected for analysis

Bladder ultrasound (bladder scan): Noninvasive use of a portable ultrasound device to measure the amount of retained urine

Blood urea nitrogen (BUN): Lab value used to measure kidney function, based on nitrogen levels in the blood

Culture and sensitivity (C&S): Process of growing microorganisms, then exposing them to antimicrobial drugs to determine which ones kill them most effectively

Cystoscopy: Visual examination of the bladder lining with a cystoscope (see Fig. 10-12)

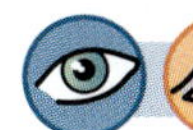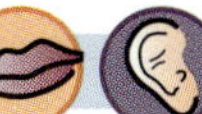 **Learning Style Tip**

Work with study buddies to create written mnemonics and acronyms to help you remember abbreviations and definitions of pathology terms. Say them aloud repeatedly.

Extracorporeal shock wave lithotripsy: Procedure in which shock waves or sound waves crush stones in the kidneys or urinary tract (see Fig. 10-13)

Hemodialysis: Filtration of wastes and fluid from blood as it passes through selectively permeable membranes; also called *dialysis* (see Fig. 10-4)

Intravenous pyelogram (IVP): X-ray examination of the kidneys, ureters, and bladder after injection of a contrast medium

KUB: Radiological imaging (x-ray) of the abdomen, specifically the kidneys, ureters, and bladder

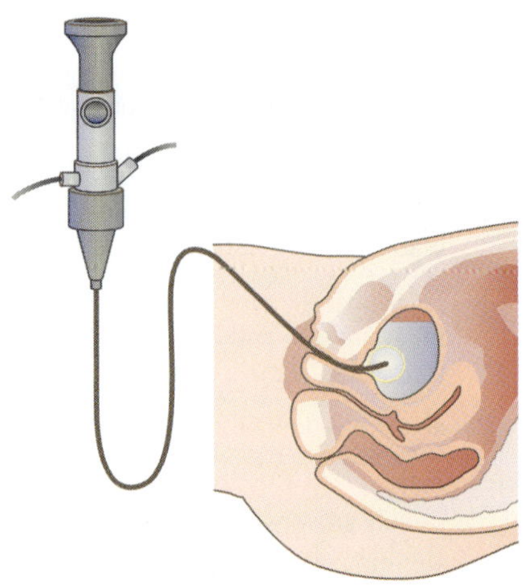

FIGURE 10-12 **Cystoscopy**

Peritoneal dialysis: Filtration of fluid and wastes from the blood using the lining of the patient's peritoneal cavity as a dialyzing membrane (see Fig. 10-5)

Serum creatinine: Lab value used to measure kidney function that is more specific than BUN

Urinalysis (UA): Visual and microscopic analysis of a urine specimen (see Table 10-4)

Urinary catheterization: Insertion of a tube into the bladder via the urethra to drain urine, obtain a urine specimen, or instill medication (see Fig. 10-14)

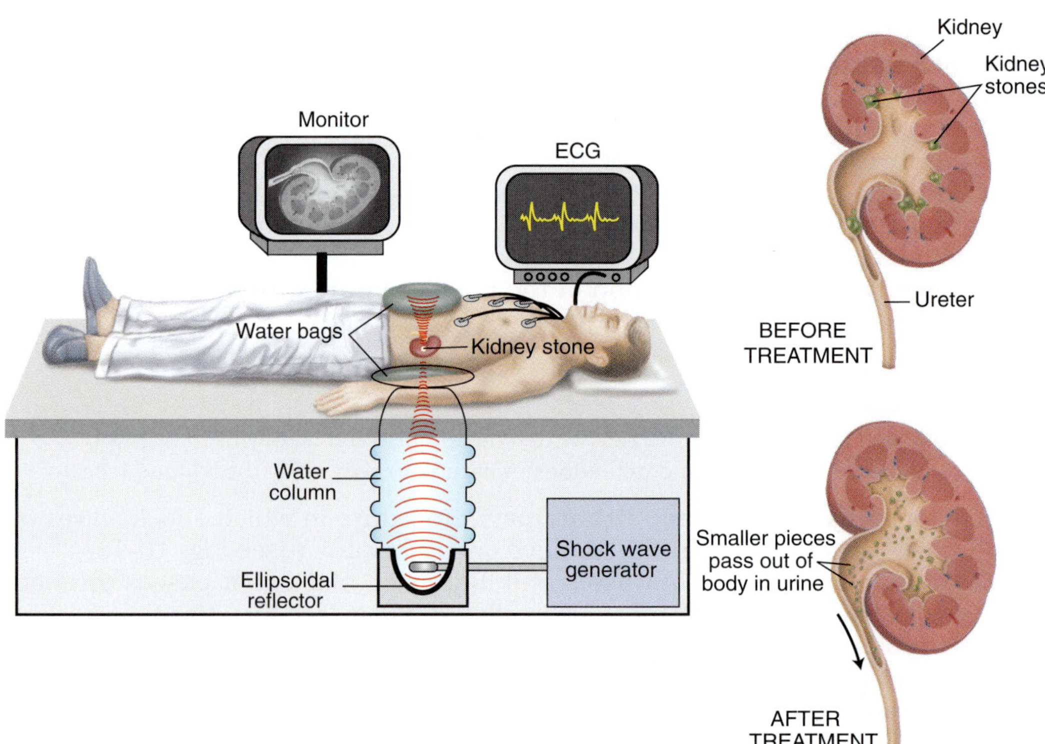

FIGURE 10-13 **Extracorporeal shock wave lithotripsy** (From Eagle, S, et al.: *The Professional Medical Assistant.* F.A. Davis, Philadelphia, 2009, p. 581; with permission)

TABLE 10-4
NORMAL VALUES OF A URINALYSIS

Chem Stick		Microscope	
Color	Light yellow or straw	**Epithelial cells**	3-4
Appearance	Clear	**WBCs**	0-1
S.G.	1.010-1.030	**RBCs**	0
pH	5-8	**Bacteria**	0
Protein	Neg		
Glucose	Neg		
Ketones	Neg		
Bilirubin	Neg		
Blood	Neg		
Nitrites	Neg		

Voiding cystourethrography (VCUG): Radiological examination of the bladder and urethra during urination

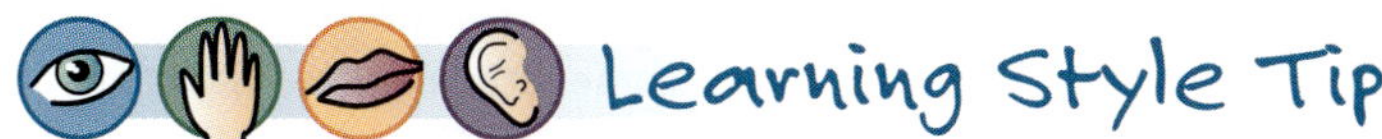

After reading aloud the brief definition of each test or procedure from this book, look each one up in a medical dictionary and read the expanded definition found there. Then reread aloud the brief definition in this book.

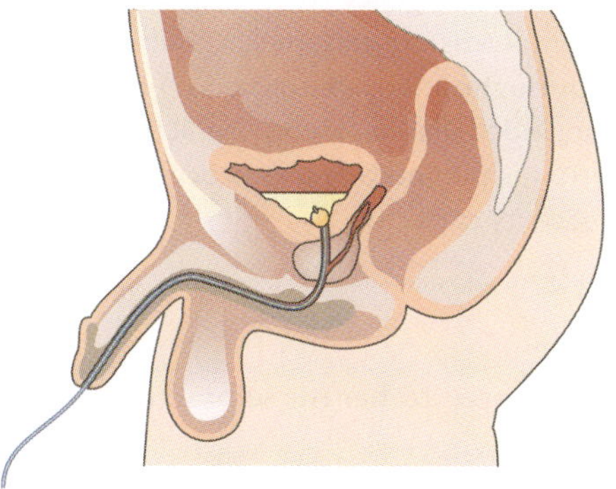

FIGURE 10-14 **Urinary catheterization**

CASE STUDY

Read the case study and answer the questions that follow. Most of the terms are included in this chapter. Refer to the glossaries (Appendixes B and D) or to your medical dictionary for the other terms.

Interstitial Cystitis

Lisa Galerno is a 32-year-old woman who came to her nurse practitioner 2 months ago with c/o frequency, urgency, dysuria, and low back and pelvic pain. A urine specimen was collected and analyzed. The findings were normal except for a small number of RBCs. Because of her symptoms, Ms. Galerno was treated for a possible UTI and was put on a course of antibiotics. She returned a week later with her symptoms unchanged. A second urine specimen was tested, with the same results as the first time. Then Lisa was put on a different antibiotic. When she returned a week later, with still no improvement in Sx, she was referred to a urologist for further evaluation.

After an initial consultation with the urologist, a cystoscopy was done under general anesthesia and tissue collected for a Bx. The cytology report revealed that the specimen was benign; however, visual inspection during the cystoscopy confirmed the presence of hemorrhagic lesions and ulcerations, as well as smaller-than-normal bladder capacity. Based on these findings, a Dx of interstitial cystitis was confirmed. A bladder distention was performed at that time.

Interstitial cystitis (IC) is a disorder of the bladder lining that affects approximately 1 million people in the United States; mostly women. The cause has not been clearly identified, although severe stress appears to be a contributor. There is also some speculation that it may be autoimmune in nature. There is no known cure, and treatments are few and provide variable results.

People with IC manage their disease most effectively by noticing what seems to trigger or worsen their symptoms and what brings relief. It is essentially a process of trial and error; the results are not the same for everyone. Dietary triggers may include caffeine, alcohol, chocolate, or acidic foods such as citrus fruits; therefore, the usual remedy of drinking cranberry juice for a bladder infection is **not** helpful, and may exacerbate symptoms. Some interventions that may bring relief include taking Elmiron (the only medication approved so far for IC), taking NSAIDs such as ibuprofen or naproxen, and applying heat. People with IC generally notice wide fluctuations in symptoms, and will have good days and bad days. They may need to adopt lifestyle modifications and avoid activities that seem to increase their pain.

Common symptoms of IC include low back and pelvic pain, **frequency** (the need to urinate often, caused by bladder irritation), **urgency** (the need to urinate *now*), and **dysuria** (pain or burning on urination). The symptoms are extremely variable in duration and intensity and may fluctuate dramatically throughout any given day.

Definitive diagnosis is concluded via cystoscopy, which may be performed under general anesthesia if bladder distention is planned. In this procedure, the bladder is filled with sterile saline to stretch it and increase its capacity.

Flashpoint

During cystoscopy the physician closely examines the inner bladder wall.

Case Study Questions

1. Ms. Galerno initially presented to her nurse practitioner with which of the following symptoms?
- **a.** Nausea
- **b.** Diarrhea
- **c.** Fever
- **d.** Pelvic pain

2. Both times that a urinalysis was performed, the findings confirmed the presence of:
- **a.** Pus
- **b.** Bacteria
- **c.** Blood
- **d.** Protein

3. Ms. Galerno was referred to a physician who specializes in the treatment of:
   a. Female disorders
   b. Urinary-tract disorders
   c. Colorectal disorders
   d. Endocrine disorders

4. The urologist performed which of the following procedures?
   a. Surgical removal of the bladder
   b. Surgical incision into the bladder
   c. Visual examination of the bladder
   d. Surgical fixation of the bladder

5. Which of the following abnormal findings were noted during the cystoscopy?
   a. Small cracks and sores that bleed
   b. Presence of cancerous lesions
   c. Presence of an infection
   d. Large bladder capacity

6. During the cystoscopy, the urologist also:
   a. Injected antibiotics into the bladder
   b. Used sterile salt water to stretch the bladder
   c. Applied medication to the bladder lining
   d. Cauterized the lesions to stop the bleeding

7. Which of the following statements is true about IC?
   a. It affects men more often than women
   b. It is a very common disorder
   c. The cause is clearly understood
   d. There is no known cure

8. Which of the following statements is true about IC?
   a. Each person with IC must learn by trial and error what makes symptoms better or worse
   b. All people with IC experience the same symptoms
   c. The same treatments are effective for everyone with IC
   d. The course of IC is predictable

9. Common symptoms of IC include:
   a. Urinary incontinence
   b. Fever
   c. Need to empty the bladder often
   d. Urinary retention

Answers to Case Study Questions

1. d
2. c
3. b
4. c
5. a
6. b
7. d
8. a
9. c

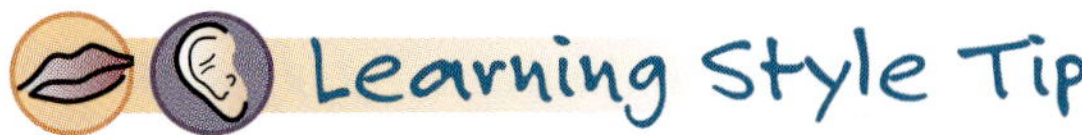

Arrange to meet regularly with a study buddy (a minimum of three times per week). If you cannot get together in person, arrange to have virtual study sessions using a web camera or, at the very least, by telephone.

Websites

Please go to the F.A. Davis website at http://davisplus.fadavis.com/eagle/medterm to view resource websites for the urinary system.

Practice Exercises

Deciphering Terms

Write the correct meaning of these medical terms. Check Appendix G for the correct answers.

Exercise 2

1. renopathy ____________________
2. urethropexy ____________________
3. periurethral ____________________
4. cystectomy ____________________
5. nephrotomy ____________________
6. ureterostomy ____________________
7. glomerulonephritis ____________________
8. polydipsia ____________________
9. nephrectomy ____________________
10. nocturia ____________________
11. bacteriuria ____________________
12. hematuria ____________________
13. nephrolith ____________________
14. anuric ____________________
15. cystomegaly ____________________

Fill in the Blanks

Fill in the blanks below. Check Appendix G for the correct answers.

Exercise 3

1. Three terms that mean *sugar in the urine* are ______________________, ______________________, and ______________________.

2. The abbreviation that refers to the final phase of kidney disease is ______________________.

3. The abbreviation that refers to an infection in the bladder is ______________________.

4. The term that refers to involuntary urination during sleep is ______________________.

5. The term ______________________ means *narrowing or stricture of the foreskin opening.*

6. The term ______________________ refers to an increased level of urea or other waste in the blood.

7. The term ______________________ refers to an abnormal secretion of large amounts of urine.

8. The term that indicates a chronic condition of inflammation of the bladder lining is ______________________ ______________________.

9. A condition in which the glomeruli suffer gradual, progressive, destructive changes, with a resulting loss of kidney function, is ______________________ ______________________.

10. The term ______________________ refers to inflammation and infection caused by bacterial growth in the renal pelvis and kidney.

11. When the person is unable to urinate or completely empty the bladder, the condition is known as ______________________ ______________________.

12. Leakage of urine when one coughs or sneezes is known as ______________________ ______________________.

13. Two terms that indicate visual examination of the bladder are ______________________ and ______________________.

14. The term ______________________ ______________________ refers to pathological changes in renal tissue that destroy nephrons and impair kidney function.

15. The term that indicates the presence of nitrogenous compounds in the urine is ______________________.

16. The abbreviation that indicates testing done to identify sensitivity to antimicrobial medication in a urine specimen is ______________________.

17. A patient suffering from urinary retention may have a ______________________ ______________________ performed to measure the quantity of retained urine prior to catheterization.

18. ______________________ ______________________ is the radiological examination of the bladder and urethra during urination.

19. The abbreviation used when measuring the patient's total liquid intake and total liquid output is ______________________.

20. A ______________________ may be used to measure an opening.

Multiple Choice

Select the one best answer to the following multiple-choice questions. Check Appendix G for the correct answers.

Exercise 4

1. During her annual health check with her nurse practitioner, Mrs. Tran states that she has recently been experiencing involuntary leakage of urine when she laughs, coughs, or sneezes. Her symptoms are most consistent with which of the following disorders?

   a. Enuresis

   b. Polyuria

   c. Stress incontinence

   d. Nocturia

2. Mrs. Fernandez tells her physician that she has been having pain in her abdomen and lower pelvic area. To gather further information, the physician orders a KUB, an x-ray procedure that specifically looks at the:

   a. Kidney, uterus, and bowel

   b. Kidney stones, urine, and blood

   c. Kyphosis, uremia, and bones

   d. Kidney, ureter, and bladder

3. Mr. Stadnick is a 73-year-old man who complains of increasing episodes of nocturia and frequency. Examination and testing reveal that he is not emptying his bladder completely when he urinates. The physician determines that he has a noncancerous enlargement of his prostate, abbreviated:

   a. TURP

   b. BPH

   c. RP

   d. IVP

4. Ms. Johansen has had chronic complaints of frequency, urgency, dysuria, and intermittent low back and pelvic pain. She was initially treated with antibiotics for a presumed UTI, without any relief. A cystoscopy reveals that she has chronic inflammation of her bladder lining. This is most consistent with which of the following diagnoses?

   a. Urinary retention

   b. Interstitial cystitis

   c. Interstitial nephritis

   d. Uremia

5. Which of the following terms means *a measuring instrument for urine?*

   a. Urogram

   b. Urinoscopy

   c. Urinometer

   d. Urotome

Word Building

*Using **only** the word parts in the lists provided, create medical terms with the indicated meanings. Check Appendix G for the correct answers.*

Exercise 5

Prefixes	**Combining Forms**	**Suffixes**
an-	azot/o	-al
dys-	bacteri/o	-algia
poly-	cyst/o	-ary
	glomerul/o	-dynia
	hemat/o	-ectomy
	lith/o	-gram
	nephr/o	-iasis
	noct/o	-ic
	olig/o	-itis
	py/o	-lith
	pyel/o	-logist
	ren/o	-plasty

Continued

Combining Forms	Suffixes
ureter/o	-scopy
urethr/o	-uria
ur/o	
urin/o	
vesic/o	

1. absence of urination ______
2. much urination ______
3. pus in the urine ______
4. bad, painful, or difficult urination ______
5. pertaining to deficient urination ______
6. pain of the urethra ______
7. visual examination of the bladder ______
8. blood in the urine ______
9. condition of a kidney stone ______
10. urination at night ______
11. bacteria in the urine ______
12. excision or surgical removal of a ureter ______
13. abnormal movement of urine from the bladder into the ureters ______
14. record of the urethra and bladder ______
15. pertaining to urine ______
16. surgical repair of the bladder ______
17. pertaining to the kidneys ______
18. inflammation of the glomerulus and kidney ______
19. nitrogenous compounds in the urine ______
20. specialist in urine (study and treatment of urinary disorders)

______

True or False

Decide whether the following statements are true or false. Check Appendix G for the correct answers.

Exercise 6

1. True False The term **enuresis** indicates involuntary urination during sleep.
2. True False The term **ureterodynia** indicates pain of the urethra.
3. True False The term **oliguric** indicates absence of urination.
4. True False The abbreviation **UTI** stands for *urinary tract infection.*
5. True False The combining form **ureter/o** refers to the urethra.
6. True False The term **diuresis** indicates deficient urination.
7. True False The abbreviation **ESRD** stands for *end-stage renal disease.*
8. True False The term **phimosis** refers to stenosis or narrowing of the foreskin opening of the penis.
9. True False **Interstitial cystitis** is a chronic condition of inflammation of the bladder lining.
10. True False The abbreviation **IVP** stands for *intravenous pyelogram.*

Deciphering Terms

Write the correct meaning of these medical terms. Check Appendix G for the correct answers.

Exercise 7

1. retroperitoneal ____________________
2. meatodilation ____________________
3. cystourethropexy ____________________
4. lithotripsy ____________________
5. urogenic ____________________
6. urostasis ____________________
7. polyuresis ____________________
8. ureterospasm ____________________
9. cystocele ____________________
10. nephromegaly ____________________

Multiple Choice

Select the one best answer to the following multiple-choice questions. Check Appendix G for the correct answers.

Exercise 8

1. Which of the following terms means *involuntary urination during sleep?*
   a. Enuresis
   b. Diuresis
   c. Glycosuria
   d. Uremia

2. A patient with which of the following conditions will typically complain of pain?
   a. Neurogenic bladder
   b. Renal colic
   c. Diuresis
   d. Enuresis

3. Which of the following conditions involves inflammation or infection?
   a. Bacterial cystitis
   b. Pyelonephritis
   c. Glomerulonephritis
   d. All of these

4. Which of the following conditions involves a disruption in urine flow?
   a. Glomerulonephritis
   b. Phimosis
   c. Hydronephrosis
   d. Wilms tumor

5. All of the following abbreviations indicate a procedure **except**:
   a. HD
   b. IVP
   c. VCUG
   d. BNO

6. All of the following abbreviations indicate a urinary-tract disorder **except**:
   a. ATN
   b. BUN
   c. VUR
   d. UTI

7. Which of the following procedures involves microscopic examination of the urine?
   a. AGN
   b. UA
   c. TURP
   d. PKD

8. A patient with kidney stones may benefit from which of the following tests or procedures?
   a. Culture and sensitivity
   b. Extracorporeal shock wave lithotripsy
   c. Urinary catheterization
   d. Voiding cystourethrography

9. Which of the following tests will most accurately help with the diagnosis of urinary retention?
   a. Bladder ultrasound
   b. Blood urea nitrogen
   c. Hemodialysis
   d. Intravenous pyelogram

10. Which of the following terms means *blood in the urine?*
    a. Bacteriuria
    b. Hematuria
    c. Pyuria
    d. Oliguria

11. Which of the following terms means *sugar in the blood?*
    a. Glycosuria
    b. Glucogenesis
    c. Glomerulosis
    d. Glycemia

12. Which of the following terms indicates absence of urination?
    a. Oliguria
    b. Anuria
    c. Polyuria
    d. Nocturia

13. Which of the following terms means *pertaining to the bladder and urethra?*
    a. Cystoureteral
    b. Vesicourethroid
    c. Cholecystic
    d. None of these

14. All of the following combining forms indicate sugar **except**:
    a. Gluc/o
    b. Glyc/o
    c. Glomerul/o
    d. Glycos/o

15. Which of the following combining forms refers to pus?
    a. Pyel/o
    b. Peritone/o
    c. Py/o
    d. None of these

16. Which of the following combining forms means *stone?*
    a. Lith/o
    b. Azot/o
    c. Cyst/o
    d. None of these

17. Which of the following combining forms means *deficiency?*
    a. Nephr/o
    b. Vesic/o
    c. Pyel/o
    d. Olig/o

18. The term *urostasis* means:
    a. Absence of urination
    b. Cessation or stopping of urine
    c. Movement of urine
    d. Resembling urine

19. The term *ureteroscope* means:
    a. Visualization of the urethra
    b. Viewing instrument for the ureter
    c. Mouthlike opening into the ureter
    d. None of these

20. The term *nephrocentesis* means:
    a. Surgical puncture of the kidney
    b. Hernia of the kidney
    c. Behind the kidney
    d. None of these

11 REPRODUCTIVE SYSTEM

Structure and Function

The major function of the male and female reproductive systems is procreation. They work together in a complementary fashion to join a sperm and an egg at the moment of conception to create a new human being.

Male Reproductive System

The male reproductive system shares some structures with other body systems, including the penis and urethra, shared by the urinary system, and the testes, shared by the endocrine system. Other structures within the male reproductive system include the prostate gland, the scrotum, and a series of ducts and glands (see Fig. 11-1).

Flashpoint
Male sperm cells contain half of the genetic material needed to form a new human being.

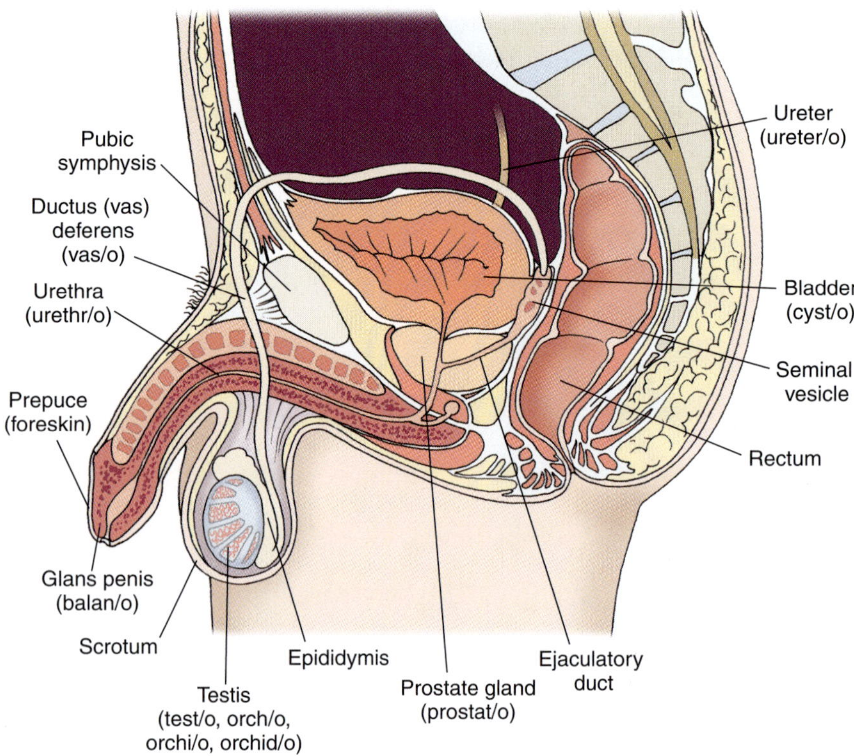

FIGURE 11-1 The male reproductive system

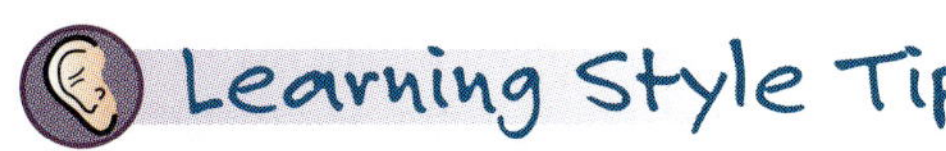

If you are a strong auditory learner, you may notice that you take incomplete lecture notes because you focus more energy on listening than writing. If this is the case, consider getting the notes from a classmate who is a more thorough note taker. Or better yet, ask for your instructor's permission to record lectures to play back at a later time, with the purpose of filling in the gaps in your own notes.

The **testes** are located within the **scrotum**. They are oval-shaped structures composed of an outer capsule, made of thick, white connective tissue, and an inner part divided into 200 to 300 lobules, which contain the seminiferous tubules. Spermatogenesis (creation of sperm cells) occurs here. Spermatocytes are the male reproductive cells, which carry half of the genetic material needed to form a new human being. They are sensitive to heat and must live within an environment that is slightly below normal body temperature.

Therefore, prior to birth, the testes in the male fetus normally descend from the lower abdomen into the scrotum. The scrotum is composed of two internal compartments surrounded by loose connective tissue and a smooth muscle layer. A second muscle group, called the cremasters, extends from the abdomen into the scrotum. The structures of the scrotum are designed to maintain an optimal temperature for spermatogenesis. In a cold environment, the smooth muscle of the scrotum and the cremaster muscles contract, bringing the scrotum and testes closer to the body to keep them warmer. In a warm environment, the same muscles relax and allow the scrotum and testes to descend away from the body to keep them cooler. When spermatocytes have reached a sufficient stage of maturity, they exit the testes through a series of ducts beginning with the **seminiferous tubules,** then the **rete testis, efferent ductules, epididymis, vas deferens,** and finally the **ejaculatory duct,** which joins with the **urethra.** From there they exit the body during ejaculation.

The penis is composed of three sections of erectile tissue and a distal, rounded end, which is the glans penis. A fold of skin commonly called the **foreskin** covers the glans penis. In many cultures, a procedure called circumcision is commonly practiced, in which part or all of the foreskin is removed.

The urethra serves a dual purpose, as the exit passageway for both urine and semen; however, both do not exit at the same time. During sexual activity, the internal urinary sphincter contracts to keep semen from entering the bladder and to keep urine from exiting the bladder.

Flashpoint

Circumcision is a procedure in which part or all of the foreskin is removed.

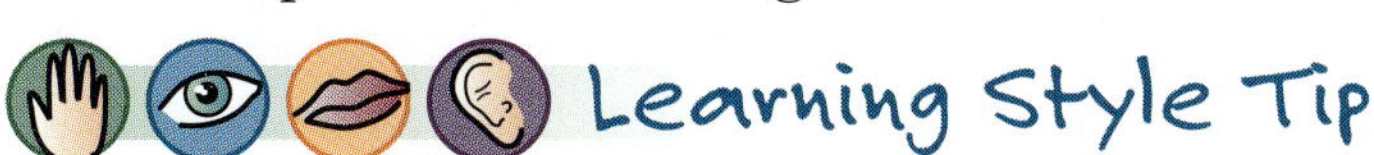

Complete the interactive activities on the student disc that accompanies this text. They provide a fun way to practice your new medical terminology while appealing to all learning styles.

During arousal, the erectile tissue of the penis becomes engorged with blood and the penis becomes firm and erect, to facilitate sexual intercourse and ejaculation. The state of erection ends with ejaculation, also known as semen or seminal fluid, or when sexual arousal diminishes.

Secretions from a variety of sources contribute to the seminal fluid. Mucous secretions from the **bulbourethral glands** and the inner urethral wall lubricate the urethra and neutralize its normally acidic environment. **Seminal vesicles** secrete fructose and other nutrients for sperm cells. They also secrete a substance called prostaglandin, which stimulates smooth muscle contractions in the female reproductive tract. This is thought to help move sperm through that environment. The prostate gland secretes prostatic fluid that flows through a number of ducts to the urethra and helps to create a more alkaline environment, which is important to sperm motility.

Flashpoint
In males, the urethra serves a dual purpose, as a route for both urine and semen.

Female Reproductive System

The female reproductive system is made of internal and external structures. The primary function of the female reproductive system is to bear offspring, or produce another human being. The internal and external organs and structures of the female reproductive system all function toward achieving this ultimate goal. The female reproductive system also manufactures hormones (chemicals secreted into the bloodstream that cause bodily reactions) that are necessary for the development and functioning of reproductive organs.

Internal organs and structures of the female reproductive system include the ovaries, fallopian tubes, uterus, cervix, and vagina (see Fig. 11-2).

Flashpoint
The ovaries and the testes are somewhat round in shape, like the letter O. Terms associated with the ovaries and testes usually have lots of Os in them: *ovari/o, oophor/o, orch/o, orchi/o, orchid/o,* and so on.

The **ovaries** are oval-shaped structures located on each side of the uterus in the lower abdominal cavity, attached to the broad ligament. They are the primary sex organs in females. They contain graafian follicles, in which are immature ova, or eggs. Approximately every 28 days one of the ovaries produces a mature ovum, which contains one half of the necessary components of a new life. The ovaries also produce the two female hormones estrogen and progesterone. Estrogen acts to develop the female reproductive organs during puberty, produces secondary sexual characteristics such as breasts and pubic hair, and prepares the uterus for a fertilized egg. Progesterone is responsible for the changes in the endometrium (uterine lining) in preparation for implantation of a developing embryo.

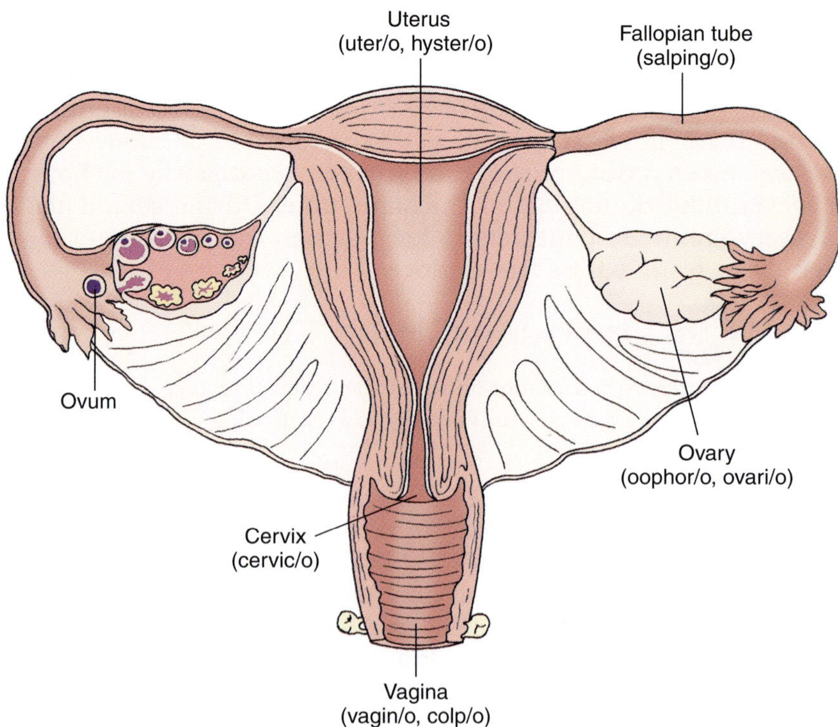

FIGURE 11-2 **The female reproductive system**

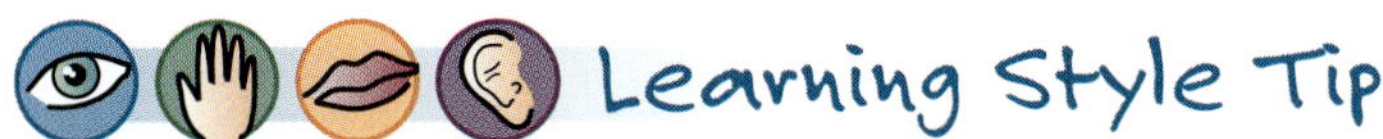

Study Figures 11-1 and 11-2 and then draw them as accurately as you can from memory. Add anatomical labels and related combining forms. If you are a verbal or an auditory learner, be sure to speak aloud as you do so. Next, check your work against the book illustrations and make any needed corrections.

The two fallopian tubes extend approximately 4 inches from the sides of the uterus toward the ovaries. Although the fallopian tubes do not connect to the ovaries directly, they are attached to the broad ligament for stability. Each fallopian tube ends with structures called **fimbriae**. They move in a wavelike fashion to help direct the ovum into the tube through which it travels on its way to the uterus. As the ovum travels down the fallopian tube, the ovary secretes estrogen and progesterone, which act to change the endometrial lining of the uterus to become more receptive to implantation.

Flashpoint
The fimbriae help direct the ovum into the fallopian tubes.

The **uterus** is a thick-walled, muscular organ located behind the urinary bladder and in front of the rectum. It consists of the **fundus**, the rounded upper portion; the **corpus**, the body of the uterus; and the **cervix**, the narrowed section that opens into the vagina. The cavity of the uterus is triangular in shape; the innermost lining is called the **endometrium**. The myometrium, or muscular wall of the uterus, consists of muscle fibers that run in many directions, including circular, longitudinal, and diagonal. During pregnancy, the cervix and uterus house and protect the developing fetus. The muscular tissue of the uterus is able to expand during pregnancy to accommodate the growing fetus. The cervix dilates during the birth process to allow delivery of the fetus. The multidirectional muscles of the myometrium also enable forceful contraction of the uterus during the birth process. The **vagina** connects the cervix with the external surface. It acts as the passageway for the penis during sexual intercourse and as the birth canal during the birth process.

The external structures of the female reproductive system, also called the **vulva**, include the clitoris, urethral meatus, labia, mons pubis, and Bartholin glands (see Fig. 11-3). This area in men and women is also called the **perineum**.

The **clitoris**, made up of elongated erectile tissue, is located beneath the anterior portion of the labia. It responds to stimulation, causing orgasm. The urethral meatus, located posterior to the clitoris and anterior to the vaginal opening, is the opening to the urinary bladder. The **labia** consist of two layers, covering and protecting the clitoris, urethral meatus, and vaginal opening. The inner labia minora extends from the anterior clitoris to the posterior aspect of the vaginal opening. The outer labia majora forms the lateral borders of the vulva. The labia majora and mons pubis, the pad of fatty tissue that covers the pubic symphysis (or **pubic bone**), are covered in coarse hair.

During puberty, increased secretion of estrogen causes **breast** development (see Fig. 11-4). The center surface of each breast has a region of pigmented tissue called the **areola**. At the center of the areola is the **nipple**. Inside each breast are 15 to 20 lobes of glandular tissue, including mammary glands, which are milk-producing glands in a female. This glandular tissue is surrounded by connective tissue, which provides support, and adipose tissue, which provides insulation. The amount and distribution of adipose tissue determine the size and shape of the breasts. The role of the breasts in reproduction is nourishing the neonate, or newborn baby, with the mother's breast milk, a process called **lactation**.

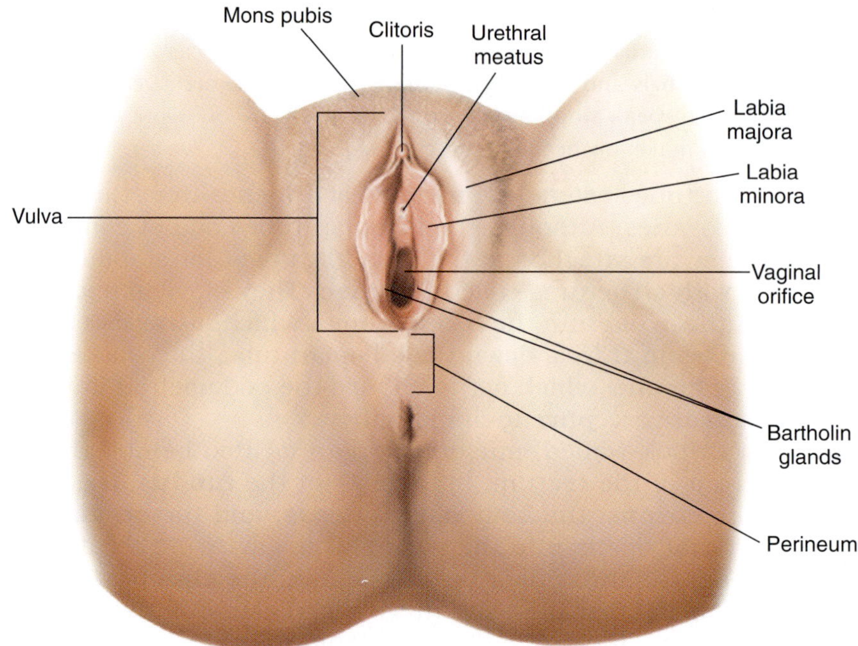

FIGURE 11-3 **External structures of the female reproductive system** (From Eagle, S, et al.: *The Professional Medical Assistant.* F.A. Davis, Philadelphia, 2009, p. 602; with permission)

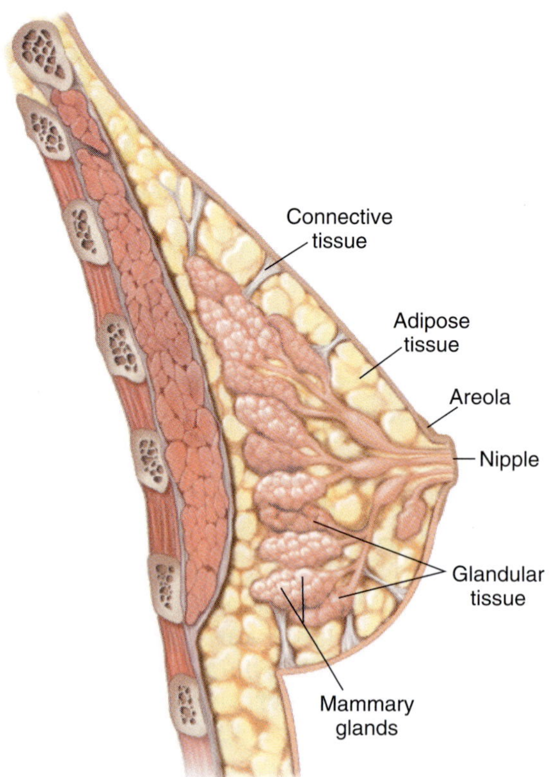

FIGURE 11-4 **Female breast** (From Eagle, S, et al.: *The Professional Medical Assistant.* F.A. Davis, Philadelphia, 2009, p. 602; with permission)

The mammary glands of the breasts produce milk in response to the later part of pregnancy and after giving birth. During pregnancy, the breasts respond to four different hormones: Estrogen increases breast size, progesterone stimulates the development of the duct system (for lactation), prolactin stimulates milk production, and oxytocin promotes the flow of milk from the glands.

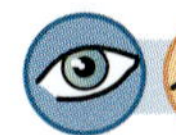 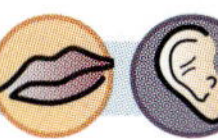 Learning Style Tip

Arrange with your study group or study buddy to each write at least 10 medical-terminology "test" questions. For variety, write several multiple-choice, several true-false, and a couple fill-in-the-blank questions. Don't make them too easy. Next, get together with your group and challenge each other with your questions.

Female Reproductive Cycle

The female reproductive system follows a cycle that parallels the lifespan. The cycle includes menarche, menstruation, pregnancy and childbirth (for some women), and menopause.

Menarche (onset of menstruation) varies widely in adolescent females, with the average age of onset being 13 years. Menstruation, also called the **menstrual cycle** or **menses**, occurs approximately every 28 days, but this timing varies. During menstruation, the uterus sheds the layer of endometrial tissue that develops each month in preparation for pregnancy. Phases of the 28-day cycle include the follicular, luteal, and menstrual phases.

During the **follicular phase**, the hypothalamus of the brain secretes gonadotropin-releasing hormone (GnRH), which stimulates the anterior pituitary gland to secrete follicle-stimulating hormone (FSH) and luteinizing hormone (LH). These hormones act on the graafian follicles within the ovaries to secrete estrogen, which stimulates the growth and thickening of the endometrium. Between day 9 and day 14, the ripened graafian follicle ruptures out of the ovarian wall and begins to secrete the hormone progesterone. Some women know when they are ovulating because they experience mild to moderately sharp pain on the side of the ovulating ovary. The next month they may notice similar pain on their other side.

During the **luteal phase**, the ovum (egg cell) is propelled toward the fallopian tube by the wavelike action of the fimbriae. During this phase, progesterone produced by the corpus luteum, the remainder of the follicle after a woman ovulates, continues to cause extensive growth of the functional layer of the endometrium. If fertilization of the ovum, also called **conception**, occurs, the corpus luteum will secrete human chorionic gonadotropin (HCG). If no conception occurs, the corpus luteum does not secrete HCG, but instead atrophies into a mass of fibrous tissue called the **corpus albicans**. In the absence of HCG and with decreasing progesterone levels, the endometrium begins to deteriorate, and menstruation begins.

Flashpoint

Several hormones act together to trigger ovulation and prepare the uterus for potential pregnancy.

The third and final phase of the menstrual cycle is the **menstrual phase**. In this phase, the uterus sheds the unneeded endometrial lining. The menstrual phase lasts between 5 and 7 days, after which the follicular phase begins again (see Fig. 11-5).

 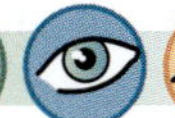 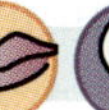 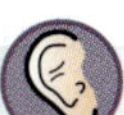 Learning Style Tip

Study with a study buddy. Take turns challenging each other by using the flash cards provided in this book. Show just one side of the card while your partner guesses the information contained on the other side. After you've each taken a turn, repeat the process with the cards flipped to the other side.

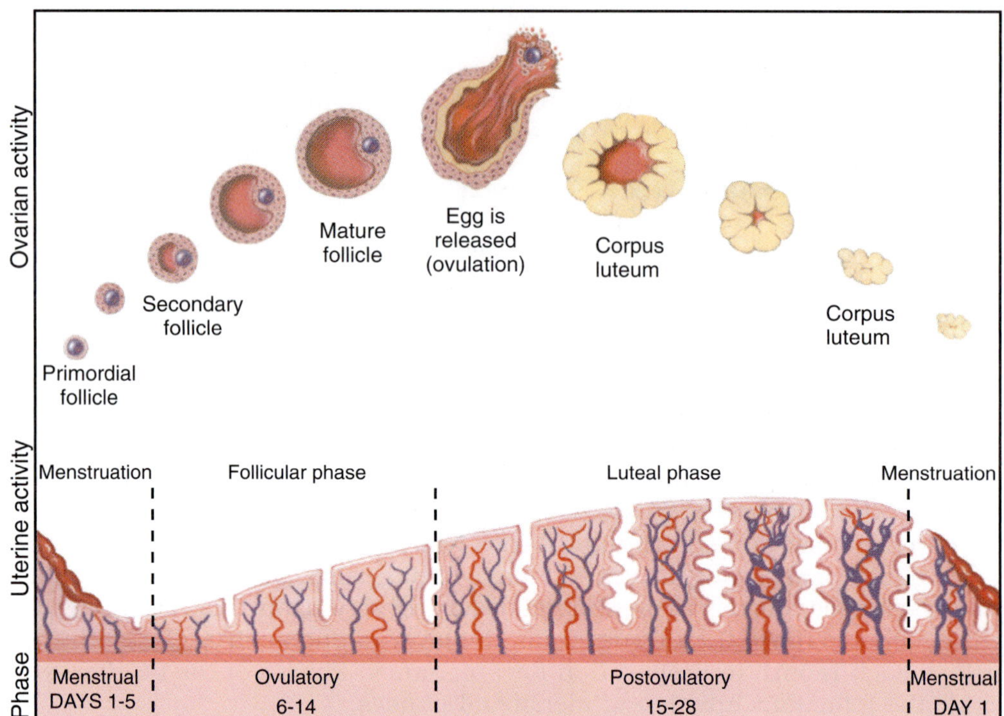

FIGURE 11-5 **Phases of the menstrual cycle** (From Eagle, S, et al.: *The Professional Medical Assistant.* F.A. Davis, Philadelphia, 2009, p. 605; with permission)

Pregnancy

Fertilization occurs when one sperm penetrates an egg and forms a zygote. The resulting zygote has 23 chromosomes from the ovum and 23 chromosomes from the sperm. The zygote immediately begins growing and multiplying as it travels down the fallopian tube. When it reaches the uterus in 4 to 6 days, it implants into the uterine wall. Implantation of the zygote causes a change in the menstrual cycle: The ovaries respond to implantation by releasing high levels of estrogen and progesterone, which increases the endometrium's receptivity to implantation. The corpus luteum secretes a substance called inhibin. As its name implies, inhibin acts to inhibit secretion of FSH in the anterior pituitary gland. It also causes the secretion of relaxin, which prevents uterine contraction, increasing the likelihood of successful zygote implantation. The resulting low level of FSH, along with low levels of LH, prevents stimulation of a new follicle and disrupts the 28-day menstrual cycle. After implantation, the placenta, the organ of nutrition for the growing zygote, forms within the wall of the uterus.

As the zygote develops into an **embryo** and then a **fetus**, the placenta also grows to provide nourishment and oxygen. The placenta begins forming early after conception and is completely formed by 12 weeks. The mature, disk-shaped placenta is approximately 7 inches in diameter. It adheres to the wall of the uterus and connects to the developing fetus through the umbilical cord. The umbilical cord contains two arteries and one vein; the arteries supply oxygen and nutrients to the fetus while the vein removes carbon dioxide and wastes. The corpus luteum secretes human chorionic gonadotropin (HCG), a hormone that stimulates the maternal ovary so that it will continue to secrete estrogen and progesterone. As the placenta increases in size, it secretes estrogen and progesterone itself, and HCG levels in the bloodstream drop. Estrogen prevents the secretion of FSH and LH (in the anterior pituitary gland), which prevents the normal menstrual cycle. Progesterone prevents contractions of the uterus that could result in a miscarriage.

Pregnancy, also called **gestation**, is broken into three equal time periods called **trimesters**. The first trimester lasts to 12 weeks. During this period, the zygote becomes an **embryo** and develops all its tissues and organs. At 9 weeks, the embryo is called a **fetus**. Symptoms commonly experienced by the pregnant woman during the first trimester include fatigue, nausea, vomiting, breast tenderness, urinary frequency, constipation, and insomnia.

Flashpoint

The placenta delivers nutrients and oxygen to the developing fetus.

The second trimester begins around week 13. At 15 to 28 weeks, the uterus expands to above the umbilicus, and the expectant mother can feel the first fetal movements. By 20 weeks the fetus can open its eyes, and by 24 weeks it can hear sounds made outside the uterus. As the second trimester progresses, fetal movements become more vigorous, and the mother may be aware of when the fetus is sleeping or awake. This is a time of rapid growth, during which the fetus develops eyelashes, eyebrows, and subcutaneous fat deposits. Even so, the fetus still weighs less than 2 pounds and is not yet ready for birth.

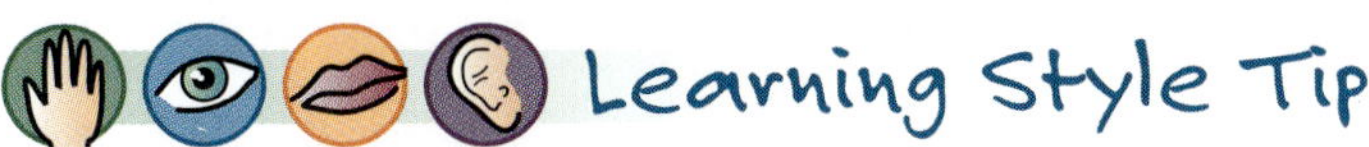

Meet your friend for a study date. Take turns looking up pathological conditions in a medical dictionary and reading the definition aloud to each other.

During the third trimester, the fetus adds more subcutaneous fat, the lungs grow toward full development, and the testes descend in males. Maternal weight gain can be in excess of 1 pound per week. During this trimester, the mother may experience low back pain and fatigue, due to increasing fetal size and quantity of amniotic fluid. By the end of the seventh month, or 28 weeks, the fetus has typically moved into the head-down position in anticipation of birth. At full term, 38 to 40 weeks, average fetal weight is around 3,400 grams ($7^1/_2$ pounds) (see Fig. 11-6).

Flashpoint

Pregnancy lasts about 40 weeks, and average newborn infants typically weigh about 7 pounds.

Birth Process

Toward the end of gestation, the placental secretion of progesterone decreases, while the levels of estrogen remain high. The uterus begins to gently contract at irregular intervals. These early **Braxton Hicks contractions** are sometimes called *false labor.* The beginning of labor and delivery is usually signaled by the expulsion of the mucous plug that develops in the cervix to protect the fetus from organisms in the vagina. After expulsion of the mucous plug, amniotic fluid may begin to leak slowly or may flow quickly. The uterus begins more rhythmic contractions due to the drop in the secretion of progesterone from the placenta.

The first stage of active labor begins with dilation (expansion or opening) and effacement (thinning) of the cervix. The degree of cervical dilation is measured in centimeters, from 1 to 10 centimeters. At 10 centimeters, the cervix is large enough to accommodate delivery. Uterine contractions increase in frequency and intensity in this stage, which can last from 1 to 24 hours.

The second stage of labor involves delivery of the infant. In this stage, the posterior pituitary gland secretes oxytocin, a powerful hormone that causes even more forceful contraction of the uterus. During these contractions, the woman typically feels the need to "push," or bear down. Eventually the top of the infant's head appears at the cervical opening, a process called **crowning**. As soon as the infant's head delivers, it rotates to the side, and then the shoulders are delivered, followed by the rest of the body.

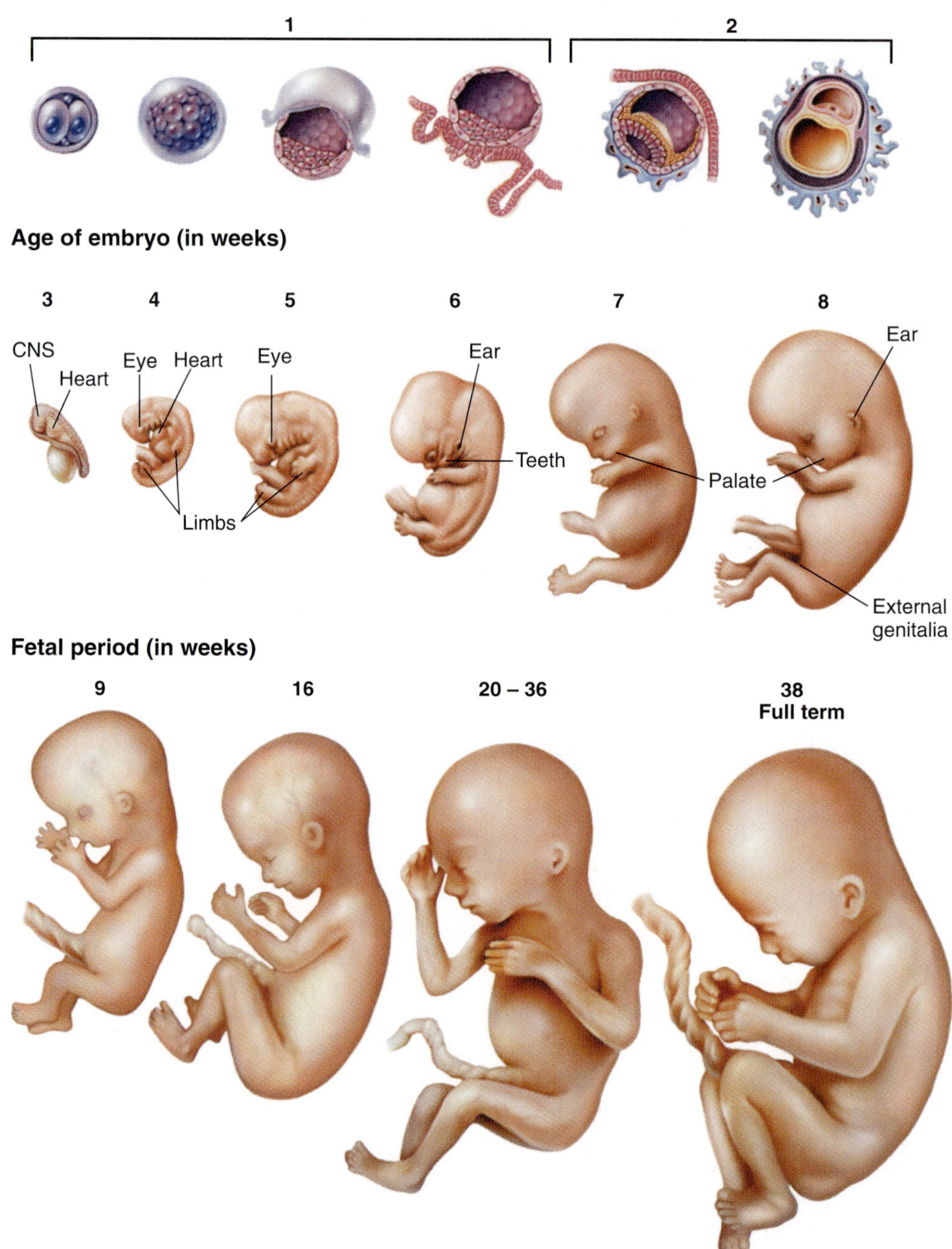

FIGURE 11-6 **Stages of embryonic and fetal development** (From Eagle, S, et al.: *The Professional Medical Assistant.* F.A. Davis, Philadelphia, 2009, p. 606; with permission)

In the third stage of labor, the placenta detaches from the uterine wall and is expelled from the body, usually with a few more uterine contractions. The uterus continues to contract after delivery, to constrict blood vessels and control bleeding.

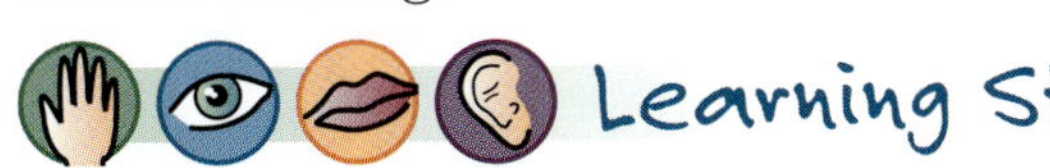

Learning Style Tip

Identify whether there are museums in your area with anatomical displays. One that allows you to touch the displays would be especially useful. Visit and study the models. Touch the displays only if allowed to do so.

Menopause

The menstrual cycle continues throughout a woman's life until a period called **menopause**, the normal cessation of menses. Menopause occurs naturally in most women approximately 40 years after menarche. Menses may stop suddenly, or the flow and frequency of menses may decrease gradually.

Symptoms of menopause begin soon after the ovaries stop functioning, vary widely in severity, and may last from a few months to several years. Common signs and symptoms of menopause include hot flashes, chills, night sweats, mood swings, and insomnia. Treatment of menopausal symptoms may include hormone replacement therapy (HRT). However, because there are some associated risks, each woman should consult with her health-care provider to determine whether or not HRT is a viable option for her.

Flashpoint

Menopause typically occurs about 40 years after menarche.

Combining Forms

Tables 11-1 and 11-2 contain combining forms that pertain to the male and female reproductive systems, respectively, along with examples of terms that utilize the combining forms, and a pronunciation guide. Read aloud to yourself as you move from left to right across the table. Be sure to use the pronunciation guide so that you can learn to say the terms correctly.

TABLE 11-1
COMBINING FORMS RELATED TO THE MALE REPRODUCTIVE SYSTEM

Combining Form	Meaning	Example (Pronunciation)	Meaning of New Term
andr/o	male	androgynous (ăn-DRŎJ-ĭ-nŭs)	pertaining to male and female
balan/o	glans penis	balanitis (băl-ă-NĪ-tĭs)	inflammation of the glans penis
crypt/o	hidden	cryptorchidism (krĭpt-OR-kĭd-ĭ-zum)	condition of hidden testes
epididym/o	epididymis	epididymitis (ĕp-ĭ-dĭd-ĭ-MĪ-tĭs)	inflammation of the epididymis

Continued

TABLE 11-1

COMBINING FORMS RELATED TO THE MALE REPRODUCTIVE SYSTEM—cont'd

Combining Form	Meaning	Example (Pronunciation)	Meaning of New Term
orch/o	testis	orchiopathy (ōr-kē-OP-ă-thē)	disease of a testis
orchi/o		orchiectomy (ŏr-kē-ĔK-tō-mē)	surgical removal of a testis
orchid/o		orchidopexy (ŎR-kĭ-dō-pĕk-sē)	surgical fixation of a testis
test/o		testomegaly (tĕs-tō-MĔG-ă-lē)	enlargement of a testis
testicul/o		testicular (tĕs-TĬK-ū-lăr)	pertaining to the testes
phall/i	penis	phalloid (FĂL-oyd)	resembling a penis
prostat/o	prostate	prostatoplasty (PRŎS-tă-tō-plăs-tē)	surgical repair of the prostate
semin/o	sperm	seminuria (sē-mĭn-Ū-rē-ă)	semen in the urine
sperm/o		aspermia (ă-SPĔR-mē-ă)	condition of no sperm
spermat/o		spermatogenesis (spĕr-măt-ō-JĔN-ĕ-sĭs)	production of sperm
vas/o	vessel	vasotomy (văs-ŎT-ō-mē)	cutting into or incision of a vessel

TABLE 11-2

COMBINING FORMS RELATED TO THE FEMALE REPRODUCTIVE SYSTEM

Combining Form	Meaning	Example (Pronunciation)	Meaning of New Term
amni/o	amnion (amniotic sac), amniotic fluid	amniocentesis (ăm-nē-ō-sĕn-TĒ-sĭs)	surgical puncture of the amnion
cervic/o	cervix	cervical (SĔR-vĭ-kăl)	pertaining to the cervix
colp/o	vagina	colposcopy (kŏl-PŎS-kō-pē)	visual examination of the vagina
vagin/o		vaginopexy (VĂJ-ĭn-ō-pĕk-sē)	surgical fixation of the vagina
embry/o	embryo	embryonic (ĕm-brē-ŎN-ĭk)	pertaining to an embryo
episi/o	vulva	episiotomy (ĕ-pĭz-ē-ŎT-ō-mē)	cutting into or incision of the vulva (perineum)
vulv/o		vulvodynia (vŭl-vō-DĬN-ē-ă)	pain of the vulva

TABLE 11-2

COMBINING FORMS RELATED TO THE FEMALE REPRODUCTIVE SYSTEM—cont'd

Combining Form	Meaning	Example (Pronunciation)	Meaning of New Term
fet/o	fetus	fetotoxic (fē-tō-TŎK-sĭk)	poisonous to a fetus
galact/o	milk	galactorrhea (gă-lăk-tō-RĒ-ă)	flow or discharge of milk
lact/o		lactotherapy (lăk-tō-THĔR-ă-pē)	milk therapy
gonad/o	gonads	gonadectomy (gŏn-ă-DĔK-tō-mē)	surgical removal of a gonad
gynec/o	woman, female	gynecology (gī-nĕ-KŎL-ō-jē)	study of female (disorders)
hyster/o	uterus	hysterotomy (hĭs-tĕr-ŎT-ō-mē)	cutting into or incision of the uterus
metr/o		metrocarcinoma (MET-ro-kärs-ă-nō-mă)	cancerous tumor of the uterus
uter/o		uterocervical (ū-tĕr-ō-SĔR-vĭ-kăl)	pertaining to the uterus and cervix
lapar/o	abdomen, abdominal wall	laparoscopy (lăp-ăr-ŎS-kō-pē)	visual examination of the abdomen
mamm/o	breast	mammoplasty (MĂM-ō-plăs-tē)	surgical repair of a breast
mast/o		mastectomy (măs-TĔK-tō-mē)	surgical removal of a breast
men/o	menses	dysmenorrhea (dĭs-mĕn-ō-RĒ-ă)	bad, painful, or difficult menstrual flow
nat/o	birth	natal (NĀ-tăl)	pertaining to birth
oophor/o	ovary	oophorectomy (ō-ŏf-ō-RĔK-tō-mē)	surgical removal of an ovary
ovari/o		ovarioptosis (ō-vă-rē-ŏp-TŌ-sĭs)	prolapse of an ovary
ov/o	ovum	ovogenesis (ō-vō-JĔN-ĕ-sĭs)	creation of an ovum
perine/o	perineum	perineoplasty (pĕr-ĭ-NĒ-ō-plăs-tē)	surgical repair of the perineum
placent/o	placenta	placental (plă-SĔN-tăl)	pertaining to the placenta
salping/o	tube (fallopian or eustachian)	salpingitis (săl-pĭn-JĪ-tĭs)	inflammation of a fallopian tube
son/o	sound	sonorous (sun-ŌR-ŭs)	full and loud in sound
vagin/a	vagina	vaginapexy (vă-JĪ-nă-pexē)	surgical fixation of the vagina

STOP HERE.
Select the Combining Form Flash Cards for Chapter 11 and run through them at least three times before you continue.

Practice Exercises

Fill in the Blanks

Fill in the blanks below using Table 11-1. Check Appendix G for the correct answers.

Exercise 1

1. resembling a penis ______________________
2. surgical removal of a testis ______________________
3. cutting into or incision of a vessel ______________________
4. pertaining to male and female ______________________
5. inflammation of the glans penis ______________________
6. production of sperm ______________________
7. condition of hidden testes ______________________
8. surgical fixation of a testis ______________________
9. inflammation of the epididymis ______________________
10. enlargement of a testis ______________________
11. disease of a testis ______________________
12. surgical repair of the prostate ______________________
13. pertaining to the penis and scrotum ______________________
14. condition of no sperm ______________________
15. pertaining to the testes ______________________
16. semen in the urine ______________________
17. **Fill in the blanks in Figure 11-7 with the appropriate anatomical terms and combining forms.**

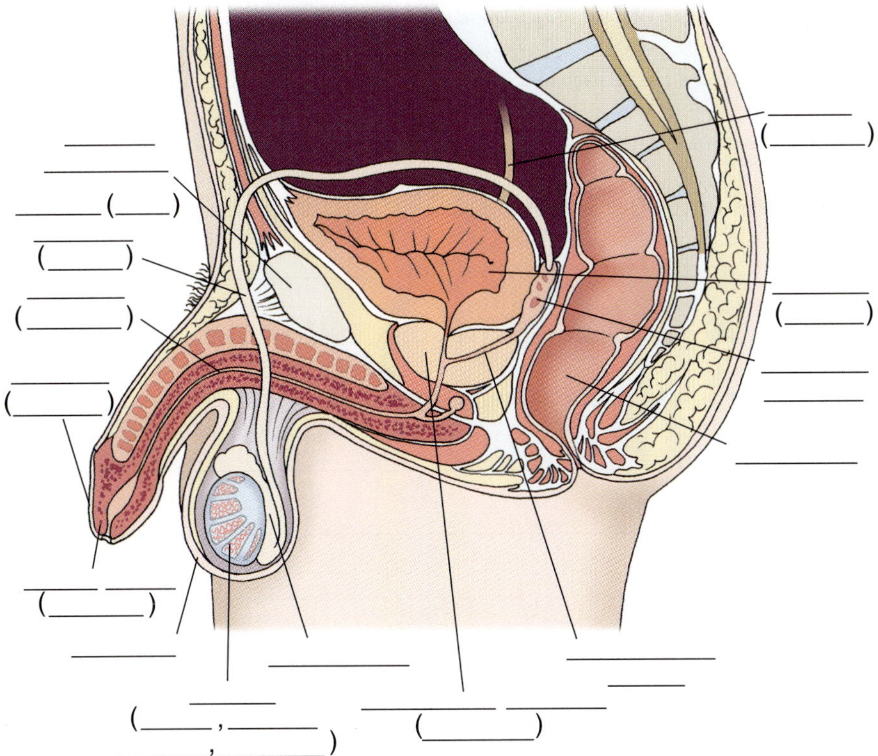

FIGURE 11-7 **Male reproductive system with blanks**

Fill in the Blanks

Fill in the blanks below using Table 11-2. Check Appendix G for the correct answers.

Exercise 2

1. surgical puncture of the amnion ______________________________
2. prolapse of the ovary ______________________________
3. pertaining to the embryo ______________________________
4. pertaining to the cervix ______________________________
5. poisonous to the fetus ______________________________
6. surgical removal of an ovary ______________________________
7. flow or discharge of milk ______________________________
8. pertaining to the uterus ______________________________
9. milk therapy ______________________________

10. visual examination of the vagina ______

11. surgical removal of a gonad ______

12. surgical repair of a breast ______

13. cancerous tumor of the uterus ______

14. bad, painful, or difficult menstrual flow ______

15. pertaining to the uterus and cervix ______

16. cutting into or incision of the vulva (perineum) ______

17. creation of an ovum ______

18. pain of the vulva ______

19. prolapse of the ovary ______

20. cutting into or incision of the uterus ______

21. surgical repair of the perineum ______

22. visual examination of the abdomen ______

23. pertaining to the placenta ______

24. inflammation of a fallopian tube ______

25. full or loud in sound ______

26. surgical removal of a breast ______

27. study of female (disorders) ______

28. pertaining to birth ______

29. surgical fixation of the vagina ______

30. **Fill in the blanks in Figure 11-8 with the appropriate anatomical terms and combining forms.**

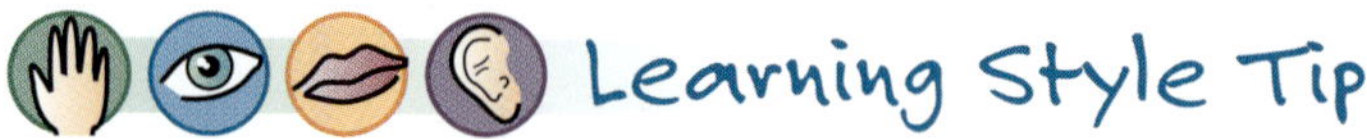

Trace your finger across the terms as you read them and the definitions aloud. Then close your eyes, visualize each term, and say it and its corresponding definition aloud again.

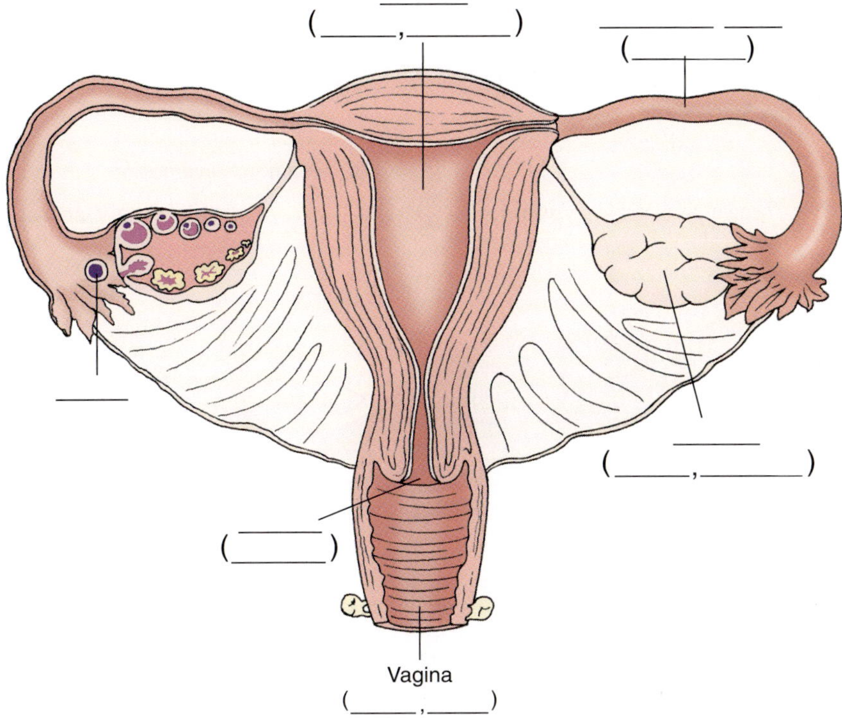

FIGURE 11-8 **Female reproductive system with blanks**

Abbreviations

Table 11-3 lists some of the most common abbreviations related to the reproductive system, as well as others often used in medical documentation.

TABLE 11-3
ABBREVIATIONS

Female Reproductive System			
♀	female	L&D	labor and delivery
AB	abortion	LMP	last menstrual period
BSE	breast self-examination	OB-GYN	obstetrics and gynecology
C-section	cesarean section	OC	oral contraceptive
D&C	dilation and curettage	Pap	Papanicolaou smear
EDC	estimated date of confinement (due date)	PID	pelvic inflammatory disease
ERT, HRT	estrogen replacement therapy, hormone replacement therapy	PMS	premenstrual syndrome
FHR	fetal heart rate	TAH	total abdominal hysterectomy
GYN	gynecology	TAH-BSO	total abdominal hysterectomy, bilateral salpingo-oophorectomy
IUD	intrauterine device	TSS	toxic shock syndrome
IVF	in vitro fertilization		

Continued

TABLE 11-3

ABBREVIATIONS—cont'd

Male Reproductive System

♂	male	CIRC, circum	circumcision
BPH	benign prostatic hypertrophy; also called *benign prostatic hyperplasia* (see Fig. 11-9)	DRE	digital rectal examination

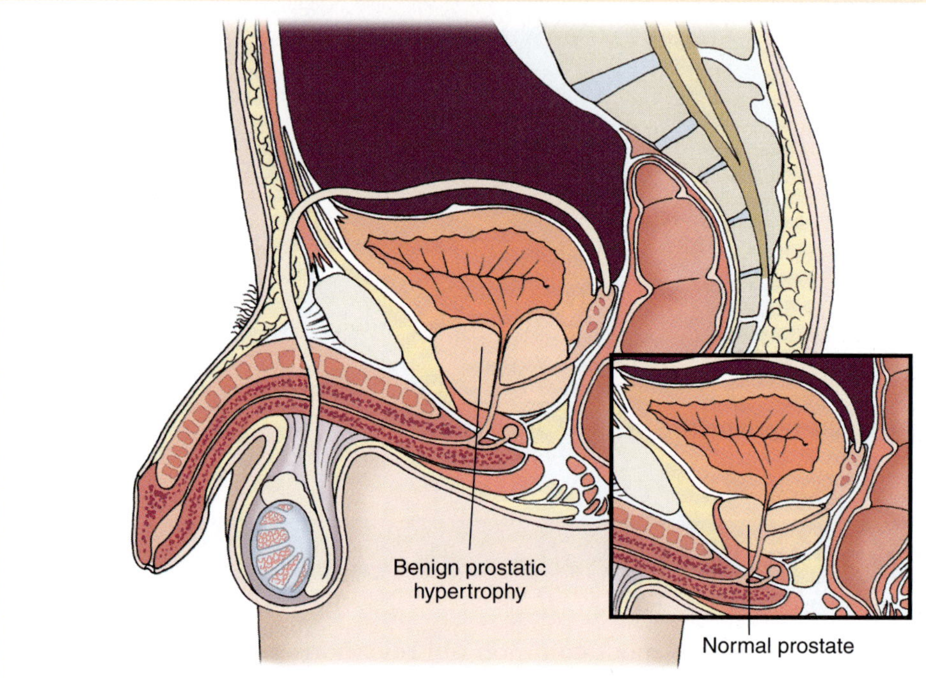

FIGURE 11-9 **Benign prostatic hypertrophy**

ED	erectile dysfunction	TSE	testicular self-examination
PSA	prostate-specific antigen	TURP	transurethral resection of the prostate

Male and Female Reproductive Systems

GC	gonorrhea	Trich	Trichomoniasis
GU	genitourinary	VD	venereal disease; sexually transmitted disease
HPV	human papilloma virus		
STD, STI	sexually transmitted disease, sexually transmitted infection		

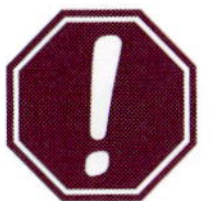

STOP HERE.
Select the Abbreviation Flash Cards for Chapter 11 and run through them at least three times before you continue.

Pathology Terms

Table 11-4 includes terms that relate to diseases or abnormalities of the reproductive system. Use the pronunciation guide and say the terms aloud as you read them. This will help you get in the habit of saying them properly.

TABLE 11-4
PATHOLOGY TERMS

Female Reproductive System	
amenorrhea (ă-mĕn-ō-RĒ-ă)	absence of menses in a woman between the ages of 16 and 40
Bartholin gland cyst (BĂR-tō-lĭn glănd sĭst)	blockage of one or both of the Bartholin glands, causing inflammation and tenderness (see Fig. 11-10)

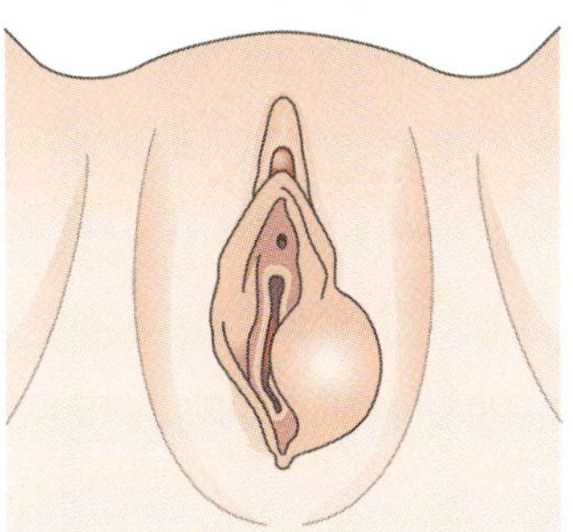

FIGURE 11-10 **Bartholin gland cyst**

candidiasis (kăn-dĭ-DĪ-ă-sĭs)	vaginal fungal infection caused by *Candida albicans,* with key Sx including itching, burning, and a thick, curdy discharge; also known as a vaginal *yeast infection* (see Fig. 11-11)

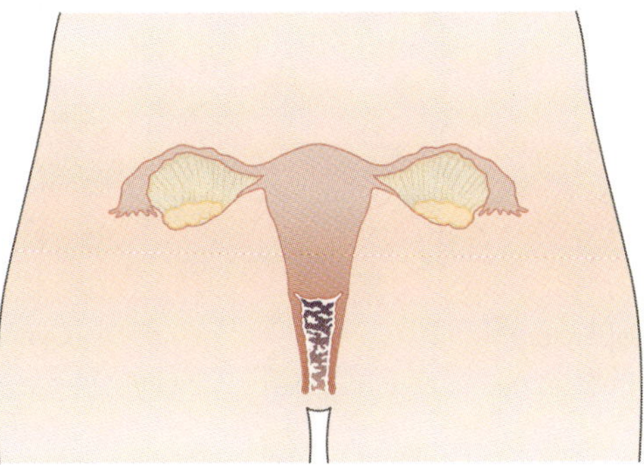

FIGURE 11-11 ***Candida albicans*** **(vaginal yeast infection)**

Continued

TABLE 11-4

PATHOLOGY TERMS—cont'd

Female Reproductive System	
dysmenorrhea (dĭs-mĕn-ō-RĒ-ă)	pain in the lower abdominopelvic area and other discomfort associated with menses
ectopic pregnancy (ĕk-TŎ-pĭk PRĔG-năn-sē)	implantation of a fertilized ovum outside of the uterus, often in the fallopian tube; also called *tubal pregnancy* (see Fig. 11-12)

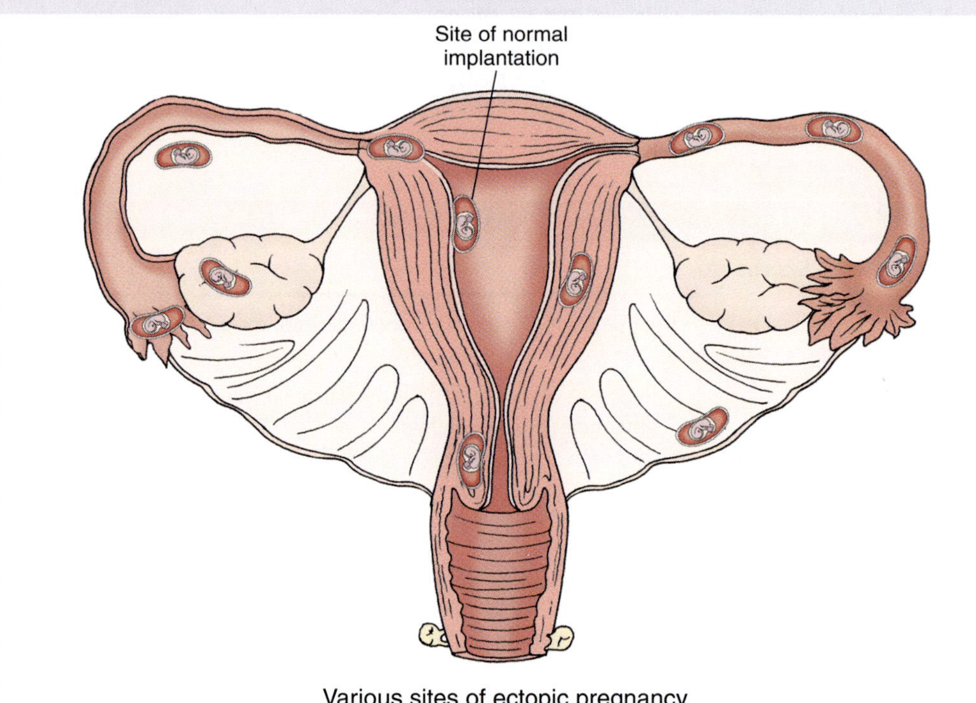

FIGURE 11-12 **Ectopic pregnancy**

endometriosis (ĕn-dō-mē-trē-Ō-sĭs)	growth of endometrial tissue in abnormal sites in the lower abdominopelvic area (see Fig. 11-13)

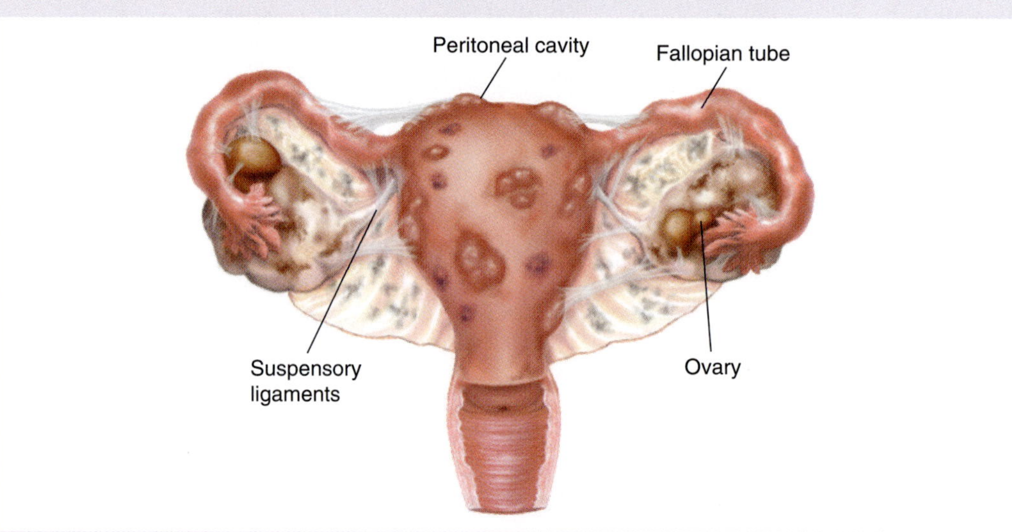

FIGURE 11-13 **Endometriosis** (From Eagle, S, et al.: *The Professional Medical Assistant.* F.A. Davis, Philadelphia, 2009, p. 616; with permission)

TABLE 11-4
PATHOLOGY TERMS—cont'd

Female Reproductive System	
fibrocystic breast disease (fī-brō-SĬS-tĭk brĕst dĭ-ZĒZ)	presence of multiple lumps in the breast, consisting of fibrous tumors or fluid-filled cysts (see Fig. 11-14)

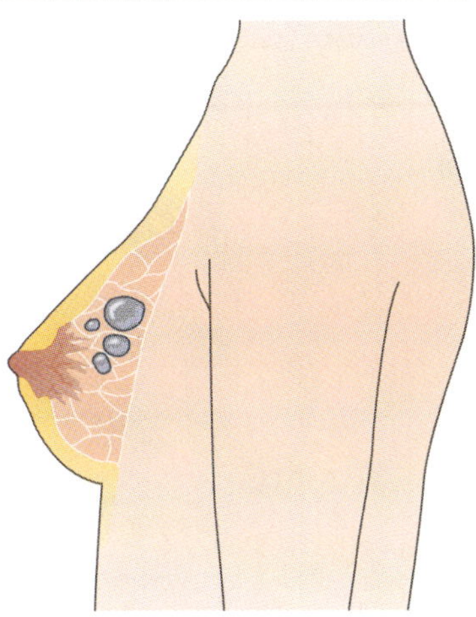

FIGURE 11-14 Fibrocystic breast disease

infertility (ĭn-fĕr-TIL-ĭ-tē)	inability to achieve pregnancy after trying to conceive for a period of 1 year or more; may be primary, which is an inability to conceive a first child, or secondary, which is infertility in a woman who has previously conceived
ovarian cyst (ō-VĀ-rē-ăn sĭst)	sac of fluid or semisolid mass that grows within the ovary (see Fig. 11-15)

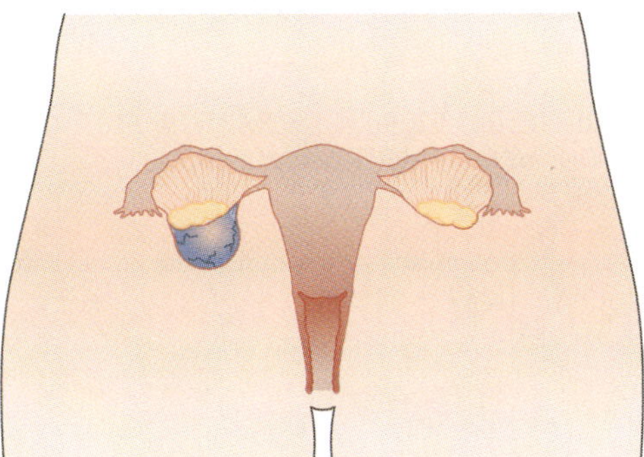

FIGURE 11-15 Ovarian cyst

pelvic inflammatory disease (PID) (PĔL-vĭk ĭn-FLĂ-mă-tōr-ē dĭ-ZĒZ)	any acute or chronic infection of the female reproductive system, including the uterus, fallopian tubes, and ovaries
premenstrual syndrome (prē-MĔN-stroo-ăl SĬN-drōm)	range of symptoms occurring 7 to 14 days before menstruation, including fluid retention, bloating, temporary weight gain, breast tenderness, headaches, depression, irritability, diarrhea, constipation, and appetite changes

Continued

TABLE 11-4 PATHOLOGY TERMS—cont'd	
Female Reproductive System	
toxic shock syndrome (TSS) (TŎKS-ĭk shŏk SĬN-drōm)	rare disorder caused by bacterial exotoxins; most commonly occurs in young women who use tampons
uterine fibroids (Ū -tĕr-ĭn FĪ-broyds)	benign, smooth tumors made of muscle and fat; also called *leiomyomas* (see Fig. 11-16)

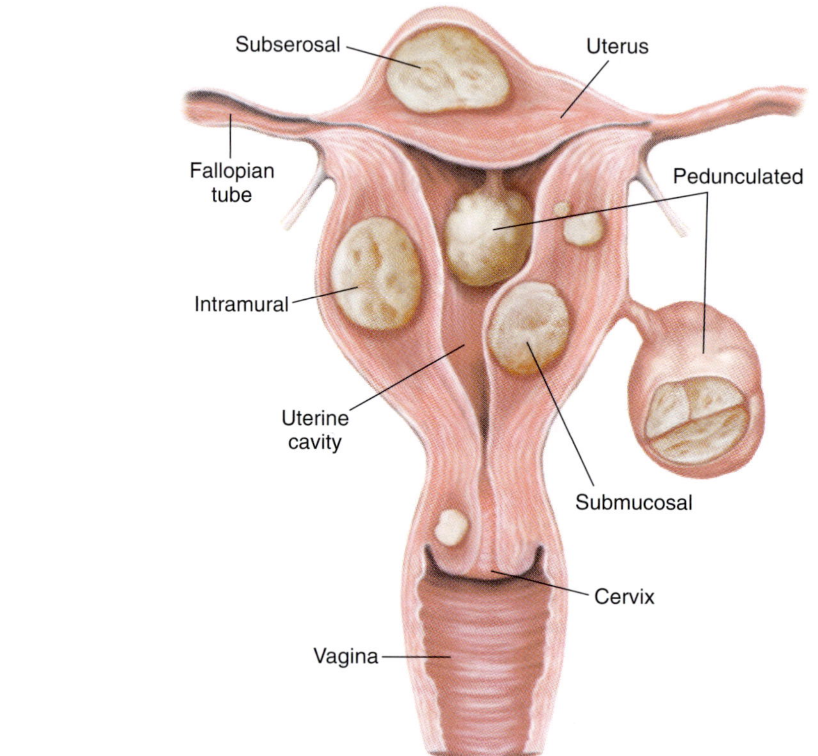

FIGURE 11-16 **Uterine fibroids** (From Eagle, S, et al.: *The Professional Medical Assistant.* F.A. Davis, Philadelphia, 2009, p. 617; with permission)

uterine prolapse (Ū-tĕr-ĭn PRŌ-lăps)	downward protrusion of the uterus into the vaginal opening (see Fig. 11-17)

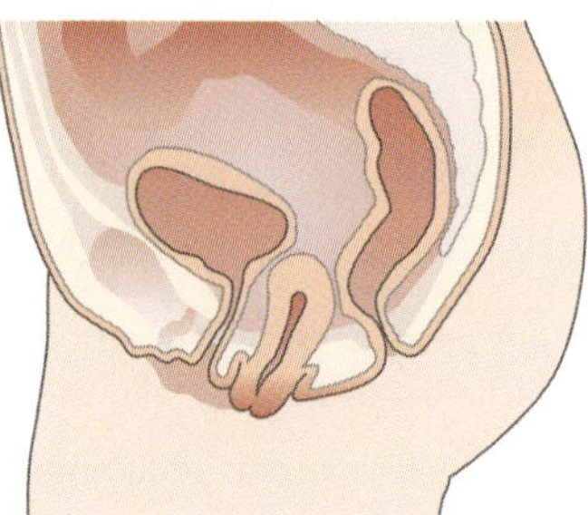

FIGURE 11-17 **Uterine prolapse**

TABLE 11-4

PATHOLOGY TERMS—cont'd

Complications of Pregnancy	
abortion (ă-BOR-shŭn)	spontaneous or therapeutic loss of a pregnancy at less than 20 weeks; also called *miscarriage*
abruptio placentae (ă-BRŬP-shē-ō plă-SĔN-tă)	sudden, premature detachment of the placenta from the uterine wall (see Fig. 11-18)

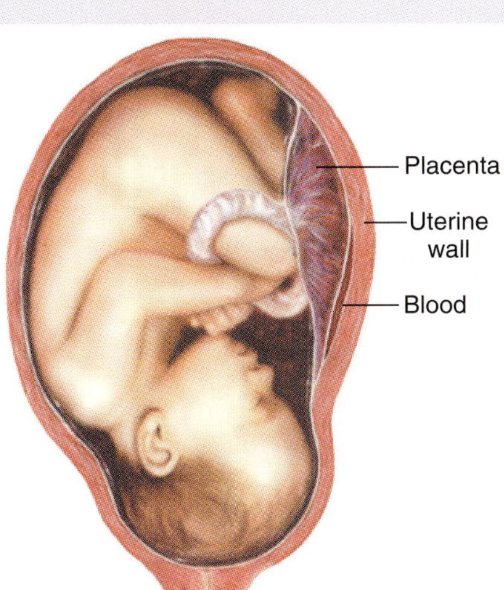

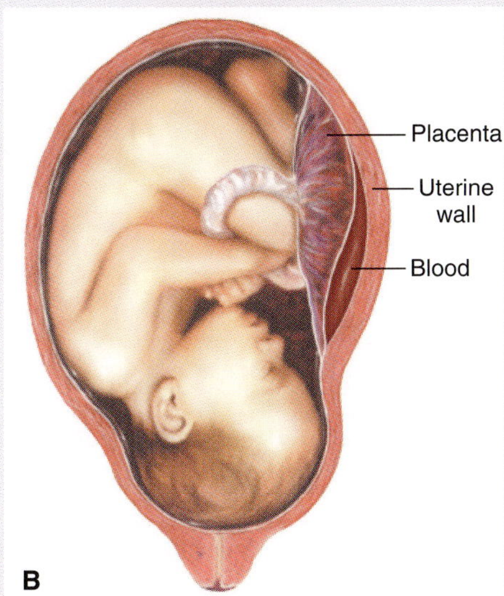

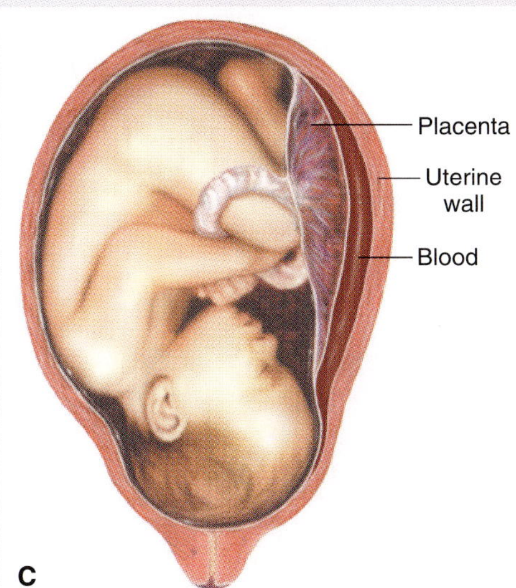

FIGURE 11-18 **Abruptio placentae: (A) Grade 1, (B) Grade 2, (C) Grade 3** (From Eagle, S. et al.: *The Professional Medical Assistant.* F.A. Davis, Philadelphia, 2009, p. 620; with permission)

Continued

TABLE 11-4

PATHOLOGY TERMS—cont'd

Complications of Pregnancy	
eclampsia (ĕ-KLĂMP-sē-ă)	complication of pregnancy characterized by severe hypertension, seizures, and possible coma
ectopic pregnancy (ĕk-TŎP-ik PRĔG-năn-sē)	implantation of a fertilized ovum somewhere other than in the uterus (see Fig. 11-19)

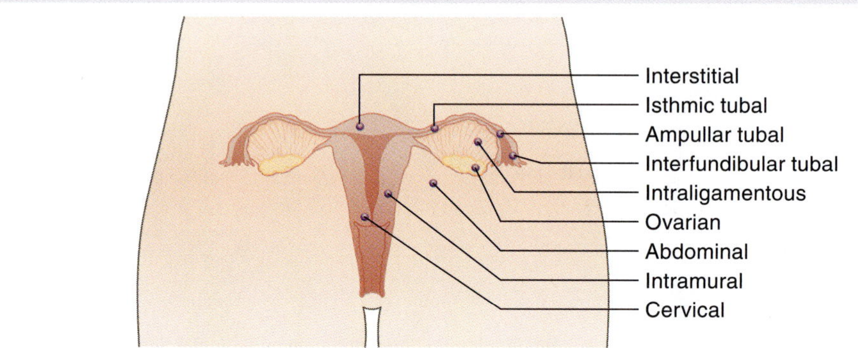

FIGURE 11-19 **Implantation sites of ectopic pregnancy**

gestational diabetes (jĕs-TĀ-shŭn-ăl dī-ă-BĒ-tēz)	development of type 2 diabetes mellitus in a pregnant woman who did not have diabetes before becoming pregnant
placenta previa (plă-SĔN-tă PRĒ-vē-ă)	implantation of the placenta in the lower uterine segment rather than the central or upper portion of the uterine wall, which may cause maternal hemorrhage during labor (see Fig. 11-20)

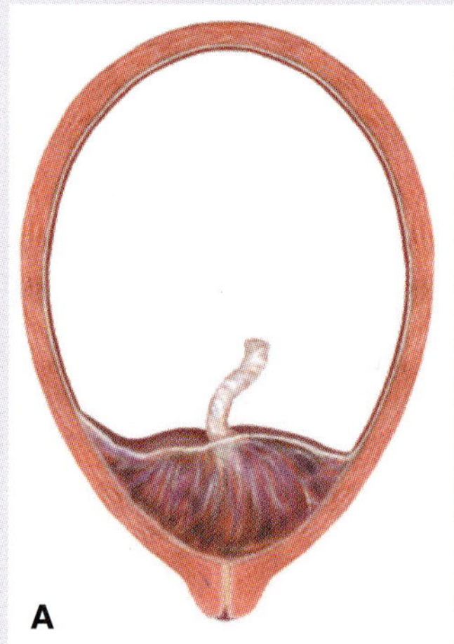

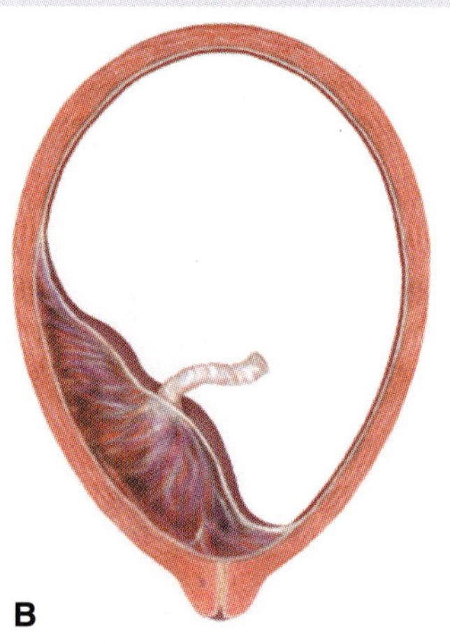

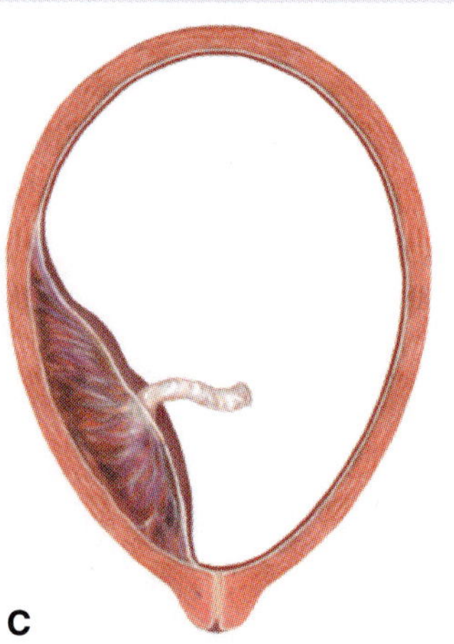

FIGURE 11-20 **Placenta previa: (A) Centralis, (B) Marginalis, (C) Lateralis** (From Eagle, S, et al.: *The Professional Medical Assistant.* F.A. Davis, Philadelphia, 2009, p. 620; with permission)

TABLE 11-4

PATHOLOGY TERMS—cont'd

Male Reproductive System	
balanoposthitis (băl-ă-nō-pŏs-THĪ-tĭs)	inflammation of the glans penis and foreskin covering the glans penis; also called *balanitis*
benign prostatic hypertrophy (BPH) (bē-NĪN prŏs-TĂT-ĭc hī-PĔR-trŏ-fē)	noncancerous enlargement of the prostate gland, common in elderly men (see Fig. 11-21)

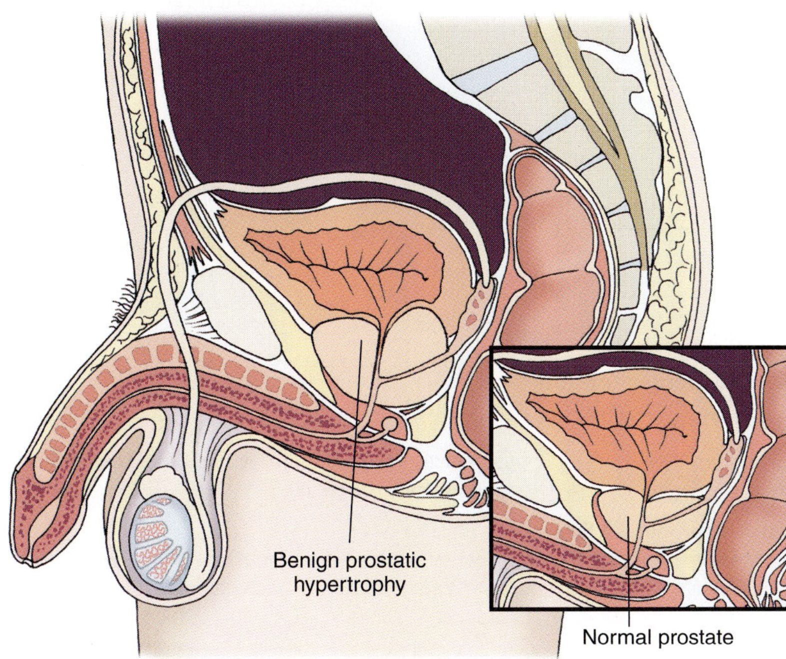

FIGURE 11-21 **Benign prostatic hypertrophy**

cryptorchidism (krĭpt-ŎR-kĭd-ĭ-zum)	failure of one or both testes to descend into the scrotum
epididymitis (ĕp-ĭ-dĭd-ĭ-MĪ-tĭs)	acute or chronic inflammation or infection of the epididymis, a tubular structure on the posterior surface of the testicle
erectile dysfunction (ED) (ĕ-RĔK-tīl dĭs-FŬNK-shŭn)	general term that describes a number of disorders, all of which impact the ability of a man to attain an erection adequate to achieve a satisfactory sexual experience; also called *impotence*
impotence (ĬM-pŏ-tĕns)	inability of a male to achieve or maintain an erection
orchitis (or-KĪ-tĭs)	acute or chronic condition of inflammation of one or both testicles, caused by (usually viral) infection
prostatitis (prŏs-tă-TĪ-tĭs)	acute or chronic inflammation of the prostate gland

Continued

TABLE 11-4

PATHOLOGY TERMS—cont'd

Male Reproductive System	
testicular torsion (tĕs-TĬK-ū-lăr TŌR-shŭn)	condition in which the testicles become twisted and the spermatic cord, blood vessels, nerves, and vas deferens become strangled (see Fig. 11-22)

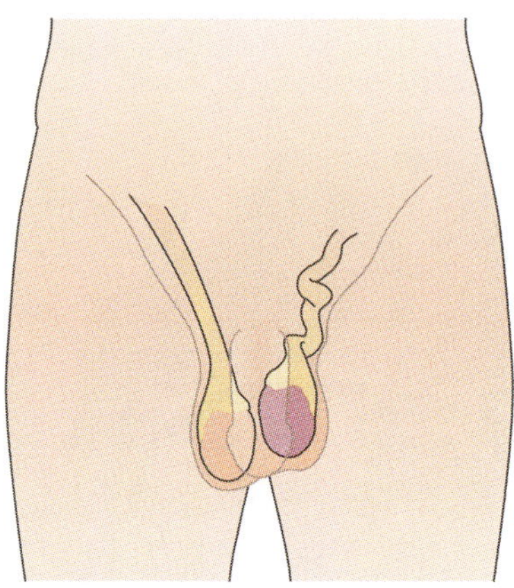

FIGURE 11-22 **Testicular torsion**

varicocele (VĂR-ĭ-kō-sēl)	enlargement and dilation or herniation of the veins of the spermatic cord that drain the testis
Male and Female Reproductive Systems	
chlamydia (klă-MĬD-ē-ă)	the most common STI, a bacterial infection caused by *Chlamydia trachomatis*
gonorrhea (gŏn-ō-RĒ-ă)	STI caused by *Neisseria gonorrhoeae* that results in inflammation of mucous membranes
herpes genitalis (HĔRP-ēs jĕn-ĭ-TĂL-ĭs)	STI caused by herpes simplex virus type 2 that results in painful vesicles; commonly called *genital herpes* (see Fig. 11-23)

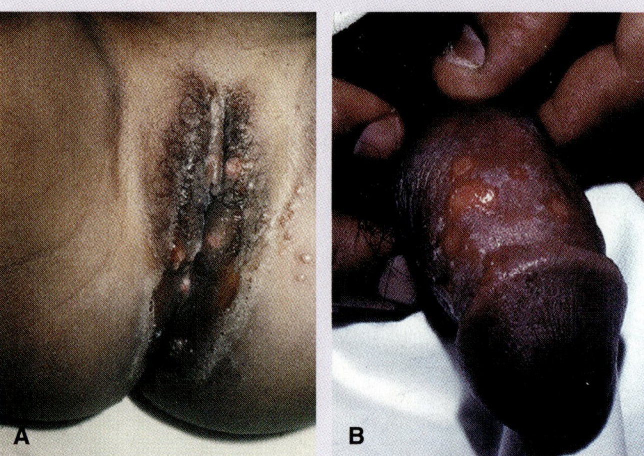

FIGURE 11-23 **Herpes genitalis as manifested in female (A) and male (B) patients.** (From Dillon, PM: *Nursing Health Assessment.* F.A. Davis, Philadelphia, 2008, pp. 543 and 577; with permission)

TABLE 11-4

PATHOLOGY TERMS—cont'd

Male and Female Reproductive Systems	
human papilloma virus (HŪ-măn păp-ĭ-LŌ-mă VĪ-rŭs)	STI caused by human papilloma virus that results in painless, cauliflower-like warts; a cause of cervical cancer in women
sterility (stĕr-ĬL-ĭ-tē)	inability to produce offspring
syphilis (SĬF-ĭ-lĭs)	multistage STI caused by the spirochete *Treponema pallidum,* with key Sx including skin lesions; eventually fatal unless treated
trichomoniasis (trĭk-ō-mō-NĪ-ă-sĭs)	STI infestation with *Trichomonas vaginalis* parasites; key Sx include vaginitis, urethritis, and cystitis

STOP HERE.
Select the Pathology Terms Flash Cards for Chapter 11 and run through them at least three times before you continue.

Common Diagnostic Tests and Procedures

Cryosurgery: Destruction of abnormal tissue by freezing

Dilation and curettage (D&C): Dilation of the cervix followed by scraping of the endometrial lining

Needle biopsy: Aspiration of tissue or fluid through a large-gauge needle for analysis (see Fig. 11-24)

Papanicolaou smear: Removal of tissue cells from the cervix for analysis

Pelvic sonography: Ultrasound imaging of the structures in the female pelvis

Prostate-specific antigen (PSA): Blood test used to screen for prostate cancer

Transurethral resection of the prostate (TURP): Removal of tissue from the prostate gland with an endoscope, via the urethra

Tubal ligation: Sterilization procedure in which fallopian tubes are cut and ligated (see Fig. 11-25)

Uterine ablation: Procedure that destroys the entire surface of the endometrium and superficial myometrium

Vasectomy: Sterilization procedure in which a small section of the vas deferens is removed (see Fig. 11-26)

Flashpoint
The Papanicolaou smear is often called the **Pap test**, and is an important test to screen for cervical and uterine cancer.

CASE STUDY

Read the case study and answer the questions that follow. Most of the terms are included in this chapter. Refer to the glossaries (Appendixes B and D) or to your medical dictionary for the other terms.

Endometriosis

Susan Brownlee is a 32-year-old woman with a history of dysmenorrhea since the age of 13. Her primary symptoms include pelvic pain and cramping prior to and during her menses. Severity of Sx caused her to occasionally miss 1 or 2 days of school each month when she was young. Over time, her symptoms have slowly worsened, currently causing her to miss an average of 2 or 3 days of work each month. Treatment with acetaminophen and NSAIDs provided only partial relief, so she was eventually started on hormonal therapy.

Mrs. Brownlee has been married for 8 years and has been trying to get pregnant for the past 5 years. During evaluation and treatment for infertility, a laparoscopy was performed and a diagnosis of endometriosis confirmed. Surgical treatment was performed at the same time, in which endometrial implants and cysts were removed from the outer surface of her ovaries and fallopian tubes. She was informed that this procedure might reduce her dysmenorrhea symptoms and increase the chance of a successful pregnancy but that the only definitive treatment for endometriosis is a total hysterosalpingo-oophorectomy. Mrs. Brownlee stated that she understood this but wanted to postpone that decision because of her wish to have children.

Endometriosis occurs in 10% to 15% of all women of reproductive age, and in 50% of infertile women. The cause is not clearly understood, but there seems to be a genetic predisposition. One theory involves the implantation of endometrial cells from menstrual flow, which moves up the fallopian tubes and into the pelvic cavity. Another theory involves the spread of endometrial cells through blood and lymphatic vessels. Other theories list possible immunological factors. A presumptive diagnosis is made based on history and symptoms, but a definitive diagnosis is made by the performance of a laparoscopy, which allows direct visualization of the reproductive organs and surrounding structures. Treatment depends on the severity of the symptoms; options include analgesics, hormone therapy, and surgery.

Case Study Questions

1. Since the age of 13, Mrs. Brownlee has experienced:
   a. Painful or difficult menstrual flow
   b. Absence of menses
   c. Excessive menstrual flow
   d. Fear of menses

2. Treatment for her dysmenorrhea has included:
   a. Cystoscopy with bladder distention
   b. Steroids
   c. Nonsteroidal anti-inflammatory drugs
   d. Hysterectomy

3. The diagnosis of endometriosis was confirmed by:
   a. Visual examination of the bladder
   b. Incision into the abdomen
   c. Visual examination of the abdomen
   d. Visual examination of the vagina and cervix

4. What was removed from Mrs. Brownlee's abdomen during her laparoscopy?
   a. Her uterus
   b. Her fallopian tubes
   c. Cancerous growths
   d. Endometrial tissue

5. As a result of the surgical procedure, Mrs. Brownlee understands that:
   a. Her endometriosis is probably cured
   b. Her symptoms of dysmenorrhea will likely worsen
   c. Her chances of becoming pregnant have increased
   d. The only reliable cure for her endometriosis is surgical removal of her fallopian tubes

6. Which of the following statements is true regarding endometriosis?
   a. It is common among women
   b. There is no relationship to infertility
   c. Severity of symptoms tends to remain constant over time
   d. Endometrial tissue proliferates in abnormal areas

7. Which of the following statements is true regarding endometriosis?
   a. The most effective permanent treatment is complete removal of uterus, fallopian tubes, and ovaries
   b. A definite diagnosis can be made based on history and current symptoms
   c. Standard treatment for endometriosis involves the use of steroids
   d. Symptoms tend to improve as the woman ages

Answers to Case Study Questions

1. a
2. c
3. c
4. d
5. c
6. d
7. a

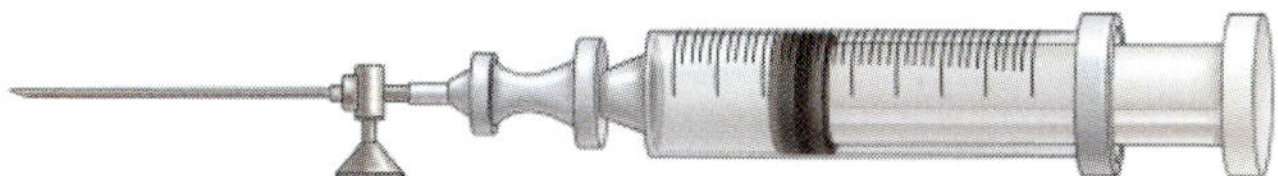

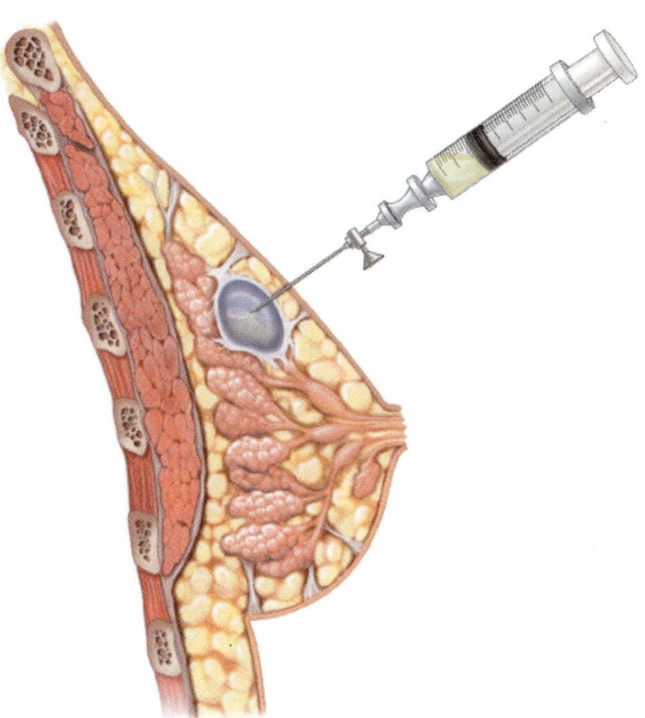

FIGURE 11-24 **Needle biopsy** (From Eagle, S, et al.: *The Professional Medical Assistant.* F.A. Davis, Philadelphia, 2009, p. 387; with permission)

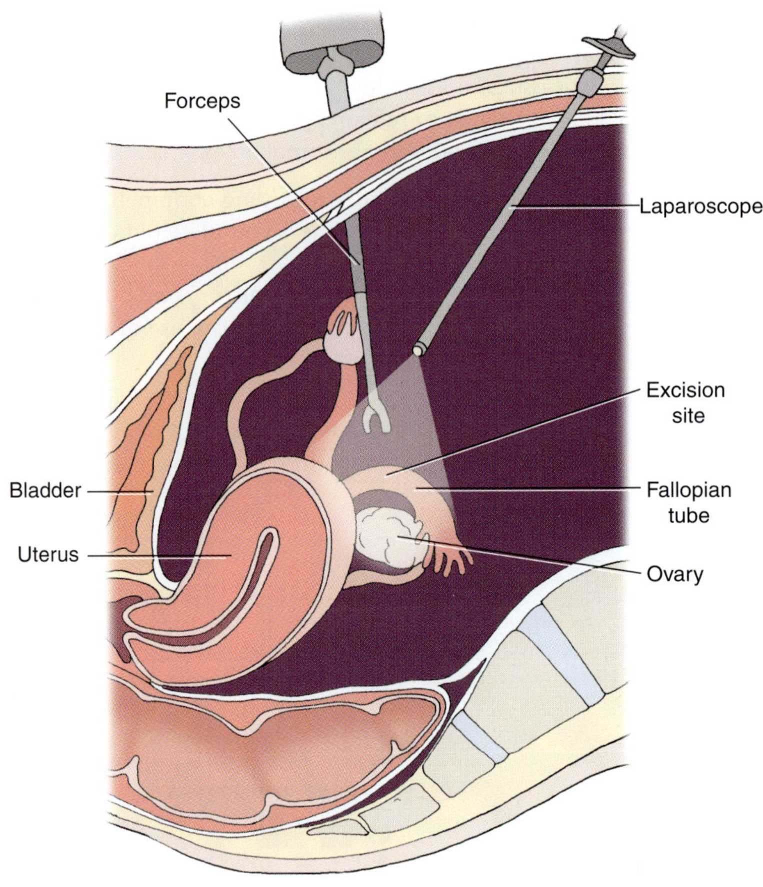

FIGURE 11-25 **Tubal ligation**

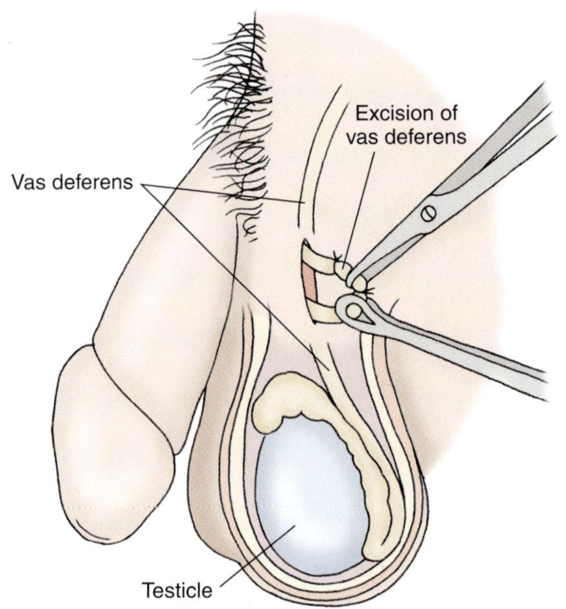

FIGURE 11-26 **Vasectomy**

Websites

Please go to the F.A. Davis website at http://davisplus.fadavis.com/eagle/medterm to view resource websites for the reproductive system.

Practice Exercises

Fill in the Blanks

Write the correct meaning of these medical terms. Check Appendix G for the correct answers.

Exercise 3

1. The abbreviation *Gyn* stands for ____________________.
2. Uterine fibroids are ____________________.
3. *OC* stands for ____________________.
4. Ectopic pregnancy occurs when ____________________.
5. The abbreviation *TURP* stands for ____________________.
6. Endometriosis occurs when ____________________.
7. The abbreviation *TAH-BSO* stands for ____________________.
8. The term *trichomoniasis* is a(n) ____________________.
9. The term *orchiectasis* means ____________________.
10. The term *salpingo-oophorectomy* means ____________________.
11. The term *balanoplasty* means ____________________.
12. The term *dysplasia* means ____________________.
13. The term *neoplastic* means ____________________.
14. The term *mammography* means ____________________.
15. The term *laparoscopy* means ____________________.

Fill in the Blanks

Fill in the blanks below. Check Appendix G for the correct answers.

Exercise 4

1. When a fertilized ovum is implanted outside of the uterus, it is called an ____________ pregnancy.
2. Lacey has dysmenorrhea due to endometrial tissue growth in her abdominopelvic area. This condition is known as ____________.
3. ____________ is an STI that is eventually fatal if not treated.
4. Olga is a 54-year-old woman who underwent a ____________ ____________ ____________, abbreviated *TAH*, due to noncancerous uterine tumors also known as ____________.
5. Marcella will see her OB-GYN physician every week during her 9th month of pregnancy. *OB-GYN* stands for ____________ ____________ ____________.
6. ____________ is an STI infestation caused by a parasite.
7. The abbreviation for oral contraceptive is ____________.
8. Danielle's nurse practitioner recommends that she have a Pap test once a year. *Pap* is an abbreviation that stands for ____________.
9. ____________ is the inability to produce offspring.
10. Carla and her husband have tried unsuccessfully for 4 years to have a baby. They are now considering IVF, which is ____________ ____________ ____________.
11. The abbreviation for a total abdominal hysterectomy, bilateral salpingo-oophorectomy is ____________ ____________.
12. Nicholas is a 65-year-old man with BPH, or ____________ ____________ ____________.
13. Nicholas will undergo a procedure known as a TURP, or ____________ ____________ ____________ ____________ ____________.

14. The inability of a man to achieve or maintain erection is known as ______________________.

15. The term *seminuria* means ______________________.

16. The term *galactorrhea* means ______________________.

17. The term *ovogenesis* means ______________________.

18. The term *phalloid* means ______________________.

19. The definition of cryptorchidism is ______________________.

20. The term *sonorous* means ______________________.

Multiple Choice

Select the one best answer to the following multiple-choice questions. Check Appendix G for the correct answers.

Exercise 5

1. Ms. Andretti came to the clinic today complaining of severe menstrual pain and cramping. Which of the following medical terms best describes her complaint?
   a. Menitis
   b. Vaginorrhea
   c. Dysmenorrhea
   d. Cervicitis

2. Mrs. Ramirez had a painful ovarian cyst on her left side. The ovary and the cyst were surgically removed through her lower abdomen with a small endoscope. The proper name for this procedure is a:
   a. Laparoscopic oophorectomy
   b. Colposcopic oophorotomy
   c. Vaginoscopic salpingo-oophorectomy
   d. Laparoscopic hysterectomy

3. Mr. Smyth had to be circumcised due to chronic balanitis. He had:
   a. A continual prostate infection
   b. Constant inflammation of his testes
   c. Constant inflammation of his glans penis
   d. Continual pain of his vas deferens

4. Mrs. Brown is 6 months pregnant and sees her physician each month for care. This type of care is known as:
   a. Prenatal care
   b. Perinatal care
   c. Postnatal care
   d. Circumnatal care

5. Which of the following combining forms does **not** mean testis?
   a. Test/o
   b. Orchi/o
   c. Orchid/o
   d. Oophor/o

Word Building

*Using **only** the word parts in the lists provided, create medical terms with the indicated meanings. Check Appendix G for the correct answers.*

Exercise 6

Prefixes	Combining Forms	Suffixes
an-	balan/o	-al
dys-	cervic/o	-algia
neo-	colp/o	-dynia
oligo-	episi/o	-ectomy
peri-	gynec/o	-esthesia
retro-	hyster/o	-gram
	lapar/o	-ia
	mamm/o	-ism
	mast/o	-itis
	men/o	-logist
	nat/o	-pause
	orchid/o	-pexy
	prostat/o	-plasia
	sperm/o	-plasm
	vagin/o	-rrhaphy
	vas/o	-scope
		-stenosis
		-tomy

1. inflammation of the glans penis ____________________
2. cutting into or incision of the vulva (perineum) ____________________
3. condition of absent testes ____________________
4. surgical fixation of a testis ____________________
5. condition of deficient sperm ____________________

6. pertaining to near (the time of) birth ______________________

7. bad, painful, or difficult formation or growth ______________________

8. new formation or growth ______________________

9. pertaining to behind the vagina ______________________

10. absence of sensation ______________________

11. narrowing or stricture of a vessel ______________________

12. pain of the prostate ______________________

13. inflammation of the cervix ______________________

14. suturing of the vagina ______________________

15. specialist in the study of female (disorders) ______________________

16. viewing instrument for the abdomen ______________________

17. excision or surgical removal of the uterus ______________________

18. record (x-ray) of a breast ______________________

19. surgical fixation of a breast ______________________

20. cessation or stopping of menses ______________________

True or False

Decide whether the following statements are true or false. Check Appendix G for the correct answers.

Exercise 7

1. True False **Herpes genitalis** is caused by herpes simplex virus type 2.
2. True False The abbreviation **PID** stands for *pelvic invasive disorder.*
3. True False The key symptoms of **candidiasis** are itching, burning, and a thick curdy discharge.
4. True False The abbreviation **IUD** stands for *inter-urinary disorder.*
5. True False **Uterine prolapse** is a herniation of the vaginal wall.
6. True False **VD** and **STD** are the same thing.
7. True False The symbol for male is ♂.
8. True False The symbol for female is ♀.

9. True False The abbreviation **GU** stands for *gonorrhea.*

10. True False **Cryptorchidism** is the absence of testes.

Deciphering Terms

Write the correct meaning of these medical terms. Check Appendix G for the correct answers.

Exercise 8

1. orchidorrhaphy ____________________
2. cervicocolpitis ____________________
3. multigravida ____________________
4. gynecomastia ____________________
5. menopause ____________________
6. phallodynia ____________________
7. hyperplasia ____________________
8. spermolytic ____________________
9. prostatocele ____________________
10. cryptomenorrhea ____________________

Multiple Choice

Select the one best answer to the following multiple-choice questions. Check Appendix G for the correct answers.

Exercise 9

1. The term *android* means:
   - a. Resembling female
   - b. Resembling amnion
   - c. Resembling male
   - d. None of these

2. The term *salpingolysis* means:
   - a. Process of recording sound
   - b. Pertaining to the destruction of sperm
   - c. Destruction of a tube
   - d. None of these

3. The term *uteropexy* means:
   a. Surgical fixation of the uterus
   b. Suturing of the uterus
   c. Slight or partial paralysis of the uterus
   d. None of these

4. The term *balanic* means:
   a. Condition of the penis
   b. Pertaining to the glans penis
   c. Disease of the prostate
   d. None of these

5. The term *sonography* means:
   a. Process of recording sound
   b. Record of sound
   c. Instrument used to record sound
   d. None of these

6. All of the following abbreviations indicate a type of sexually transmitted infection **except**:
   a. HPV
   b. GC
   c. Trich
   d. TSS

7. All of the following are matched with the correct definition **except**:
   a. ♀: male
   b. PMS: premenstrual syndrome
   c. TSS: toxic shock syndrome
   d. ED: erectile dysfunction

8. Which of the following statements is true?
   a. The abbreviations *STI* and *STD* mean the same thing
   b. EDC is a type of contraceptive device
   c. The abbreviation *OC* stands for ovarian cyst
   d. The abbreviation *FHR* stands for female hormone

9. Which of the following abbreviations pertains to the male reproductive system?
   a. TSE
   b. BSE
   c. D&C
   d. PID

10. Which of the following abbreviations pertains to the female reproductive system?
    a. PSA
    b. HRT
    c. DRE
    d. TURP

11. All of the following abbreviations indicate a type of procedure **except**:
    a. AB
    b. TAH
    c. GU
    d. DRE

12. All of the following abbreviations indicate a type of disease or disorder **except**:
    a. PID
    b. BPH
    c. STI
    d. OC

13. All of the following terms are matched with the correct definition **except**:
    a. Endometriosis: tissue growth in abnormal sites in lower abdominopelvic area
    b. Eclampsia: condition marked by severe hypertension, seizures, and possible coma
    c. Abruptio placentae: implantation of the placenta in the lower uterine segment rather than the central or upper portion of the uterine wall
    d. Uterine fibroids: benign, smooth tumors made of muscle and fat

14. All of the following terms are matched with the correct definition **except**:
    a. Cryptorchidism: failure of one or both testes to descend into the scrotum
    b. Impotence: inability to produce offspring
    c. Varicocele: enlargement and dilation of veins of the spermatic cord
    d. Testicular torsion: condition in which the testicles become twisted and the spermatic cord, blood vessels, nerves, and vas deferens become strangled

15. Balanoposthitis is:
    a. Inflammation caused by blockage of one or both of the Bartholin glands
    b. Protrusion of the uterus through the vaginal opening
    c. Inflammation of the glans penis and foreskin
    d. Pain in the lower abdominal and pelvic area, associated with menses

16. Which of the following procedures destroys the entire surface of the endometrium and superficial myometrium?
    a. Cryosurgery
    b. Ablation
    c. Dilation and curettage
    d. None of these

17. Which of the following procedures involves freezing of tissue?
    a. Cryosurgery
    b. Needle biopsy
    c. Ablation
    d. Prostate-specific antigen

18. Which of the following combining forms means *sound?*
    a. Salping/o
    b. Son/o
    c. Semin/o
    d. None of these

19. Which of the following combining forms means *vulva?*
    a. Andr/o
    b. Episi/o
    c. Colp/o
    d. None of these

20. The combining form *phall/i* means:
    a. Hidden
    b. Amnion
    c. Fetus
    d. None of these

12 ENDOCRINE SYSTEM

Structure and Function

The endocrine system is made up of all the major glands, which act to regulate hormones in the body. Various endocrine organs produce and secrete these hormones in order to maintain homeostasis, which is defined as the state of dynamic equilibrium (see Fig. 12-1). In other words, they act together to keep the body's internal environment healthy. Some hormones act directly on target organs; others stimulate certain glands to secrete yet different hormones.

Hormone levels in the blood may vary according to bodily functions. Hormones usually work in pairs to maintain a healthy balance, with one acting to raise levels of other substances when needed and the other acting to lower levels when needed. For example, the hormones **calcitonin** and **parathyroid hormone** function in an opposite, yet complementary, fashion to maintain a healthy level of calcium in the blood. Endocrine glands are responsible for the sexual maturation of individuals from childhood to adolescence and into adulthood. Endocrine glands also play a role in the body's ability to metabolize food and store energy.

The **pituitary gland** is a small, round, pea-sized structure attached to the lower surface of the hypothalamus in the brain. It is commonly called the **master gland** because it controls all of the other glands in the body. Even so, it is actually controlled by the hypothalamus. The pituitary gland is divided into an anterior lobe and a posterior lobe. These two parts function separately to produce many different hormones (see Fig. 12-2). The anterior lobe is responsible for secreting the following six hormones:

Growth hormone (GH) promotes the growth of body structures, such as bones.

Thyroid-stimulating hormone (TSH) affects the growth and functioning of the thyroid gland.

Follicle-stimulating hormone (FSH) and **luteinizing hormone (LH)** are referred to as gonadotropins because they act on the gonads—the ovaries in the female, to produce an ovum, and the testes in the male, to produce sperm.

Prolactin acts on the mammary glands to produce milk.

Adrenocorticotropic hormone (ACTH) acts on the adrenal glands to secrete glucocorticoids, including cortisol.

The posterior lobe of the pituitary gland secretes the following two hormones:

Oxytocin acts on the uterus to promote contractions during labor and delivery.

Antidiuretic hormone (ADH) acts on the kidneys to increase the absorption of water.

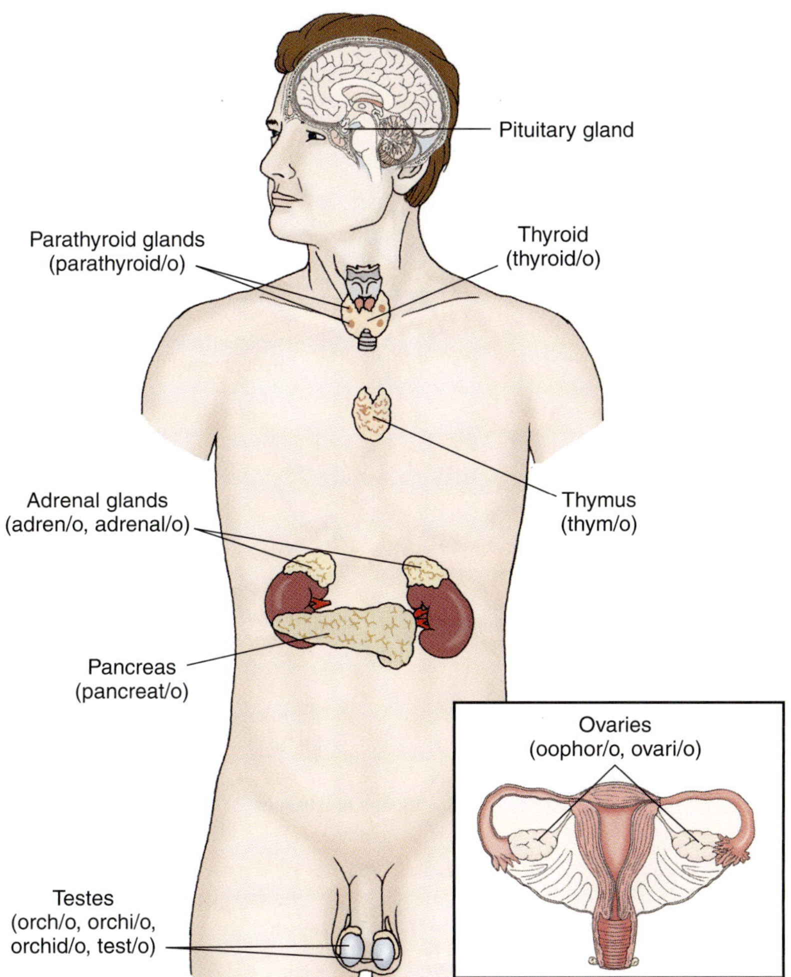

FIGURE 12-1 **The endocrine system**

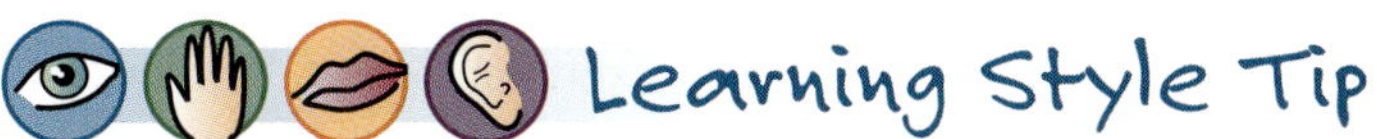

Study Figure 12-1 and then create a fun and colorful 3-D model which similarly illustrates the pituitary gland, the hormones it produces, and the target organs the hormones affect. An example might be a hanging mobile with the pituitary gland at the top and labeled "hormone" strings that each dangle their respective target organs. Once you've completed it, show and explain your model to a friend.

The tiny **pineal gland** is sometimes referred to as the **pineal body**. It is shaped like a pine cone and is located in the brain, above and behind the thalamus. It produces the hormone **melatonin**, which influences the body's natural circadian rhythm, or sleep-wake cycle.

Flashpoint
The pituitary gland is nicknamed the "master gland" because it controls all other glands in the body.

The **thyroid gland** is one of the largest endocrine glands; it is highly vascular and is located in the base of the neck. It is shaped similarly to the letter H and has two lobes total, one located on each side of the trachea, which are connected by a narrow band. It produces the two thyroid hormones, **triiodothyronine (T3)** and **thyroxine (T4)**, which are responsible for growth throughout childhood and regulation of body metabolism. For the thyroid gland to function properly, iodine must be obtained in the diet. The thyroid gland also secretes

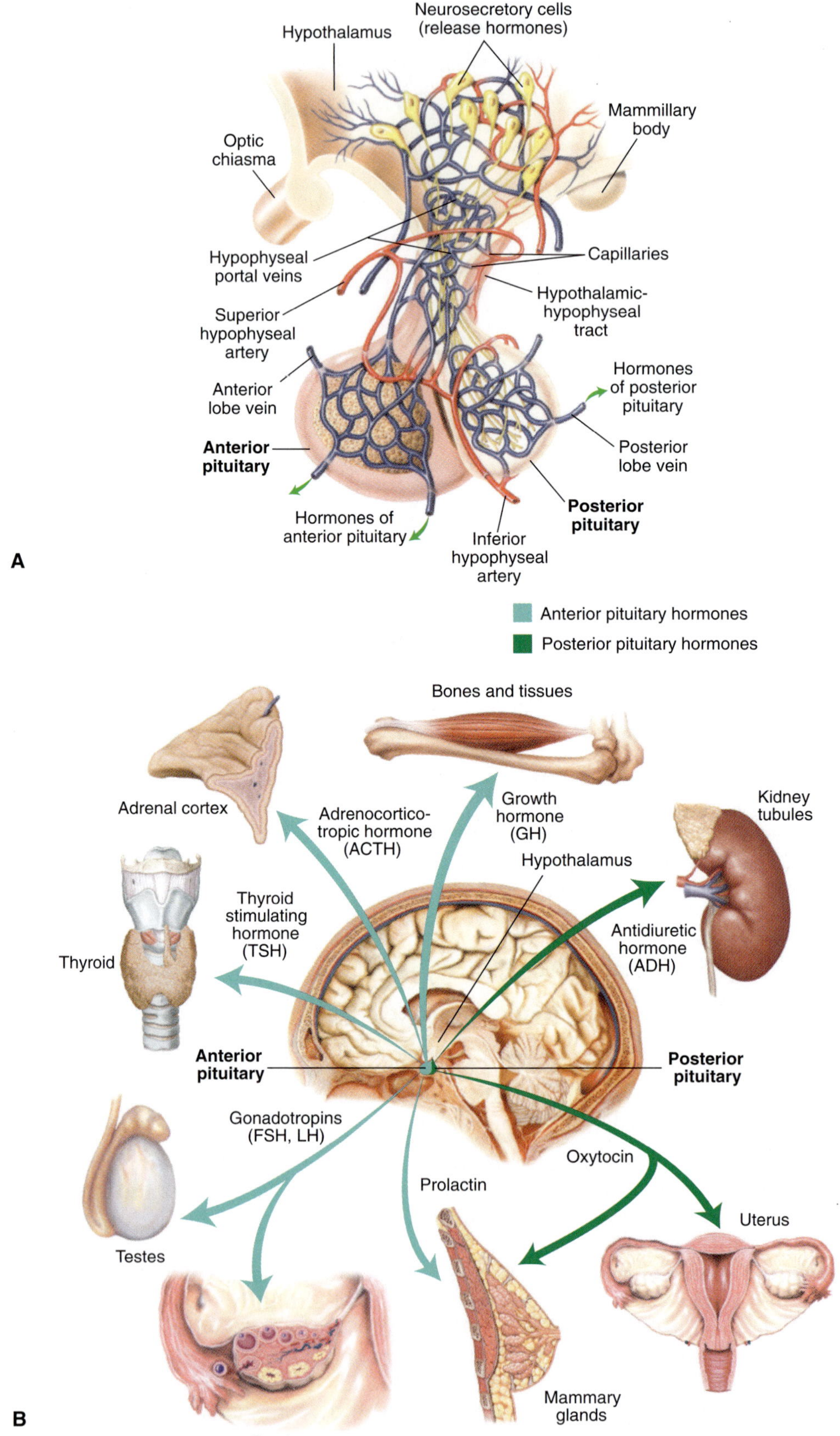

FIGURE 12-2 **Pituitary gland: (A) anterior and posterior view, (B) Hormones and target glands** (From Eagle, S, et al.: *The Professional Medical Assistant.* F.A. Davis, Philadelphia, 2009, p. 523; with permission)

the hormone calcitonin, which is responsible for regulating calcium and phosphorus levels in the blood.

Four tiny **parathyroid glands** lie on the posterior surface of the thyroid gland, within its connective tissue. They secrete parathormone (PTH), also called parathyroid hormone, which also helps regulate calcium and phosphorus levels in the blood.

The two **adrenal glands** are triangular in shape and are located on top of each kidney, within the retroperitoneal cavity (behind the abdomen). They are made up of an outer layer called the *adrenal cortex* and an inner part called the *adrenal medulla.* The adrenal glands secrete several hormones:

Epinephrine, also known as *adrenaline*, is released during the fight-or-flight response, which increases your ability to cope with stress or trauma. Epinephrine enables the body to respond to stressful situations by converting glycogen into glucose for quick energy, dilating the pupils, opening the airways, and decreasing peristalsis.

Aldosterone plays a role in regulating and maintaining the body's water, sodium, and electrolyte balance.

Cortisol is the body's natural steroid and works to decrease inflammation.

Androgens are responsible for secondary sexual characteristics in females and males.

The **pancreas** is a long, somewhat flat organ located in the upper left quadrant of the abdomen. It plays an active role in the digestive system as well as the endocrine system. The endocrine portion of the pancreas includes the pancreatic islets, also called the *islets of Langerhans.* The beta cells of the pancreas secrete **insulin** after food is eaten, to metabolize carbohydrates and break them down into glucose. Insulin also stimulates cells to take up glucose from the blood so that it can be delivered to tissue cells for energy. As a result, blood glucose levels decrease. The alpha cells of the pancreas secrete **glucagon**, which acts on the liver to convert **glycogen** into glucose. (Glycogen is also stored in the muscles.) Glycogen is converted into glucose to meet energy needs, such as during exercise or prolonged periods without meals. Normally, pancreatic hormones work cooperatively to maintain healthy blood glucose levels. However, when dysregulation occurs, as with **diabetes mellitus**, blood glucose levels may widely fluctuate, resulting in hyperglycemia (high blood sugar) or hypoglycemia (low blood sugar). The classic signs of new onset of undiagnosed diabetes are the three "poly"s: **polydipsia** (much thirst), **polyphagia** (much eating, which indicates an increased appetite), and **polyuria** (much urination). In spite of eating more, a diabetic may lose weight because of faulty carbohydrate metabolism; in spite of drinking more, a diabetic may become dehydrated due to polyuria. In severe cases, as these symptoms worsen and blood glucose levels rise, lethargy may progress to loss of consciousness. This is called **diabetic ketoacidosis (DKA)**, otherwise known as a *diabetic coma.* Treatment includes admission to the hospital for fluid rehydration and insulin therapy.

Flashpoint

If you feel threatened or frightened, your adrenal glands give you a dose of epinephrine, which prepares you for action. This response is known as the fright, fight, or flight response. It stimulates your adrenal glands to secrete cortisol and epinephrine (adrenaline), which increase your heart rate, blood pressure, blood glucose, and respiratory rate.

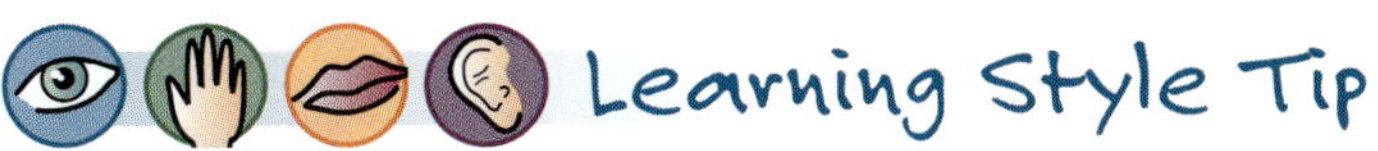

As you read the text, challenge yourself to think like the instructor and underline or highlight information you believe is most likely to be used in exam questions. Then read the information aloud until you fully understand and remember it.

The **thymus gland** consists of two symmetrical lobes located in the mediastinum (mid-chest area). It is proportionately larger in infants and children and shrinks in size as people age. The main function of the thymus gland is to produce T lymphocytes that are necessary for the immune system. It plays an active role in the immune system in childhood, but shrinks and becomes less active as a person ages.

The **reproductive glands**, sometimes called the **gonads**, are the ovaries and testes. The ovaries are small, oval-shaped structures located on each side of the uterus in the lower abdominal cavity, attached to the broad ligament. The ovaries contain graafian follicles, in which are immature ova, or eggs. The ovaries produce an ovum during each menstrual cycle and secrete **estrogen** and **progesterone**. Estrogen helps develop secondary sexual characteristics in the female, including breasts and pubic hair. It also plays a vital role in the menstrual cycle and is important in the prevention of osteoporosis in post-menopausal women. Progesterone is necessary to prepare and maintain the uterus for a fertilized ovum.

The testes are egg-shaped glands located in the scrotum of the male reproductive tract. The testes secrete **testosterone**, which is responsible for the development of male secondary sexual characteristics during puberty, such as deepening of the voice, growth of facial and pubic hair, and increased muscle development. It is also necessary in the production of sperm.

Within the endocrine system, glands and hormones work together to maintain homeostasis in the body by utilizing a **negative feedback system**. The system is called "negative" because it works by opposites to maintain a healthy balance of certain substances in the body. Each gland produces a hormone that serves to oppose another substance. The gland may increase or decrease production of the hormone to stimulate a corresponding decrease or increase of that substance. Thus, this system works much like a thermostat functions, activating the production of heat in response to falling temperatures (a decrease in the normal level) or decreasing heat production in response to normal or above-normal heat levels.

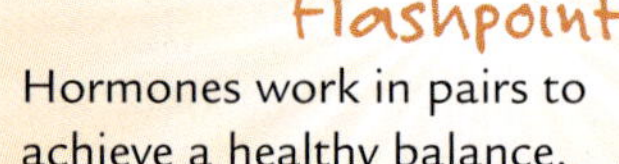

Hormones work in pairs to achieve a healthy balance.

Almost all endocrine glands operate in a negative feedback system. For example, the parathyroid glands secrete parathyroid hormone, which regulates blood calcium levels. A decrease in blood calcium level stimulates the parathyroid glands to secrete more parathyroid hormone; parathyroid hormone stimulates the bones to release more calcium into the blood and facilitates calcium uptake from the kidneys into the bloodstream. Thus, blood calcium levels are restored to normal. On the other hand, if blood calcium levels increase (above normal), the parathyroid glands decrease production of parathyroid hormone. Either way, the response of the parathyroid glands is a negative (opposite) response to the stimulus of a decrease or increase in blood calcium levels.

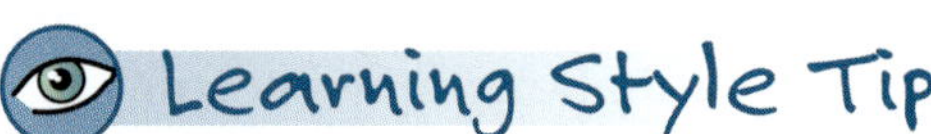

Noticing data patterns helps you recall them later. For example, note that the chemistry abbreviations for electrolytes can be grouped into the pattern below:

		higher level	lower level
potassium:	K	hyper**k**alemia	hypo**k**alemia
sodium:	Na	hyper**na**tremia	hypo**na**tremia
calcium:	Ca	hyper**ca**lcemia	hypo**ca**lcemia

Also remember: *hyper-* means *excessive or above*

hypo- means *below or beneath*

-emia means *a condition of the blood*

Combining Forms

Table 12-1 contains combining forms that pertain to the endocrine system, along with examples of terms that utilize the combining forms, and a pronunciation guide. Read aloud to yourself as you move from left to right across the table. Be sure to use the pronunciation guide so that you learn to say the terms correctly.

TABLE 12-1
COMBINING FORMS

Combining Form	Meaning	Example (Pronunciation)	Meaning of New Term
acr/o	extremities	acroanesthesia (ăk-rō-ăn-ĕs-THĒ-zē-ă)	absence of sensation in the extremities
aden/o	gland	adenopathy (ăd-ĕ-NŎP-ă-thē)	disease of a gland
adren/o	adrenal gland	adrenal (ăd-rē-năl)	pertaining to the adrenal gland
adrenal/o		adrenalectomy (ăd-rē-năl-ĔK-tō-mē)	excision or surgical removal of an adrenal gland
calc/o	calcium	hypercalcemia (hī-pĕr-kăl-SĒ-mē-ă)	condition of excessive calcium in the blood
gluc/o	glucose, sugar, sweet	glucogenesis (gloo-kō-JĔN-ĕ-sĭs)	creation of glucose
glucos/o		glucosuria (gloo-kō-SŪR-ē-ă)	sugar in the urine
glyc/o		glycemia (glī-SĒ-mē-ă)	sugar in the blood
glycos/o		glycosuria (glī-kō-SŪ-rē-ă)	sugar in the urine
home/o	same, unchanging	homeostasis (hō-mē-ō-STĀ-sĭs)	unchanging, stopping (maintenance of equilibrium)
hydr/o	water	hydrolysis (hī-DRŎL-ĭ-sĭs)	destruction of water
kal/i	potassium	hyperkalemia (hī-pĕr-kă-LĒ-mē-ă)	condition of excessive potassium in the blood
natr/o	sodium	natremia (nă-TRĒ-mē-ă)	condition of sodium in the blood
pancreat/o	pancreas	pancreatography (păn-krē-ă-TŎG-ră-fē)	process of recording the pancreas
parathyroid/o	parathyroid	parathyroidectomy (păr-ă-thī-royd-ĔK-tō-mē)	excision or surgical removal of a parathyroid gland
thym/o	thymus	thymoma (thī-MŌ-mă)	tumor of the thymus
thyr/o	thyroid	thyrotoxicosis (thī-rō-tŏks-ĭ-KŌ-sĭs)	abnormal condition of poison in the thyroid
thyroid/o		thyroiditis (thī-royd-Ī-tĭs)	inflammation of the thyroid
toxic/o	toxin, poison	toxicologist (tŏks-ĭ-KŎL-ō-jĭst)	specialist in the study of toxins

STOP HERE.
Select the Combining Form Flash Cards for Chapter 12 and run through them at least three times before you continue.

Practice Exercises

Fill in the Blanks

Fill in the blanks below using Table 12-1. Check Appendix G for the correct answers.

Exercise 1

1. excision or surgical removal of a parathyroid gland ____________________
2. excision or surgical removal of an adrenal gland ____________________
3. disease of a gland ____________________
4. specialist in the study of toxins ____________________
5. condition of excessive calcium in the blood ____________________
6. creation of glucose ____________________
7. destruction of water ____________________
8. tumor of the thymus ____________________
9. sugar in the urine ____________________
10. pertaining to the adrenal gland ____________________
11. inflammation of the thyroid ____________________
12. process of recording the pancreas ____________________
13. absence of sensation in the extremities ____________________
14. unchanging, stopping (maintenance of equilibrium) ____________________
15. condition of excessive potassium in the blood ____________________
16. condition of sodium in the blood ____________________
17. abnormal condition of poison in the thyroid ____________________
18. **Fill in the blanks in Figure 12-3 with the appropriate anatomical terms and combining forms.**

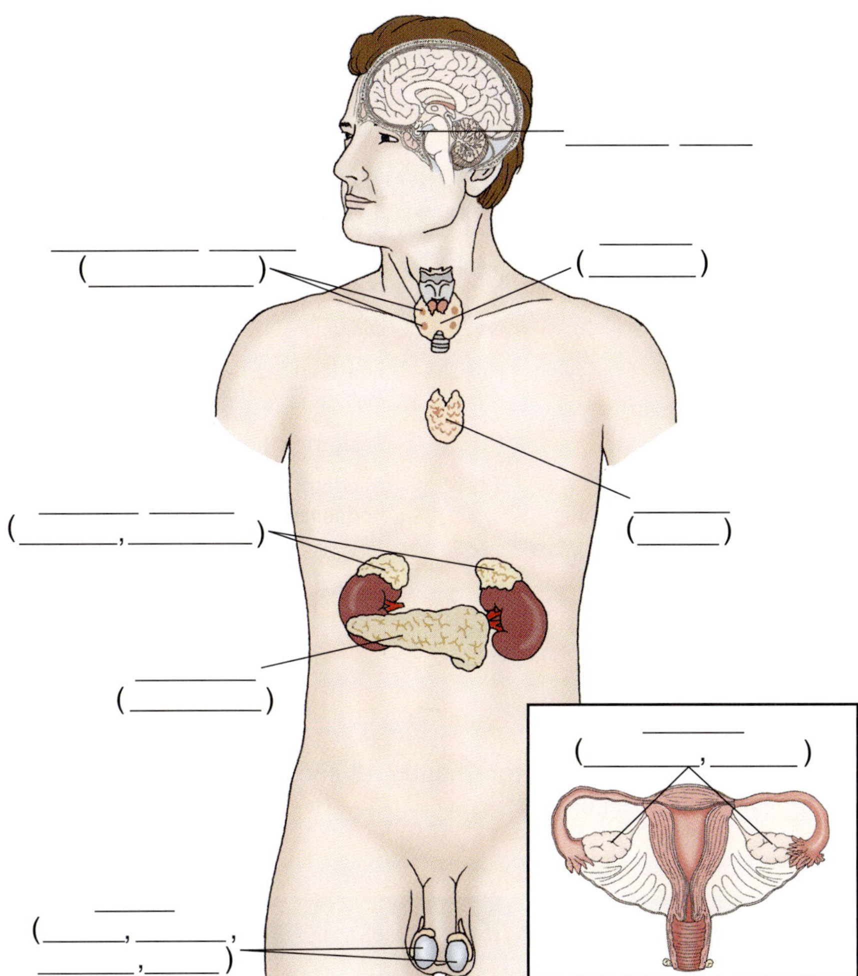

FIGURE 12-3 **Endocrine system with blanks**

Abbreviations

Table 12-2 lists some of the most common abbreviations related to the endocrine system, as well as others often used in medical documentation.

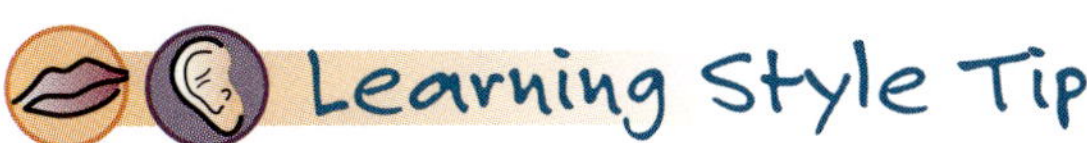

Learning Style Tip

With your study buddy, create a fun "abbreviation conversation" in which two people are talking in code by using as many medical abbreviations as possible from this and other chapters. Take turns reciting the conversation and review the meaning of any abbreviations you have forgotten.

TABLE 12-2
ABBREVIATIONS

ADH	antidiuretic hormone	GH	growth hormone
BG, BS	blood glucose, blood sugar	GTT	glucose tolerance test
BMI	body mass index	HRT	hormone replacement therapy
BMR	basal metabolic rate	IDDM	insulin-dependent diabetes mellitus (type 1 diabetes)
Ca	calcium	K	potassium
CA	cancer	Na	sodium
DI	diabetes insipidus	NIDDM	non-insulin-dependent diabetes mellitus (type 2 diabetes)
DKA	diabetic ketoacidosis	PTH	parathyroid hormone
DM	diabetes mellitus	T3, T4	triiodothyronine, thyroxine (thyroid hormones)
FBG, FBS	fasting blood glucose, fasting blood sugar	TSH	thyroid-stimulating hormone
fsbs	finger stick blood sugar		

STOP HERE.
Select the Abbreviation Flash Cards for Chapter 12 and run through them at least three times before you continue.

Pathology Terms

Table 12-3 includes terms that relate to diseases or abnormalities of the endocrine system. Use the pronunciation guide and say the terms aloud as you read them. This will help you get in the habit of saying them properly.

TABLE 12-3
PATHOLOGY TERMS

acromegaly (ăk-rō-MĔG-ă-lē)	type of hyperpituitarism in which an overactive pituitary gland after adulthood causes abnormal continued growth of bones and tissues of the face and extremities
Addison disease (ĂD-ĭ-sŭn dĭ-ZĒZ)	illness characterized by gradual adrenal-gland failure, resulting in insufficient production of steroid hormones and the need for hormone replacement therapy; also called *hypoadrenalism*
congenital hypothyroidism (kŏn-JĔN-ĭ-tăl hī-pō-THĪ-royd-ĭ-zum)	congenital condition of thyroid hormone deficiency, characterized by arrested physical and mental development; formerly called *cretinism* (see Fig. 12-4)

TABLE 12-3

PATHOLOGY TERMS—cont'd

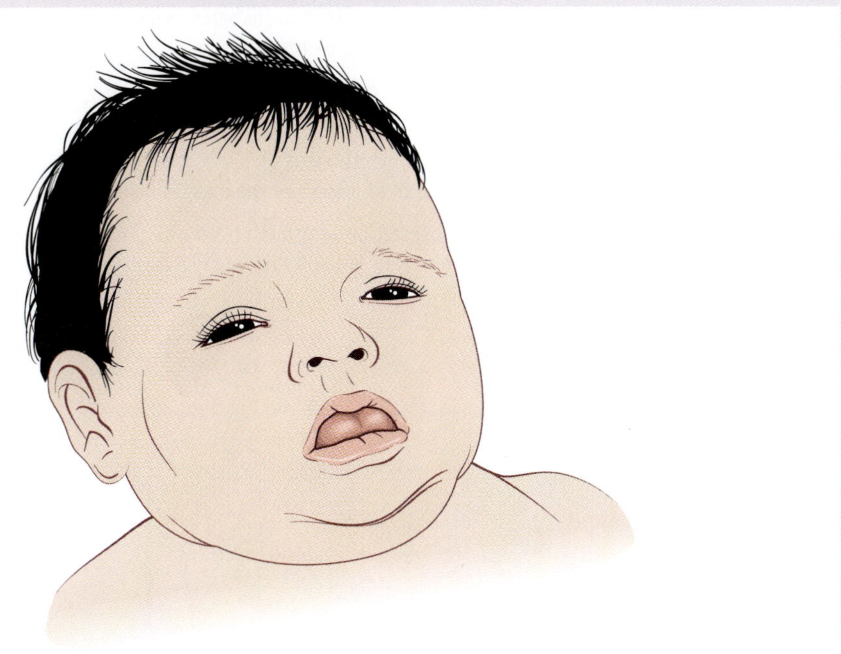

FIGURE 12-4 **Congenital hypothyroidism**

Cushing disease (KOOSH-ĭng dĭ-ZĒZ)	disorder caused by hypersecretion of cortisol by the adrenal gland, resulting in altered fat distribution and muscle weakness; also called *hypercortisolism*, and *hyperadrenalism* (see Fig. 12-5)

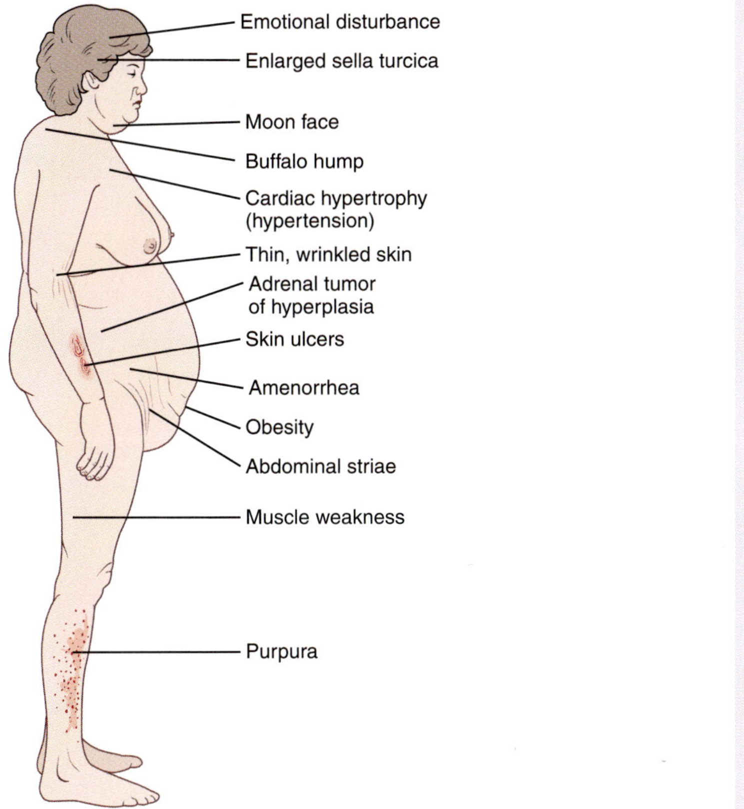

FIGURE 12-5 **Cushing disease**

Continued

TABLE 12-3

PATHOLOGY TERMS—cont'd

Term	Definition
diabetes insipidus (dī-ă-BĒ-tēz ĭn-SĬP-ĭ-dŭs)	disorder unrelated to diabetes mellitus, characterized by excessive output of dilute urine
diabetic ketoacidosis (dī-ă-BĔT-ĭk kē-tō-ă-sĭ-DŌ-sĭs)	condition of severe hyperglycemia
diabetes mellitus (DM) (dī-ă-BĒ-tēz mĕl-Ī-tŭs)	chronic metabolic disorder in which the pancreas secretes insufficient amounts of insulin or the body is insulin resistant
dwarfism (DWĂRF-i-zum)	hyposecretion of growth hormone during childhood, resulting in an abnormally small adult (see Fig. 12-6)

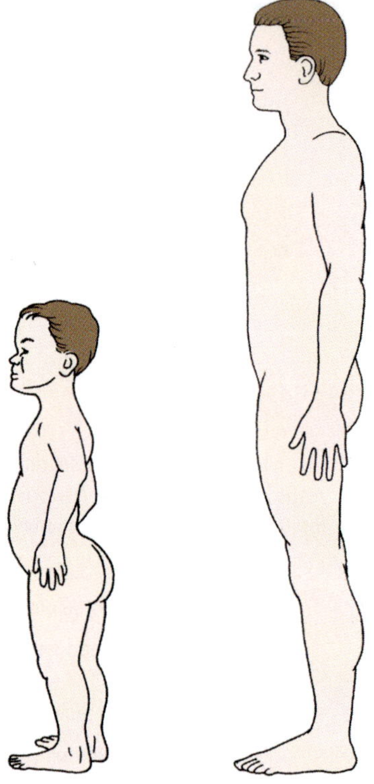

FIGURE 12-6 **Dwarfism**

TABLE 12-3
PATHOLOGY TERMS—cont'd

exophthalmos (ĕks-ŏf-THĂL-mōs)	abnormal protrusion of the eyeballs (see Fig. 12-7)

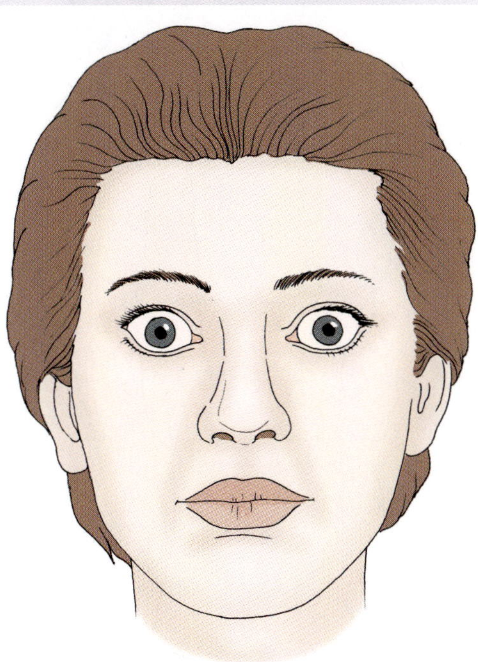

FIGURE 12-7 **Exophthalmos**

gestational diabetes (jĕs-TĀ-shŭn-ăl dī-ă-BĒ-tēz)	diabetes that begins during pregnancy due to insulin resistance and altered glucose metabolism
giantism (JĪ-ăn-tĭ-zum)	type of hyperpituitarism that causes hypersecretion of growth hormone during childhood, resulting in an abnormally large adult (see Fig. 12-8)

Continued

TABLE 12-3
PATHOLOGY TERMS—cont'd

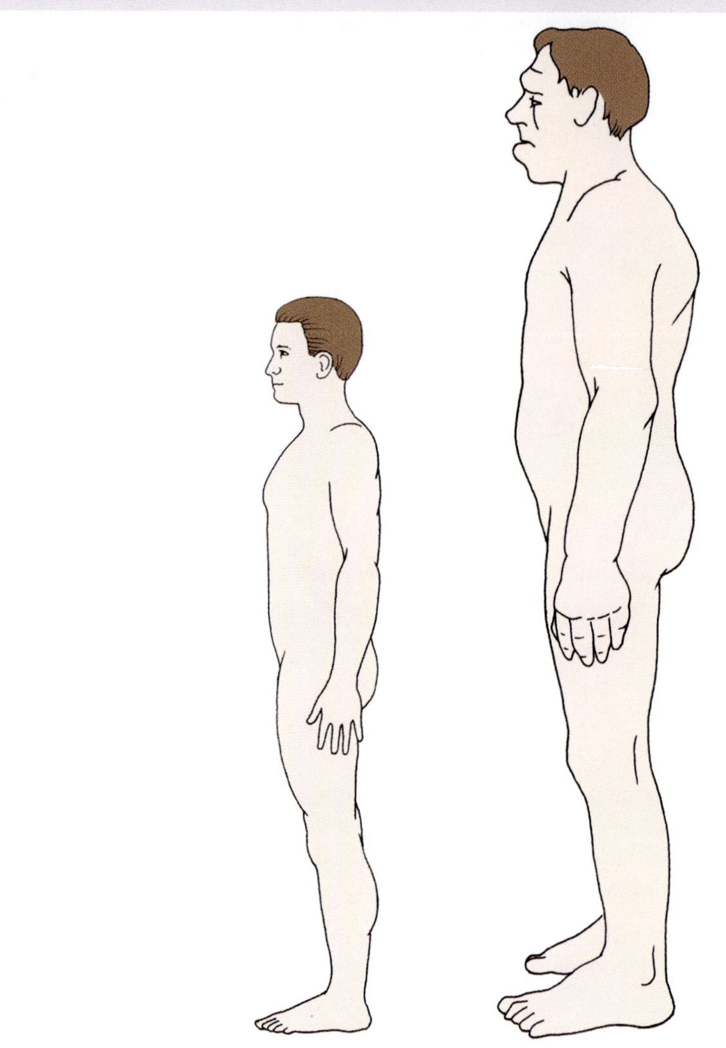

FIGURE 12-8 **Giantism**

goiter (GOY-tĕr)	enlarged thyroid gland
Graves disease (grāvz dĭ-ZĒZ)	hyperthyroidism caused by an autoimmune response, which may cause exophthalmos
Hashimoto disease (hă-shē-MŌ-tō dĭ-ZĒZ)	chronic, inflammatory condition that leads to the most common type of thyroiditis; also called *chronic lymphocytic thyroiditis*
hirsutism (HŬR-sūt-ĭ-zum)	male pattern of body-hair development in females
hyperaldosteronism (hī-pĕr-ăl-dō-STĔR-ōn-ĭ-zum)	condition in which adrenal glands release excessive aldosterone; also called *Conn syndrome*
hyperparathyroidism (hī-pĕr-păr-ă-THĪ-royd-ĭ-zum)	condition in which the parathyroid glands produce an excessive amount of parathyroid hormone (PTH)

TABLE 12-3

PATHOLOGY TERMS—cont'd	
hypoparathyroidism (hī-pō-păr-ă-THĪ-royd-ĭ-zum)	condition in which the parathyroid glands are hypoactive and as a result the level of parathyroid hormones (PTH) is too low
myxedema (mĭks-ĕ-DĒ-mă)	severe form of hypothyroidism that develops in the older child or adult, causing nonpitting edema in connective tissue
nondiabetic hypoglycemia (nŏn-dī-ă-BĔT-ĭk hī-pō-glī-SĒ-mē-ă)	condition in which a nondiabetic person experiences mild symptoms associated with low blood glucose
panhypopituitarism (păn-hī-pō-pĭ-TŪ-ĭ-tăr-ĭ-zum)	condition resulting from diminished secretion of pituitary hormones; also called *underactive pituitary gland*
pheochromocytoma (fē-ō-krō-mō-sī-TŌ-mă)	tumor of the adrenal medulla (central part of the adrenal gland), usually benign but sometimes causing fluctuation of stress hormones like adrenaline
pituitary dwarfism (pĭ-TŪ-ĭ-tăr-ē dwărf-ĭ-zum)	type of hypopituitarism in which reduced growth and development occur due to deficiency of growth hormone in childhood
polydipsia (pŏl-ē-DĬP-sē-ă)	much (increased) thirst
polyphagia (pŏl-ē-FĀ-jē-ă)	much (increased) appetite
polyuria (pŏl-ē-Ū-rē-ă)	much (increased) urination
precocious puberty (prē-KŌ-shŭs PŪ-bĕr-tē)	premature onset of puberty with the appearance of secondary sex characteristics in young children
retinopathy (rĕt-ĭn-ŎP-ă-thē)	disease of the retina, often caused by diabetes
thyrotoxicosis (thī-rō-tŏks-ĭ-KŌ-sĭs)	severe episode of worsening symptoms of hyperthyroidism

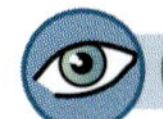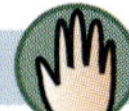

Learning Style Tip

Choose several terms that interest you from Table 12-3 and enter them, one at a time, into an Internet image search engine such as Google Images. Examine the interesting variety of photos and illustrations that you find and see what you can learn from them.

STOP HERE.
Select the Pathology Terms Flash Cards for Chapter 12 and run through them at least three times before you continue.

Common Diagnostic Tests and Procedures

Fasting blood glucose (FBG): Test of blood glucose levels after a fast of 8 to 12 hours, used to screen for diabetes; also called *FBS*, or *fasting blood sugar*

Finger stick blood sugar (fsbs): Test of blood glucose from a drop of capillary blood obtained by pricking the finger; also called *finger stick blood glucose (FSBG)*

Glycosylated hemoglobin (Hb A1c): Reflection of the average blood glucose level over the past 3 to 4 months

Radioactive iodine uptake: Nuclear medicine study which measures how rapidly radioactive iodine is taken up from the blood after oral or intravenous administration

Thyroid function test: Reflection of thyroid function by measuring levels of thyroid-stimulating hormone (TSH), triiodothyronine (T3), and thyroxine (T4)

Thyroid scan: Radiographic evaluation of the thyroid after a radioactive substance is injected; identifies thyroid size, shape, position, and function

Thyroid-stimulating hormone (TSH): Measure of the ability of the thyroid gland to concentrate and retain circulating iodine for synthesis of thyroid hormone

A common area of confusion is between finger stick blood sugar (fsbs) and fasting blood sugar (FBS). Please note the following differences:

FBS: The person has fasted (not eaten anything) for a designated time, usually 8 to 12 hours. Blood is drawn from a vein with a needle and syringe or with a device called a Vacutainer (a needle attached to a vacuum-sealed tube). The blood specimen is tested in the laboratory.

fsbs: Blood sugar may be checked at any time, but is usually checked just prior to meals. A drop of capillary blood is obtained by poking the tip of the finger with a lancet (tiny, sharp blade). The blood is tested immediately using an instrument called a glucometer (see Fig. 12-9).

Flashpoint

FBS requires an 8-to-12-hour fast. Fsbs is often checked just prior to meals

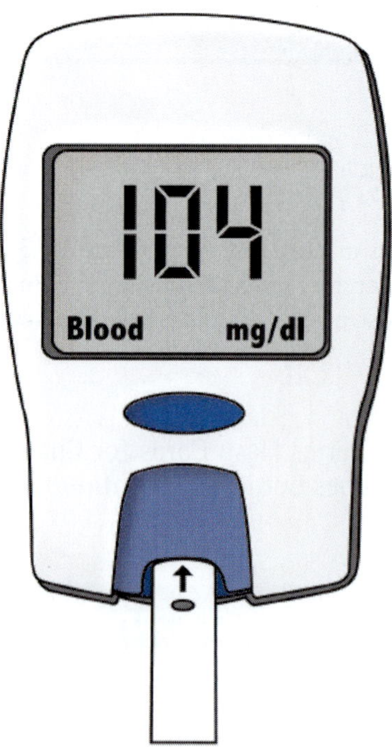

FIGURE 12-9 **Glucometer** (From Eagle, S, et al.: *The Professional Medical Assistant.* F.A. Davis, Philadelphia, 2009, p. 535; with permission)

CASE STUDY

Read the case study and answer the questions that follow. Most of the terms are included in this chapter. Refer to the glossaries (Appendixes B and D) or to your medical dictionary for the other terms.

Diabetes

Marsha Bloom is a 43-year-old female with a history of good health other than mild obesity. She reported a recent 25-pound weight loss over 3 months without dieting. She described an increased appetite and states that she has been eating more than usual. She has also had polydipsia, polyphagia, and polyuria. Ms. Bloom complained of increasing fatigue in spite of getting 8 to 9 hours of sleep each night. Her greatest concern was a recent realization that her vision has worsened significantly. She described being unable to recognize her friend at the grocery store until she was just a few feet away from her. This is what prompted her to seek medical attention.

Ms. Bloom underwent a random blood glucose level test, a fasting blood glucose level test, and a glycosylated hemoglobin test. Diagnosis of diabetes is usually confirmed based on the classic symptoms and two separate fasting glucose levels of more than 126 mg/dl or a random glucose level over 200 mg/dl. In Ms. Bloom's case, the results of all three tests were elevated. Because of this, her physician started her on oral agents to control her blood glucose levels and referred her to a diabetic educator to learn more about her disease and develop a food and exercise plan.

Three months later, after meeting with the diabetic educator and being evaluated by her ophthalmologist, Ms. Bloom began a regular exercise program and made some positive changes in her diet. Over the past 3 months, she has lost another 20 pounds, has noted an improvement in her vision, and commented that her "poly" symptoms have resolved. Best of all, she states that her energy level has increased dramatically.

Non-insulin-dependent diabetes mellitus (NIDDM), also known as **type 2 diabetes**, is the most common form of diabetes, affecting an estimated 20 million Americans. Typical onset occurs after the age of 40, which explains why it has also been known as *adult onset diabetes.* There appears to be a genetic tendency, because it runs in families. Sadly, the incidence of type 2 diabetes is rapidly growing in this country. This is thought to be due to childhood and adult obesity as well as sedentary lifestyle.

Symptoms begin gradually and include the three "poly"s: **polydipsia, polyuria,** and **polyphagia.** Obesity is a common factor, yet as blood sugar skyrockets out of control, individuals may begin to note an ability to eat more yet lose weight. They may also experience delayed wound healing. In NIDDM, the pancreas still produces some insulin; the problem may be a deficiency of insulin production or resistance to the insulin that is produced.

Case Study Questions

1. Ms. Bloom experienced which of the following symptoms prior to diagnosis?
   - **a.** Decreased appetite
   - **b.** Decreased urination
   - **c.** Decreased visual acuity
   - **d.** Weight gain
2. Ms. Bloom's diagnosis of type 2 diabetes was confirmed by:
   - **a.** A test that reveals the average blood glucose level over the past 3 to 4 months
   - **b.** A test of a drop of capillary blood obtained by pricking her finger
   - **c.** A test of her blood after a 1-hour fast
   - **d.** All of these

3. Which of the following statements is true regarding NIDDM?
   a. It is the second most common form of diabetes
   b. Onset is usually before the age of 40 years
   c. Obesity is uncommon
   d. There may be a genetic component

4. Which of the following statements is true regarding NIDDM?
   a. The pancreas fails to produce insulin
   b. The body may be resistant to the insulin that is produced
   c. Exercise is not recommended for disease management
   d. The primary form of treatment is injection of insulin

Answers to Case Study Questions

1. c
2. a
3. d
4. b

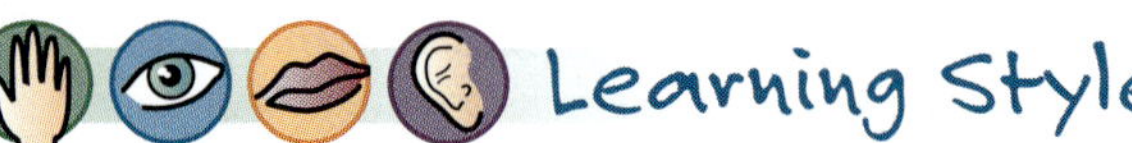

If your instructor provides exam reviews, be sure to attend. They are your opportunity to review and reinforce information, identify correct answers on questions you missed, and ask questions.

Websites

Please go to the F.A. Davis website at http://davisplus.fadavis.com/eagle/medterm to view resource websites for the endocrine system.

Practice Exercises

Deciphering Terms

Write the correct meaning of these medical terms. Check Appendix G for the correct answers.

Exercise 2

1. pancreatic ____________________

2. acromicria ____________________

3. homeotherapy ____________________

4. adrenopathy ______________________________

5. hyperkalemia ______________________________

6. euglycemia ______________________________

7. dysthymic ______________________________

8. thyroidorrhexis ______________________________

9. adenopathy ______________________________

10. glucopenia ______________________________

11. hypoglycemia ______________________________

12. hypernatremia ______________________________

13. glycosuria ______________________________

14. toxicologist ______________________________

15. hydrophobia ______________________________

Fill in the Blanks

Fill in the blanks below. Check Appendix G for the correct answers.

Exercise 3

1. The abbreviation *BS* stands for ____________________ ____________________.

2. Chester has a condition caused by hyposecretion of growth hormone during his childhood. He has ____________________.

3. The abbreviation *CA* stands for ____________________.

4. The abbreviation *Ca* stands for ____________________.

5. The thyroid hormones include ____________________ and ____________________.

6. The abbreviation for diabetes mellitus is ____________________.

7. There are two major forms of diabetes. One is NIDDM, which stands for ____________________ ____________________ ____________________ ____________________.

8. Another form of diabetes is IDDM, which stands for ______ ______ ______ ______.

9. The abbreviation *GH* stands for ______ ______.

10. Abnormal protrusion of the eyeballs is known as ______.

11. Lonnie has a condition caused by hypersecretion of growth hormone during his childhood. He has ______.

12. Adreanna has exophthalmos caused by hyperthyroidism. She has ______ ______.

13. ______ ______ is a condition caused by hypersecretion of cortisol by the adrenal gland, which results in altered fat distribution and muscle weakness.

14. Benito has developed a severe form of hypothyroidism that causes nonpitting edema in connective tissue. He has ______.

15. Julia has ______ disease, in which gradual adrenal gland failure causes insufficient production of steroid hormones and the need for hormone replacement therapy.

16. ______ ______ is a congenital condition of thyroid hormone deficiency, characterized by arrested physical and mental development.

17. The hormone ______ plays a role in regulating and maintaining the body's water, sodium, and electrolyte balance.

18. ______ is the body's natural steroid and works to decrease inflammation.

19. ______ reflects the average blood glucose level over the past 3 to 4 months.

20. The abbreviation *DKA* stands for ______ ______.

Multiple Choice

Select the one best answer to the following multiple-choice questions. Check Appendix G for the correct answers.

Exercise 4

1. Annette Vizzetti has insulin-dependent diabetes mellitus (IDDM). She is a regular patient at Valley Clinic and has come in today for a regular health check. The physician is interested in knowing what Ms. Vizzetti's average blood glucose levels have been for the last 3 to 4 months. Which of the following tests is the physician most likely to order?

   a. TSH

   b. GTT

   c. Hb A1c

   d. Fasting blood glucose

2. When Ms. Vizzetti was first diagnosed with IDDM, she complained to her physician of the three "poly"s, the classic signs of diabetes. Which of the following is **not** one of them?

   a. Polyphagia

   b. Polydipsia

   c. Polyphasia

   d. Polyuria

3. Normal blood glucose level is 60 to 99. When Ms. Vizzetti checks her glucose today, she notes that the result is 172. The correct medical term for this condition is:

   a. Hypercalcemia

   b. Hyperglycemia

   c. Hyperkalemia

   d. Hypernatremia

4. Ms. Singh has been ill for the past 2 days with stomach flu. Her symptoms include diarrhea and vomiting. She has not been able to keep food or fluids down and has become moderately dehydrated. Because of her diarrhea and poor intake, her blood potassium level is below normal. The correct term for this is:

   a. Hyponatremia

   b. Hypocalcemia

   c. Hypokalemia

   d. Hypoglycemia

5. Because Ms. Singh is dehydrated, her blood sodium level is higher than normal. The correct term for this is:
   a. Hypernatremia
   b. Hypercalcemia
   c. Hyperkalemia
   d. Hyperglycemia

Word Building

*Using **only** the word parts in the lists provided, create medical terms with the indicated meanings. Check Appendix G for the correct answers.*

Exercise 5

Prefixes	**Combining Forms**	**Suffixes**
eu-	acr/o	-centesis
hyper-	aden/o	-ectomy
hypo-	adrenal/o	-emia
	calc/o	-ic
	cyan/o	-ism
	dermat/o	-itis
	gluc/o	-kinesia
	hydr/o	-logy
	kal/i	-megaly
	natr/o	-meter
	pancreat/o	-oma
	parathyroid/o	-osis
	thym/o	-pathy
	thyr/o	-ptosis
	thyroid/o	-therapy
	toxic/o	

1. study of poison __________
2. tumor of a gland __________
3. below-normal parathyroid (hormone) __________
4. adrenal disease __________
5. condition of excessive calcium in the blood __________
6. measuring instrument for glucose __________
7. water treatment __________
8. abnormal condition of blueness of the extremities __________
9. condition of excessive potassium in the blood __________

10. inflammation of the pancreas ________________

11. pertaining to a good or normal thymus ________________

12. condition of excessive thyroid ________________

13. inflammation of the skin of the extremities ________________

14. condition of below-normal sodium in the blood ________________

15. excision or surgical removal of the thymus ________________

16. surgical puncture of the pancreas ________________

17. prolapse of the pancreas ________________

18. tumor of the thymus ________________

19. enlargement of the thyroid ________________

20. movement of the extremities ________________

True or False

Decide whether the following statements are true or false. Check Appendix G for the correct answers.

Exercise 6

1. True False The abbreviation **TSH** stands for *thyroid-stimulating hormone.*

2. True False The abbreviation **ADH** stands for *adenopathy.*

3. True False The abbreviation **K** stands for *kidney.*

4. True False A **FBS** measures blood glucose levels after the patient has fasted for 8 to 12 hours.

5. True False The abbreviation **Na** stands for *natural.*

6. True False A **glycosylated hemoglobin** test reveals the average blood glucose level over the past 9 months.

7. True False The abbreviation **fsbs** stands for *fasting blood sugar.*

8. True False A **TSH** level may be drawn to check for hypothyroidism.

9. True False The abbreviation **PTH** stands for *parathyroid hormone.*

10. True False A **fasting blood sugar** is drawn after an 8-to-12-hour fast.

Deciphering Terms

Write the correct meaning of these medical terms. Check Appendix G for the correct answers.

Exercise 7

1. polyphagia ______________________
2. thyrotoxicosis ______________________
3. parathyroidomegaly ______________________
4. polydipsia ______________________
5. glycolysis ______________________
6. pancreatorrhexis ______________________
7. hydrogenic ______________________
8. polyuria ______________________
9. pancreatopathy ______________________
10. microthymic ______________________

Multiple Choice

Select the one best answer to the following multiple-choice questions. Check Appendix G for the correct answers.

Exercise 8

1. Which of the following combining forms means *poison?*
   a. Thyr/o
   b. Thym/o
   c. Toxic/o
   d. Thyroid/o
2. Which of the following combining forms means *extremities?*
   a. Kal/i
   b. Calc/o
   c. Acr/o
   d. None of these

3. Which of the following combining forms means *sodium?*

   a. Natr/o

   b. Kal/i

   c. Acr/o

   d. None of these

4. Which of the following combining forms means *same, unchanging?*

   a. Thym/o

   b. Hydr/o

   c. Aden/o

   d. None of these

5. Which of the following combining forms refers to the adrenal gland?

   a. Aden/o

   b. Thyroid/o

   c. Adren/o

   d. Acr/o

6. Which of the following abbreviations is related to body size?

   a. BMR

   b. BS

   c. BMI

   d. None of these

7. Which of the following abbreviations represents a hormone?

   a. GH

   b. HRT

   c. DI

   d. DKA

8. All of the following abbreviations represent electrolytes **except**:

   a. Na

   b. K

   c. T3

   d. Ca

9. Which of the following tests might be done to measure a patient's current blood sugar?
    a. DM
    b. Fsbs
    c. TSH
    d. ADH

10. An individual suffering from a low hormone level may be administered:
    a. CA
    b. FBS
    c. HRT
    d. IDDM

11. A severe form of hypothyroidism that develops in the older child or adult and causes nonpitting edema in connective tissue is:
    a. Myxedema
    b. Addison disease
    c. Cushing disease
    d. Hirsutism

12. A condition of thyroid hormone deficiency characterized by arrested physical and mental development and formerly known as *cretinism* is:
    a. Congenital hypothyroidism
    b. Hashimoto disease
    c. Acromegaly
    d. Dwarfism

13. A condition of severe hyperglycemia potentially leading to coma is:
    a. Diabetes mellitus
    b. Diabetes insipidus
    c. Diabetic ketoacidosis
    d. Nondiabetic hypoglycemia

14. A tumor of the adrenal medulla that is usually benign but may cause fluctuation of stress hormones like adrenaline is:
    a. Exophthalmos
    b. Pheochromocytoma
    c. Goiter
    d. Thyrotoxicosis

15. All of the following diagnostic tests are matched with the correct definition **except**:

    a. Glycosylated hemoglobin: Reflection of the average blood glucose level over the past 3 to 4 months

    b. Thyroid scan: Radiographic evaluation of the thyroid after a radioactive substance is injected; identifies thyroid size, shape, position, and function

    c. Fasting blood glucose: Test of blood glucose from a drop of capillary blood obtained by pricking the finger

    d. Thyroid function test: Reflection thyroid function by measuring levels of thyroid-stimulating hormone (TSH), triiodothyronine (T3), and thyroxine (T4)

16. Which of the following terms means *excessive sensation in the extremities?*

    a. Acroanesthesia

    b. Adrenalodynia

    c. Anacusis

    d. Hyperacroesthesia

17. Which of the following terms means *creation of sugar?*

    a. Glycolysis

    b. Glucogenic

    c. Glycogenesis

    d. Glucokinesia

18. The term *adenopathy* means:

    a. Disease of a gland

    b. Pertaining to the adrenal gland

    c. Abnormal condition of a gland

    d. None of these

19. The term *hyperkalemia* means:

    a. Condition of excessive calcium in the blood

    b. Condition of excessive potassium in the blood

    c. Condition of excessive sodium in the blood

    d. Condition of excessive iron in the blood

20. Breakdown by the body of water molecules may be called:

    a. Hydrogenesis

    b. Hydrolysis

    c. Hydrokinesis

    d. Hydrophobia

13 SKELETAL AND MUSCULAR SYSTEMS

Structure and Function

The skeletal and muscular systems work together in a complementary fashion to make movement possible. Neither one would be effective without the other: Bones of the skeletal system provide a strong framework for the muscles that are attached to them. When the muscles contract and relax in different combinations, they create a pulling effect on the bones that results in movement.

The Skeletal System

Structures of the skeletal system include bones, tendons, and ligaments (see Fig. 13-1). **Bones** are composed of dense connective tissue, which includes bone cells in a matrix of the mineral calcium and collagen fibers. They are dynamic, living, ever-changing structures. Unlike the white, dry, dead bones you may have seen, living bones have a rich supply of blood vessels and nerves. If injured, they may hurt and bleed. The most common injuries to bones are fractures. This also means they have the ability to heal themselves. Important to the healing process is the development of **osteocytes**, new bone cells, which are constantly created through **osteogenesis**. New cells replace older ones that are injured or broken down as they age. Because bones are able to remodel themselves in this way, certain activities, such as weight lifting or weight-bearing exercise like jogging and walking, stimulate bones to become stronger and denser.

The skeletal system functions to provide protection, movement, and a framework for the body. An example of bones that provide protection are those that make up the **cranium**. They are fused together to create a strong protective container for the brain. Another example is the bones of the **vertebral column**, which protect the spinal cord and combine with the **sternum** and **ribs** to create the **thorax**, which protects the heart, great vessels, and lungs (see Fig. 13-2).

The skeletal system also plays important roles in blood production and mineral regulation. Bone marrow within bone performs **hematopoiesis**, or the production of red and white blood cells. This explains why a bone marrow transplant may be necessary for someone with a blood disorder such as leukemia.

Flashpoint
Weight-bearing exercise helps bones become stronger.

Flashpoint
The skeletal system protects soft tissues and organs.

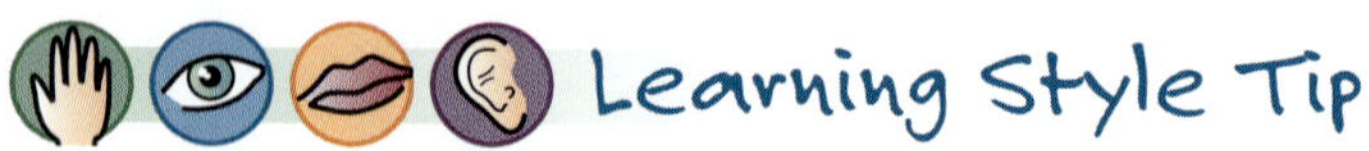

Rewrite explanations, concepts, and definitions from this chapter in your own words. This forces you to think about what they really mean, and to put them into simpler terms that you will remember. For verbal and auditory benefit, read aloud to yourself as you do this.

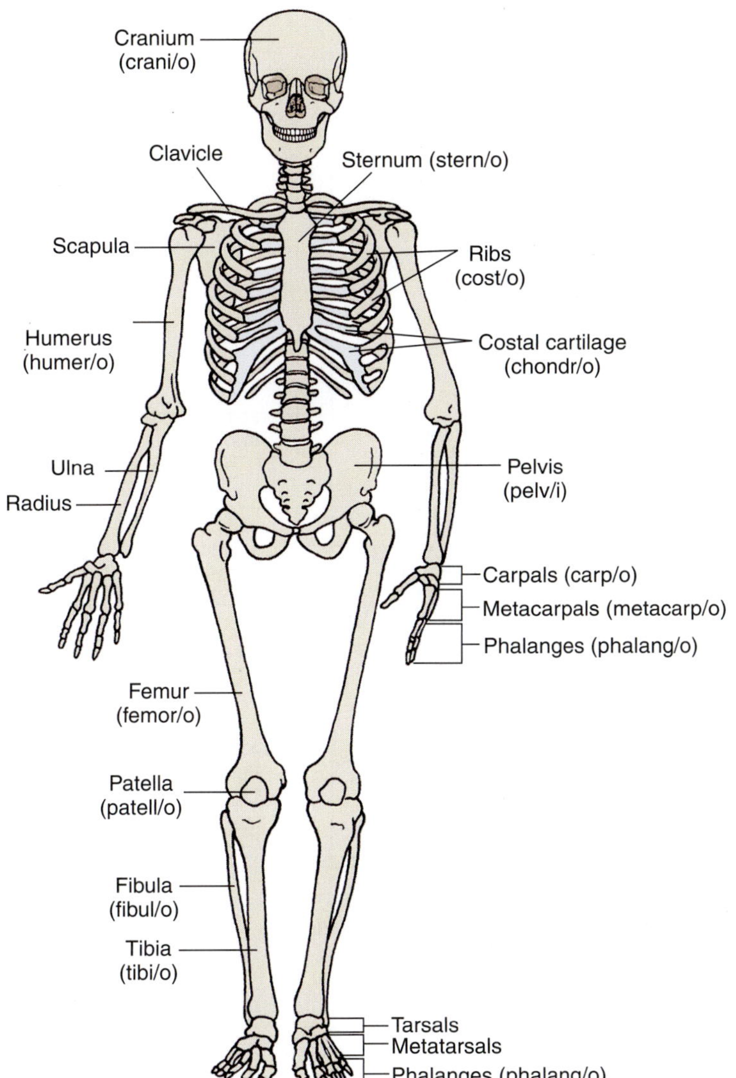

FIGURE 13-1 **The skeletal system**

Bones store essential minerals such as calcium, phosphorus, and magnesium. These minerals are largely responsible for providing bones with strength and hardness. These same minerals are also necessary for nerve and muscle function, so they must be present in these tissues as well as in the blood. When dietary mineral intake is inadequate or the need for these minerals increases, as in puberty or pregnancy, the bones release their stores of minerals into the bloodstream for use. This may result in decreased bone strength and density. If sufficient minerals are not replenished, the result is a disorder known as **osteoporosis**.

Tendons are cords of fibrous connective tissue that attach muscles to bones. A tendon that attaches to a larger area of a bone is called an **aponeurosis**. This structure is flat or ribbonlike, and larger than a typical tendon. Tendons do not contract or lengthen when muscles contract or relax, but they help to enable the bone's movement.

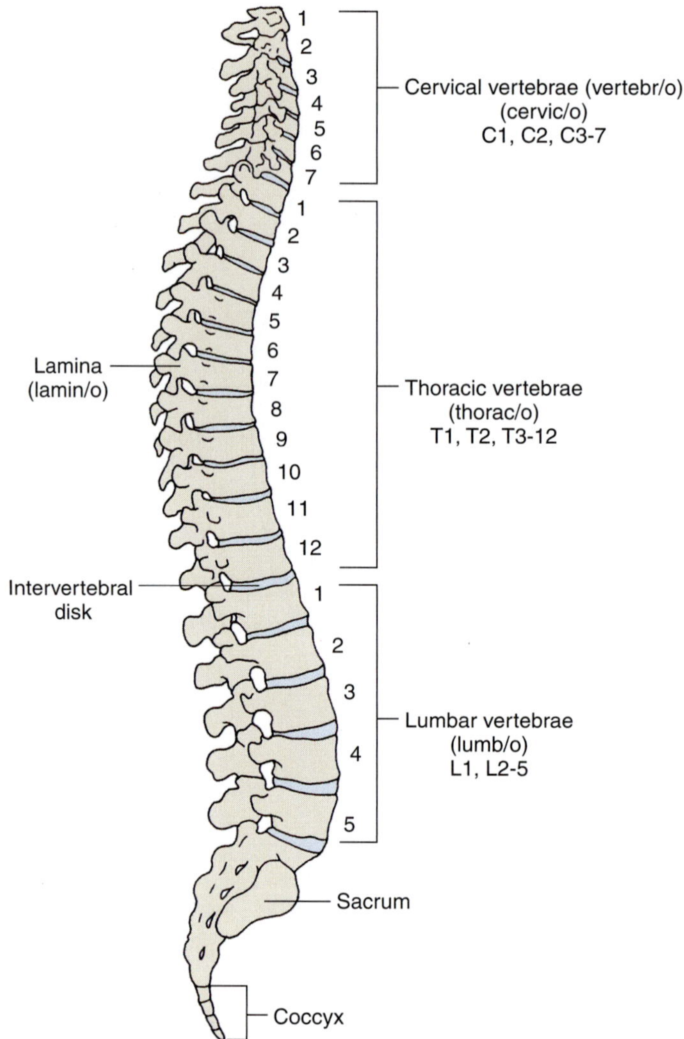

FIGURE 13-2 **The vertebral column**

Ligaments are bands or sheets of strong, fibrous connective tissue that connect bones to other bones across joints. They provide joint stability and limit joint motion. They essentially hold joints together, allowing the attached muscles to move bones upon contraction while preventing the joint from falling apart.

Flashpoint
Ligaments give our joints their stability.

A **joint** is a place where two bones meet. Bones enable movement at joints through attachments to muscles and tendons. There are three types of bone joint, sometimes called *articulations:*

Synarthrosis—an immovable joint, such as the sutures of the skull
Amphiarthrosis—a slightly movable joint, such as a vertebra
Diarthrosis—a freely movable joint, such as the knee joint

Some joints allow for a great deal of movement, such as the shoulder joint. Some allow no movement, such as those between the bones of the skull. The movable joints are similar to each other and include structures located within a **joint capsule** (see Fig. 13-3). These structures include the **articular cartilage**,

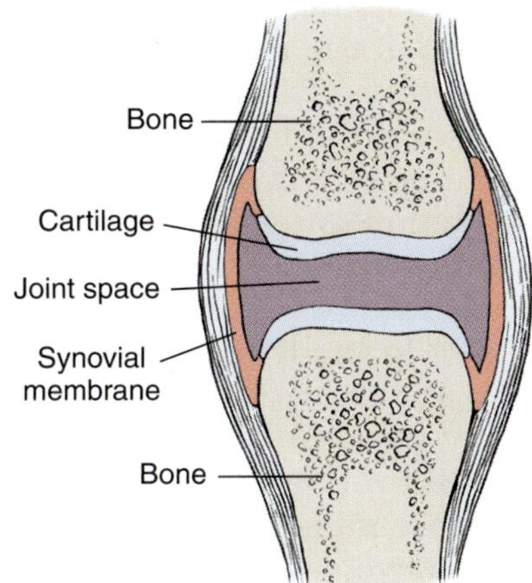

FIGURE 13-3 **Synovial joint**

the **synovial membrane**, and the **synovial fluid**. They protect bone ends and facilitate movement. A common disorder of these joints is called **osteoarthritis**, also known as **degenerative joint disease (DJD)**; it causes erosion of these structures, resulting in inflammation, pain, and decreased movement.

The Muscular System

Muscles are connective tissues made up of contractile fibers. They are covered by a fibrous membrane called a **fascia**, which is connective tissue arranged in sheets or bands. The fascia covers, separates, and supports muscle. Because muscle and fascia are connected, these structures are commonly referred to as one structure: **myofascia**.

There are three types of muscle: striated (skeletal) muscle, sometimes called *voluntary muscle;* smooth muscle, sometimes called *involuntary muscle;* and cardiac muscle (see Fig. 13-4).

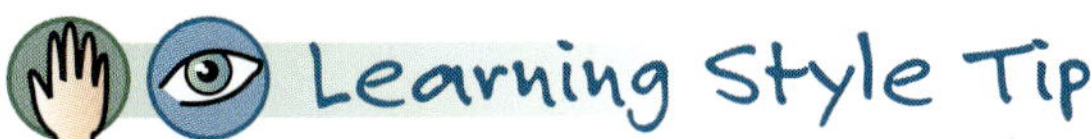

Translate key sections of text or definitions of terms from this chapter into pictures, symbols, or diagrams. Without looking at the original text, attempt to translate your symbolic writing back into words. Then check the original text to see how close you came.

Striated muscles are found in all skeletal muscles and also in the tongue, pharynx, and upper portion of the esophagus. The striations, or stripes, in this type of muscle are due to the bundled structure of the muscle fibers and its appearance under the microscope. This type of muscle is also sometimes called

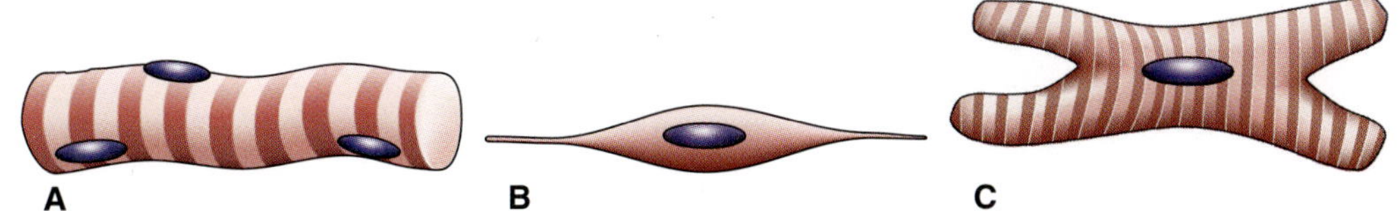

FIGURE 13-4 **Three types of muscle: (A) Skeletal, (B) Smooth, (C) Cardiac**

voluntary muscle because we are usually able to consciously move and control it. Skeletal muscles are involved in the movement of body parts, reflexive movements, and maintenance of posture. Examples of skeletal muscles are those that move bones, the eyeballs, and the tongue. Skeletal muscles contract to create movement. The type and force of movement depends on the type of muscle and the force of muscle contraction. Muscle groups often work together to achieve movement and stabilization. For example, the quadriceps femoris, or "quads," as they are commonly known, work together to extend the leg. While this is occurring, other muscles in the trunk of the body maintain enough contraction to keep the body in a stable, upright position. They work with tendons and ligaments to help the body move under the control of the brain and spinal cord. Nerves at motor points within the muscle tissue receive signals from the brain and spinal cord and initiate muscle movement (see Fig. 13-5). Skeletal muscles are required for such movement as walking. A person's **gait**, or the manner and style in which the person walks, is coordinated by the skeletal muscles of the back, trunk, and legs. Skeletal muscle responds to exercise by increasing in strength, size, and definition. Skeletal muscles that are not used (for example, in a comatose patient), will **atrophy**, or decrease in size. Figure 13-6 illustrates the major muscles of the body.

Flashpoint

Muscles and bones work together so that we can move.

In addition to fostering movement and providing support, skeletal muscles also produce heat as a by-product of their function. This is why a person feels hot and begins to perspire while exercising: The body has produced more heat than is needed, and natural cooling mechanisms kick in. This same principle works when a person is exposed to a cold environment and more body heat is needed. Without adequate clothing, body temperature drops and shivering begins. Shivering is an involuntary increase in muscle activity that produces heat energy as a by-product, which warms the body.

Flashpoint

Heat is a natural by-product of muscle activity.

Smooth muscle is found principally in the internal organs of the digestive tract, respiratory passages, the urinary bladder, and the walls of blood vessels. No cross striations appear on these muscle fibers. This type of muscle

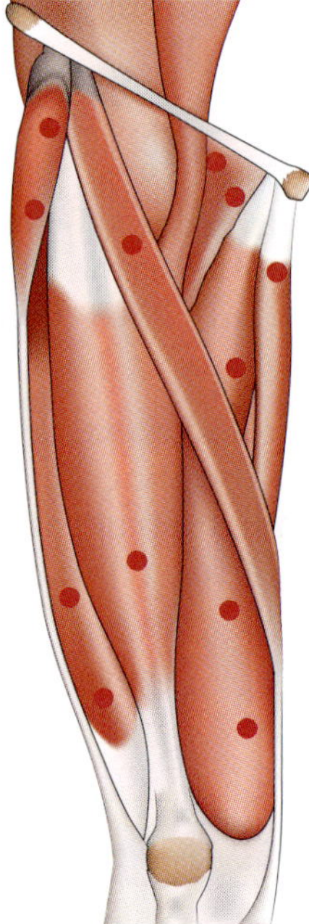

FIGURE 13-5 Motor point of muscle

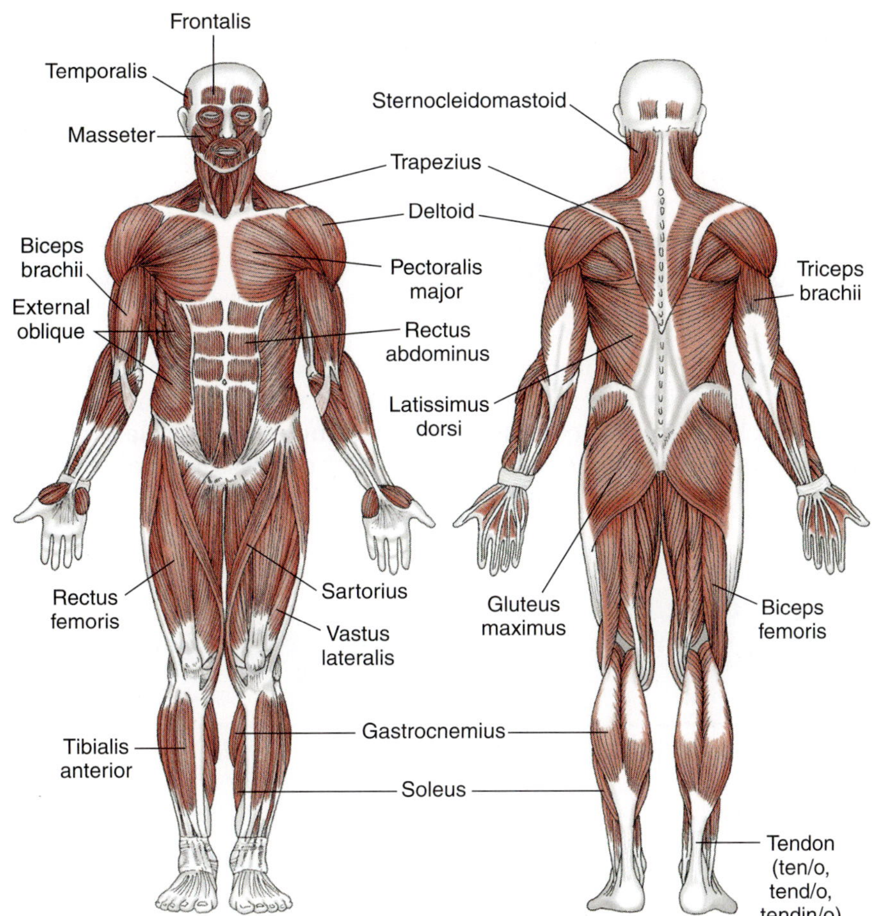

FIGURE 13-6 **The muscular system**

is arranged in sheets or layers. It is considered involuntary because it functions without the need for conscious thought. In the digestive tract, smooth muscle contracts to propel food through the alimentary canal to be broken down for digestion and absorption. In the walls of blood vessels, smooth muscle moves blood through the vessels to various parts of the body. Unlike skeletal muscle, smooth muscle's size and strength cannot be affected by exercise.

Cardiac (heart) muscle cells contain striations that appear similar to skeletal muscle cells. However, these muscle fibers are arranged in branching networks, rather than linear bundles. The branched structure allows them to connect with one another in a continuous network. Located at the connections are *intercalated disks,* which increase the efficiency of electrical impulse transmission throughout the heart. Cardiac muscle works to pump blood through the heart and out to the body. Strong contractions of the heart muscle push blood through the circulatory system, supplying blood and oxygen to all the tissues of the body. Blood returns to the right side of the heart—which pumps it to the lungs, where it is reoxygenated—and then returns back to the left side of the heart. As with skeletal muscles, cardiac muscle's efficiency improves with use. Exercise that increases the heart rate increases the efficiency of the cardiac muscle.

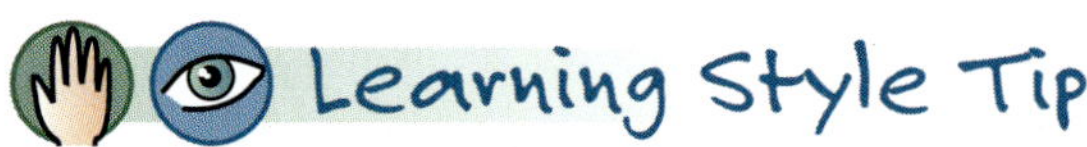

Purchase an anatomy coloring book and color the bone illustrations with bright colors. Write the associated combining forms in the same colors next to each bone as you color it.

Combining Forms

Table 13-1 contains combining forms that pertain to the musculoskeletal system, a combination of the skeletal and muscular systems, along with examples of terms which utilize the combining forms, and a pronunciation guide. Read aloud to yourself as you move from left to right across the table. Be sure to use the pronunciation guide so that you can learn to say the terms correctly.

Flashpoint

Write the following numbers in a vertical pattern: 7, 12, 5, 5, 4. Repeat the numbers aloud until you have them memorized. Second, write the following terms next to each number from top to bottom: cervical, thoracic, lumbar, sacral, coccygeal. Third, repeat the numbers with each term top to bottom until you have them memorized. You have just memorized 33 bones of the body: the vertebrae— seven cervical, twelve thoracic, five lumbar, five sacral, and four coccyx.

TABLE 13-1
COMBINING FORMS

Combining Form	Meaning	Example (Pronunciation)	Meaning of New Term
ankyl/o	stiff joint	ankylosis (ăng-kĭ-LŌ-sĭs)	abnormal condition of a stiff joint
arthr/o	joint	arthrocentesis (ăr-thrō-sĕn-TĒ-sĭs)	surgical puncture of a joint
articul/o		articular (ăr-TĬK-ū-lăr)	pertaining to a joint
burs/o	bursa, sac	bursitis (bŭr-SĪ-tĭs)	inflammation of a bursa
carp/o	carpus	carpectomy (kăr-PĔK-tō-mē)	excision or surgical removal of a carpus
cervic/o	neck	cervicodynia (sĕr-vĭ-kō-DĬN-ē-ă)	pain of the neck
chondr/o	cartilage	chondrodysplasia (kŏn-drō-dĭs-PLĀ-zē-ă)	bad, painful, or difficult formation or growth of cartilage
cost/o	ribs	costochondritis (kŏs-tō-kŏn-DRĪ-tĭs)	inflammation of the ribs and cartilage
crani/o	cranium	craniocerebral (krā-nē-ō-sĕ-RĒ-brăl)	pertaining to the cranium and brain
fasci/o	fascia	fasciodesis (făsh-ē-ŎD-ĕ-sĭs)	binding or surgical fixation of a fascia
femor/o	femur	femorotibial (fĕm-ō-rō-TĬB-ē-ăl)	pertaining to the femur and tibia
fibul/o	fibula	fibular (FĬB-ū-lăr)	pertaining to the fibula
humer/o	humerus	humeral (HŪ-mĕr-ăl)	pertaining to the humerus

TABLE 13-1
COMBINING FORMS—cont'd

Combining Form	Meaning	Example (Pronunciation)	Meaning of New Term
ili/o	ilium	iliolumbar (ĭl-ē-ō-LŬM-bar)	pertaining to the ilium and lower back
kinesi/o	movement	kinesiology (kĭ-nē-zē-ŎL-ō-jē)	study of movement
kyph/o	hump	kyphosis (kī-FŌ-sĭs)	abnormal condition of a hump
lamin/o	lamina	laminectomy (lăm-ĭ-NĔK-tō-mē)	excision or surgical removal of a lamina
lord/o	bent backward	lordoscoliosis (lōr-dō-skō-lē-Ō-sĭs)	abnormal condition of crookedness and backward bend
lumb/o	lower back	lumbodynia (lŭm-bō-DĬN-ē-ă)	pain of the lower back
menisc/o	meniscus	meniscectomy (mĕn-ĭ-SĔK-tō-mē)	excision or surgical removal of a meniscus
metacarp/o	metacarpus	metacarpectomy (mĕt-ă-kăr-PĔK-tō-mē)	excision or surgical removal of a metacarpus
metatars/o	metatarsals, ankle	metatarsophalangeal (mĕt-ă-tăr-sō-fă-LĂN-jē-ăl)	pertaining to the ankle, metatarsals, and phalanges
muscul/o	muscle	musculoskeletal (mŭs-kū-lō-SKĔL-ĕ-tăl)	pertaining to the muscles and skeleton
my/o		myocardial (mī-ō-KĂR-dē-ăl)	pertaining to heart muscle
myel/o	spinal cord, bone marrow	myeloplegia (mī-ĕl-ō-PLĒ-jē-ă)	paralysis of the spinal cord
orth/o	straight	orthopnea (or-THŎP-nē-ă)	breathing in the straight position
oste/o	bone	osteolytic (ŏs-tē-ō-LĬT-ĭk)	pertaining to the destruction of bone
patell/a	patella	patellapexy (pă-TĔL-ă-pĕk-sē)	surgical fixation of the patella
patell/o		patelloptosis (pă-TĔL-ŏpt-ō-sis)	prolapse of the patella
pelv/i	pelvis	pelvimeter (pĕl-VĬM-ĕ-tĕr)	measuring instrument for the pelvis
phalang/o	phalanges	phalangitis (făl-ăn-JĪ-tĭs)	inflammation of the phalanges
pub/o	pubis	pubofemoral (pū-bō-FĔM-ōr-ăl)	pertaining to the pubis and femur
radi/o	radius	radioulnar (rā-dē-ō-ŬL-năr)	pertaining to the radius and ulna
sacr/o	sacrum	sacrodynia (sā-krō-DĬN-ē-ă)	pain of the sacrum

Continued

TABLE 13-1
COMBINING FORMS—cont'd

Combining Form	Meaning	Example (Pronunciation)	Meaning of New Term
scoli/o	crooked, bent	scoliometer (skō-lē-ŎM-ĕt-ĕr)	measuring instrument for crookedness or bend
spondyl/o	vertebrae	spondylomalacia (spŏn-dĭ-lō-mă-LĀ-shē-ă)	softening of a vertebra
vertebr/o		vertebroplasty (vĕr-TĒ-brō-plăs-tē)	surgical repair of a vertebra
stern/o	sternum	sternocostal (stĕr-nō-KŎS-tăl)	pertaining to the sternum and ribs
synov/o	synovial membrane	synovectomy (sĭn-ō-VĔK-tō-mē)	surgical removal of a synovial membrane
synovi/o		synovioma (sĭn-ō-vē-Ō-mă)	tumor of a synovial membrane
tars/o	ankle (tarsal bones)	tarsometatarsal (tăr-sō-mĕt-ă-TĂR-săl)	pertaining to the ankle
ten/o	tendon	tenodynia (tĕn-ō-DĬN-ē-ă)	pain of a tendon
tend/o		tendotome (TĔN-dō-tōm)	cutting instrument for a tendon
tendin/o		tendinous (TĔN-dĭ-nŭs)	pertaining to a tendon
thorac/o	thorax	thoracolumbar (thō-răk-ō-LŬM-bar)	pertaining to the thorax and lower back
tibi/o	tibia	tibiofibular (tĭb-ē-ō-FĬB-ū-lăr)	pertaining to the tibia and fibula
uln/o	ulna	ulnocarpal (ŭl-nō-KĂR-păl)	pertaining to the ulna and carpus

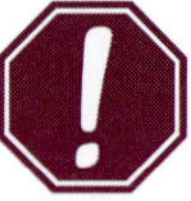

STOP HERE.
Select the Combining Form Flash Cards for Chapter 13 and run through them at least three times before you continue.

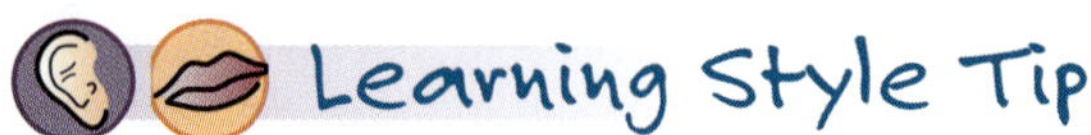

Play instrumental music (without lyrics) while studying these terms. Repeatedly sing the terms and their meanings aloud along to the music until you can remember them.

Practice Exercises

Fill in the Blanks

Fill in the blanks below using Table 13-1. Check Appendix G for the correct answers.

Exercise 1

1. pertaining to the tibia and fibula ______________________________
2. inflammation of the phalanges ______________________________
3. surgical repair of a vertebra ______________________________
4. surgical fixation of the patella ______________________________
5. pain in a tendon ______________________________
6. pertaining to the femur and tibia ______________________________
7. cutting instrument for a tendon ______________________________
8. pertaining to a tendon ______________________________
9. paralysis of the spinal cord ______________________________
10. pertaining to the destruction of bone ______________________________
11. excision or surgical removal of a metacarpus ______________________________
12. pertaining to the humerus ______________________________
13. pertaining to the sternum and ribs ______________________________
14. measuring instrument for the pelvis ______________________________
15. pertaining to the thorax and lower back ______________________________
16. breathing in the straight position ______________________________
17. pertaining to heart muscle ______________________________
18. surgical puncture of a joint ______________________________
19. excision or surgical removal of a carpus ______________________________
20. bad, painful, or difficult formation or growth of cartilage

    ____
21. inflammation of the ribs and cartilage ______________________________

22. pain of the neck ______________________

23. pertaining to the cranium and brain ______________________

24. pertaining to the fibula ______________________

25. excision or surgical removal of a lamina ______________________

26. pertaining to a joint ______________________

27. inflammation of a bursa ______________________

28. binding or surgical fixation of a fascia ______________________

29. pertaining to the ilium and lower back ______________________

30. abnormal condition of crookedness and backward bend

____

31. abnormal condition of a hump ______________________

32. pertaining to the muscles and skeleton ______________________

33. study of movement ______________________

34. measuring instrument for crookedness or bend ______________________

35. excision or surgical removal of a meniscus ______________________

36. pain of the sacrum ______________________

37. pertaining to the ulna and carpus ______________________

38. pain of the lower back ______________________

39. pertaining to the radius and ulna ______________________

40. excision or surgical removal of a synovial membrane ______________________

41. abnormal condition of a stiff joint ______________________

42. softening of a vertebra ______________________

43. pertaining to the pubis and femur ______________________

44. pertaining to the ankle ______________________

45. tumor of a synovial membrane ______________________

46. pertaining to the metatarsals and phalanges ______________________

47. **Fill in the blanks in Figure 13-7 with the appropriate anatomical terms and combining forms.**

48. **Fill in the blanks in Figure 13-8 with the appropriate anatomical terms and combining forms.**

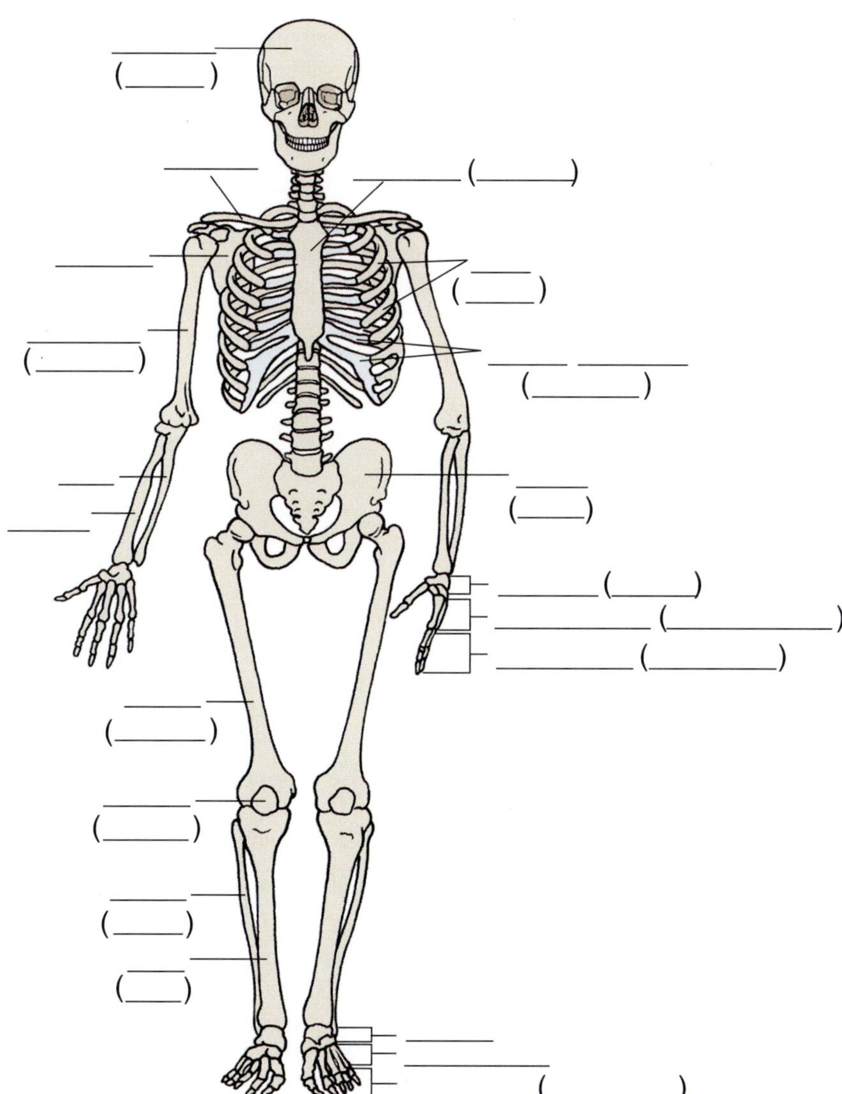

FIGURE 13-7 **Skeletal system with blanks**

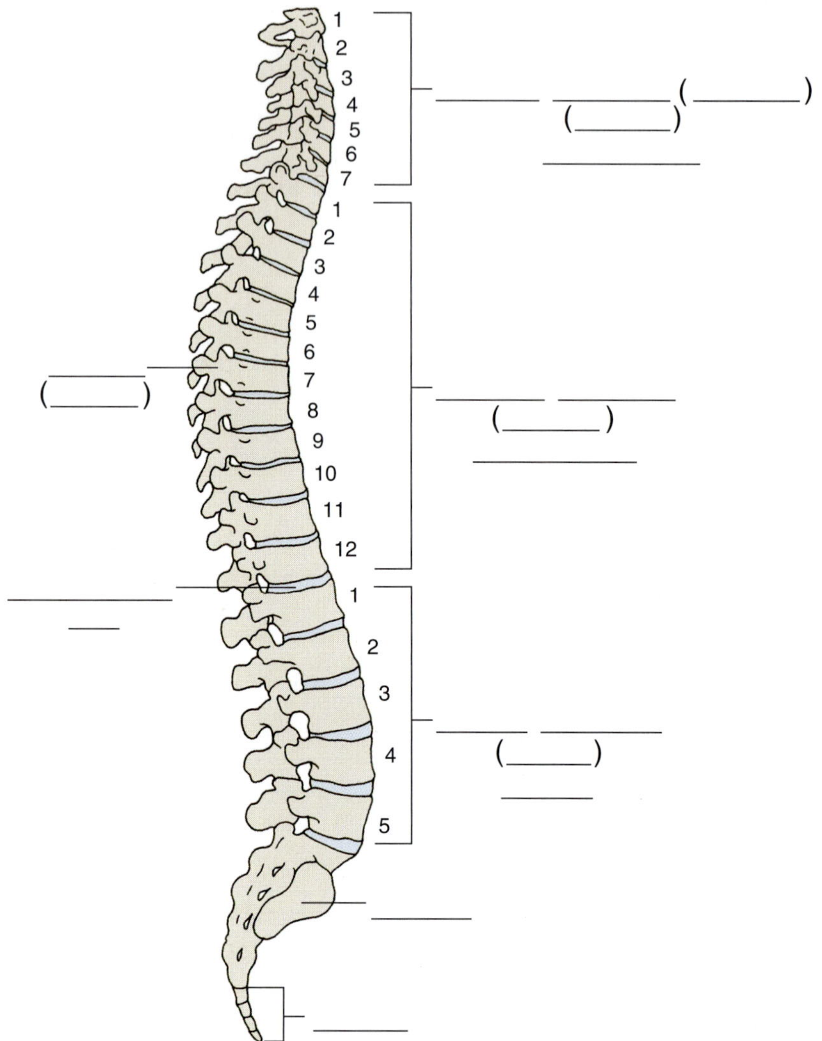

FIGURE 13-8 Vertebral column with blanks

49. Fill in the blanks in Figure 13-9 with the appropriate anatomical terms and combining forms.

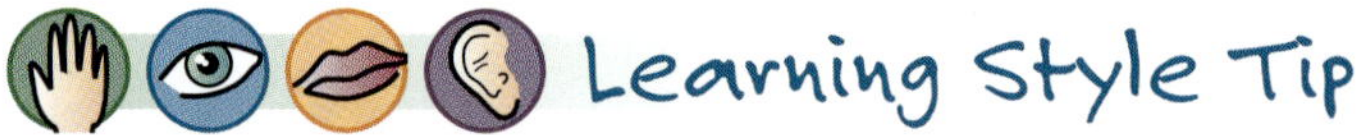

Learning Style Tip

Write out poems or sayings that include the terms and definitions from this chapter that you need to remember. The sillier they are, the more likely you are to remember them. Read them aloud and repeat them over and over until you have them memorized.

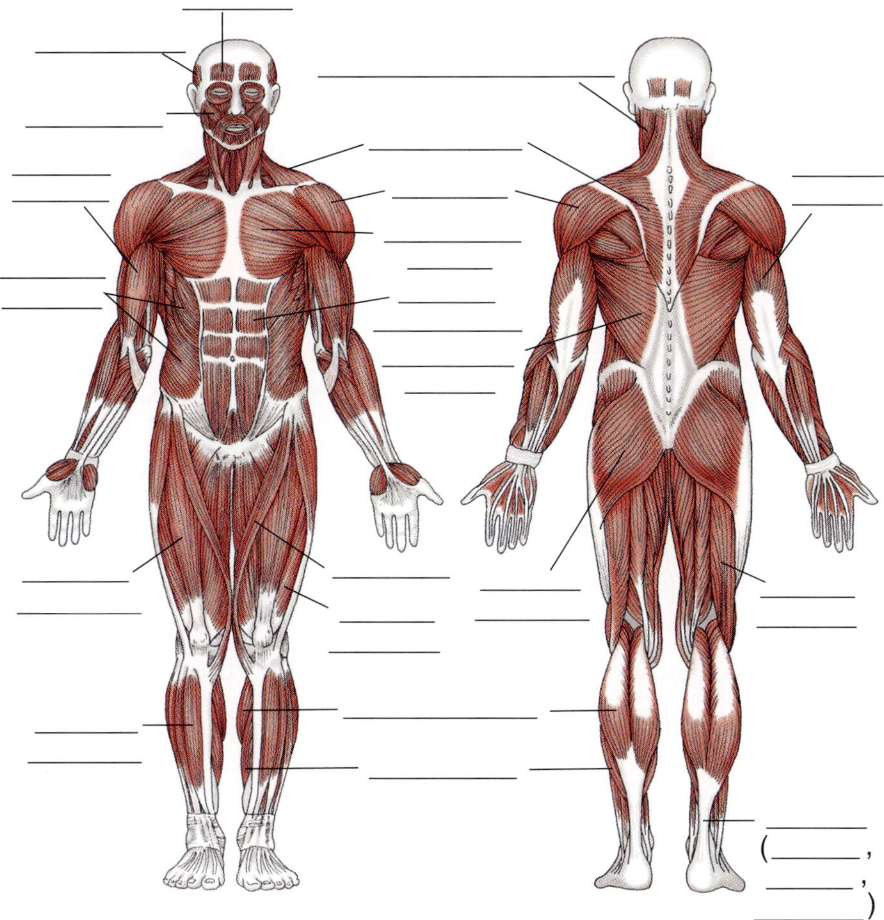

FIGURE 13-9 **Muscular system with blanks**

Abbreviations

Table 13-2 lists some of the most common abbreviations related to the musculoskeletal system, as well as others often used in medical documentation.

TABLE 13-2
ABBREVIATIONS

ACL	anterior cruciate ligament	AS	ankylosing spondylitis
ADL	activities of daily living	BE	below the elbow
AE	above the elbow	BK	below the knee
AK	above the knee	BKA	below-the-knee amputation
AKA	above-the-knee amputation	BMD	bone mineral density
AP	anteroposterior	C1-C7	first cervical vertebra, second cervical vertebra, etc.

Continued

TABLE 13-2
ABBREVIATIONS—cont'd

DJD	degenerative joint disease (osteoarthritis)	HNP	herniated nucleus pulposus
DTR	deep tendon reflex	IM	intramuscular
EMG	electromyography	JRA	juvenile rheumatoid arthritis
Fx	fracture (see Fig. 13-10)	L1-L5	first lumbar vertebra, second lumbar vertebra, etc.

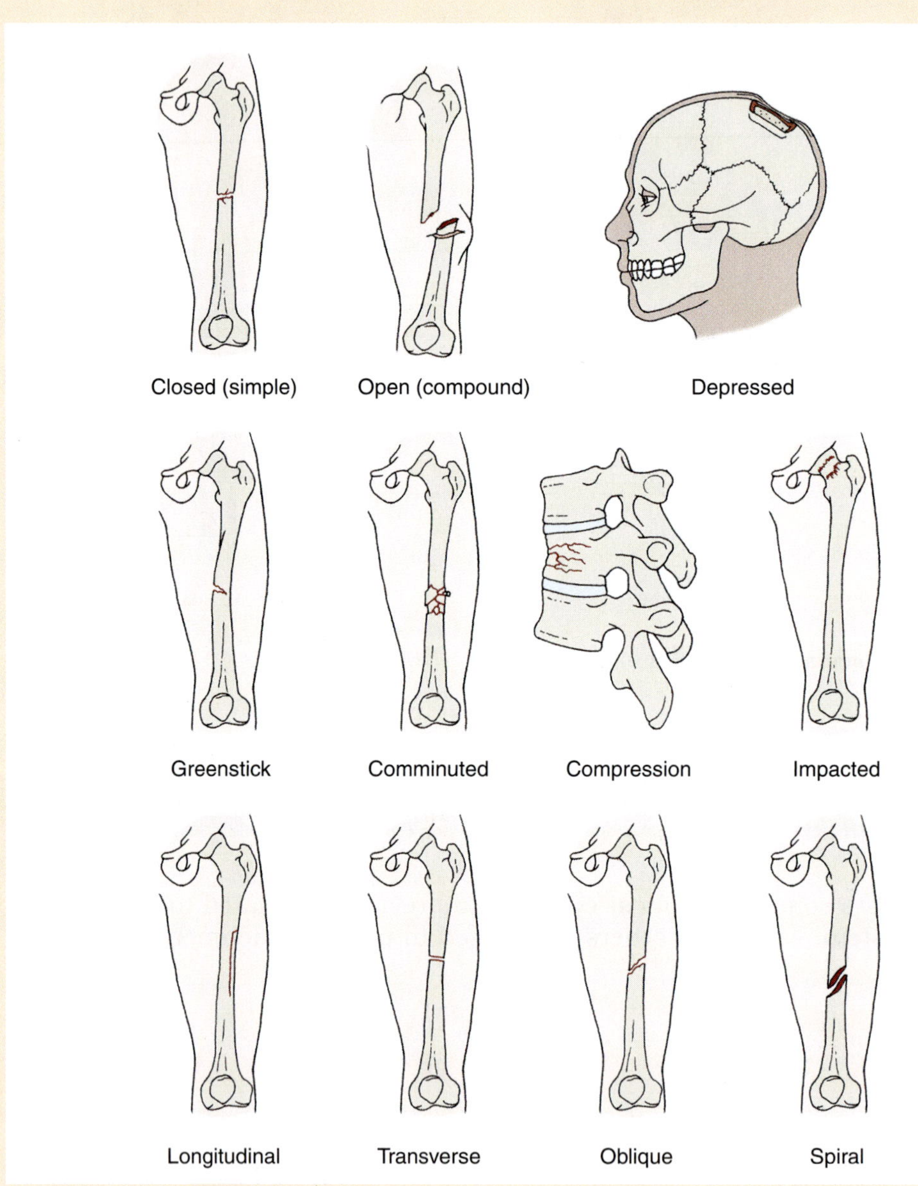

FIGURE 13-10 **Types of fractures**

TABLE 13-2
ABBREVIATIONS—cont'd

LE	lower extremity	RA	rheumatoid arthritis
LLE	left lower extremity	RLE	right lower extremity
LUE	left upper extremity	ROM	range of motion
MVA	motor vehicle accident	RUE	right upper extremity
NSAID	nonsteroidal anti-inflammatory drug	S1-S5	first sacral vertebra, second sacral vertebra, etc.
OA	osteoarthritis	T1-T12	first thoracic vertebra, second thoracic vertebra, etc.
ORIF	open reduction-internal fixation	THA, THR	total hip arthroplasty, total hip replacement
ortho	orthopedic, straight	TKR	total knee replacement
OT	occupational therapy	UE	upper extremity
PT	physical therapy		

STOP HERE.
Select the Abbreviation Flash Cards for Chapter 13 and run through them at least three times before you continue.

Pathology Terms

Table 13-3 includes terms that relate to diseases or abnormalities of the musculoskeletal system. Use the pronunciation guide and say the terms aloud as you read them. This will help you get in the habit of saying them properly.

Flashpoint
With so many people using computers, carpal tunnel syndrome (CTS) has become a common disorder.

STOP HERE.
Select the Pathology Terms Flash Cards for Chapter 13 and run through them at least three times before you continue.

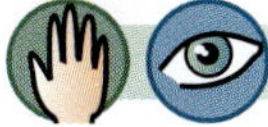

Learning Style Tip

Ask permission to spend time with your study buddy in the anatomy lab at your school. Locate the muscle and skeletal models and take turns applying temporary sticky labels to them with the appropriate names and associated combining forms.

TABLE 13-3

PATHOLOGY TERMS

adhesive capsulitis (ăd-HĒ-sĭv kăp-sū-LĪ-tĭs)	loss of range of motion in the shoulder; also called *frozen shoulder*
anterior cruciate ligament tear (ăn-TĒR-ē-ōr KROO-shē-āt LĬG-ă-mĕnt tār)	injury to one of the stabilizing ligaments of the knee, which originates on the anterior portion of the femur (see Fig. 13-11)

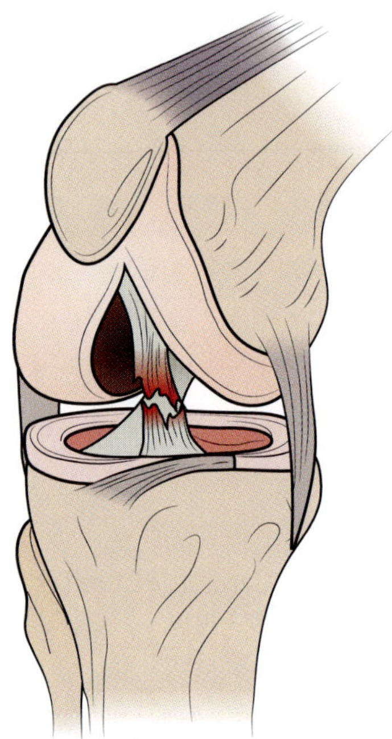

FIGURE 13-11 **Anterior cruciate ligament tear**

bursitis (bŭr-SĪ-tĭs)	condition of inflammation of the tiny fluid-filled sacs that act as cushions and provide lubrication to decrease friction and irritation between structures such as bones, tendons, muscles, and skin
carpal tunnel syndrome (CTS) (KĂR-păl TŬN-ĕl SĬN-drōm)	compression of the median nerve, causing pain or numbness in the wrist, hand, and fingers (see Fig. 13-12)

TABLE 13-3

PATHOLOGY TERMS—cont'd

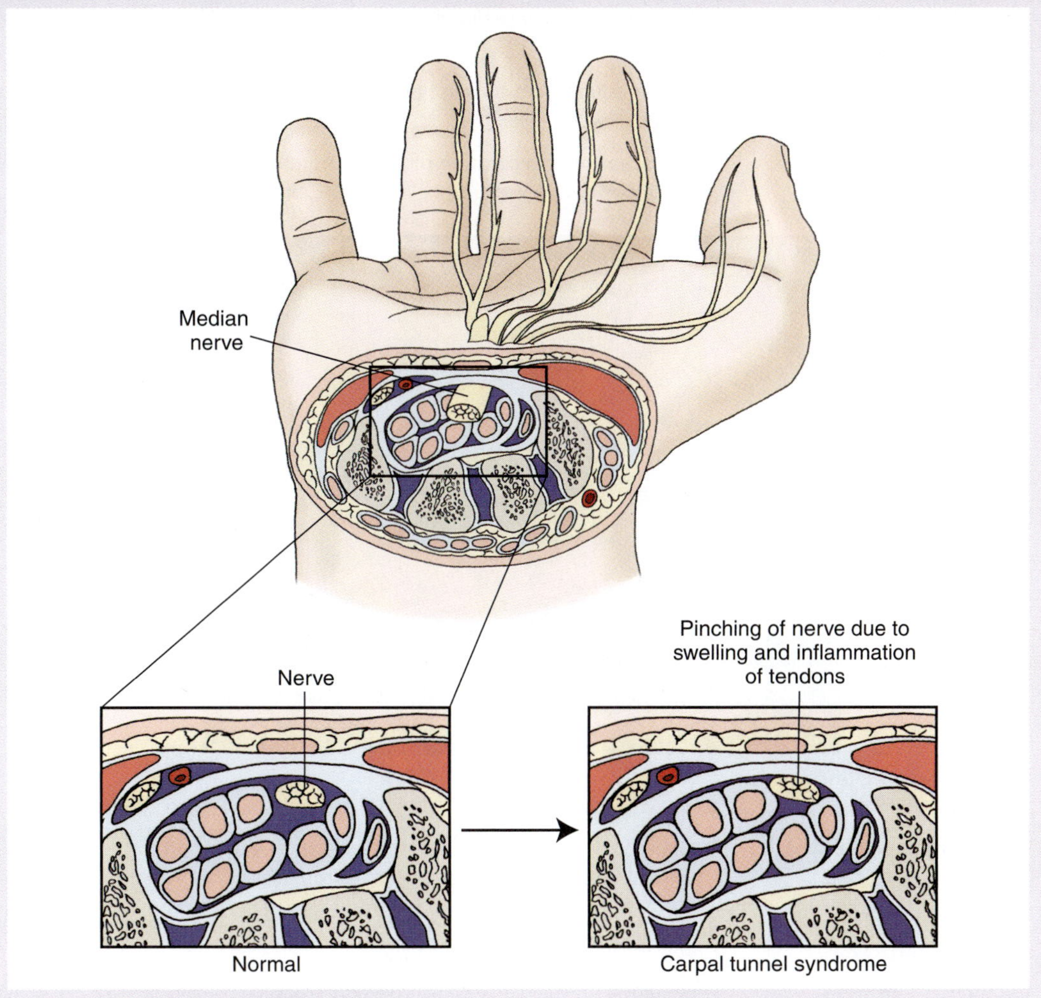

FIGURE 13-12 **Carpal tunnel syndrome**

claw toe (klaw tō)	condition in which the metatarsophalangeal (MTP) joint flexes dorsally while the other joint or joints in the toe flex toward the sole (see Fig. 13-13)

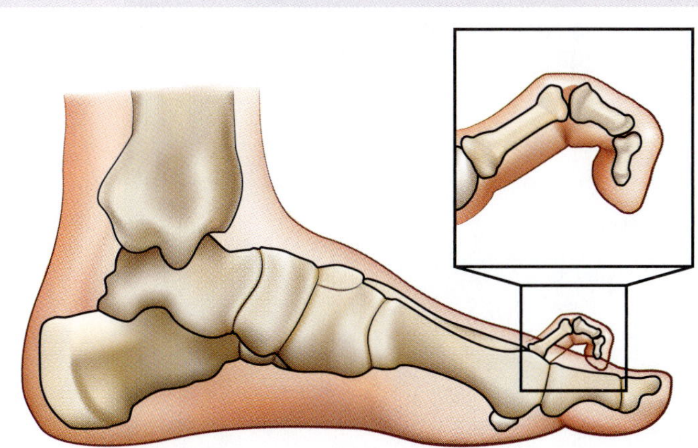

FIGURE 13-13 **Claw toe**

Continued

TABLE 13-3

PATHOLOGY TERMS—cont'd

contracture (kŏn-TRĂK-chūr)	fibrosis of connective tissue which decreases the mobility of a joint
crepitation (krĕp-ĭ-TĀ-shŭn)	grating sound from broken bones, or a clicking or crackling sound from joints
dislocation (dĭs-lō-KĀ-shŭn)	displacement or separation of a bone from its normal position where it articulates with another bone (see Fig. 13-14)

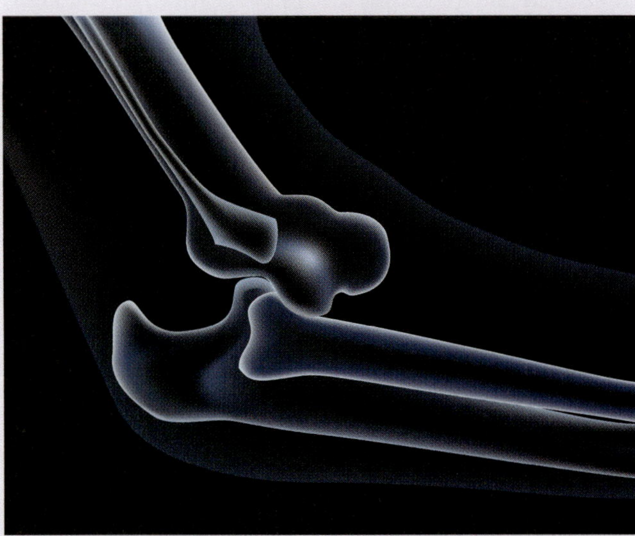

FIGURE 13-14 **Dislocation**

electromyography (EMG) (ē-LEK-trō-mī-og-ră-fē)	test used to evaluate and record the electrical activity produced by skeletal muscles; used to diagnose neuromuscular disorders
fibromyalgia (fī-brō-mī-ĂL-jē-ă)	chronic condition marked by pain in the muscles, tendons, ligaments, and soft tissues of the body
fracture (FRĂK-chūr)	condition in which a bone is broken or cracked (see Fig. 13-15)

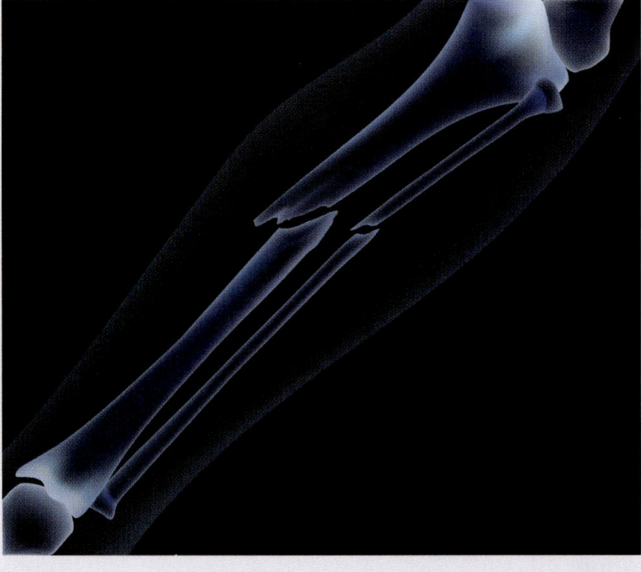

FIGURE 13-15 **Fracture**

TABLE 13-3
PATHOLOGY TERMS—cont'd

ganglion cyst (GĂNG-glē-ŏn sĭst)	condition in which one or more small, benign tumors filled with a thick, colorless, gelatinous substance develop over a joint or tendon, usually on the wrist or back of the hand; sometimes called a *Bible cyst* (see Fig. 13-16)

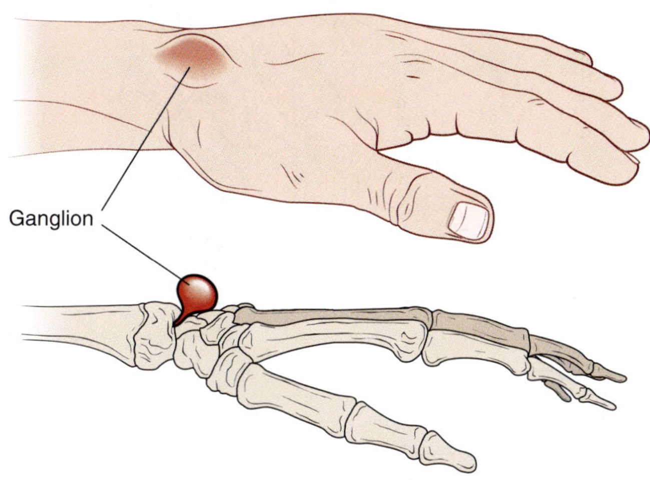

FIGURE 13-16 Ganglion cyst

gout (gowt)	hereditary form of arthritis, characterized by uric acid accumulation in the joints, especially in the great toe (see Fig. 13-17)

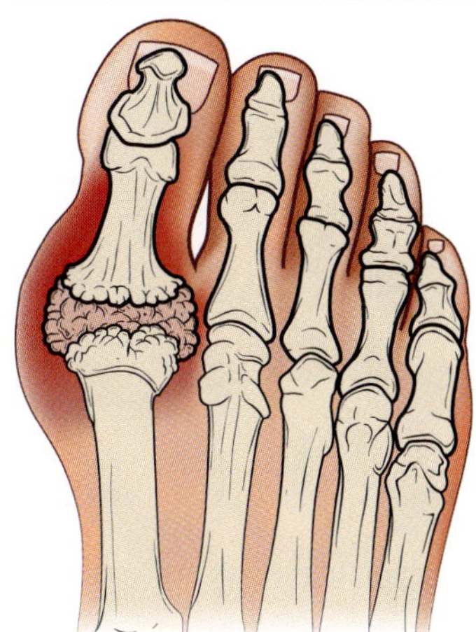

FIGURE 13-17 Gout affecting the great toe

hallux rigidus (HĂL-ŭks RĬJ-ĭ-dŭs)	condition in which degenerative arthritis affects the metatarsophalangeal (MTP) joint at the base of the big toe, causing pain and stiffness
hallux valgus (HĂL-ŭks VĂL-gŭs)	condition in which the big toe is improperly aligned, pointing laterally toward the second toe and creating a large bump on the inner edge of the foot at the base of the big toe; commonly called *bunion* (see Fig. 13-18)

Continued

TABLE 13-3
PATHOLOGY TERMS—cont'd

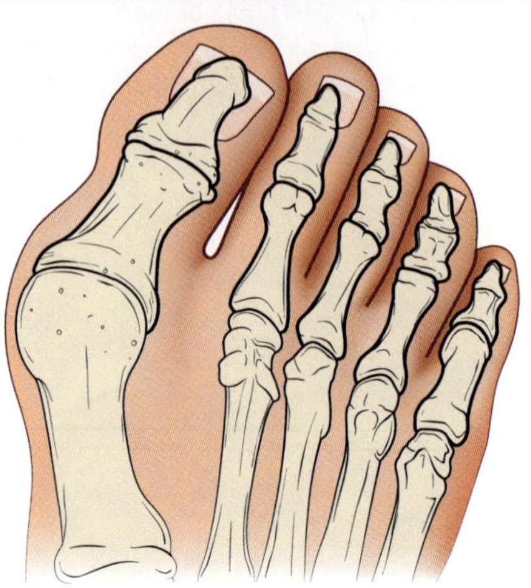

FIGURE 13-18 **Hallux valgus**

hammertoe (HĂM-ĕr-tō)	condition in which the toe is bent downward at the proximal interphalangeal (PIP) joint (see Fig. 13-19)

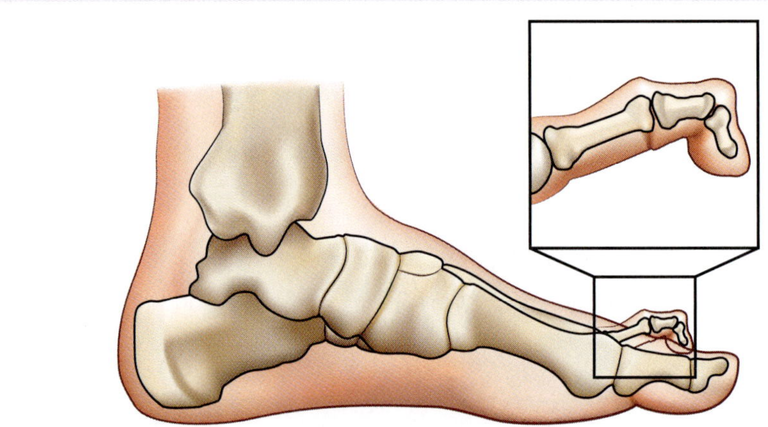

FIGURE 13-19 **Hammertoe**

herniated disk (HĔR-nē-ā-tĕd dĭsk)	herniation of the soft center of an intervertebral disk (see Fig. 13-20)

TABLE 13-3
PATHOLOGY TERMS—cont'd

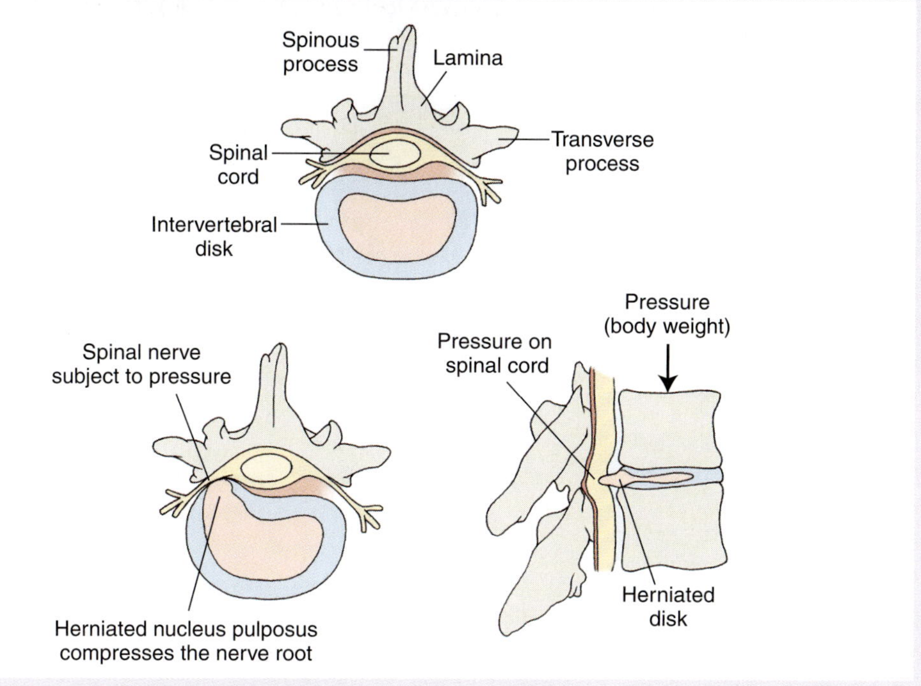

FIGURE 13-20 **Herniated lumbar disk**

juvenile rheumatoid arthritis (JRA) (JŪ-vě-nīl ROO-mă-toyd ăr-THRĪ-tĭs)	disorder similar to adult-onset RA, with earlier onset and more severe symptoms
kyphosis (kī-FŌ-sĭs)	abnormal increase in the curvature of the thoracic vertebrae, causing hunchback (see Fig. 13-21)

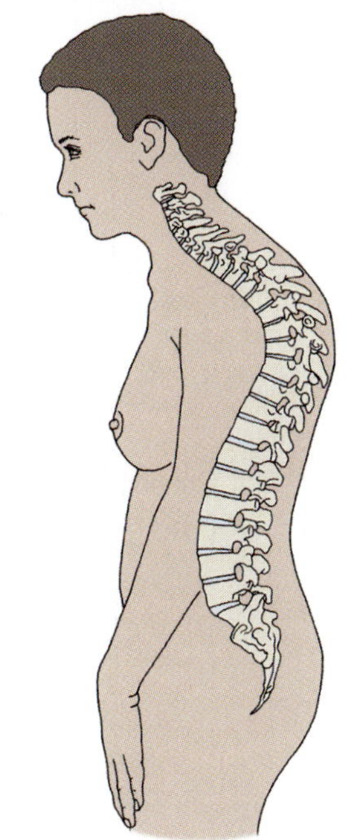

FIGURE 13-21 **Kyphosis**

Continued

TABLE 13-3 PATHOLOGY TERMS—cont'd	
lordosis (lor-DŌ-sĭs)	abnormal increase in the curvature of the lumbar vertebrae, causing swayback (see Fig. 13-22)

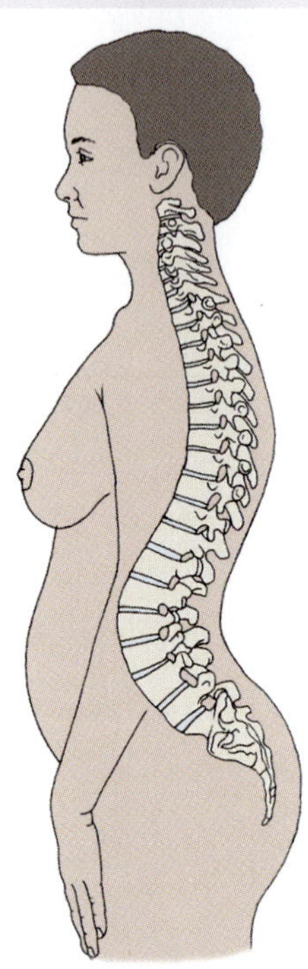

FIGURE 13-22 **Lordosis**

mallet toe (MĂL-ĕt- tō)	condition in which the toe is bent downward at the distal interphalangeal (DIP) joint (see Fig. 13-23)

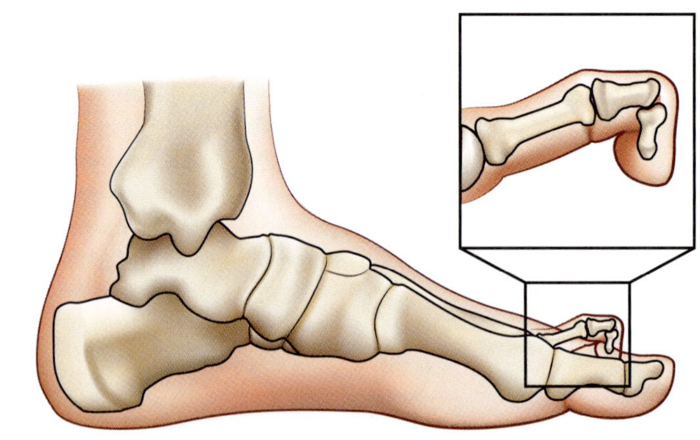

FIGURE 13-23 **Mallet toe**

TABLE 13-3

PATHOLOGY TERMS—cont'd

medial tibial syndrome (MĒ-dē-ăl TĬB-ē-ăl SĬN-drōm)	painful condition involving tiny tears in the muscles and tendons that attach to the anterior tibia (shin); commonly called *shin splints*
meniscal tear (mĕn-ĬS-kăl tār)	tear of one of the two C-shaped cartilage structures that serve to cushion and stabilize the knee joint, usually caused by a twisting force (see Fig. 13-24)

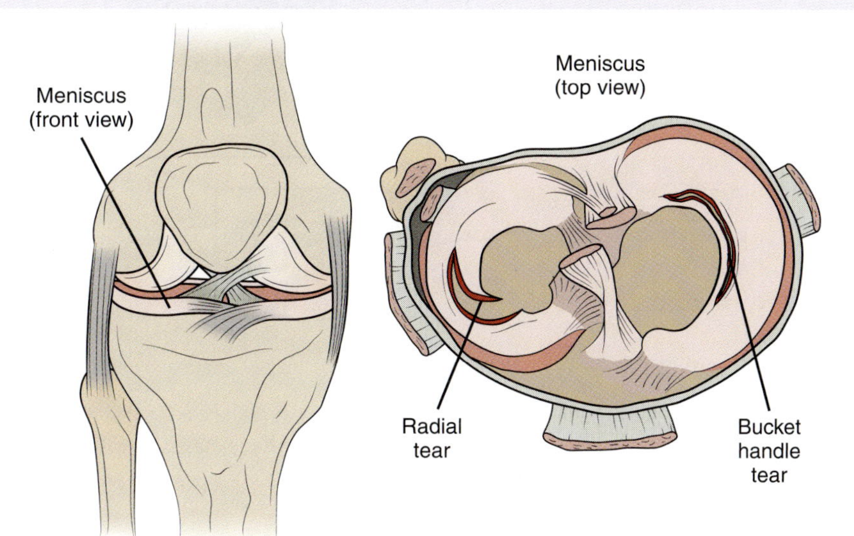

FIGURE 13-24 **Meniscal tear**

muscular dystrophy (MD) (MŬS-kū-lăr DĬS-trō-fē)	hereditary, progressive, terminal disease that causes muscle atrophy and death, usually by age 20
myasthenia gravis (mī-ăs-THĒ-nē-ă GRĂV-ĭs)	autoimmune motor disorder that causes progressive muscle fatigue and weakness
osteitis deformans (äs-tē-Ī T-ŭs dē-FŌRM-ănz)	chronic condition in which the process of bone destruction and regrowth occurs abnormally, causing weak, fragile, enlarged, and misshapen bones; also called *Paget disease*
osteoarthritis (ŏs-tē-ō-ăr-THRĪ-tĭs)	condition of cartilage deterioration and joint inflammation marked by pain, stiffness, and decreased ROM, most commonly affecting synovial weight-bearing joints and vertebrae
osteomalacia (ŏs-tē-ō-măl-Ā-shē-ă)	condition of softening and weakening of the bones; when it occurs in children, it is called *rickets*

Continued

TABLE 13-3

PATHOLOGY TERMS—cont'd

osteomyelitis (ŏs-tē-ō-mī-ĕl-Ī-tĭs)	acute or chronic infection within the bone, most commonly affecting the legs, arms, pelvis, and spine (see Fig. 13-25)

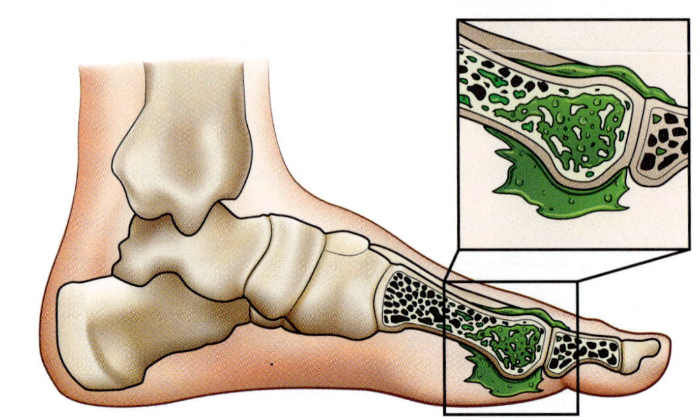

FIGURE 13-25 **Osteomyelitis**

osteoporosis (ŏs-tē-ō-pōr-Ō-sĭs)	condition characterized by loss of bone mass throughout the skeleton (see Fig. 13-26)

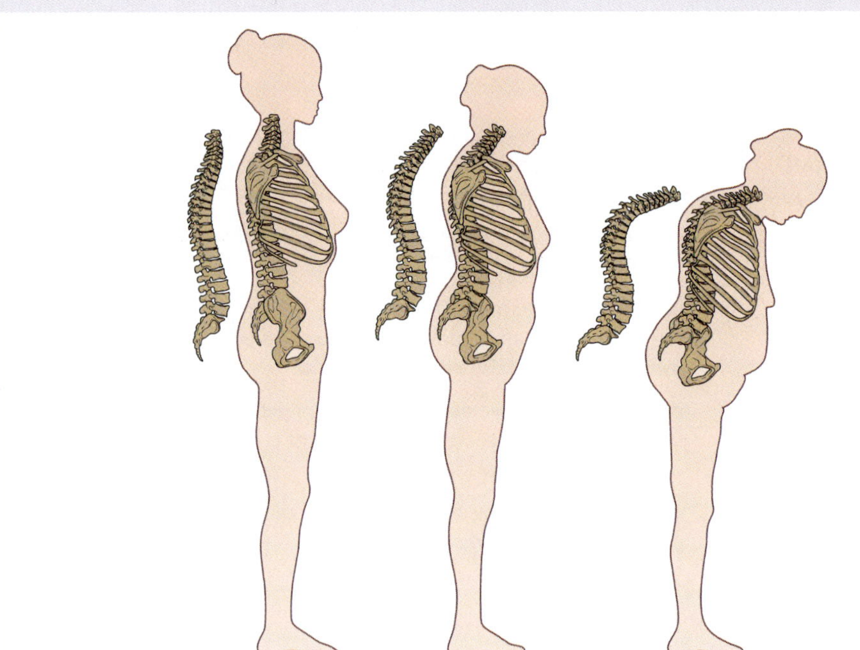

FIGURE 13-26 **Osteoporosis**

pathological fracture (păth-ō-LŎJ-ĭk-ăl FRĂK-chūr)	breaking of diseased, weakened bone from the stress of normal everyday activities

TABLE 13-3
PATHOLOGY TERMS—cont'd

plantar fasciitis (PLĂN-tăr făs-ē-Ī-tĭs)	painful condition of the supporting structures of the arch of the foot, primarily the plantar fascia, a band of tissue that connects the heel with the toes (see Fig. 13-27)

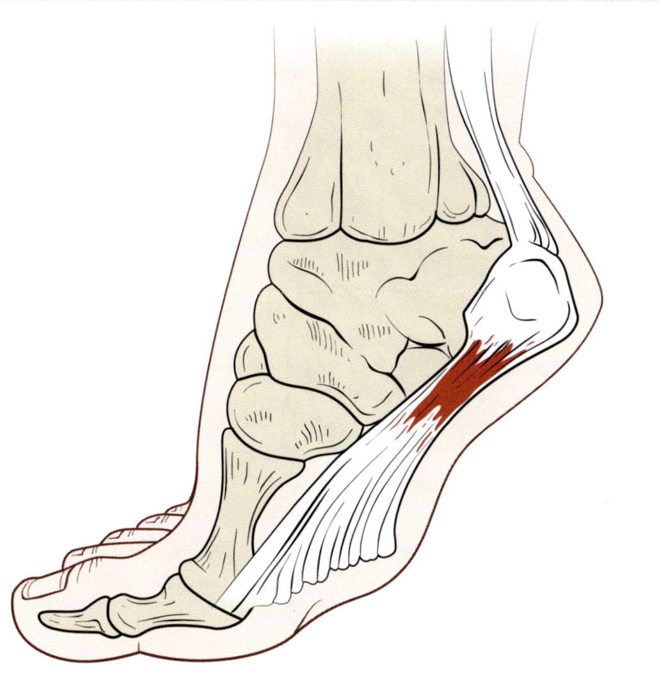

FIGURE 13-27 **Plantar fasciitis**

rheumatoid arthritis (RA) (ROO-mă-toyd ăr-THRĪ-tĭs)	autoimmune arthritis that causes progressive joint pain and deformity and may affect organ systems (see Fig. 13-28)

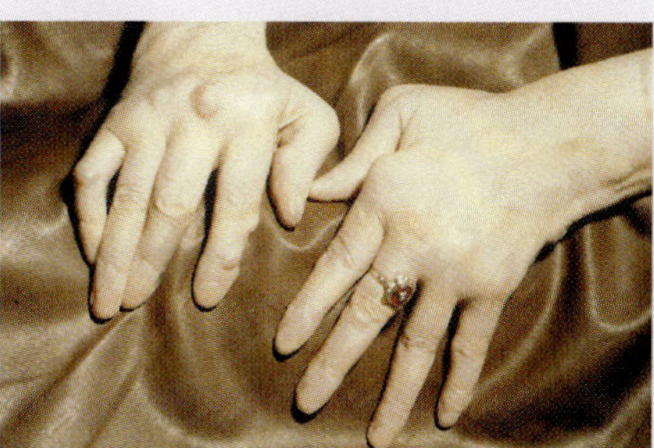

FIGURE 13-28 **Rheumatoid arthritis** (From Dillon, PM: *Nursing Health Assessment.* F.A. Davis, Philadelphia, 2008, p. 627; with permission)

Continued

TABLE 13-3

PATHOLOGY TERMS—cont'd

rotator cuff tear (RŌ-tā-tŏr kŭf tār)	traumatic rip of one or more of the muscles or tendons within the rotator cuff of the shoulder (see Fig. 13-29)

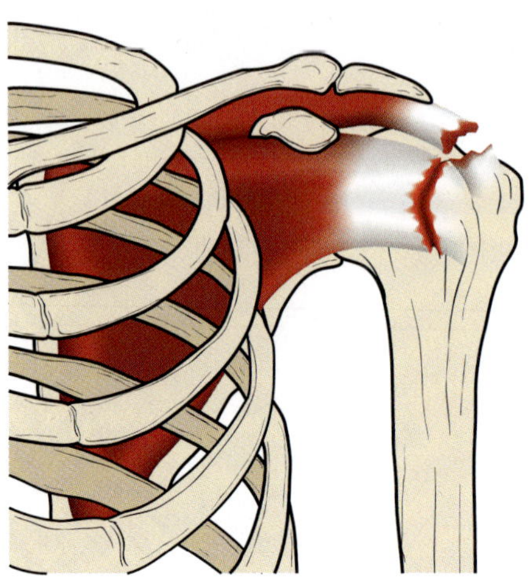

FIGURE 13-29 **Rotator cuff tear**

scoliosis (sko-lē-Ō-sĭs)	abnormal S-shaped lateral curvature of the vertebrae (see Fig. 13-30)

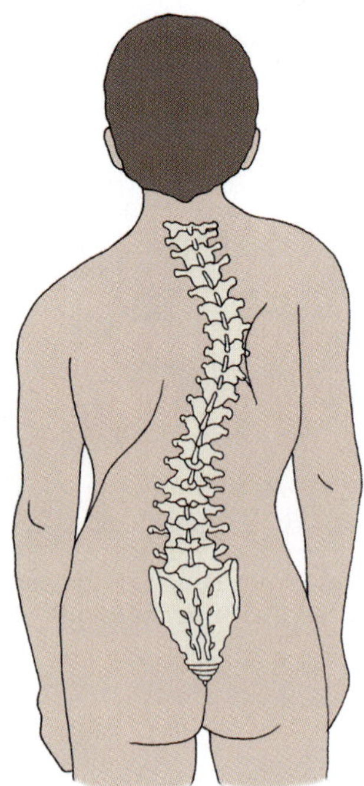

FIGURE 13-30 **Scoliosis**

TABLE 13-3

PATHOLOGY TERMS—cont'd	
sprain (sprān)	complete or incomplete tear in the ligaments around a joint
strain (strān)	trauma to a muscle, and sometimes a tendon, due to violent contraction or excessive forcible stretching
tendinitis (tĕn-dĭn-Ī-tĭs)	inflammation of a tendon due to overuse
thoracic outlet syndrome (TOS) (thō-RĂS-ĭk OWT-lĕt SĬN-drōm)	group of painful disorders involving compression of the nerves or vessels in the neck and arms (see Fig. 13-31)

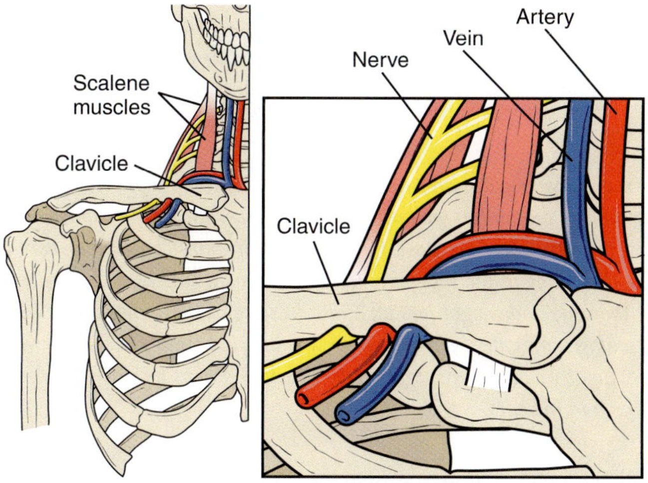

FIGURE 13-31 **Thoracic outlet syndrome**

Common Diagnostic Tests and Procedures

Arthrography: Radiological examination of a joint after injection of a contrast fluid into the joint space

Bone marrow aspiration: Removal of a bone marrow specimen from the cortex of a flat bone for analysis

Bone scan: Use of a gamma camera to detect abnormalities in bone density after injection of radioactive material

Creatine kinase (CK): Test to measure isoenzyme released by skeletal and cardiac muscle into the blood when they are damaged

Cryotherapy: Application of cold, such as with ice compresses, to decrease inflammation and pain

Dual-energy x-ray absorptiometry (DXA): Radiological evaluation of bone density to detect osteoporosis

Electromyogram (EMG): Record of skeletal-muscle electrical activity, used to diagnose neuromuscular disorders

Erythrocyte sedimentation rate (ESR, sed rate: Rate at which red blood cells settle in a tube of unclotted blood; an elevated ESR indicates inflammation

Rheumatoid factor: Blood test used to identify rheumatoid arthritis and other disorders

Total hip replacement (THR): Procedure to replace an arthritic hip with a prosthetic device to restore mobility and function; also referred to as total hip arthroplasty

Transcutaneous electrical nerve stimulation (TENS): Delivery of a mild electrical current to a painful area, to disrupt transmission of pain signals between the body and brain

CASE STUDY

Read the case study and answer the questions that follow. Most of the terms are included in this chapter. Refer to the glossaries (Appendixes B and D) or to your medical dictionary for the other terms.

Osteoarthritis

Michael Mayhew is a 59-year-old man with osteoarthritis of the knees. He has a history of bilateral knee injuries from college football as well as a 33-year career in construction. He has noticed a slow onset of symptoms, primarily over the past 10 years. His primary complaints were arthralgia and stiffness, especially first thing in the morning. Initial treatment was conservative and included rest, NSAIDs, physical therapy, and weight loss of 25 lb. In spite of these measures, Mr. Mayhew continued to experience worsening symptoms over the next few years. Eventually, he underwent bilateral TKRs.

Follow-up note: Eight weeks after surgery, Mr. Mayhew stated he was pain free and had better use of his knees than he had in years.

Osteoarthritis, also known as **degenerative joint disease (DJD)**, is the most common form of noninflammatory joint disease. The key feature of osteoarthritis is the wearing down and loss of cartilage in synovial joints. Osteoarthritis occurs most often after the age of 40, and involves joints that have had prior injuries or heavy chronic wear and tear. The most common joints involved are those of the hips, knees, hands, and spine. Pathological features include erosion of the articular cartilage, sclerosis of the bone beneath the cartilage, and formation of bone spurs. The primary symptom is joint pain on weight-bearing. Management of osteoarthritis includes rest, NSAIDs, glucosamine supplements, physical therapy, and weight loss (obesity is a common factor). If necessary, the patient may rely on a cane, crutches, or a walker. Surgery may eventually be necessary.

Case Study Questions

1. Which of the following statements is true regarding Mr. Mayhew's experience?
   a. He had arthritis in his right knee only
   b. The onset of his arthritis was sudden and severe
   c. His symptoms were worse in the evening
   d. He experienced stiffness in his knees in the mornings
2. What type of surgery did Mr. Mayhew have?
   a. Repair of both knee joints
   b. Replacement of both knee joints
   c. Fixation of both knee joints
   d. Fusion of both knee joints

3. Mr. Mayhew's primary symptom was arthralgia. This means:
   a. Pain of a joint
   b. Inflammation of a joint
   c. Destruction of a joint
   d. Softening of a joint

4. Which of the following statements is true regarding osteoarthritis?
   a. It is an uncommon form of arthritis
   b. It is characterized by demineralization of the bones
   c. It affects joints that have had prior injuries or heavy chronic wear and tear
   d. It most commonly involves the shoulders, elbows, and wrists

Answers to Case Study Questions

1. d
2. b
3. a
4. c

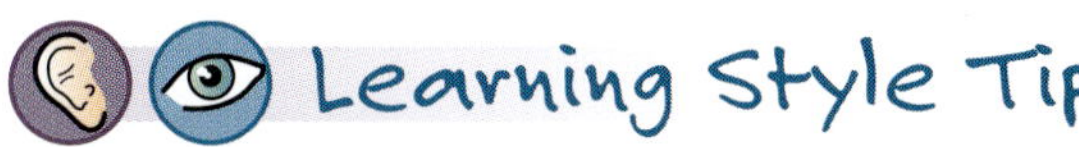

Stress and anxiety can impair your ability to concentrate and remember what you study. Therefore, try beginning and ending your study sessions with a few minutes of soothing, relaxing music. As you listen, visualize yourself passing your exams with an alert mind, perfect recall, and clear focus. Visualize the grade you earn and how good you feel about your accomplishment.

Websites

Please go to the F.A. Davis website at http://davisplus.fadavis.com/eagle/medterm to view resource websites for the skeletal and muscular systems.

Practice Exercises

Deciphering Terms

Write the correct meaning of these medical terms. Check Appendix G for the correct answers.

Exercise 2

1. paravertebral ______________________________
2. supratibial ______________________________
3. thoracic ______________________________

4. tendolysis ______________________________

5. sternotomy ______________________________

6. phalangeal ______________________________

7. patelloptosis ______________________________

8. osteotomy ______________________________

9. myopathy ______________________________

10. myelosclerosis ______________________________

11. lumbar ______________________________

12. laminotome ______________________________

13. femorodynia ______________________________

14. cranioplasty ______________________________

15. costochondritis ______________________________

Fill in the Blanks

Fill in the blanks below. Check Appendix G for the correct answers.

Exercise 3

1. When the lower leg is removed below the knee, the procedure is known as a ______________ ______________, abbreviated ______________.

2. Suzanne has an abnormal S-shaped, lateral curvature of her spine. This condition is known as ______________.

3. Another name for degenerative joint disease is ______________.

4. A ______________ is one kind of injury to a muscle or tendon.

5. Joseph has ______________, an inflammatory condition that affects the tiny fluid-filled sacs located between structures such as bones, tendons, muscles, and skin.

6. The cervical vertebrae are abbreviated ______________.

7. When Howard climbs the stairs, his knees creak. This crackling sound is known as ______________.

8. Lorinda spends much of her workday at a computer; as a result, she has developed __________ __________ __________, which causes pain and numbness in her wrists, hands, and fingers due to compression of the median nerve.

9. The abbreviation for Lorinda's disorder is __________.

10. Two different names for hip replacement are __________ __________ __________ and __________ __________ __________.

11. The sacral vertebrae are abbreviated __________.

12. The combining form *orth/o* means __________ or __________.

13. Pablo had a __________ of his radius and ulna and had to have his forearm in a cast for several weeks. The abbreviation for this injury is __________.

14. The physician ordered an __________ x-ray, which will aim from front to back. This is abbreviated __________.

15. The lumbar vertebrae are abbreviated __________.

16. A(n) __________ records electrical activity of skeletal muscles. It is used to diagnose neuromuscular disorders.

17. An autoimmune form of arthritis that causes pain and deformity of joints and may involve organ systems is __________ arthritis.

18. When the leg is surgically removed from above the knee, it is known as a(n) __________ __________, abbreviated __________.

19. Herniation of the soft center of an intervertebral disk is known as __________.

Multiple Choice

Select the one best answer to the following multiple-choice questions. Check Appendix G for the correct answers.

Exercise 4

1. Which of the following conditions is caused by compression of the median nerve, resulting in pain or numbness in the wrist, hand, and fingers?
   a. Herniated disk
   b. Myasthenia gravis
   c. Gout
   d. Carpal tunnel syndrome

2. Which of the following conditions is an autoimmune motor disorder that causes progressive muscle fatigue and weakness?
   a. Myasthenia gravis
   b. Gout
   c. Carpal tunnel syndrome
   d. Kyphosis

3. Martha Snyder has been diagnosed with rheumatoid arthritis. She most likely has which of the following complaints?
   a. Arthralgia
   b. Osteoplegia
   c. Patelloptosis
   d. Metacarpotome

4. The application of cold, such as with ice compresses, to decrease inflammation and pain is known as:
   a. Arthrography
   b. Cryotherapy
   c. Dual-energy absorptiometry
   d. Transcutaneous electrical nerve stimulation

5. Ilka Heidrick has myasthenia gravis. Which of the following is she most likely to experience?
   a. Increased energy level after exercise
   b. Progressive dementia
   c. Arthralgia
   d. Progressive fatigue

Word Building

*Using **only** the word parts in the lists provided, create medical terms with the indicated meanings. Check Appendix G for the correct answers.*

Exercise 5

Prefixes	Combining Forms	Suffixes
inter-	arthr/o	-al
para-	carp/o	-algia
sub-	cervic/o	-ar
	chondr/o	-dynia
	cost/o	-ectomy
	crani/o	-itis
	femor/o	-metry
	humer/o	-oma
	lamin/o	-pathy
	lumb/o	-penia
	metacarp/o	-plasty
	my/o	-plegia
	myel/o	-pnea
	orth/o	-tome
	oste/o	
	patell/o	
	pelv/i	
	stern/o	
	vertebr/o	

1. pertaining to the ribs and vertebrae ______________________
2. inflammation of a bone and joint ______________________
3. pertaining to a carpus ______________________
4. pertaining to beside or near the neck ______________________
5. pain of the cartilage ______________________
6. cutting instrument for a lamina ______________________
7. pertaining to between the ribs ______________________
8. surgical repair of the cranium ______________________
9. pertaining to the femur ______________________
10. disease of the humerus ______________________
11. pertaining to straight or upright ______________________
12. pain of the lower back ______________________
13. inflammation of a metacarpus ______________________
14. tumor of the bone marrow or spinal cord ______________________
15. paralysis of a muscle ______________________
16. pertaining to beneath the sternum ______________________

17. disease of a bone ______________________

18. excision or surgical removal of a patella ______________________

19. measurement of the pelvis ______________________

20. deficiency of bone ______________________

True or False

Decide whether the following statements are true or false. Check Appendix G for the correct answers.

Exercise 6

1. True False **BKA** is an abbreviation for *broken.*
2. True False **Gout** is a hereditary from of arthritis characterized by uric acid accumulation in the joints, especially in the great toe.
3. True False The abbreviation **IM** stands for *immobility.*
4. True False **Contracture** is fibrosis of connective tissue, which decreases mobility of a joint.
5. True False **Muscular dystrophy** is a hereditary, progressive, terminal disease that causes muscle atrophy and death.
6. True False **Lordosis** is an abnormal increase in the curvature of the lumbar vertebrae, causing swayback.
7. True False The abbreviation **RA** stands for *rheumatoid arthritis.*
8. True False A **sprain** is an injury to a muscle or tendon.
9. True False **Kyphosis** is an abnormal increase in the curvature of the thoracic vertebrae, causing hunchback.
10. True False **Myasthenia gravis** is a grating sound from broken bones or a clicking or crackling sound from joints.

Deciphering Terms

Write the correct meaning of these medical terms. Check Appendix G for the correct answers.

Exercise 7

1. cervicitis ______________________

2. carpocentesis ______________________

3. arthralgia ______________________________

4. osteoclasis ______________________________

5. extratibial ______________________________

6. thoracolumbar ______________________________

7. kinesimeter ______________________________

8. meniscal ______________________________

9. muscular ______________________________

10. puborectal ______________________________

Multiple Choice

Select the one best answer to the following multiple-choice questions. Check Appendix G for the correct answers.

Exercise 8

1. Which of the following terms means *treatment (using) movement?*
   a. Kinesiotherapy
   b. Kyphoplasty
   c. Tarsokinesia
   d. Tetrakinesis

2. Which of the following terms means *abnormal condition of pus in the vertebrae?*
   a. Vertebromyelosis
   b. Spondylopyosis
   c. Pubovertebrosis
   d. Pyelospondylosis

3. Which of the following terms means *drooping or prolapse of the tarsus?*
   a. Dystocia
   b. Tarsatrophy
   c. Thoracopexy
   d. Tarsoptosis

4. Which of the following terms means *pertaining to muscle and skin?*
   a. Dermatomycosis
   b. Myelocutaneous
   c. Sternomyosis
   d. None of these

5. Which of the following terms means *pertaining to the sternum and around the heart?*
   a. Sternopericardial
   b. Retrosternocardial
   c. Transcardiac
   d. Anticardiosternal

6. The term *lordosis* indicates:
   a. Back pain of the lower back
   b. A pathological condition of the upper back
   c. An abnormal condition of the cervical and lumbar areas of the back
   d. Inflammation of the cervical and lumbar areas of the back

7. The term *meniscocyte* indicates:
   a. A condition of fungus
   b. Softening of the cartilage
   c. A hernia of a meniscus
   d. None of these

8. The term *puboprostatic* means:
   a. Pertaining to the back of the pelvis
   b. Pertaining to behind the patella
   c. Pertaining to the pubis and prostate
   d. Pertaining to disease of the prostate

9. Scoliokyphosis is:
   a. A pathological condition of back curvature
   b. An abnormal condition involving crookedness and a hump
   c. A condition of crooked movement
   d. None of these

10. The term *costochondrosis* indicates:
    a. A painful condition of the ribs
    b. Surgical puncture of the skin and ribs
    c. Cancer of the carpus
    d. An abnormal condition of the ribs and cartilage

11. Which of the following tests will most likely identify the presence of inflammation?
    a. Erythrocyte sedimentation rate
    b. Creatine kinase
    c. Electromyogram
    d. Rheumatoid factor

12. Which of the following tests is most likely to identify osteoporosis?
    a. Bone marrow aspiration
    b. Dual-energy absorptiometry
    c. Bone scan
    d. Arthrography

13. Which of the following conditions causes loss of range of motion in the shoulder?
    a. Crepitation
    b. Hallux rigidus
    c. Adhesive capsulitis
    d. Osteitis deformans

14. All of the following disorders involve the feet **except**:
    a. Gout
    b. Plantar fasciitis
    c. Hallux valgus
    d. Ganglion cyst

15. All of the following disorders involve the arm or shoulder **except**:
    a. Carpal tunnel syndrome
    b. Adhesive capsulitis
    c. Kyphosis
    d. Rotator cuff tear

16. Which of the following abbreviations indicates a location on the lower extremities?

    a. AP

    b. AK

    c. BE

    d. AS

17. Which of the following abbreviations indicates an anatomical location?

    a. DTR

    b. IM

    c. UE

    d. OT

18. All of the following abbreviations indicate a surgical procedure **except**:

    a. TKR

    b. ADL

    c. AKA

    d. ORIF

19. All of the following abbreviations indicate a disease or disorder **except**:

    a. ROM

    b. DJD

    c. HNP

    d. Fx

20. All of the following abbreviations pertain to a type of arthritis **except**:

    a. OA

    b. RA

    c. JRA

    d. BKA

SPECIAL SENSES (EYES AND EARS) 14

Structure and Function of the Eye

The eye is the sensory organ of sight. It is located within the orbital cavity of the face and is surrounded by protective structures including the eyebrows, eyelashes, and eyelids, which help keep foreign objects out of the eye.

The **eyeball** is a globe-shaped organ that consists of three layers (see Fig. 14-1). These are the sclera, the outer portion; the choroid, the middle portion; and the retina, the inner portion. Each of these layers functions to protect the eye, provide vision, or communicate vision to the brain.

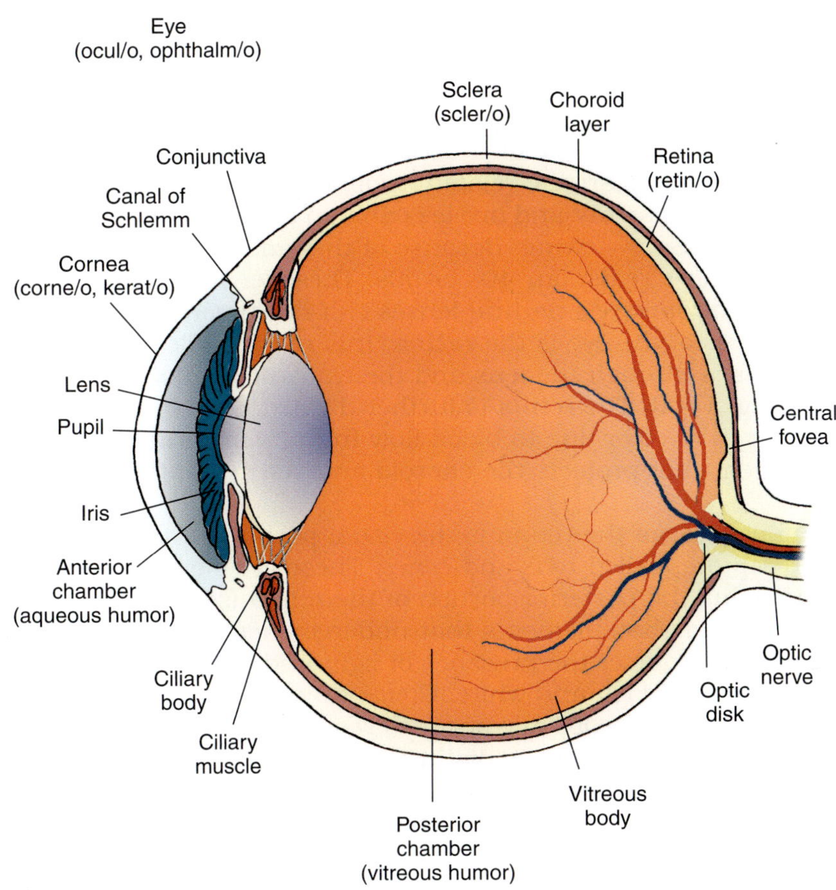

FIGURE 14-1 The eyeball

The outermost layer of the eye includes the **sclera** and **cornea**. The sclera has a distinctive white color. It provides strength, structure, and shape to the eye. At the front of the eye, the sclera bulges forward to become the cornea, which is transparent and allows light into the eye. A thin mucous membrane called the **conjunctiva** covers the outer surface of the eye and lines the eyelids. The conjunctiva contains many tiny blood vessels and secretory glands. These glands produce a clear, watery mucus that allows the eyelid to slide smoothly over the eye when you blink. When the eye is irritated, the tiny blood vessels dilate (enlarge) and become more prominent. This makes the whites of the eye appear bloodshot or reddened.

The middle layer of the eyeball is the **choroid layer**. It is a dark-blue vascular layer between the sclera and retina that supplies blood to the entire eye. The **optic nerve**, which is attached to the retina, exits the posterior eye through an opening in the choroid and extends to the brain, where visual messages are delivered.

Other structures in the choroid include the iris, ciliary body, lens, and suspensory ligaments. The **iris** is a circular structure that surrounds the pupil and gives your eyes their typical color. The **pupil** functions as an adjustable window that lets light into the inner structures of the eye. The iris contracts in low lighting, thereby dilating the pupil and making it appear bigger. This allows more light into the eye. In brightly lit environments the iris expands, causing the pupil to constrict and appear smaller. This decreases the amount of light entering the eye. The **ciliary body** includes several ciliary muscles, including a circular muscle that lies posterior to the iris. It is attached to the **lens** by the **suspensory ligaments**. The lens is a clear, firm, transparent disk. With the help of **ciliary muscles**, it continually changes shape, enabling us to focus clearly on objects we are viewing. For near vision, the ciliary muscles contract, causing increased rounding of the lens; for far vision, they expand, causing flattening of the lens. This process is called *accommodation.* As we age, most of us develop *presbyopia,* which is an age-related decline in visual acuity. As this occurs, our lenses lose elasticity and are less able to accommodate for distance changes, especially close-up viewing. Because of this, many of us need corrective lenses by the time we reach our 40s or 50s. These lenses are mostly able to help make up for what our eye's natural lenses can no longer do.

Flashpoint

The eye's natural lens loses elasticity with age, causing loss of visual acuity.

The innermost layer of the eye is the **retina**. It is responsible for the reception of visual impulses through the lens and the transmission of these impulses to the brain (see Fig. 14-2). The retina is further divided into two layers. The thin outer layer is red in color due to blood flow from its main central artery. It also contains pigment that protects the choroid and sclera from light at the back of the eye.

The thicker inner layer of the retina is the visual portion. It contains two types of visual receptors, called *rods* and *cones.* These are elongated nerve cells that are lined up along the posterior portion of the retina (see Fig. 14-3). These visual receptors contain photopigments that undergo chemical changes when light strikes them. Rods detect the presence of light and function in dim lighting to produce images in black and white. Cones function in more brightly lit situations and detect color. Deficiency of cones results in *color deficiency,* often called *color blindness*—the inability to distinguish colors. As light waves from the anterior portion of the eye hit the retina, they stimulate rods and cones, which direct visual information to **optic nerve** fibers located on the inner surface of the thick inner layer of the retina.

Optic nerve fibers transmit visual information via ganglion neurons, which converge at the optic disc. The optic disc, commonly called the *blind spot,*

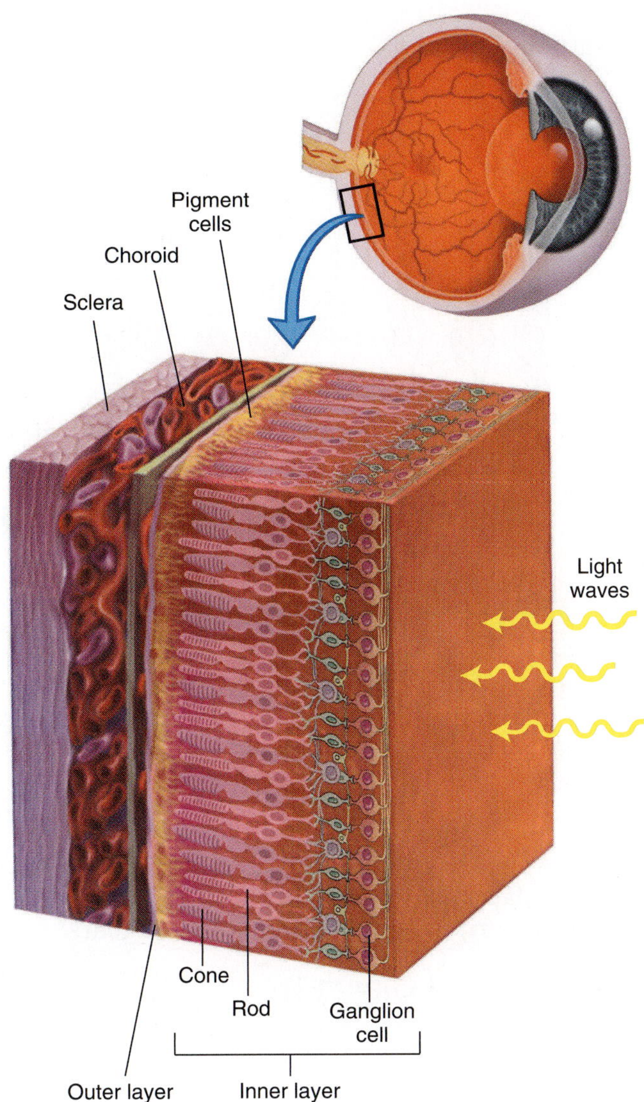

FIGURE 14-2 **Microscopic structures of the retina** (From Eagle, S, et al.: *The Professional Medical Assistant.* F.A. Davis, Philadelphia, 2009, p. 748; with permission)

contains no rods or cones. The optic nerve gathers visual stimuli from the ganglion neurons and transmits this information to the brain for interpretation.

The eye contains two fluids, historically called humors. **Aqueous humor** is found in the **posterior** and **anterior chambers**. In the anterior chamber it provides nourishment for the lens and cornea. It drains through a small opening called the **canal of Schlemm**. In addition to aqueous humor, the posterior chamber also contains **vitreous humor**. Vitreous humor is a jellylike substance that fills the posterior chamber and gives shape to the eye. The aqueous humor, vitreous humor, and lens are all refractory structures that bend light rays to focus them sharply onto the retina.

Lacrimal glands are located on the superolateral (upper outer) side of the eye and open through the lacrimal duct at the medial (inner) side, next to the nose. They bathe, moisten, and lubricate the eye by producing tears that flow over the eye's surface. Tears also serve a protective role, containing a bacteria-killing

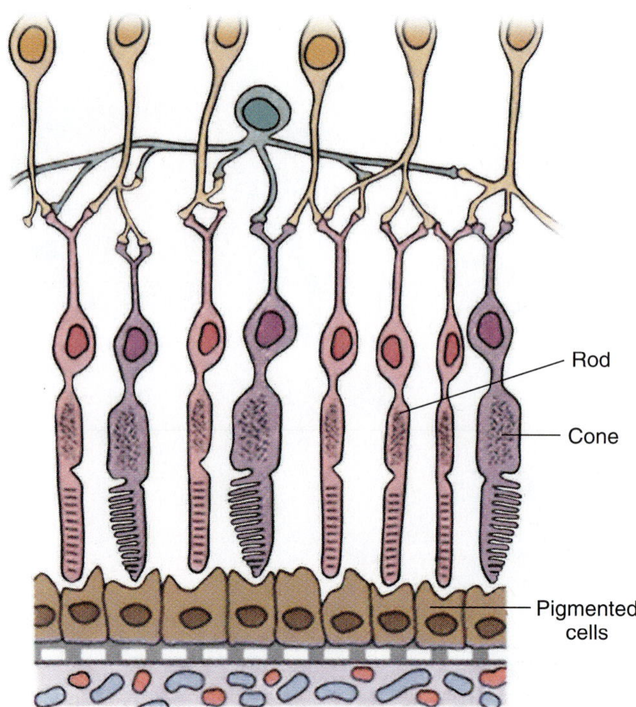

FIGURE 14-3 **Rods and cones** (From Eagle, S, et al.: *The Professional Medical Assistant.* F.A. Davis, Philadelphia, 2009, p. 748; with permission)

enzyme, and wash away foreign debris. The lacrimal gland is connected to the nose through the nasolacrimal duct and drains into the nasal cavity. This explains why our noses drip when our eyes produce tears.

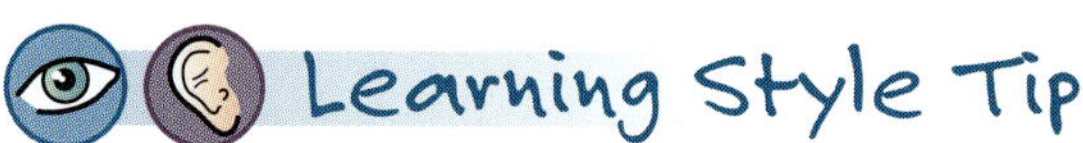

Learning Style Tip

Inquire whether medical-terminology videos, audio tapes, or CDs are available for checkout at your college library. They will most likely present information in a different manner than your classroom instructor did. By repeatedly exposing yourself to medical terms, in a variety of different ways, you increase your ability to learn and remember.

Structure and Function of the Ear

The ear is responsible for hearing, balance, and equilibrium. The structures of the ear are located in three main areas: the external, middle, and internal ear (see Fig. 14-4).

> **Flashpoint**
> Swimmer's ear, also known as *otitis externa,* is an infection of the external ear canal.

The **external ear** is composed of the **auricle**, or **pinna**, which is the outer structure. It is made up of cartilage covered with skin, and sits visibly outside of the head. It collects sound waves and channels them into the **external auditory canal**, which is a slender tube that leads to the middle ear. The canal is lined with modified sweat glands called *ceruminous glands* that secrete **cerumen**, a waxy substance that traps tiny foreign particles and prevents them from entering the deeper structures. Infections of the external ear are called **otitis**

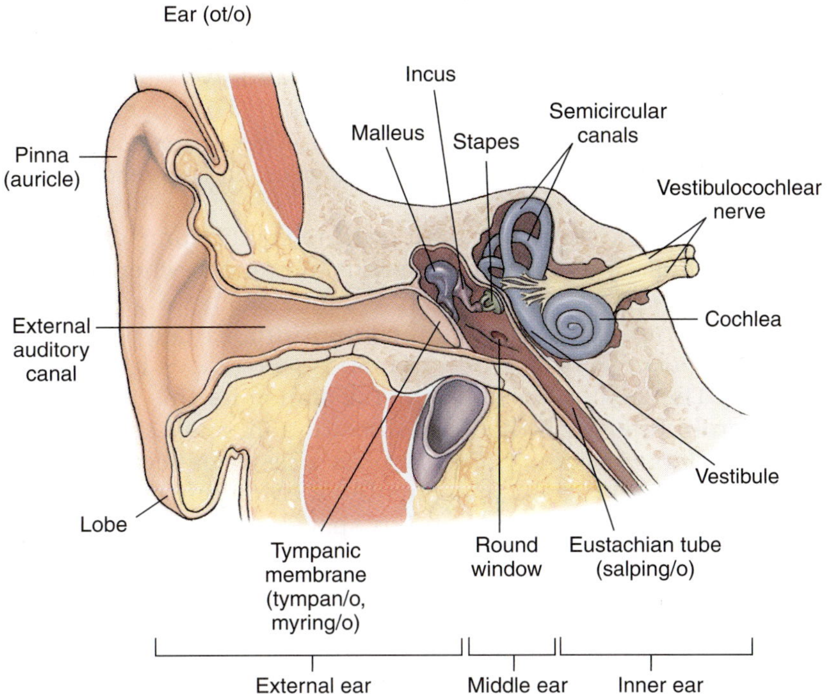

FIGURE 14-4 **The ear**

externa, also known as *swimmer's ear,* and are common in children who spend a great deal of time in the water. When the ear canal harbors moisture, it creates a warm, hospitable environment conducive to fungal and bacterial growth.

At the inner end of the auditory canal is the **tympanic membrane**, which is a thin, flat, irregularly shaped membrane commonly known as the *eardrum.* It creates a wall between the external and **middle ear**. Located within the middle ear is a downward-sloping canal called the **eustachian tube** that connects the middle ear to the throat. It allows air movement between the inner ear and outer atmosphere. When the eustachian tube is closed and the middle-ear pressure is greater or less than atmospheric pressure, we may describe our ears as feeling plugged. The pressure is relieved when the eustachian tube opens to allow air through. This is a common experience with altitude changes, and explains the ear-popping sensation we experience when we travel over the mountains or ride in an airplane.

The tympanic membrane is connected to the *malleus* (hammer), the first of three tiny ossicles (bones) also including the *incus* (anvil) and *stapes* (stirrup). The tympanic membrane vibrates in response to sound waves, which causes movement of the ossicles. This in turn sends vibrations to the inner ear.

The anatomy of the inner ear is quite complex, with a mazelike design of twists and turns. Because of this, the inner ear is sometimes also called a **labyrinth**. The first structure of the **inner ear** is the **cochlea**, a tiny, circular, snail-shaped structure filled with fluid called *perilymph.* The inner surface of the cochlea is lined with a highly sensitive hearing structure called the *organ of Corti.* It contains nerve endings called *hair cells,* which are long, hairlike fibers that transmit impulses to the **vestibulocochlear (auditory) nerve**.

> **Flashpoint**
> When your ears pop, air is moving through the eustachian tube to equalize pressure.

The cochlea receives vibration from the stapes through the **oval window**. These vibrations cause a disturbance of the perilymph, which in turn disturbs hair cells on the organ of Corti. The hair cells transmit impulses to the auditory nerve, where they are interpreted as sound. The **round window** is an opening in the lower part of the temporal bone, covered with a thin membrane. The **semicircular canals**, located behind the ossicles and two windows, contain perilymph and endolymph, a pale, transparent fluid. Together with the cochlea, these structures make up the vestibular system. They translate sound vibrations into nerve impulses that are sent to the brain via the vestibulocochlear nerve.

Another function of the inner ear is to provide *equilibrium*, which is the sense of balance. *Static equilibrium* is feeling a sense of balance when we are at rest; *dynamic equilibrium* refers to our sense of balance when we are in motion. The vestibular system controls both forms of equilibrium. Endolymph, the pale transparent fluid within the labyrinth, responds to changes in body position based on gravity. The vestibulocochlear nerve transmits this information to the brain, and the brain interprets the body's position in space. Inflammation of the inner ear is called *labyrinthitis*. It often causes a disturbance in the inner ear's ability to maintain equilibrium. Consequently, a common symptom is *vertigo*, which is the sensation of moving around in space.

Flashpoint

Vertigo is an unpleasant sensation of spinning or moving in space.

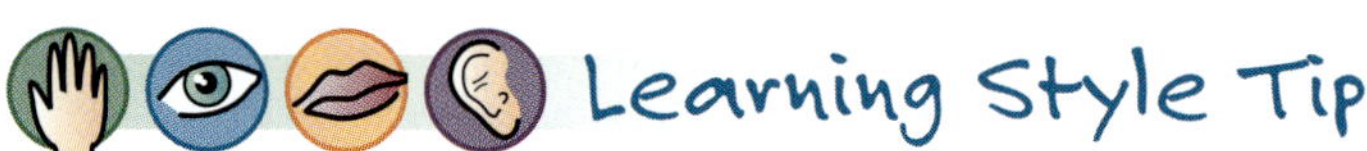

Draw a vertical line down a sheet of paper. Write a series of "exam" questions on one side with the answers on the other. Cover the answer side so that you can't see it. Review the questions, looking at your answers only if you can't remember them. Repeat the process until you know all of the answers by heart. Remember to verbalize aloud if you are an auditory or verbal learner. Now repeat the process with new questions on a clean sheet of paper.

Combining Forms

Table 14-1 contains combining forms that pertain to vision and hearing, along with examples of terms that utilize the combining forms, and a pronunciation guide. Read aloud to yourself as you move from left to right across the table. Be sure to use the pronunciation guide so you can learn to say the terms correctly.

TABLE 14-1
COMBINING FORMS

Combining Form	Meaning	Example (Pronunciation)	Meaning of New Term
acous/o	hearing	acoustic (ă-KOOS-tĭk)	pertaining to hearing
audi/o		audiometry (aw-dē-ŎM-ĕ-trē)	measurement of hearing
blephar/o	eyelid	blepharoptosis (blĕf-ă-rō-TŌ-sĭs)	drooping or prolapse of the eyelid
conjunctiv/o	conjunctiva	conjunctivitis (kŏn-jŭnk-tĭ-VĪ-tĭs)	inflammation of the conjunctiva
corne/o	cornea	corneous (KŌR-nē-ŭs)	pertaining to the cornea

TABLE 14-1
COMBINING FORMS—cont'd

Combining Form	Meaning	Example (Pronunciation)	Meaning of New Term
dacry/o	tear	dacryopyorrhea (dăk-rē-ō-pī-ō-RĒ-ă)	flow or discharge of pus in the tears
dipl/o	double	diploid (DĬP-loyd)	resembling double
ir/o	iris	irotomy (ī-RŎT-ō-mē)	cutting into or incision of the iris
irid/o		iridectome (ĭr-ĭ-DĔK-tōm)	cutting instrument for the iris
kerat/o	cornea, keratinized tissue	keratocele (kĕr-ĂT-ō-sēl)	hernia of the cornea
lacrim/o	lacrimal gland	lacrimal (LĂK-rĭm-ăl)	pertaining to the lacrimal glands
myring/o	tympanic membrane	myringoplasty (mĭr-ĬN-gō-plăst-ē)	surgical repair of the tympanic membrane
tympan/o		tympanosclerosis (tĭm-pă-nō-sklĕ-RŌ-sĭs)	hardening of the tympanic membrane
ocul/o	eye	oculomycosis (ŏk-ū-lō-mī-KŌ-sĭs)	abnormal condition of eye fungus
ophthalm/o		ophthalmorrhexis (ŏf-thăl-mō-RĔK-sĭs)	rupture of the eye
optic/o		optician (ŏp-TĬSH-ăn)	specialist in eyes
ot/o	ear	otorrhea (ō-tō-RĒ-ă)	flow or discharge from the ear
phac/o	lens	phacotoxic (făk-ō-TŎK-sĭk)	poisonous to the lens
phak/o		phakolysis (făk-ŎL-ĭ-sĭs)	destruction of the lens
presby/o	old age	presbycusis (prĕz-bĭ-KŪ-sĭs)	old-age hearing
retin/o	retina	retinopexy (rĕt-Ĭ-nō-pĕk-sē)	surgical fixation of the retina
salping/o	tube (eustachian or fallopian)	salpingopharyngeal (săl-pĭng-gō-fă-RĬN-jē-ăl)	pertaining to the eustachian tube and pharynx
scler/o	sclera, hardening	scleral (sklĕr-ăl)	pertaining to the sclera

STOP HERE.
Select the Combining Form Flash Cards for Chapter 14 and run through them at least three times before you continue.

Practice Exercises

Fill in the Blanks

Fill in the blanks below using Table 14-1. Check Appendix G for the correct answers.

Exercise 1

1. flow or discharge from the ear ______________________________
2. rupture of the eye ______________________________
3. abnormal condition of eye fungus ______________________________
4. hardening of the tympanic membrane ______________________________
5. pertaining to hearing ______________________________
6. measurement of hearing ______________________________
7. hernia of the cornea ______________________________
8. surgical fixation of the retina ______________________________
9. pertaining to the sclera ______________________________
10. drooping or prolapse of the eyelid ______________________________
11. pertaining to the eustachian tube and pharynx ______________________________
12. pertaining to the cornea ______________________________
13. resembling double ______________________________
14. surgical repair of the tympanic membrane ______________________________
15. cutting into or incision of the iris ______________________________
16. cutting instrument for the iris ______________________________
17. poisonous to the lens ______________________________
18. inflammation of the conjunctiva ______________________________
19. pertaining to the lacrimal glands ______________________________
20. flow or discharge of pus in the tears ______________________________

21. specialist in eyes ______________________________

22. destruction of the lens ______________________________

23. old-age hearing ______________________________

24. **Fill in the blanks in Figure 14-5 with the appropriate anatomical terms and combining forms.**

25. **Fill in the blanks in Figure 14-6 with the appropriate anatomical terms and combining forms.**

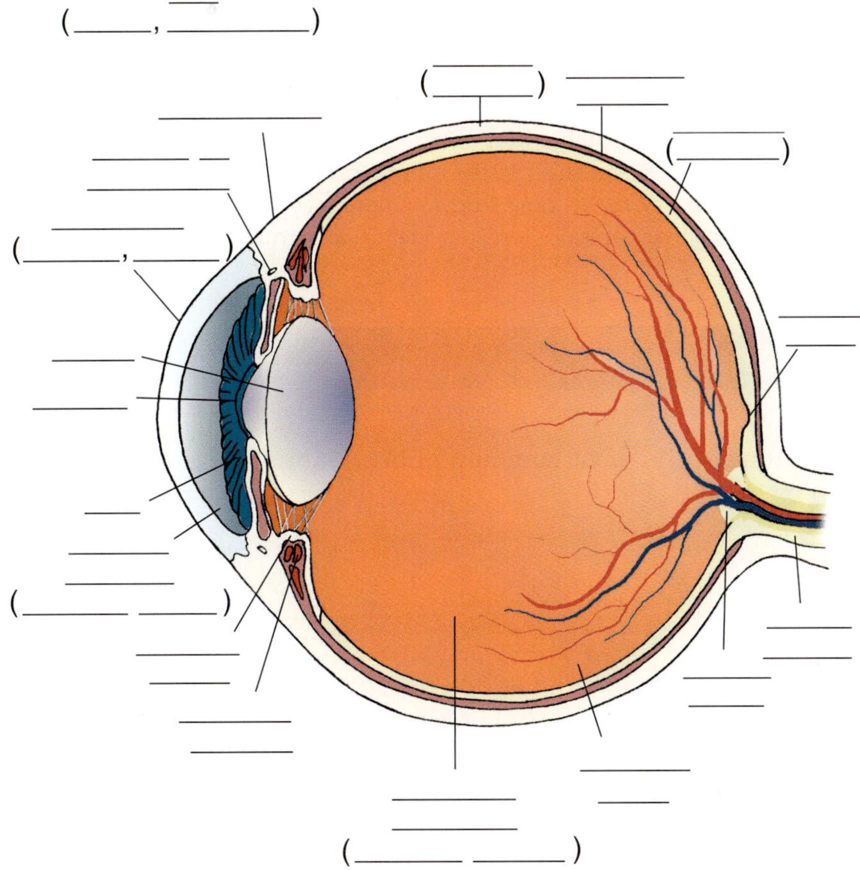

FIGURE 14-5 **Eyeball with blanks**

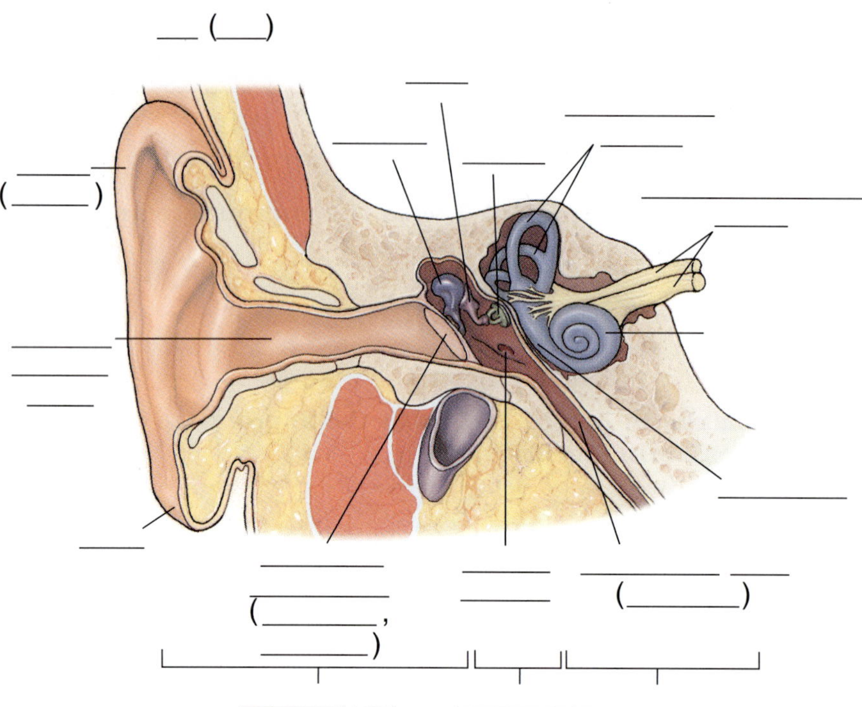

FIGURE 14-6 **Ear with blanks**

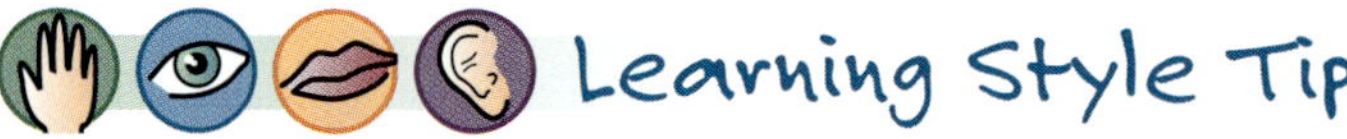

Identify the time of the day you are best able to grasp and understand complex material. For most people this is first thing in the morning, when they are rested. Spend at least 30 minutes each day at this time studying material you find most challenging. Be sure to use strategies that capitalize on your identified learning style.

Abbreviations

Table 14-2 lists some of the most common abbreviations related to vision and hearing.

TABLE 14-2
ABBREVIATIONS

Eye			
AS, Ast	astigmatism	MD	macular degeneration
CAT	cataract	PERRLA	pupils are equal, round, reactive to light and accommodation
EM, em	emmetropia	RD	retinal detachment
EOM	extraocular movement	RK	radial keratotomy
G, glc	glaucoma	V, VA	visual acuity
LASIK	laser-assisted in-situ keratomileusis		

TABLE 14-2			
ABBREVIATIONS—cont'd			
Ear			
AOM	acute otitis media	ENT	ears, nose, and throat
EENT	eyes, ears, nose, and throat	TM	tympanic membrane

STOP HERE.
Select the Abbreviation Flash Cards for Chapter 14 and run through them at least three times before you continue.

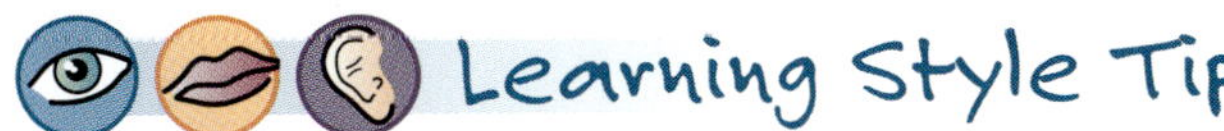

Associate visual images with terms you need to remember. Then link that visual image with the meaning of the term. For example, to remember the term *-centesis,* try picturing a penny (cent) with a large needle punctured through it. Share your images with your study buddies and ask them to share theirs with you.

Pathology Terms

Table 14-3 includes terms that relate to diseases or abnormalities of vision or hearing. Use the pronunciation guide and say the terms aloud as you read them. This will help you get in the habit of saying them properly.

Flashpoint
Diabetic retinopathy is a leading cause of blindness.

TABLE 14-3	
PATHOLOGY TERMS	
Eye	
amblyopia (ăm-blē-Ō-pē-ă)	disorder in which the brain disregards images from the weaker eye and relies on those from the stronger eye; sometimes called *lazy eye*
astigmatism (ă-STĬG-mă-tĭ-zum)	abnormal curvature of the cornea that distorts the visual image (see Fig. 14-7)

A Normal eye

FIGURE 14-7 **Eyeball shape affects where the image is projected: (A) Normal—on the retina**

Continued

TABLE 14-3

PATHOLOGY TERMS—cont'd

Eye

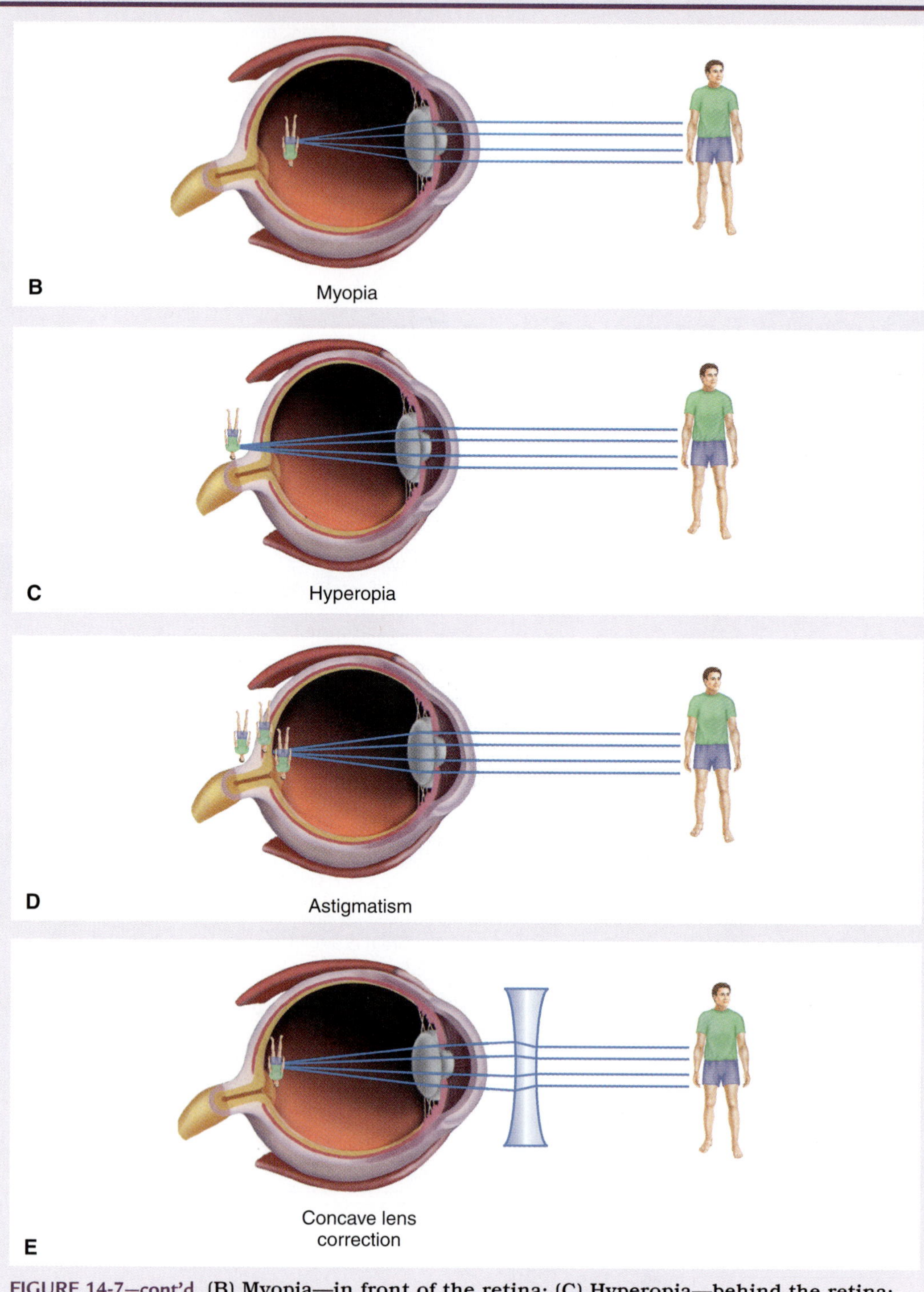

FIGURE 14-7—cont'd (B) Myopia—in front of the retina; (C) Hyperopia—behind the retina; (D) Astigmatism—multiple images on the retina; (E) Concave lens correction for myopia

TABLE 14-3

PATHOLOGY TERMS—cont'd

Eye

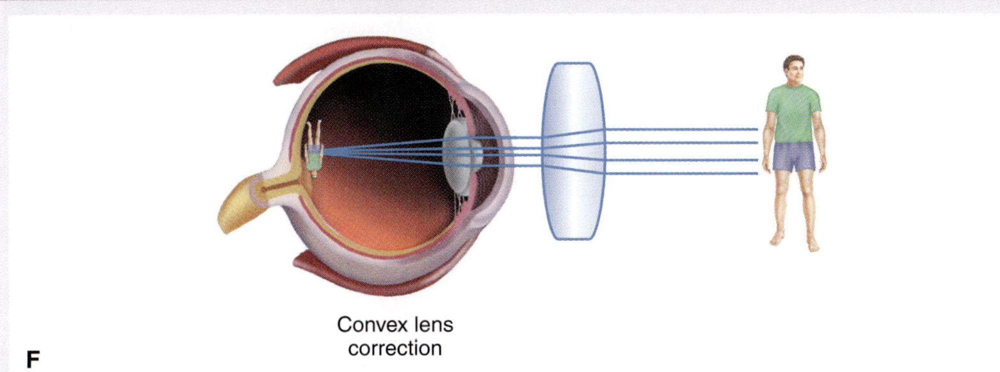

FIGURE 14-7—cont'd (F) **Convex lens correction for hyperopia** (From Eagle, S, et al.: *The Professional Medical Assistant.* F.A. Davis, Philadelphia, 2009, p. 757; with permission)

blepharitis (blĕf-ăr-Ī-tĭs)	noncontagious inflammation of the eyelash follicles and tiny oil glands along the margins of the eyelids (see Fig. 14-8)

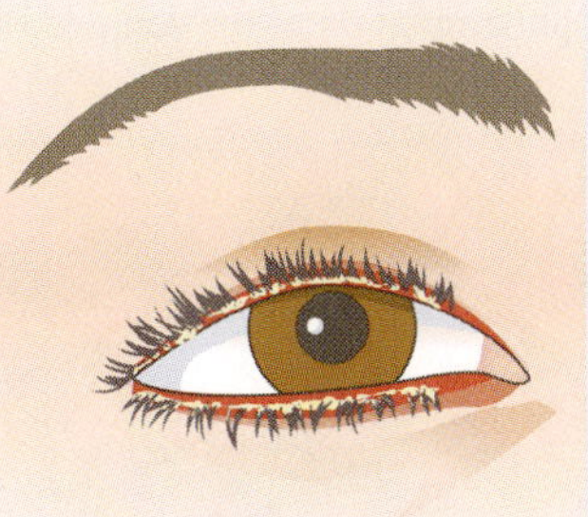

FIGURE 14-8 **Blepharitis**

cataract (KĂT-ă-răkt)	cloudiness of the lens due to protein deposits as a result of aging, disease, or trauma, or as a side effect of tobacco use or certain medications (see Fig. 14-9)

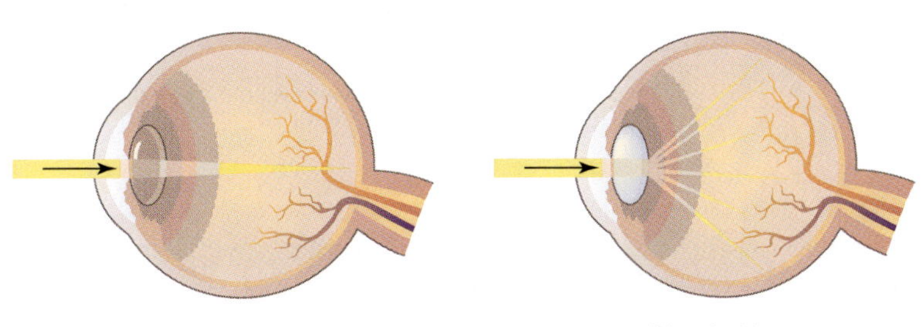

FIGURE 14-9 **Cataracts**

Continued

TABLE 14-3

PATHOLOGY TERMS—cont'd	
Eye	
central scotoma (SĔN-trăl skō-TŌ-mă)	blind spot in the center of the visual field surrounded by an area of normal vision
chalazion (kă-LĀ-zē-ōn)	small benign cyst in the eyelid formed by the distention of a meibomian gland (sebaceous gland of the eye) with secretions (see Fig. 14-10) 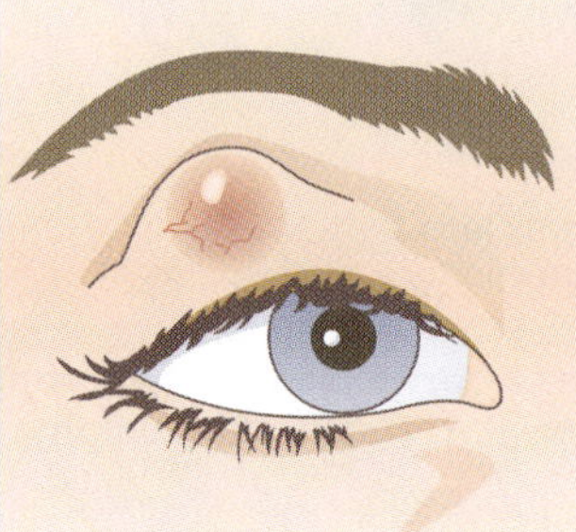 FIGURE 14-10 Chalazion
conjunctivitis (kŏn-jŭnk-tĭ-VĪ-tĭs)	inflammation of the conjunctiva; also called *pinkeye* (see Fig. 14-11) 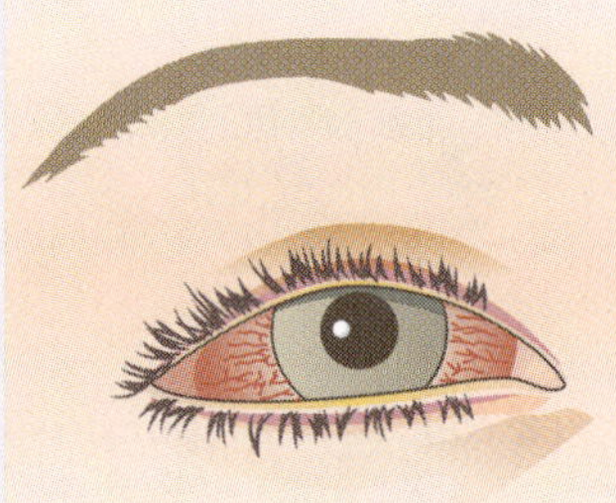 FIGURE 14-11 Conjunctivitis
diabetic retinopathy (dī-ă-BĔT-ĭk rĕt-ĭn-ŎP-ă-thē)	progressive damage to microscopic vessels and other structures of the retina in patients with longstanding diabetes mellitus, which may result in blindness
ectropion (ĕk-TRŌ-pē-ŏn)	condition in which the lower eyelid is turned outward and droops more with aging (see Fig. 14-12) 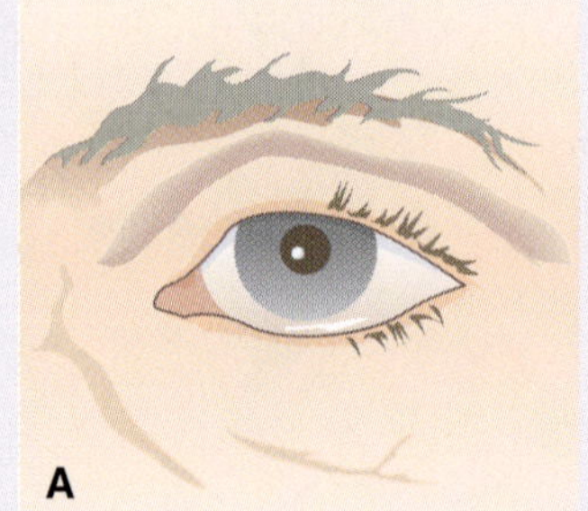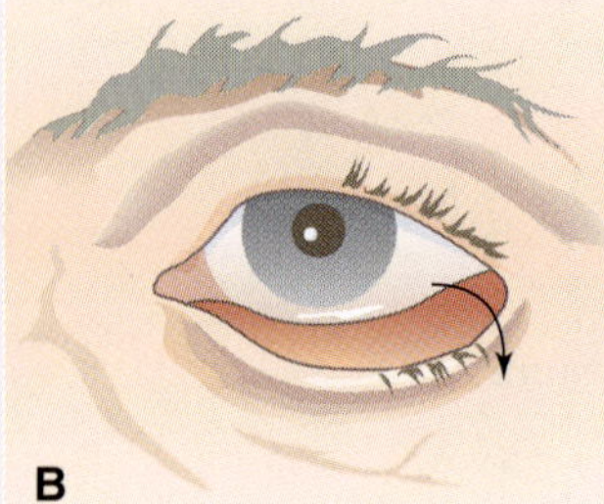 FIGURE 14-12 (A) Normal eyelid, (B) Ectropion

TABLE 14-3

PATHOLOGY TERMS—cont'd

Eye	
entropion (ĕn-TRŌ-pē-ŏn)	condition in which the eyelid edges are turned inward and rub against the surface of the eye, usually affecting the lower eyelid (see Fig. 14-13)

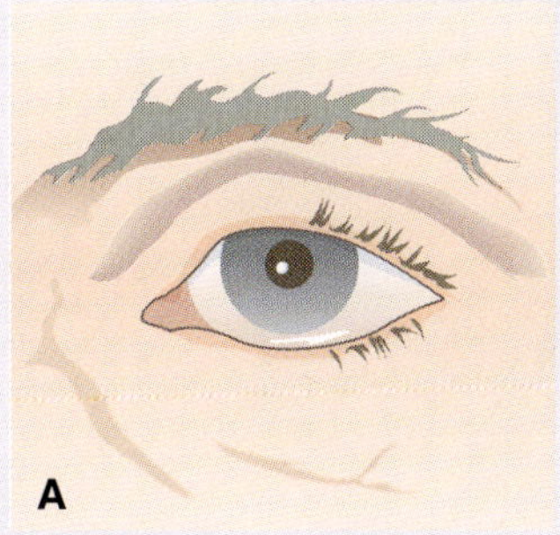

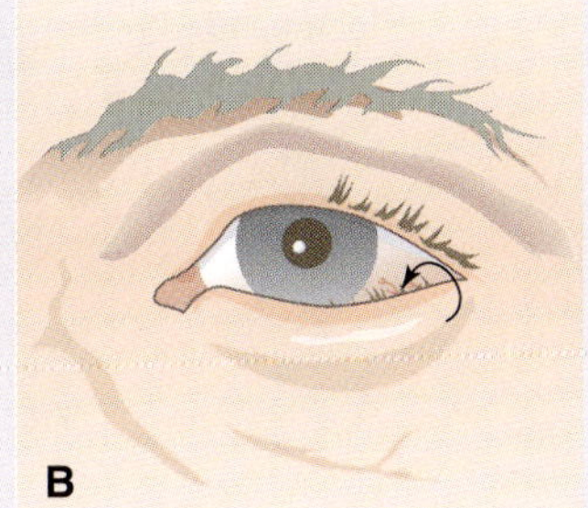

FIGURE 14-13 **(A) Normal eyelid, (B) Entropion**

glaucoma (acute) [glaw-KŌ-mă (a-KYŪT)]	type of glaucoma in which a sudden blockage of aqueous-humor outflow causes a rapid increase in intraocular pressure; can cause vision loss; also called *closed-angle glaucoma* (see Fig. 14-14)

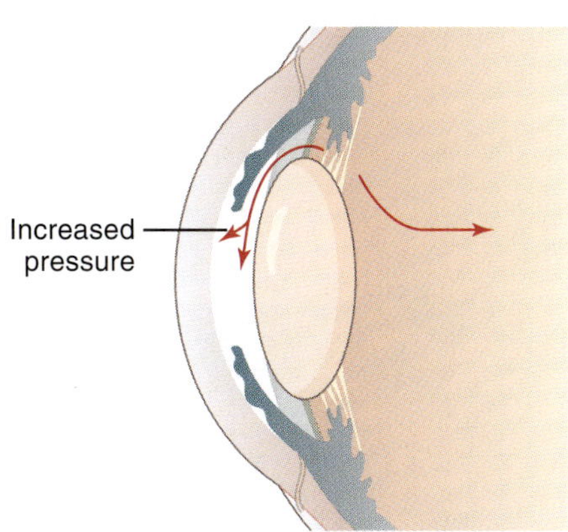

FIGURE 14-14 **Glaucoma (acute)**

glaucoma (chronic) [glaw-KŌ-mă (KRĂ-nik)]	type of glaucoma in which the aqueous humor drains too slowly, leading to increasing intraocular pressure; can cause vision loss; also called *primary open-angle glaucoma* (see Fig. 14-15)

Continued

TABLE 14-3

PATHOLOGY TERMS—cont'd

Eye

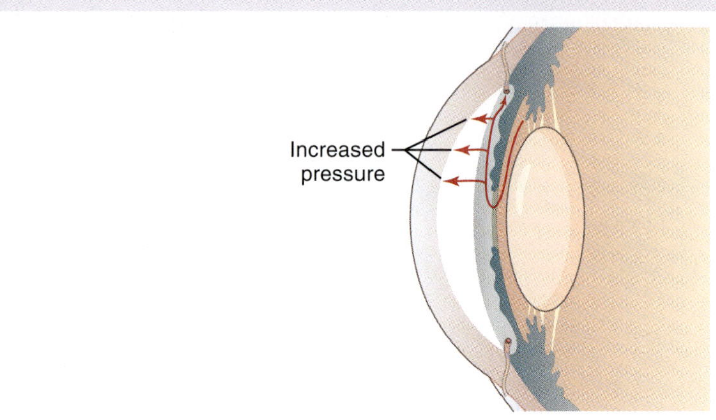

FIGURE 14-15 **Glaucoma (chronic)**

hordeolum (hor-DĒ-ō-lŭm)	infection of a sebaceous gland of the eyelid; also called a *stye* (see Fig. 14-16)

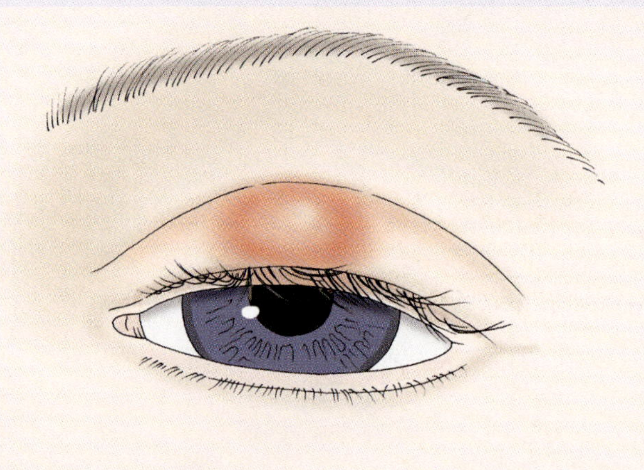

FIGURE 14-16 **Hordeolum (stye)**

hyperopia (hī-pĕr-Ō-pē-ă)	vision defect in which parallel rays focus behind the retina as a result of flattening of the globe of the eye or of an error in refraction; commonly called *farsightedness* (see Fig. 14-17)

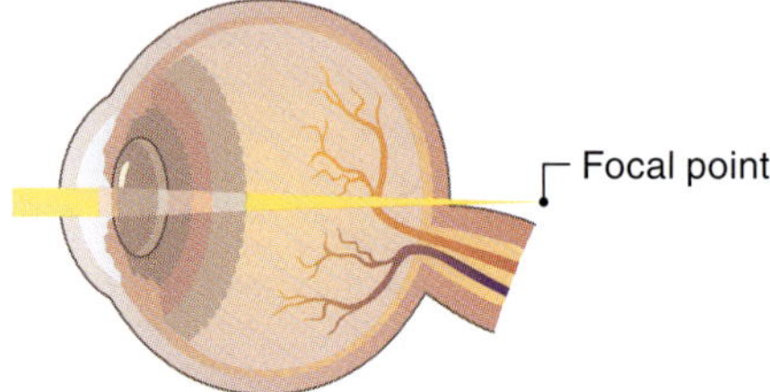

FIGURE 14-17 **Hyperopia**

TABLE 14-3 PATHOLOGY TERMS—cont'd	
Eye	
hypertensive retinopathy (hī-pĕr-TĔN-sĭv rĕt-ĭn-ŎP-ă-thē)	destructive retinal changes caused by hypertension (see Fig. 14-18)

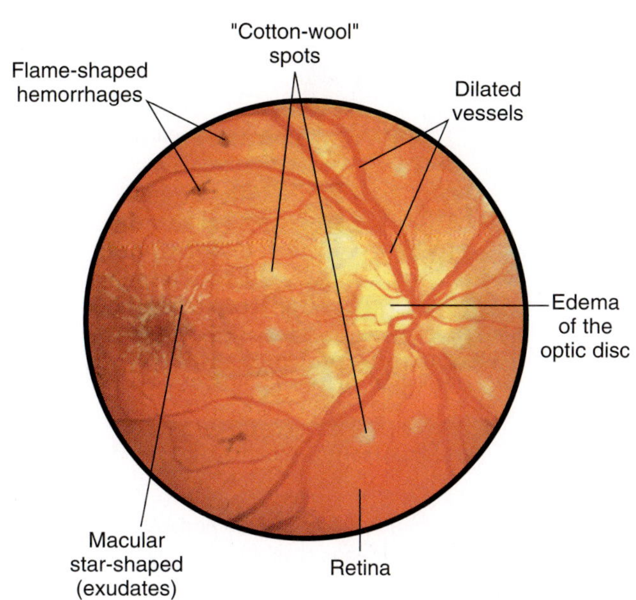

FIGURE 14-18 **Hypertensive retinopathy** (From Eagle, S, et al.: *The Professional Medical Assistant.* F.A. Davis, Philadelphia, 2009, p. 756; with permission)

keratitis (kĕr-ă-TĪ-tĭs)	inflammation of the cornea, usually associated with decreased visual acuity, which may, if untreated, result in blindness
legal blindness (LĒ-gul BLĪND-nis)	loss in visual acuity that prevents a person from performing work requiring eyesight; defined as corrected visual acuity of 20/200 or less or a visual field of 20 degrees or less in the better eye
macular degeneration (MĂK-ū-lăr dĭ-jen-er-Ā-shŭn)	macular deterioration resulting in central vision loss, categorized as either atrophic (dry) or exudative (wet) (see Fig. 14-19)

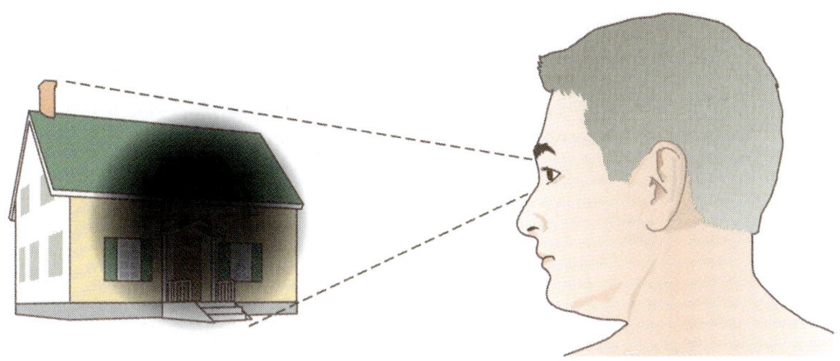

FIGURE 14-19 **Macular degeneration**

Continued

TABLE 14-3

PATHOLOGY TERMS—cont'd

Eye	
myopia (mī-Ō-pē-ă)	error of refraction in which light rays focus in front of the retina, enabling the person to see distinctly for only a short distance; commonly called *nearsightedness* (see Fig. 14-20)
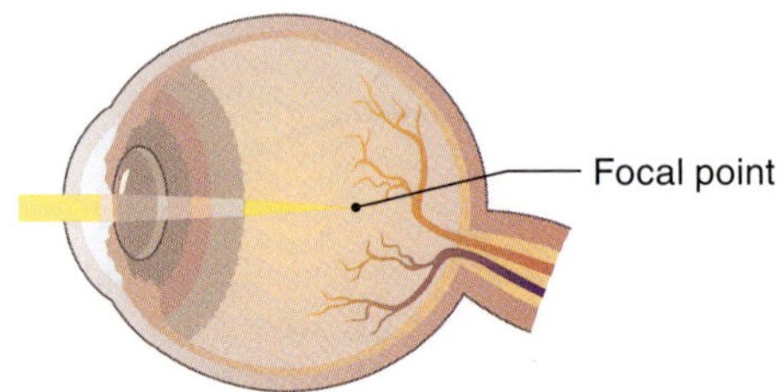 FIGURE 14-20 **Myopia**	
nystagmus (nĭs-TĂG-mŭs)	involuntary back-and-forth or cyclical movements of the eyes
ophthalmology (ŎP-thuh-mäl-ŭ-jē)	study of the structure, functions, and diseases of the eye
presbyopia (prĕz-bē-Ō-pē-ă)	permanent loss of accommodation of the lens of the eye that occurs as people enter their 40s, causing a marked inability to maintain focus on near objects
retinal detachment (RĔT-ĭ-năl dĭ-TACH-mŭnt)	separation of the inner sensory layer of the retina from the outer pigment layer, caused by a break in the inner layer that permits vitreous fluid to leak under the retina and lift off its innermost layer; may cause blindness (see Fig. 14-21)
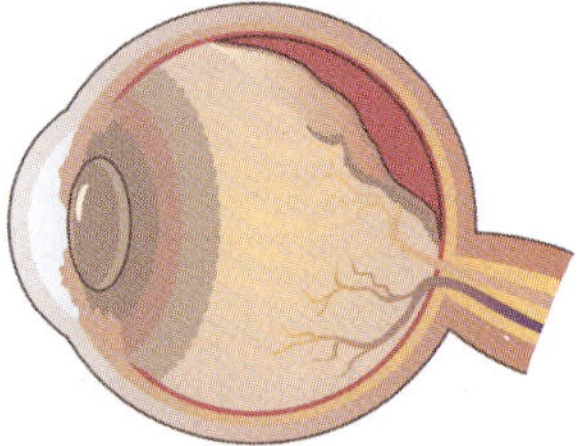 FIGURE 14-21 **Retinal detachment**	
strabismus (stră-BĬZ-mŭs)	deviation or misalignment of eyes that may adversely affect depth perception; types include *exotropia* (eyes turned outward), *esotropia* (eyes turned inward), *hypertropia* (eyes turned upward), and *hypotropia* (eyes turned downward) (see Fig. 14-22)

TABLE 14-3

PATHOLOGY TERMS—cont'd

Eye	
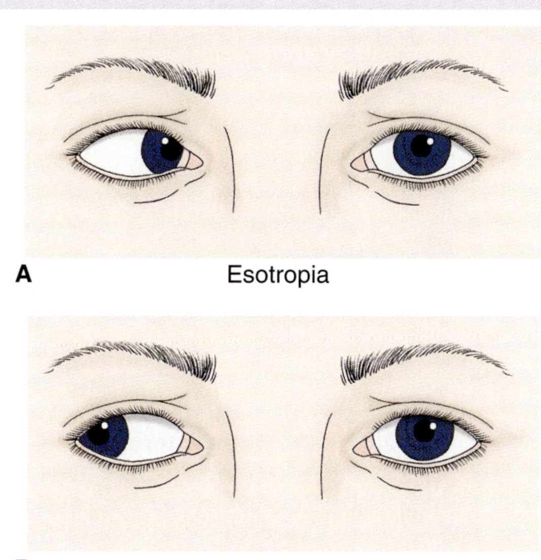 FIGURE 14-22 **Strabismus: (A) Esotropia, (B) Exotropia**	
uveitis (ū-vē-Ī-tĭs)	nonspecific term for any intraocular inflammatory disorder, which may affect the iris, ciliary body, choroid, or other parts of the eye
Ear	
anacusis (ăn-ă-KŪ-sĭs)	total deafness
cholesteatoma (kō-lē-stē-ă-TŌ-mă)	condition in which a cyst develops in the middle ear (see Fig. 14-23)
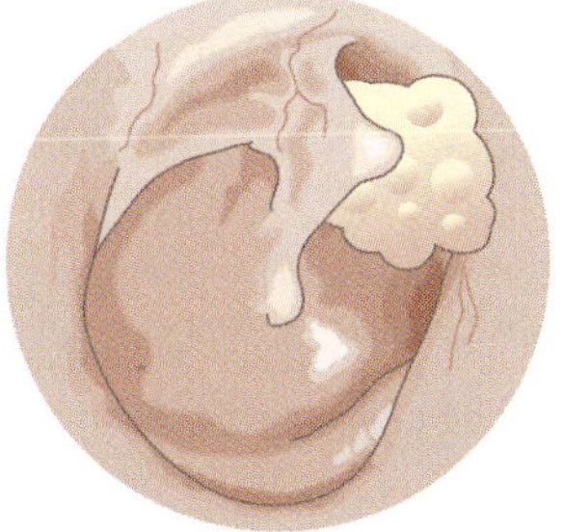 FIGURE 14-23 **Cholesteatoma**	
labyrinthitis (lăb-ĭ-rĭn-THĪ-tĭs)	inflammation of the labyrinth within the inner ear; also called *otitis interna*
Ménière disease (mān-ē-ĀR dĭ-ZĒZ)	chronic, noncontagious disorder of the labyrinth that leads to progressive hearing loss, vertigo, and tinnitus

Continued

TABLE 14-3
PATHOLOGY TERMS—cont'd

Ear	
otitis externa (ō-TĪ-tĭs ĕks-TĔR-nă)	acute inflammation or infection of the external auditory canal; also called *swimmer's ear* (see Fig. 14-24)

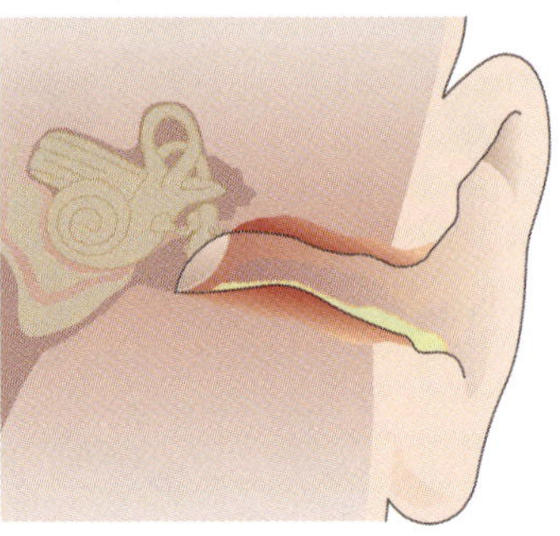

FIGURE 14-24 **Otitis externa**

otitis media (ō-TĪ-tĭs MĒ-dē-ă)	inflammation or infection of the middle ear (see Fig. 14-25)

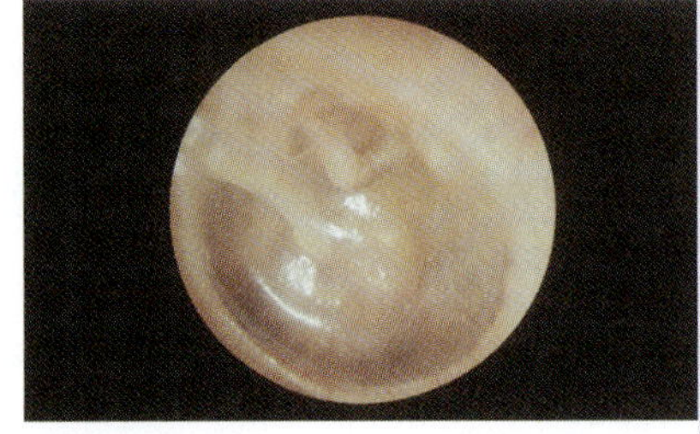

A Healthy tympanic membrane

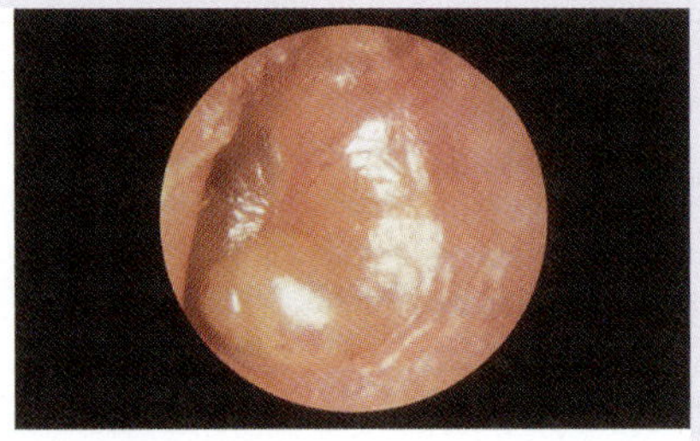

B Infected tympanic membrane

FIGURE 14-25 **Otitis media**

otosclerosis (ō-tō-sklē-RŌ-sĭs)	chronic progressive deafness caused by spongy bone formation around the oval window with resulting ankylosis of the stapes
presbycusis (prĕz-bĭ-KŪ-sĭs)	progressive loss of hearing with aging
tinnitus (tĭn-Ī-tŭs)	perception of ringing, buzzing, tinkling, or hissing sound in the ear
vertigo (VĔR-tĭ-gō)	feeling of spinning or moving in space

STOP HERE.
Select the Pathology Terms Flash Cards for Chapter 14 and run through them at least three times before you continue.

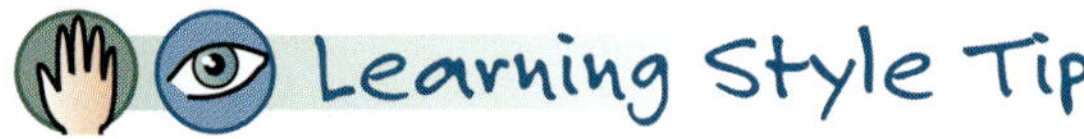

Spend time in the anatomy lab (with permission) studying 3-D models of the eye and ear. Label the parts using removable sticky notes. Include the anatomical term and the associated combining forms.

Common Diagnostic Tests and Procedures

Audiometry: Detailed measurement of hearing with an audiometer

Cochlear implant: Surgical insertion into the cochlea of a device that receives sound and transmits signals to electrodes implanted within the cochlea, allowing hearing-impaired persons to perceive sound

Color vision tests: Use of multicolored charts to evaluate the patient's ability to recognize color (see Fig. 14-26)

Corneal transplant (keratoplasty): Surgical replacement of a diseased cornea with a healthy one from a donor

Enucleation: Surgical removal of the entire eyeball

Laser-assisted in-situ keratomileusis (LASIK): Procedure in which a laser is used to alter the shape of the deep corneal layer after a top flap in the surface is opened

Laser photocoagulation: Destruction of areas of the retina with a laser beam

Phacoemulsification: Removal of the lens with an ultrasonic device to treat cataracts

Radial keratotomy: Incision into the outer portion of the cornea to flatten it and help correct nearsightedness

Refractive error test: Evaluation of the eye's ability to focus an image

Rinne test: Hearing test that compares bone conduction to air conduction, using a tuning fork (see Fig. 14-27)

Scleral buckling: Placement of a band of silicone around the eyeball to stabilize a detaching retina

Slit-lamp microscopy: Examination of the posterior surface of the cornea with a slit lamp

Tonometry: Measurement of intraocular tension to detect glaucoma

Tympanometry: Procedure for evaluation of the mobility and patency of the eardrum, detection of middle-ear disorders, and evaluation of the patency of the eustachian tube

Tympanoplasty: Reconstruction of a perforated tympanic membrane (see Fig. 14-28)

Visual acuity test: Examination that identifies the smallest letters that can be correctly identified on a standardized Snellen vision chart from 20 feet (see Fig. 14-29)

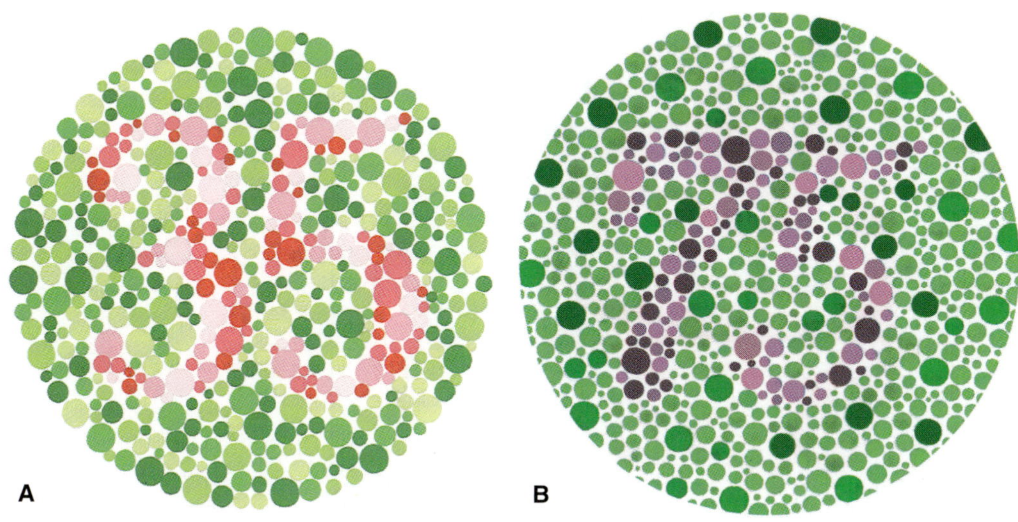

FIGURE 14-26 Color vision test

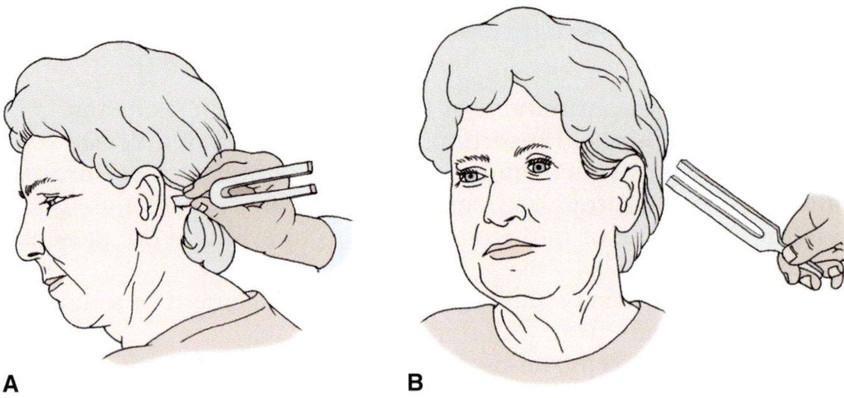

FIGURE 14-27 Rinne test

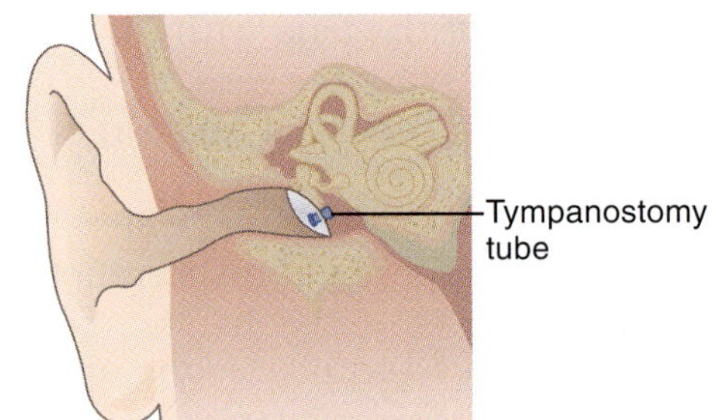

FIGURE 14-28 Tympanoplasty

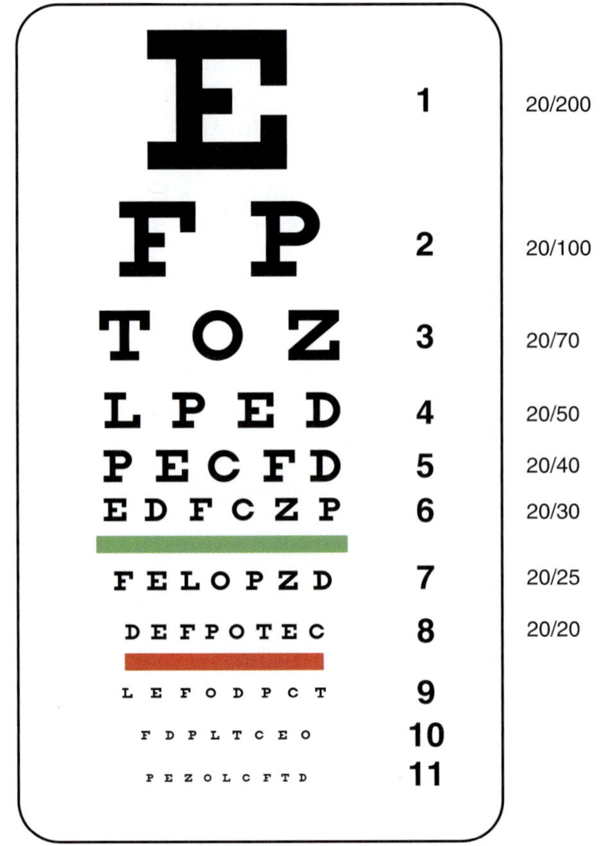

FIGURE 14-29 Visual acuity test: (A) Snellen chart with letters

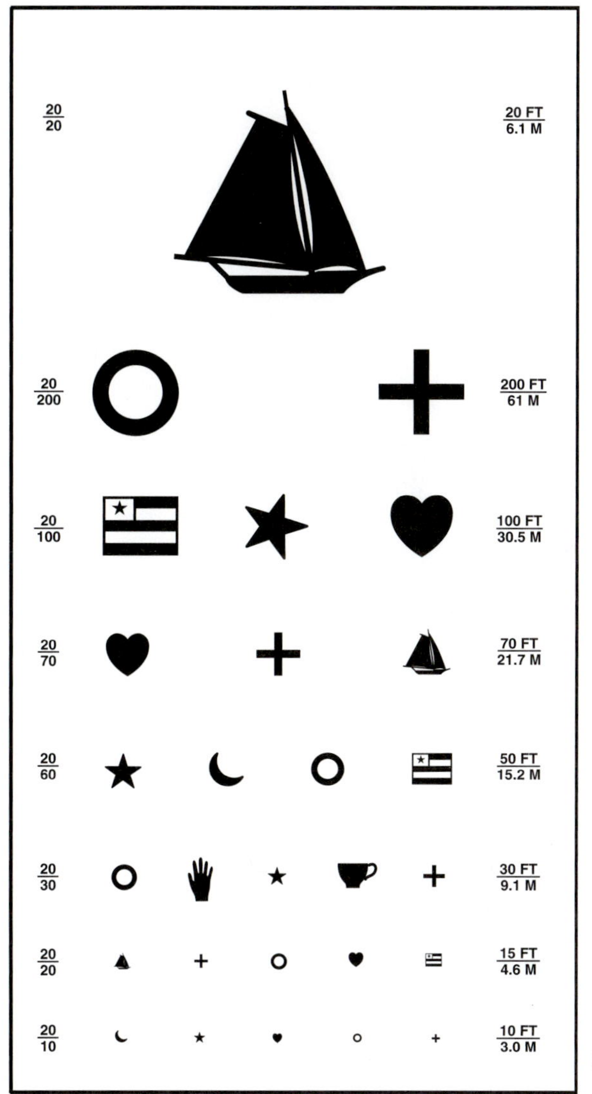

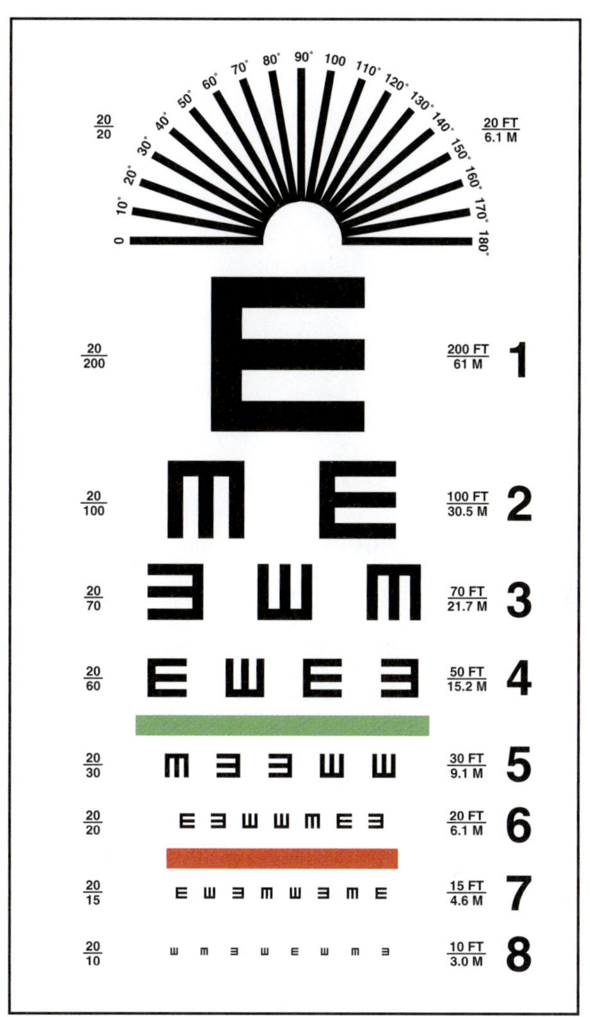

FIGURE 14-29—cont'd (B) Snellen chart with objects, (C) Rotating "E" chart

Weber test: Hearing test that evaluates bone conduction using a tuning fork (see Fig. 14-30)

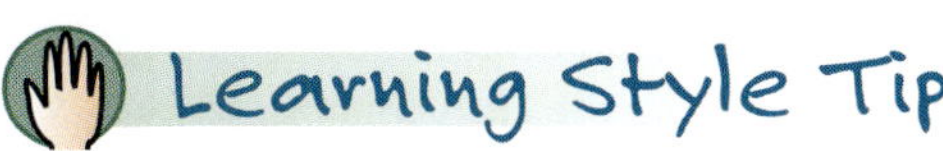

Take timed (5-to-10 minute) study breaks every 20 to 30 minutes, during which you exercise. This satisfies your need for physical movement and keeps you awake.

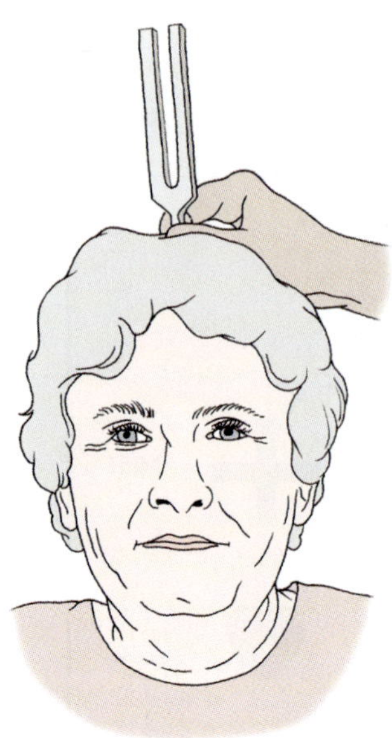

FIGURE 14-30 **Weber test**

CASE STUDY

Read the case study and answer the questions that follow. Most of the terms are included in this chapter. Refer to the glossaries (Appendixes B and D) or to your medical dictionary for the other terms.

Acute Otitis Media

Brad Stephens is a 5-year-old child with a Hx of chronic otitis media. With his first ear infection at 9 months of age, his symptoms were quite pronounced. He spiked a 104.5°F fever, ate and slept poorly, and was extremely fussy. However, with repeated episodes of AOM as he has aged, his symptoms have lessened significantly, making it difficult for his parents to know when he has an ear infection. Often his only symptom is fussiness. Brad has responded reasonably well in the past to antibiotics and decongestants, yet the infections frequently recur a short time later. At the age of 5, he still has one to two episodes of AOM each month. This raises concerns about hearing loss, so he was referred to an ENT specialist for consultation. The result was the decision to perform bilateral tympanotomy with tube placement.

Acute otitis media (AOM), the most common infection in infants and children, occurs when bacteria make their way from the oropharynx into the middle ear via the eustachian tube. Infections such as AOM often occur near the end of an upper respiratory infection (URI). Tissues are inflamed and edematous, and secretions are copious. Other risk factors for AOM include allergies and sinusitis. As infection sets in, the middle ear becomes inflamed, which causes edema and pressure in the middle ear. Serous fluid usually accumulates behind the tympanic membrane (TM) as well. In some children, the eustachian tube does not readily open to allow passage of air or fluid to relieve this pressure. As a result, the TM begins to bulge outward. This pressure, along with inflammation, causes pain and a sensation of the ear being plugged. Hearing is temporarily impaired at this point. In severe cases, the TM becomes blistered or even ruptures, which results in scarring and varying amounts of hearing loss.

With mild cases of AOM, treatment may focus on relieving pain with analgesics, such as acetaminophen, and treating congestion. More severe cases are treated with antibiotics. In the case of chronic AOM, surgery is considered. Surgery is generally a last resort, and serves the purpose of buying time while the child grows and matures. In many cases, a child will outgrow ear infections as the structures of the middle ear and throat further develop and the eustachian tubes begin to work more effectively.

When a tympanotomy is performed, tiny tubes are inserted into the TM, which creates a windowlike opening between the middle and outer ear. This does not prevent AOM from occurring, but it does allow fluid and air to escape, reducing pressure in the middle ear and preventing rupture of the TM. This reduces the risk of permanent damage or hearing loss. An added advantage is that it becomes easier to recognize an infection, because drainage from the ear is easily observed. This allows for earlier treatment. The tiny tubes remain in place for 6 months to 2 years, eventually working their way out into the ear canal, at which time the TM heals itself.

Flashpoint

Small children can experience ear pain on an airplane due to the effects of changing air pressure on their developing eustachian tubes.

Case Study Questions

1. Which of the following statements is true regarding Brad's experience?
   a. His symptoms worsened over time
   b. Brad was referred to a physician who specialized in disorders of the ears, nose, and throat
   c. Brad did not respond well to antibiotic therapy
   d. His parents could easily tell when Brad had an ear infection
2. Brad underwent a bilateral tympanotomy with tube placement. This procedure involves:
   a. Excision and removal of the eardrums
   b. Replacing the eardrums with tubes
   c. Creation of a mouthlike opening into the eustachian tube
   d. Cutting into the eardrums to place tubes
3. Which of the following statements is true regarding AOM?
   a. It is an uncommon type of infection in infants and children
   b. It is contagious
   c. It is caused when a virus attacks the middle ear
   d. It is caused by bacterial growth in the middle ear
4. Which of the following factors contributes to the development of AOM?
   a. A dry environment
   b. Failure of the outer ear canal to develop and work properly
   c. Allergies and sinusitis
   d. Accumulation of fluid in front of the TM
5. Which of the following statements is true regarding treatment of AOM?
   a. Antibiotics are always prescribed
   b. Decongestants may be used
   c. Surgery is common
   d. Analgesics are seldom used
6. Which of the following statements is true regarding the surgical procedure that Brad underwent?
   a. The purpose was to buy some time while the structures in his ear and throat further developed
   b. The purpose was to repair the defect in his middle ear and cure his problem
   c. The purpose was to restore his lost hearing
   d. The purpose was to prevent the occurrence of AOM

7. Which of the following statements is true regarding the tubes that are placed in the TM?
   a. They will be surgically removed once the ear has healed
   b. They allow for the escape of fluid or air
   c. They force the eustachian tube to work properly
   d. They usually remain in place for 5 years

Answers to Case Study Questions

1. b
2. d
3. d
4. c
5. b
6. a
7. b

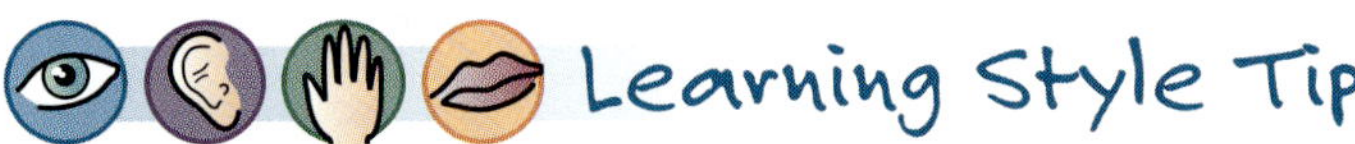

Watch medical dramas on TV or rent medical-themed movies, and write down medical terms as you hear them used. Keep this book and a medical dictionary handy to look up any terms you don't know. Read the definitions aloud.

Websites

Please go to the F.A. Davis website at http://davisplus.fadavis.com/eagle/medterm to view resource websites for the sensory system.

Practice Exercises

Deciphering Terms

Write the correct meaning of these medical terms. Check Appendix G for the correct answers.

Exercise 2

1. keratoid ______________________________
2. neoplasia ______________________________
3. myringomycosis ______________________________
4. tympanometry ______________________________
5. retro-ocular ______________________________
6. ophthalmoplegia ______________________________

7. otoplasty ______________________________

8. oculonasal ______________________________

9. tympanic ______________________________

10. keratotomy ______________________________

11. blepharoptosis ______________________________

12. ophthalmokinesia ______________________________

13. intraocular ______________________________

14. lacrimotome ______________________________

15. phacosclerosis ______________________________

Fill in the Blanks

Fill in the blanks below. Check Appendix G for the correct answers.

Exercise 3

1. Dr. Strouse specializes in treating EENT disorders. Therefore, she treats disorders of the ____________, ____________, ____________, and ____________.

2. When Dr. Strouse charts *PERRLA*, it means ____________ ____________ ____________, ____________, ____________ ____________ ____________, and ____________.

3. Kari wears corrective lenses because she has an abnormal curvature of the cornea that distorts her visual image. This is known as an ____________.

4. Herbert has total deafness. The term for this is ____________.

5. Hilda has hearing loss due to her advanced age. The term for this is ____________.

6. Jack has ____________ ____________, which is a chronic, noncontagious disorder of the labyrinth that leads to progressive hearing loss, vertigo, and tinnitus.

7. ______________ ______________ is a condition of sudden blockage of aqueous-humor outflow that causes a rapid increase in intraocular pressure.

8. David is a farmer who has developed cloudiness of the lens due to protein deposits as a result of aging and tobacco use. This is called ______________.

9. Monty has been a diabetic for 20 years and is developing the signs of ______________ ______________, which is vision loss due to his diabetes.

10. Blake has a condition that is causing central vision loss because of deterioration. This is known as ______________ ______________.

11. Louise has an infection of a sebaceous gland of the eyelid. This is known as ______________.

12. Dennis is experiencing vision loss in his left eye caused by a separation of the inner retinal layer from the outer layer. This is known as ______________ ______________.

13. ______________ is a form of strabismus in which one or both eyes are turned outward.

14. ______________ is a nonspecific term for any intraocular inflammatory disorder that may affect the iris, ciliary body, choroid, or other parts of the eye.

15. The abbreviations *Ast* and *AS* stand for ______________.

16. ______________ is a condition of inflammation of the conjunctiva.

17. The type of vision loss associated with advancing age is ______________.

18. ______________ is a small benign cyst in the eyelid formed by the distention of a meibomian gland with secretions.

19. ______________ is a cyst that develops in the middle ear.

20. A condition that causes involuntary back-and-forth or cyclical movements of the eyes is ______________.

Multiple Choice

Select the one best answer to the following multiple-choice questions. Check Appendix G for the correct answers.

Exercise 4

1. Which of the following conditions does **not** result in vision loss?
   a. Presbycusis
   b. Diabetic retinopathy
   c. Retinal detachment
   d. Glaucoma

2. Which of the following conditions results in an abnormal curvature of the cornea, distorting the visual image?
   a. Presbycusis
   b. Astigmatism
   c. Cataract
   d. Hordeolum

3. Albert Mills is an elderly man who experiences diminished hearing because of advanced age. This condition is known as:
   a. Photophobia
   b. Glaucoma
   c. Presbycusis
   d. Hordeolum

4. A type of blindness caused by diabetes is known as diabetic ________________.
   a. Retinopathy
   b. Cataract
   c. Macular degeneration
   d. Ménière disease

5. Onset of blindness caused by increased intraocular pressure is known as:
   a. Cataract
   b. Macular degeneration
   c. Hordeolum
   d. Glaucoma

Word Building

*Using **only** the word parts in the lists provided, create medical terms with the indicated meanings. Check Appendix G for the correct answers.*

Exercise 5

Prefixes	Combining Forms	Suffixes
an-	acous/o	-al
hyper-	audi/o	-ar
	blephar/o	-ectomy
	conjunctiv/o	-edema
	dipl/o	-ic
	irid/o	-itis
	kerat/o	-logy
	lacrim/o	-malacia
	myring/o	-metry
	nas/o	-oma
	ocul/o	-opia
	ophthalm/o	-osis
	ot/o	-pathy
	phac/o	-plasty
	retin/o	-plegia
	scler/o	-scope
	tympan/o	-tic
		-tomy

1. pertaining to absence of hearing ____________
2. pertaining to the eye ____________
3. swelling of the eyelid ____________
4. excessive vision or far vision ____________
5. study of the eye ____________
6. inflammation of the cornea ____________
7. double vision ____________
8. cutting into or incision of the tympanic membrane ____________
9. viewing instrument for the eye ____________
10. disease of the retina ____________
11. surgical repair of the sclera ____________
12. surgical repair of the eye ____________
13. pertaining to the ear ____________

14. pertaining to the lacrimal gland and nose ______________________

15. softening of the lens ______________________

16. abnormal condition of the retina ______________________

17. tumor of the conjunctiva ______________________

18. excision or surgical removal of the iris ______________________

19. measurement of hearing ______________________

20. paralysis of the eye ______________________

True or False

Decide whether the following statements are true or false. Check Appendix G for the correct answers.

Exercise 6

1. True False The abbreviation **ENT** stands for *eyes, ears, nose, and throat.*
2. True False **Conjunctivitis** is a condition of inflammation of the conjunctiva.
3. True False The abbreviation **EM** stands for *extraocular movement.*
4. True False **Tinnitus** is a feeling of dizziness or vertigo.
5. True False **Strabismus** is a condition of blindness.
6. True False **Otosclerosis** causes progressive hearing loss.
7. True False **Vertigo** is ringing in the ears.
8. True False **Acute otitis media** is an infection of the outer ear.
9. True False The abbreviation **Ast** stands for *acoustic.*
10. True False **LASIK** is a procedure that improves vision.

Deciphering Terms

Write the correct meaning of these medical terms. Check Appendix G for the correct answers.

Exercise 7

1. dacryohemorrhea ______________________

2. iridosis ______________________

3. lacrimotomy ____________________
4. phacoid ____________________
5. presbycusis ____________________
6. retinopathy ____________________
7. dacryadenalgia ____________________
8. blepharospasm ____________________
9. iridoplegia ____________________
10. phakoma ____________________

Multiple Choice

Select the one best answer to the following multiple-choice questions. Check Appendix G for the correct answers.

Exercise 8

1. Which of the following terms means *absence of smell or odor?*
   a. Anosmia
   b. Anacusia
   c. Anopia
   d. None of these

2. Which of the following terms means *excision or surgical removal of the tear gland?*
   a. Dacryotome
   b. Dacryoadenectomy
   c. Lacrimotomy
   d. Lacrimostomy

3. Which of the following terms means *disease of the lens?*
   a. Phakopathy
   b. Phacopathy
   c. Both a and b
   d. None of these

4. Which of the following terms means *specialist in the study of sound?*
   a. Acoustic
   b. Audiology
   c. Otonasorhinologist
   d. None of these

5. Which of the following terms means *abnormal condition of hardening of the ear drum?*
   a. Myringostenosis
   b. Tympanosclerosis
   c. Salpingoconstriction
   d. Otodilation

6. Which of the following terms means *sudden involuntary contraction of the eustachian tube?*
   a. Tympanostenosis
   b. Salpingospasm
   c. Myringosclerosis
   d. Irostomy

7. The patient who needs a vision examination will visit an:
   a. Ophthalmology
   b. Optician
   c. Ocular
   d. Otologist

8. The term *hemiopia* means:
   a. Half vision
   b. Double vision
   c. Far or beyond vision
   d. Good or normal vision

9. The term *dysosmia* means:
   a. Much thirst
   b. Abnormal vision
   c. Bad, painful, or difficult smell or odor
   d. Bad, painful, or difficult feeling

10. The term *microblepharism* means:
    a. Condition of farsightedness
    b. Abnormal condition of large eyes
    c. Having same or equal eyelids
    d. Condition of small eyelids

11. The term *dacryoid* means:
    a. Resembling double
    b. Resembling tears
    c. Resembling sound
    d. None of these

12. The term *diplopia* means:
    a. Near image
    b. Far view
    c. Double vision
    d. Two eyes

13. All of the following abbreviations pertain to conditions that cause vision loss or impairment **except**:
    a. Glc
    b. MD
    c. EOM
    d. RD

14. Which of the following abbreviations refers to a procedure that improves vision?
    a. AS
    b. LASIK
    c. CAT
    d. VA

15. All of the following abbreviations refer to the eyes **except**:
    a. ENT
    b. EM
    c. RK
    d. RD

16. Which of the following is a disorder in which the brain disregards images from a weaker eye and relies on those from the stronger eye?
    a. Amblyopia
    b. Astigmatism
    c. Chalazion
    d. Ectropion

17. Which of the following is an infection of a sebaceous gland of the eyelid?
    a. Hordeolum
    b. Keratitis
    c. Cholesteatoma
    d. Labyrinthitis

18. Which of the following is a feeling of spinning or moving in space?
    a. Vertigo
    b. Tinnitus
    c. Otosclerosis
    d. Ménière disease

19. An error in refraction is:
    a. Myopia
    b. Hyperoptism
    c. Presbyopia
    d. Hypopia

20. Glaucoma has which of the following effects on the eye?
    a. Cloudiness of the lens
    b. Inflammation of the lid and eyelash follicles
    c. Increased intraocular pressure
    d. Loss of central vision

ABBREVIATIONS

APPENDIX

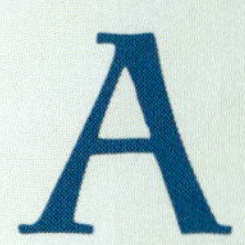

SYMBOLS

♂	male
♀	female
c̄	with
s̄	without

A

AB	antibody, abortion
Abd	abdomen
ABGs	arterial blood gases
ACL	anterior cruciate ligament
ADH	antidiuretic hormone
ADHD	attention-deficit hyperactivity disorder
ADL	activities of daily living
AE	above the elbow
AED	automated external defibrillator
AF, A-fib	atrial fibrillation
AFB	acid-fast bacillus
AG, Ag	antigen
AGN	acute glomerulonephritis
AICD	automatic implanted cardioverter defibrillator
AIDS	acquired immune deficiency syndrome
AK	above the knee
AKA	above-the-knee amputation
ALS	amyotrophic lateral sclerosis (Lou Gehrig disease)
ANS	autonomic nervous system
AP	anteroposterior
ARDS	acute respiratory distress syndrome
ARF	acute renal failure
AS	ankylosing spondylitis, astigmatism
ASHD	arteriosclerotic heart disease
Ast	astigmatism
ATN	acute tubular necrosis
AV, A-V	atrioventricular

B

BCC	basal cell carcinoma
BE	below the elbow
BG, BS	blood glucose, blood sugar
bid, b.i.d.	twice a day
BK	below the knee
BKA	below-the-knee amputation
BM	bowel movement
BMD	bone mineral density
BMI	body mass index
BMR	basal metabolic rate
BNO	bladder neck obstruction
BP	blood pressure
BPH	benign prostatic hypertrophy (benign prostatic hyperplasia)
bpm	beats per minute
BRP	bathroom privileges
BSE	breast self-examination
BUN	blood urea nitrogen
Bx, bx	biopsy

C

C&S	culture and sensitivity
C1–C7	first cervical vertebra, second cervical vertebra, etc.
Ca	calcium
CA	cancer, carcinoma
CABG	coronary artery bypass graft
CAD	coronary artery disease
CAT	cataract
Cath	catheterization, catheter
CCU	coronary care unit
CF	cystic fibrosis
CFS	chronic fatigue syndrome
CIRC, circum	circumcision

CK	creatine kinase
CMC	chronic mucocutaneous candidiasis
CNS	central nervous system
c/o	complain(ed/ing/s/t) of
CO_2	carbon dioxide
COPD	chronic obstructive pulmonary disease
CP	cerebral palsy, chest pain
CPAP	continuous positive airway pressure
CPR	cardiopulmonary resuscitation
CRF	chronic renal failure
C-section	cesarean section
CSF	cerebrospinal fluid
CT	computed tomography
CTS	carpal tunnel syndrome
CV	cardiovascular
CVA	cerebrovascular accident
CWP	coal worker's pneumoconiosis
CXR	chest x-ray
Cysto	cystoscopy

D

D&C	dilation and curettage
decub	decubitus ulcer
derm	dermatology
DEXA	dual-energy x-ray absorptiometry
DI	diabetes insipidus
DIC	disseminated intravascular coagulation
DJD	degenerative joint disease (osteoarthritis)
DKA	diabetic ketoacidosis
DM	diabetes mellitus
DOE	dyspnea on exertion
DRE	digital rectal examination
DTR	deep tendon reflex
DVT	deep vein thrombosis
Dx	diagnosis

E

EBV	Epstein-Barr virus
ECG, EKG	electrocardiogram
ECHO	echocardiogram
ED	erectile dysfunction
EDC	estimated date of confinement (due date)
EENT	eyes, ears, nose, and throat
EEG	electroencephalography
EGD	esophagogastroduodenoscopy
EIA	enzyme immunosorbent assay
EM, em	emmetropia
EMG	electromyogram
ENT	ears, nose, and throat
EOM	extraocular movement
ERCP	endoscopic retrograde cholangiopancreatography
ERT, HRT	estrogen replacement therapy, hormone replacement therapy
ESR, sed rate	erythrocyte sedimentation rate
ESRD	end-stage renal disease

F

FBG, FBS	fasting blood glucose, fasting blood sugar
FH	family history
FHR	fetal heart rate
fsbs	finger stick blood sugar
Fx	fracture

G

G, glc	glaucoma
GBS	Guillain-Barré syndrome
GC	gonorrhea
GERD	gastroesophageal reflux disease
GH	growth hormone
GI	gastrointestinal
GTT	glucose tolerance test
GU	genitourinary
GVHD	graft-versus-host disease
GYN	gynecology

H

h, hr	hour
H_2O	water
HD	hemodialysis

HF	heart failure
HIV	human immunodeficiency virus
HNP	herniated nucleus pulposus
HPV	human papilloma virus
HTN	hypertension (high blood pressure)
Hx	history

I

I&D	incision and drainage
I&O	intake and output
IBD	inflammatory bowel disease
IBS	irritable bowel syndrome
ICP	intracranial pressure
ICU	intensive care unit
ID	intradermal (injection)
IDDM	insulin-dependent diabetes mellitus (type 1 diabetes)
Ig	immunoglobulin
IM	intramuscular
INR	international normalized ratio
ITP	idiopathic thrombocytopenic purpura
IUD	intrauterine device
IV	intravenous
IVF	in vitro fertilization
IVP	intravenous pyelogram

J

JRA	juvenile rheumatoid arthritis

K

K	potassium
KS	Kaposi sarcoma
KUB	kidney, ureter, and bladder

L

L&D	labor and delivery
L1–L5	first lumbar vertebra, second lumbar vertebra, etc.
LA	left atrium
LASIK	laser-assisted in-situ keratomileusis
LAT	lateral
LE	lower extremity
LFT	liver function test
LLE	left lower extremity
LLQ	left lower quadrant
LMP	last menstrual period
LOC	level of consciousness, loss of consciousness
LP	lumbar puncture
LUE	left upper extremity
LUQ	left upper quadrant
LV	left ventricle

M

MD	macular degeneration, muscular dystrophy
MDI	metered dose inhaler
MET, met	metastasis, metastasize
MI	myocardial infarction
MM	malignant melanoma
MR	mitral regurgitation
MRI	magnetic resonance imaging
MS	multiple sclerosis, mitral stenosis
MVA	motor vehicle accident
MVP	mitral valve prolapse

N

N&V	nausea and vomiting
Na	sodium
NG	nasogastric
NIDDM	non–insulin-dependent diabetes mellitus (type 2 diabetes)
NPO	nothing by mouth
NSAID	nonsteroidal anti-inflammatory drug

O

O_2	oxygen
OA	osteoarthritis
OB-GYN	obstetrics and gynecology
OC	oral contraceptive
OCD	obsessive-compulsive disorder
ORIF	open reduction–internal fixation
ortho	orthopedic, straight
OSA	obstructive sleep apnea
OT	occupational therapy
OTC	over-the-counter

P

P	pulse
PA	posteroanterior
PAC	premature atrial contraction
PAD	peripheral artery disease
Pap	Papanicolaou smear
PCP	*Pneumocystis carinii* pneumonia, *Pneumocystis* pneumonia
PE	physical examination, pulmonary embolism
PERRLA	pupils are equal, round, reactive to light and accommodation
PFT	pulmonary function test
pH	potential of hydrogen (measure of acidity or alkalinity)
PID	pelvic inflammatory disease
PKD	polycystic kidney disease
PM	polymyositis
PMS	premenstrual syndrome
PND	paroxysmal nocturnal dyspnea
PNS	peripheral nervous system
PO	by mouth
PPD	purified protein derivative
PR	per rectum
PSA	prostate-specific antigen
PT	prothrombin time, physical therapy
PTCA	percutaneous transluminal coronary angioplasty
PTH	parathyroid hormone
PTT	partial thromboplastin time
PUD	peptic ulcer disease
PVC	premature ventricular contraction

Q

q	every
q2h	every 2 hours
qam	every morning
qh	every hour
qhs	each evening (hour of sleep)
qid, q.i.d.	four times a day

R

R	respiration
RA	rheumatoid arthritis, right atrium, room air
RD	retinal detachment
RK	radial keratotomy
RLE	right lower extremity
RLQ	right lower quadrant
ROM	range of motion
RP	retrograde pyelogram
RUE	right upper extremity
RUQ	right upper quadrant
RV	right ventricle

S

S1–S5	first sacral vertebra, second sacral vertebra, etc.
SBO	small bowel obstruction
SCC	squamous cell carcinoma
SCI	spinal cord injury
SG, sp. gr.	specific gravity
SIDS	sudden infant death syndrome
SLE	systemic lupus erythematosus
SOB	short(ness) of breath
SS	Sjögren syndrome
stat	immediate(ly)
STD, STI	sexually transmitted disease, sexually transmitted infection
SubQ, Sub-Q	subcutaneous
Sx	symptom(s)

T

T&A	tonsillectomy and adenoidectomy
T1–T12	first thoracic vertebra, second thoracic vertebra, etc.
T3, T4	triiodothyronine, thyroxine (thyroid hormones)
TAH	total abdominal hysterectomy
TAH-BSO	total abdominal hysterectomy, bilateral salpingo-oophorectomy
TAO	thromboangiitis obliterans
TB	tuberculosis
TEE	transesophageal echocardiography
TENS	transcutaneous electrical nerve stimulation
TGA	transient global amnesia
THA, THR	total hip arthroplasty, total hip replacement

TIA	transient ischemic attack
tid, t.i.d.	three times a day
TKR	total knee replacement
TN	trigeminal neuralgia
TOS	thoracic outlet syndrome
Trich	trichomoniasis
TSE	testicular self-examination
TSH	thyroid-stimulating hormone
TSS	toxic shock syndrome
TURP	transurethral resection of the prostate
TV	tidal volume
Tx	treatment

U

UA	urinalysis
UC	urine culture
UE	upper extremity
UGI	upper GI x-ray
ung	ointment
URI	upper respiratory infection
UTI	urinary tract infection

V

V, VA	visual acuity
VC	vital capacity
VCUG	voiding cystourethrography
V-fib	ventricular fibrillation
VS	vital signs
VT, V-tach	ventricular tachycardia
VTE	venous thromboembolism
VUR	vesicoureteral reflux

DISCONTINUED ABBREVIATIONS

The following abbreviations may be found in current medical records. However, the use of these terms is strongly discouraged because of the high rate of errors in transcription or interpretation.

Discontinued Abbreviation	Rationale	Replacement
AD: right ear	Mistaken for: AS, AU, OD, OS, OU	Write: right ear
AS: left ear	Mistaken for: AD, AU, OD, OS, OU	Write: left ear
AU: both ears	Mistaken for: U (units) when poorly written	Write: both ears
cc: cubic centimeter	Mistaken for: U (units) when poorly written	Write: ml
dc, DC, D/C: discharge or discontinue	Mistaken for: each other	Write: discharge or discontinue
IU: international unit	Mistaken for: IV	Write: international unit
$MgSO_4$: magnesium sulfate	Mistaken for: MSO_4	Write: magnesium sulfate
MS, MSO_4: morphine, morphine sulfate	Mistaken for: $MgSO_4$	Write: morphine sulfate
OD: right eye	Mistaken for: AD, AS, AU, OS, OU	Write: right eye
OS: left eye	Mistaken for: AD, AS, AU, OD, OU	Write: left eye
OU: both eyes	Mistaken for: AD, AS, AU, OD, OS	Write: both eyes
qd: every day	Mistaken for: qod	Write: daily
qod: every other day	Mistaken for: qd or qid	Write: every other day
SC, SQ: subcutaneous	Mistaken for: SL (sublingual) or 5 every	Write: subcut. or subcutaneously, SubQ or Sub-Q

Continued

Discontinued Abbreviation	Rationale	Replacement
ss: sliding scale	Mistaken for: 55	Write: sliding scale
u: unit	Mistaken for: 0, 4, or cc	Write: unit
µg: microgram	Mistaken for: mg	Write: mcg
<, >: less than, greater than	Mistaken for: each other	Write: less than or greater than
trailing zero (4.0 mg)	Decimal point may be missed, resulting in an overdose of 10 times the prescribed amount.	Never write an unnecessary zero after a decimal point
lack of leading zero (.4 mg)	Decimal point may be missed, resulting in an overdose of 10 times prescribed amount.	Always use a zero before a decimal point to indicate its presence (0.4 mg)

GLOSSARY OF PATHOLOGY TERMS

APPENDIX

B

A

abortion (ă-BOR-shŭn): spontaneous or therapeutic loss of a pregnancy at less than 20 weeks; also called *miscarriage*

abrasion (ă-BRĀ-zhŭn): scraping away of skin or mucous membranes

abruptio placentae (ă-BRŬP-shē-ō plă-SĔN-tă): sudden, premature detachment of the placenta from the uterine wall

achalasia (ăk-ă-LĀ-zē-ă): dilation and expansion of the lower esophagus, due to pressure from food accumulation

acne (ĂK-nē): disease of the sebaceous (oil) glands and hair follicles in the skin, marked by plugged pores, pimples, cysts, and nodules on the face, neck, chest, back, and other areas

acquired immune deficiency syndrome (AIDS) (ă-KWĪRD ĭm-ŪN dē-FĬSH-ĕn-sē SĬN-drōm): late-stage infection with the human immunodeficiency virus (HIV) which progressively weakens the immune system

acromegaly (ăk-rō-MĔG-ă-lē): type of hyperpituitarism in which an overactive pituitary gland after adulthood causes abnormal continued growth of bones and tissues of the face and extremities

actinic keratosis (ăk-TĬ-nĭk kĕr-ă-TŌ-sĭs): precancerous condition in which rough, scaly patches of skin develop, most commonly on sun-exposed areas such as the scalp, neck, face, ears, lips, hands, and forearms; also known as *solar keratosis*

acute bronchitis (ă-KŪT brŏng-KĪ-tĭs): infection and inflammation of bronchial airways

acute respiratory distress syndrome (ARDS) (ă-KŪT RĔS-pĭr-a-tor-ē dĭs-TRĔS SĬN-drōm): acute, life-threatening condition of lung injury that develops secondary to some other lung trauma or disorder

Addison disease (ĂD-ĭ-sŭn dĭ-ZĒZ): illness characterized by gradual adrenal-gland failure, resulting in insufficient production of steroid hormones and the need for hormone replacement therapy; also called *hypoadrenalism*

adhesive capsulitis (ăd-HĒ-sĭv kăp-sū-LĪ-tĭs): loss of range of motion in the shoulder; also called *frozen shoulder*

allergic rhinitis (ă-LĔR-jĭk rī-NĪ-tĭs): inflammation of the nasal membranes, caused by allergies

alopecia (ă-lō-PĒ-shē-ă): autoimmune disease that results in loss of hair; alopecia areata causes patchy hair loss from the scalp; alopecia totalis causes total scalp hair loss; alopecia universalis causes total body hair loss

Alzheimer disease (ĂLTS-hī-mĕr dĭ-ZĒZ): form of chronic, progressive dementia caused by the atrophy of brain tissue

amblyopia (ăm-blē-Ō-pē-ă): disorder in which the brain disregards images from the weaker eye and relies on those from the stronger eye; sometimes called *lazy eye*

amenorrhea (ă-mĕn-ō-RĒ-ă): absence of menses in a woman between the ages of 16 and 40

amyotrophic lateral sclerosis (ALS) (ă-mī-ō-TRŌ-fĭk LĂ-tĕr-ăl sklĕ-RŌ-sĭs): chronic, progressive, degenerative neuromuscular disorder that destroys motor neurons of the body; also called *Lou Gehrig disease*

anacusis (ăn-ă-KŪ-sĭs): total deafness

anaphylaxis (ăn-ă-fĭ-LĂK-sĭs): life-threatening systemic allergic reaction to a substance to which the body was previously sensitized

anemia (ă-NĒ-mē-ă): group of disorders generally defined as a reduction in the mass of circulating red blood cells

aneurysm (ĂN-ū-rĭ-zum): weakening and bulging of part of a vessel wall

angina (ăn-JĪ-nă): heart pain or other discomfort felt in the chest, shoulders, arms, jaw, or neck, caused by insufficient blood and oxygen to the heart; usually a symptom of heart disease

ankylosing spondylitis (AS) (ăng-kĭ-LŌ-sing spŏn-dĭl-Ī-tĭs): inflammatory response that causes degenerative changes in the spinal vertebrae; sacroiliac joints; and connective tissues such as tendons, ligaments, hips, shoulders, knees, feet, and ribs; and tissues of the lungs, eyes, and heart valves

anorexia nervosa (ăn-ō-RĔK-sē-ă nĕr-VŌ-să): physical and psychiatric disorder that involves a combination of an intense fear of weight gain, distorted body image, and self-imposed starvation

anterior cruciate ligament tear (ăn-TĒR-ē-ōr KROO-shē-āt LĬG-ă-mĕnt tār): injury to one of the stabilizing ligaments of the knee, which originates on the anterior portion of the femur

appendicitis (ă-pĕn-dĭ-SĪ-tĭs): inflammation of the appendix

arrhythmia (ă-RĬTH-mē-ă): loss of heart rhythm (rhythmic irregularity)

arteriosclerosis (ăr-tē-rē-ō-sklĕ-RŌ-sĭs): thickening, loss of elasticity, and loss of contractility of arterial walls; commonly called *hardening of the arteries*

asbestosis (ăs-bĕ-STŌ-sĭs): respiratory disease caused by chronic or repetitive inhalation of asbestos fibers

ascites (ă-SĪ-tēz): accumulation of serous fluid in the peritoneal (abdominal) cavity

asthma (ĂZ-mă): disease marked by episodic narrowing and inflammation of the airways, resulting in wheezing, SOB, and cough

astigmatism (ă-STĬG-mă-tĭ-zum): abnormal curvature of the cornea that distorts the visual image

atelectasis (ăt-ĕ-LĔK-tă-sĭs): partial collapse of the alveoli and tiny airways of the lung

atherosclerosis (ăth-ĕr-ō-sklĕ-RŌ-sĭs): the most common form of arteriosclerosis, marked by deposits of cholesterol, lipids, and calcium on the walls of arteries, which may restrict blood flow

atrial fibrillation (AF, A-fib) (Ā-trē-ăl fĭ-brĭl-Ā-shŭn): common irregular heart rhythm marked by uncontrolled atrial quivering and a rapid ventricular response

autoimmune hemolytic anemia (aw-tō-ĭm-MŪN hē-mō-LĬT-ĭk ă-NĒ-mē-ă): group of disorders caused when the immune system misidentifies red blood cells (RBCs) as foreign and creates autoantibodies that attack them

B

bacterial cystitis (bak-TIR-ē-ul sĭs-TĪ-tĭs): inflammation of the bladder caused by bacterial infection, commonly coexisting with bacterial urethritis, both of which together constitute a urinary tract infection (UTI), sometimes referred to as a *bladder infection*

balanoposthitis (băl-ă-nō-pŏs-THĪ-tĭs): inflammation of the glans penis and foreskin covering the glans penis; also called *balanitis*

Bartholin gland cyst (BĂR-tō-lĭn glănd sĭst): blockage of one or both of the Bartholin glands, causing inflammation and tenderness

basal cell carcinoma (BĀ-săl sĕl kăr-sĭ-NŌ-mă): common type of skin cancer that typically appears as a small, shiny papule and eventually enlarges to form a whitish border around a central depression or ulcer that may bleed

Bell palsy (bĕl PAWL-zē): form of facial paralysis, usually unilateral and temporary

benign prostatic hypertrophy (bē-NĪN prŏs-TĂT-ĭc hī-PĔR-trŏ-fē): noncancerous enlargement of the prostate gland, common in elderly men

blepharitis (blĕf-ăr-Ī-tĭs): noncontagious inflammation of the eyelash follicles and tiny oil glands along the margins of the eyelids

bowel obstruction (BOW-ĕl ŏb-STRŬK-shŭn): partial or complete blockage of the small or large intestine; common causes include volvulus, intussusception, tumors, and adhesions (scar tissue)

brain abscess (brān ĂB-sĕs): collection of pus anywhere within the brain

brain attack (brān ă-TĂK): damage or death of brain tissue caused by interruption of blood supply due to a clot or vessel rupture; also known as *stroke* or *cerebrovascular accident (CVA)*

brain tumor (brān TŪ-mŏr): any type of abnormal mass growing within the cranium

bruit (bruw-ē): soft blowing sound caused by turbulent blood flow in a vessel

bulimia nervosa (bū-LĬM-ē-ă nĕr-VŌ-să): physical and psychiatric disorder that involves a combination of obsessively eating huge quantities of food with purging behaviors

bulla (BŬ-lă): large blister or skin vesicle filled with fluid

burn (bŭrn): type of thermal injury to the skin caused by a variety of heat sources; classified according to severity as first-degree (superficial), second-degree (partial-thickness), and third-degree (full-thickness)

bursitis (bŭr-SĪ-tĭs): condition of inflammation of the tiny fluid-filled sacs that act as cushions and provide lubrication to decrease friction and irritation between structures such as bones, tendons, muscles, and skin

C

callus (KĂ-lŭs): thickened, hardened, toughened area of skin caused by frequent or chronic pressure or friction

***Campylobacter* infection (kăm-pĭ-lō-BĂK-tĕr ĭn-FĔK-shŭn):** infection with *Campylobacter* organisms via contaminated food or water, resulting in intestinal illness

candidiasis (kăn-dĭ-DĪ-ă-sĭs): vaginal fungal infection caused by *Candida albicans*, with key Sx including itching, burning, and a thick, curdy discharge; also known as a vaginal *yeast infection*

carbuncle (KĂR-bŭng-kul): very large furuncle or cluster of connected furuncles

cardiac tamponade (KĂR-dē-ăk tăm-pŏn-ĀD): serious condition in which the heart becomes compressed from an excessive collection of fluid or blood between the pericardial membrane and the heart

cardiomyopathy (kăr-dē-ō-mī-ŎP-ă-thē): group of conditions in which the heart muscle has deteriorated and functions less effectively

carpal tunnel syndrome (KĂR-păl TŬN-ĕl SĬN-drōm): compression of the median nerve, causing pain or numbness in the wrist, hand, and fingers

cataract (KĂT-ă-răkt): cloudiness of the lens due to protein deposits as a result of aging, disease, or trauma, or as a side effect of tobacco use or certain medications

celiac disease (SĒ-lē-ăk dĭ-ZĒZ): disorder in which the lining of the small intestine is damaged due to dietary factors, resulting in impaired nutrient absorption

cellulitis (sĕl-ū-LĪ-tĭs): potentially serious bacterial skin infection marked by pain, redness, edema, warmth, and fever

central scotoma (SĔN-trăl skō-TŌ-mă): blind spot in the center of the visual field surrounded by an area of normal vision

cerebral concussion (sĕ-RĒ-brăl kŏn-KŬ-shŭn): vague term referring to a brief loss of consciousness or brief episode of disorientation or confusion following a head injury

cerebral contusion (sĕ-RĒ-brăl kŏn-TOO-zhŭn): bruising of brain tissue

cerebral palsy (CP) (sĕ-RĒ-brăl PAWL-zē): group of motor-impairment syndromes caused by lesions or abnormalities of the brain arising in the early stages of development

cerebrovascular accident (CVA) (sĕr-ĕ-brō-VĂS-kū-lăr AK-sə-dənt): damage or death of brain tissue caused by interruption of blood supply due to a clot or vessel rupture; also called *stroke* or *brain attack*

chalazion (kă-LĀ-zē-ōn): small benign cyst in the eyelid formed by the distention of a meibomian gland with secretions

chlamydia (klă-MĬD-ē-ă): the most common STI, a bacterial vaginal infection caused by *Chlamydia trachomatis*

cholecystitis (kō-lē-sĭs-TĪ-tĭs): inflammation of the gallbladder, usually secondary to the presence of gallstones

cholelithiasis (kō-lă-lĭ-THĪ-ăs-ĭs): condition in which gallstones are present in the gallbladder, liver, or biliary ducts

cholesteatoma (kō-lē-stē-ă-TŌ-mă): condition in which a cyst develops in the middle ear

chronic fatigue syndrome (CFS) (KRŎN-ĭk fă-TĒG SĬN-drōm): complex chronic disorder marked by severe fatigue unrelieved by rest, often worsened by mental or physical activity; sometimes called *chronic fatigue and immune dysfunction syndrome (CFIDS)*

chronic mucocutaneous candidiasis (CMC) (KRŎN-ĭk mū-kō-kū-TĀ-nē-ŭs kăn-dĭ-DĪ-ă-sĭs): group of disorders in which persistent or recurrent *Candida* fungal infections develop on the skin, nails, or mucous membranes

chronic obstructive pulmonary disease (COPD) (KRŎN-ĭk ŏb-STRŬK-tĭv PŬL-mō-nĕ-rē dĭ-ZĒZ): group of diseases in which alveolar air sacs are destroyed and chronic, severe SOB results

cirrhosis (sĭ-RŌ-sĭs): chronic liver disease characterized by scarring and loss of normal structure

claw toe (klaw tō): condition in which the metatarsophalangeal (MTP) joint flexes dorsally while the other joint or joints in the toe flex toward the sole

coal worker's pneumoconiosis (CWP) (KŌL WER-kerz nū-mō-kō-nē-Ō-sĭs): a type of pneumoconiosis caused by inhalation of coal dust; often called *black lung*

comedo (KŎ-mē-dō): blackhead

congenital hypothyroidism (kŏn-JĔN-ĭ-tăl hī-pō-THĪ-royd-ĭ-zum): congenital condition of thyroid hormone deficiency, characterized by arrested physical and mental development; formerly called *cretinism*

conjunctivitis (kŏn-jŭnk-tĭ-VĪ-tĭs): inflammation of the conjunctiva; also called *pinkeye*

contracture (kŏn-TRĂK-chūr): fibrosis of connective tissue which decreases the mobility of a joint

contusion (kŏn-TOO-zhŭn): discoloration of the skin; bruise

cor pulmonale (kor pŭl-mă-NĂL-ē): condition of right ventricular enlargement or dilation from increased right ventricular pressure; also called *pulmonary heart disease* or *right-sided heart failure*

corn (kōrn): small callus that develops on smooth, hairless skin surfaces, such as the backs of fingers or toes, in response to pressure and friction; hard corns typically develop on the sides of feet and tops of toes; soft corns usually develop between toes

coronary artery disease (CAD) (KOR-ō-nă-rē ĂR-tĕr-ē dĭ-ZĒZ): narrowing of the lumen of heart arteries due to arteriosclerosis and atherosclerosis

coryza (kŏ-RĪ-ză): acute inflammation of the nasal mucosa; the common cold

crackles (KRĂ-kuls): abnormal crackly lung sound—like the sound of Rice Krispies—heard with a stethoscope, caused by air passing over retained secretions or by the sudden opening of collapsed airways

crepitation (krĕp-ĭ-TĀ-shŭn): grating sound from broken bones, or a clicking or crackling sound from joints

Crohn disease (krōn dĭ-ZēZ): disorder involving inflammation and edema deep into the layers of the lining of any part of the GI tract

croup (croop): acute viral disease, usually in children, marked by a barking, "seal-like" cough and respiratory distress

cryptorchidism (krĭpt-ŎR-kĭd-ĭ-zum): failure of one or both testes to descend into the scrotum

Cushing syndrome (KOOSH-ĭng SĬN-drōm): disorder caused by hypersecretion of cortisol by the adrenal gland, resulting in altered fat distribution and muscle weakness; also called *hypercortisolism* and *hyperadrenalism*

cyst (sĭst): fluid- or solid-containing pouch in or under the skin

cystic fibrosis (SĬS-tĭk fī-BRŌ-sĭs): fatal genetic disease that causes frequent respiratory infections, increased airway secretions, and COPD in children

D

decubitus ulcer (dē-KŪ-bĭ-tŭs ŬL-sĕr): area of injury and tissue death caused by unrelieved pressure which impedes circulation in the skin and underlying tissues; also called *pressure ulcer* or *bedsore*

deep vein thrombosis (DVT) (dēp vān thrŏm-BŌ-sĭs): development of a blood clot in a deep vein, usually in the legs; also known as *thrombophlebitis*

delirium (dĕ-LĬR-ē-ŭm): acute, reversible state of agitated confusion, marked by disorientation, hallucinations, or delusions

dementia (dē-MĔN-shē-ă): progressive neurological disorder, with numerous causes, in which an individual suffers an irreversible decline in cognition due to disease or brain damage; sometimes called *senility*

depression (dē-PRĔSH-ŭn): mood disorder marked by loss of interest or pleasure in living

deviated septum (DĒ-vē-ā-tĕd SĔP-tŭm): condition in which the nasal septum is displaced to the side, causing the two nares (nasal passages) to be unequal

diabetes insipidus (dī-ă-BĒ-tēz ĭn-SĬP-ĭ-dŭs): disorder unrelated to diabetes mellitus, characterized by excessive output of dilute urine

diabetes mellitus (DM) (dī-ă-BĒ-tēz mĕl-Ī-tŭs): chronic metabolic disorder in which the pancreas secretes insufficient amounts of insulin or the body is insulin resistant

diabetic ketoacidosis (dī-ă-BĔT-ĭk kē-tō-ă-sĭ-DŌ-sĭs): condition of severe hyperglycemia

diabetic nephropathy (dī-ă-BĔT-ĭk nĕ-FRŎP-ă-thē): kidney disease associated with diabetes that results in inflammation, degeneration, and sclerosis of the kidneys

diabetic retinopathy (dī-ă-BĔT-ĭk rĕt-ĭn-ŎP-ă-thē): progressive damage to microscopic vessels and other structures of the retina in patients with longstanding diabetes mellitus, which may result in blindness

dislocation (dĭs-lō-KĀ-shŭn): displacement or separation of a bone from its normal position where it articulates with another bone

disseminated intravascular coagulation (DIC) (dĭ-SEM-ĭ-nāt-ĕd ĭn-tră-VĂS-kū-lăr kō-ăg-ū-LĀ-shŭn): serious condition that arises as a complication of another disorder, in which widespread, unrestricted microvascular blood clotting occurs; primary symptom is hemorrhage

diuresis (dī-ū-RĒ-sĭs): abnormal secretion of large amounts of urine

diverticulitis (dī-vĕr-tĭk-ū-LĪ-tĭs): inflammation of one or more diverticula (tiny pouches in the intestinal wall)

diverticulosis (dī-vĕr-tĭk-ū-LŌ-sĭs): condition in which diverticula form in the intestinal wall due to increased pressure

dwarfism (DWĂRF-i-zum): hyposecretion of growth hormone during childhood, resulting in an abnormally small adult

dysmenorrhea (dĭs-mĕn-ō-RĒ-ă): pain in the lower abdominopelvic area and other discomfort associated with menses

E

***E. coli* O157:H7 infection (ē KŌ-lī ĭn-FĔK-shŭn):** dangerous strain of *Escherichia coli* that produces toxins which can severely damage the intestinal lining, resulting in bloody diarrhea

ecchymosis (ĕ-kĭ-MŌ-sĭs): discoloration of the skin; bruise

eclampsia (ĕ-KLĂMP-sē-ă): complication of pregnancy characterized by severe hypertension, seizures, and possible coma

ectopic pregnancy (ĕk-TŎ-pĭk PRĔG-năn-sē): implantation of a fertilized ovum somewhere other than in the uterus, often in the fallopian tube; also called *tubal pregnancy*

ectropion (ĕk-TRŌ-pē-ŏn): condition in which the lower eyelid is turned outward and droops more with aging

eczema (ĔK-zĕ-mă): inflammatory skin condition marked by red, hot, dry, scaly, cracked, and itchy skin

embolus (ĔM-bō-lŭs): undissolved matter floating in blood or lymph fluid that may cause an occlusion and infarct

emesis (ĔM-ĕ-sĭs): vomiting

emphysema (ĕm-fĭ-SĒ-mă): disorder marked by abnormal increase in the size of air spaces distal to the terminal bronchiole and destruction of the alveolar walls, resulting in loss of normal elasticity and progressive dyspnea

empyema (ĕm-pī-Ē-mă): collection of infected fluid (pus) between the two pleural membranes which line the lungs

encephalitis (ĕn-sĕf-ă-LĪ-tĭs): inflammation of the brain; often combined with meningitis and then called *encephalomeningitis*

endocarditis (ĕn-dō-kăr-DĪ-tĭs): infection of the inner lining of the heart that may cause vegetations to form within one or more heart chambers or valves

endometriosis (ĕn-dō-mē-trē-Ō-sĭs): growth of endometrial tissue in abnormal sites in the lower abdominopelvic area

end-stage renal disease (ESRD) (END-stāj RĒ-năl dĭ-ZĒZ): final phase of kidney disease

entropion (ĕn-TRŌ-pē-ŏn): condition in which the eyelid edges are turned inward and rub against the surface of the eye, usually affecting the lower eyelid

enuresis (ĕn-ū-RĒ-sĭs): involuntary urination during sleep; also called *bedwetting*

epidermoid cyst (ĕ-pĭ-DĔR-moyd sĭst): small sac or pouch below the skin surface containing a thick, cheesy substance; appears pale white or yellow, but can be darker in dark-skinned people

epididymitis (ĕp-ĭ-dĭd-ĭ-MĪ-tĭs): acute or chronic inflammation or infection of the epididymis, a tubular structure on the posterior surface of the testicle

epidural hematoma (ĕp-ĭ-DŪR-ăl hē-mă-TŌ-mă): collection of blood between the dura mater and the skull

epilepsy (ĔP-ĭ-lĕp-sē): chronic disorder of the brain marked by recurrent seizures, which are repetitive abnormal electrical discharges within the brain

epistaxis (ĕp-ĭ-STĂK-sĭs): episode of bleeding from the nose; commonly known as a *nosebleed*

Epstein-Barr virus (EBV) (ĔP-stēn-BĂR VĪ-rŭs): acute infection which causes sore throat, fever, fatigue, and enlarged lymph nodes; also called *mononucleosis*

erectile dysfunction (ED) (ē-RĔK-tīl dĭs-FŬNK-shŭn): general term that describes a number of disorders, all of which impact the ability of a man to attain an erection adequate to achieve a satisfactory sexual experience; also called *impotence*

esophageal varices (ē-sŏf-ă-JĒ-ăl VĂR-ĭ-sēz): varicose veins of distal end of the esophagus

esophagitis (ē-sŏf-ă-JĪ-tĭs): inflammation of the lower esophageal lining

exophthalmos (ĕks-ŏf-THĂL-mōs): abnormal protrusion of the eyeballs

F

fibrillation (fĭ-brĭl-Ā-shŭn): quivering of heart muscle fibers instead of an effective heartbeat

fibrocystic breast disease (fī-brō-SĬS-tĭk brĕst dĭ-ZĒZ): presence of multiple lumps in the breast, consisting of fibrous tumors or fluid-filled cysts

fibromyalgia (fī-brō-mī-ĂL-jē-ă): chronic condition marked by pain in the muscles, tendons, ligaments, and soft tissues of the body

fissure (FĬ-shŭr): small, cracklike break in the skin

folliculitis (fō-lĭ-kū-LĪ-tĭs): inflammation of hair follicles, marked by rash with small red bumps, pustules, tenderness, and itching; common on the neck, axillae, and groin area

food poisoning (fūd POY-zun-ing): common term for a number of illnesses caused by eating food contaminated with bacterial or toxic organisms; sometimes called *dysentery*

fracture (FRĂK-chūr): condition in which a bone is broken or cracked

frequency (FRĒ-kwun-sē): need to urinate more often than normal

frostbite (FRŎST-bīt): injury that occurs when skin tissues are exposed to temperatures cold enough to cause them to freeze

furuncle (FŪR-ŭng-kul): infection of a hair follicle and nearby tissue, also called a *boil*; more invasive than folliculitis because it involves the sebaceous gland

G

ganglion cyst (GĂNG-glē-ŏn sĭst): condition in which one or more small, benign tumors filled with a thick, colorless, gelatinous substance develop over a joint or tendon, usually on the wrist or back of the hand; sometimes called a *Bible cyst*

gastritis (găs-TRĪ-tĭs): inflammation of the stomach's mucosal lining

gastroenteritis (găs-trō-ĕn-tĕr-Ī-tĭs): inflammation of the stomach and intestines; often referred to as the *stomach flu* (although influenza is not the cause)

gastroesophageal reflux disease (GERD) (găs-trō-ĕ-sŏf-ă-JĒ-ăl RĒ-flŭks dĭ-ZĒZ): backflow of acidic gastric contents into the esophagus, causing esophagitis

gestational diabetes (jĕs-TĀ-shŭn-ăl dī-ă-BĒ-tēz): development of type 2 diabetes mellitus that begins during pregnancy in a woman who did not have diabetes before becoming pregnant; due to insulin resistance and altered glucose metabolism

giantism (JĪ-ăn-tĭ-zum): type of hyperpituitarism that causes hypersecretion of growth hormone during childhood, resulting in an abnormally large adult

glaucoma (acute) [glaw-KŌ-mă (ă-KŪT)]: type of glaucoma in which a sudden blockage of aqueous-humor outflow causes a rapid increase in intraocular pressure; also called *closed-angle glaucoma*

glaucoma (chronic) [glaw-KŌ-mă (KRŎN-ĭk)]: type of glaucoma in which the aqueous humor drains too slowly, leading to increasing intraocular pressure; also called *primary open-angle glaucoma*

glomerulonephritis (acute) [glō-mĕr-ū-lō-nĕ-FRĪ-tĭs (ă-KŪT)]: type of nephritis (kidney infection) in which the glomeruli are the key structures affected; also called *acute nephritic syndrome*

glomerulonephritis (chronic) [glō-mĕr-ū-lō-nĕ-FRĪ-tĭs (KRŎN-ĭk)]: condition in which the glomeruli suffer gradual, progressive, destructive changes, with a resulting loss of kidney function; also called *chronic nephritis*

glucosuria (gloo-kō-SŪ-rē-ă): sugar in the urine

glycosuria (glī-kō-SŪ-rē-ă): sugar in the urine

goiter (GOY-tĕr): enlarged thyroid gland

gonorrhea (gŏn-ō-RĒ-ă): STI caused by *Neisseria gonorrhoeae* that results in inflammation of mucous membranes

gout (gowt): hereditary form of arthritis, characterized by uric acid accumulation in the joints, especially in the great toe

graft-versus-host-disease (GVHD) (grăft VĔR-sŭz hōst dĭ-ZĒZ): complication of bone-marrow transplantation in which lymphoid cells from donated tissue attack the recipient and cause damage to skin, liver, GI-tract, and other tissues

Graves disease (grāvz dĭ-ZĒZ): hyperthyroidism caused by an autoimmune response, which may cause exophthalmos

Guillain-Barré syndrome (GBS) (gē-YĂ-băr-RĀ SĬN-drōm): acute inflammatory disorder that causes rapidly progressing paralysis (which is usually temporary) and sometimes also sensory symptoms; also known as *acute inflammatory demyelinating polyneuropathy*

H

hallux rigidus (HĂL-ŭks rĭ-JĬD-ŭs): condition in which degenerative arthritis affects the metatarsophalangeal (MTP) joint at the base of the big toe, causing pain and stiffness

hallux valgus (HĂL-ŭks VĂL-gŭs): condition in which the big toe is improperly aligned, pointing laterally toward the second toe and creating a large bump on the inner edge of the foot at the base of the big toe; commonly called *bunion*

hammertoe (HĂM-ĕr-tō): condition in which the toe is bent downward at the proximal interphalangeal (PIP) joint

Hashimoto disease (hă-shē-MŌ-tō dĭ-ZĒZ): chronic, inflammatory condition that leads to the most common type of thyroiditis; also called *chronic lymphocytic thyroiditis*

heart failure (HF) (hărt FĀL-yĕr): inability of the heart to pump enough blood to meet the needs of the body, resulting in lung congestion and dyspnea; formerly called *congestive heart failure*

hemoptysis (hē-MŎP-tĭ-sĭs): coughing up blood from the respiratory tract

hemorrhoids (HĔM-ō-roydz): internal or external varicose veins of the anal area

hemothorax (hē-mō-THŌ-răks): condition in which blood or bloody fluid has collected within the intrapleural space, causing lung compression and respiratory distress

hepatitis (hĕp-ă-TĪ-tĭs): chronic inflammation of the liver, caused by one of several viruses (types A, B, C, D, or E)

herpes genitalis (HĔRP-ēs jĕn-ĭ-TĂL-ĭs): STI caused by herpes simplex virus type 2 that results in painful vesicles; commonly called *genital herpes*

hernia (HĔR-nē-ă): protrusion of a structure through the wall that normally contains it

herniated disk (HĔR-nē-ā-tĕd dĭsk): herniation of the soft center of an intervertebral disk

hiatal hernia (hī-Ā-tăl HĔR-nē-ă): protrusion of a portion of the stomach through the diaphragm into the chest cavity; also called *hiatus hernia*

hirsutism (HŬR-sūt-ĭ-zum): male pattern of body-hair development in females

histoplasmosis (hĭs-tō-plăz-MŌ-sĭs): systemic respiratory disease caused by *Histoplasma capsulatum*, a fungus found in soil contaminated with bird droppings

Hodgkin disease (HŎJ-kĭn dĭ-ZĒZ): type of lymphatic cancer; also called *lymphoma*

hordeolum (hor-DĒ-ō-lŭm): infection of a sebaceous gland of the eyelid; also called a *stye*

human papilloma virus (HŪ-măn păp-ĭ-LŌ-mă VĪ-rŭs): STI caused by the human papilloma virus that results in painless, cauliflower-like warts; a cause of cervical cancer in women

Huntington disease (HUN-ting-tun dĭ-ZĒZ): hereditary, progressive, degenerative nervous disorder that leads to bizarre, involuntary movements and dementia

hydronephrosis (hī-drō-nĕf-RŌ-sĭs): condition in which the renal pelvis and calyces become distended and dilated and begin to atrophy due to urine outflow obstruction

hyperaldosteronism (hī-pĕr-ăl-dō-STĔR-ōn-ĭ-zum): condition in which adrenal glands release excessive aldosterone; also called *Conn syndrome*

hypercapnia (hī-pĕr-KĂP-nē-ă): chronic retention of CO_2, causing symptoms of mental cloudiness and lethargy

hyperopia (hī-pĕr-Ō-pē-ă): vision defect in which parallel rays focus behind the retina as a result of flattening of the globe of the eye or of an error in refraction; commonly called *farsightedness*

hyperparathyroidism (hī-pĕr-păr-ă-THĪ-royd-ĭ-zum): condition in which the parathyroid glands produce an excessive amount of parathyroid hormone (PTH)

hypertension (hī-pĕr-TĔN-shŭn): blood pressure that is consistently higher than 140 systolic, 90 diastolic, or both

hypertensive retinopathy (hī-pĕr-TĔN-sĭv rĕt-ĭn-ŎP-ă-thē): destructive retinal changes caused by hypertension

hypoparathyroidism (hī-pō-păr-ă-THĪ-royd-ĭ-zum): condition in which the parathyroid glands are hypoactive and as a result the level of parathyroid hormones (PTH) is too low

hypoxia (hī-PŎKS-ē-ă): O_2 deficiency

I

idiopathic thrombocytopenic purpura (ITP) (ĭd-ē-ō-PĂTH-ĭk thrŏm-bō-sī-tō-PĒ-nĭk PŬR-pū-ră): disorder in which a deficiency of platelets results in abnormal blood clotting, marked by tiny purple bruises (purpura) that form under the skin

impetigo (ĭm-pĕ-TĪ-gō): bacterial skin infection marked by yellow to red weeping, crusted, or pustular lesions; common in children

impotence (ĬM-pŏ-tĕns): inability of a male to achieve or maintain erection

incision (ĭn-SĬ-zhŭn): surgical cut in the flesh

infertility (ĭn-fĕr-TIL-ĭ-tē): inability to achieve pregnancy after trying to conceive for a period of 1 year or more; may be primary, which is an inability to conceive a first child, or secondary, which is infertility in a woman who has previously conceived

influenza (ĭn-floo-ĔN-ză): common, contagious, acute viral respiratory illness; commonly called the *flu*

interstitial cystitis (ĭn-tĕr-STĬSH-ăl sĭs-TĪ-tĭs): chronic inflammatory condition of the bladder lining not caused by infection or other identified pathology

interstitial nephritis (ĭn-tĕr-STĬSH-ăl nĕf-RĪ-tĭs): pathological changes in renal tissue that destroy nephrons and impair kidney function

intussusception (ĭn-tŭ-sŭ-SĔP-shŭn): slipping or telescoping of a portion of the bowel into itself

irritable bowel syndrome (ĬR-ĭt-ă-bul BOW-ĕl SĬN-drōm): chronic condition characterized by alternating episodes of constipation and diarrhea

ischemia (ĭs-KĒ-mē-ă): temporary reduction in blood supply to a localized area of tissue

J

jaundice (JAWN-dĭs): condition marked by yellow staining of body tissues and fluids as a result of excessive levels of bilirubin in the blood

juvenile rheumatoid arthritis (JRA) (JŪ-vĕ-nīl ROO-mă-toyd ăr-THRĪ-tĭs): disorder similar to adult-onset RA, with earlier onset and more severe symptoms

K

keratitis (kĕr-ă-TĪ-tĭs): inflammation of the cornea, usually associated with decreased visual acuity, which may, if untreated, result in blindness

kyphosis (kī-FŌ-sĭs): abnormal increase in the curvature of the thoracic vertebrae, causing hunchback

L

labyrinthitis (lăb-ĭ-rĭn-THĪ-tĭs): inflammation of the labyrinth within the inner ear; also called *otitis interna*

laceration (lăs-ĕ-RĀ-shŭn): cut or tear in the flesh

laryngitis (lăr-ĭn-JĪ-tĭs): condition of inflammation of the larynx, evidenced by a temporary hoarseness or loss of the voice

legal blindness (LĒ-gul BLĪND-nis): loss in visual acuity that prevents a person from performing work requiring eyesight; defined as corrected visual acuity of 20/200 or less or a visual field of 20 degrees or less in the better eye

legionellosis (lē-jŭ-nĕ-LŌ-sĭs): bacterial lung infection caused by the bacterium *Legionella pneumophila*

lordosis (lor-DŌ-sĭs): abnormal increase in the curvature of the lumbar vertebrae, causing swayback

Lyme disease (līm dĭ-ZĒZ): bacterial infection transmitted by ticks, marked by erythema migrans, a circular rash that slowly expands and enlarges; untreated disease causes multisystem symptoms

lymphosarcoma (lĭm-fō-săr-KŌ-mă): cancer of lymphatic tissue not related to Hodgkin disease

M

macular degeneration (MĂK-ū-lăr dĭ-jen-er-Ā-shŭn): macular deterioration resulting in central vision loss, categorized as either atrophic (dry) or exudative (wet)

macule (MĂ-kūl): flat, discolored spot on the skin, such as a freckle

malabsorption syndrome (măl-ăb-SŌRP-shŭn SĬN-drōm): inadequate absorption of nutrients from the intestinal tract, especially the small intestine

malignant hypertension (mă-LĬG-nănt hī-pĕr-TĔN-shŭn): rare, life-threatening type of hypertension evidenced by optic-nerve (eye) edema and extremely high systolic and diastolic blood pressure

malignant melanoma (mă-LĬG-nănt mĕ-lă-NŌ-mă): aggressive form of skin cancer that often begins as various-colored, asymmetrical lesions larger than 6 mm in size

mallet toe (măl-ĕt tō): condition in which the toe is bent downward at the distal interphalangeal (DIP) joint

malnutrition (măl-nū-TRĬ-shŭn): nutritional deficiency due to inadequate intake or absorption of protein, vitamins, minerals, or other vital nutrients

medial tibial syndrome (MĒ-dē-ăl TĬB-ē-ăl SĬN-drōm): painful condition involving tiny tears in the muscles and tendons that attach to the anterior tibia (shin); commonly called *shin splints*

melasma (mĕ-LĂZ-mă): development of irregular areas of darker-pigmented skin on the forehead, nose, cheek, and upper lip; also called *chloasma* or the *mask of pregnancy*

Ménière disease (mān-ē-ĀR dĭ-ZĒZ): chronic, noncontagious disorder of the labyrinth that leads to progressive hearing loss, vertigo, and tinnitus

meningitis (mĕn-ĭn-JĪT-ĭs): infection and inflammation of the meninges, the spinal cord, and CSF, usually caused by an infectious illness; often combined with encephalitis and then called *encephalomeningitis*

meniscal tear (mĕn-ĬS-kăl tār): tear of one of the two C-shaped cartilage structures that serve to cushion and stabilize the knee joint, usually caused by a twisting force

migraine headache (MĪ-grān HED-āk): familial disorder marked by episodes of severe throbbing headache that is commonly unilateral and sometimes disabling

mitral regurgitation (MĪ-trăl rē-gŭr-jĭ-TĀ-shŭn): condition in which the mitral valve does not close tightly, allowing blood to flow backward into the left atrium; also called *mitral insufficiency* or *mitral incompetence*

mitral stenosis (MĪ-trăl stĕ-NŌ-sĭs): condition in which the mitral valve fails to open properly, thereby impeding normal blood flow and increasing pressure within the left atrium and lungs

multiple sclerosis (MS) (MŬL-tĭ-pul sklĕ-RŌ-sĭs): disease involving progressive myelin degeneration, which results in loss of muscle strength and coordination

murmur (MŬR-mŭr): blowing or swishing sound in the heart, due to turbulent blood flow or backflow through a leaky valve

muscular dystrophy (MD) (MŬS-kū-lăr DĬS-trō-fē): hereditary, progressive, terminal disease that causes muscle atrophy and death, usually by age 20

myasthenia gravis (mī-ăs-THĒ-nē-ă GRĂV-ĭs): autoimmune motor disorder that causes progressive muscle fatigue and weakness

myocardial infarction (MI) (mī-ō-KĂR-dē-ăl ĭn-FĂRK-shŭn): death of heart-muscle cells due to occlusion of a vessel; commonly called *heart attack*

myocarditis (mī-ō-kăr-DĪ-tĭs): condition in which the middle layer of the heart wall becomes inflamed

myopia (mī-Ō-pē-ă): error of refraction in which light rays focus in front of the retina, enabling the person to see distinctly for only a short distance; commonly called *nearsightedness*

myxedema (mĭks-ĕ-DĒ-mă): severe form of hypothyroidism that develops in the older child or adult, causing nonpitting edema in connective tissue

N

nasal polyps (NĀ-zul PŎL-ĭps): rounded tissue growths on the nasal or sinus mucosa

nephrotic syndrome (nĕ-FRŎT-ĭk SĬN-drōm): uncommon disorder marked by massive proteinuria, edema, hypoalbuminemia (low blood albumin), hyperlipidemia (high blood lipids), and hypercoagulability (high tendency to form blood clots)

neural tube defect (NUR-ul TŪB dē-fekt): incomplete closure of the spinal canal, which may allow protrusion of the spinal cord and meninges at birth, leading to paralysis; also known as *spina bifida*

neurogenic bladder (nū-rō-JĔN-ĭk BLĂD-ĕr): bladder dysfunction (retention, incontinence, or altered capacity) due to disease or injury of the central nervous system or certain peripheral nerves

nondiabetic hypoglycemia (nŏn-dī-ă-BĔT-ĭk hī-pō-glī-SĒ-mē-ă): condition in which a nondiabetic person experiences mild symptoms associated with low blood glucose

non-Hodgkin lymphoma (nŏn-HŎJ-kĭn lĭm-FŌ-mă): group of more than 30 types of malignancies of B and T lymphocytes

nystagmus (nĭs-TĂG-mŭs): involuntary back-and-forth or cyclical movements of the eyes

O

obstructive sleep apnea (OSA) (ŏb-STRŬK-tĭv slēp ăp-NĒ-ă): dysfunctional breathing that occurs when the upper airway is intermittently blocked during sleep

oral herpes (OR-ăl HĔR-pēz): vesicular eruption in or on the mouth caused by herpes virus; also called *herpes labialis* or *cold sore*

oral thrush (OR-ăl thrŭsh): infection of the skin or mucous membrane with any species of candida, but mainly *Candida albicans*; also called *candidiasis*

orchitis (or-KĪ-tĭs): acute or chronic condition of inflammation of one or both testicles, caused by (usually viral) infection

orthopnea (ōr-THŎP-nē-ă): labored breathing that occurs when lying flat and improves when sitting up

osteitis deformans (ăs-tē-ĪT-ŭs dē-FŌRM-ănz): chronic condition in which the process of bone destruction and regrowth occurs abnormally, causing weak, fragile, enlarged, and misshapen bones; also called *Paget disease*

osteoarthritis (ŏs-tē-ō-ăr-THRĪ-tĭs): condition of cartilage deterioration and joint inflammation marked by pain, stiffness, and decreased ROM, most commonly affecting synovial weight-bearing joints and vertebrae

osteomalacia (ŏs-tē-ō-măl-Ā-shē-ă): condition of softening and weakening of the bones; when it occurs in children, it is called *rickets*

osteomyelitis (ŏs-tē-ō-mī-ĕl-Ī-tĭs): acute or chronic infection within the bone, most commonly affecting the legs, arms, pelvis, and spine

osteoporosis (ŏs-tē-ō-pōr-Ō-sĭs): condition characterized by loss of bone mass throughout the skeleton

otitis externa (ō-TĪ-tĭs ĕks-TĔR-nă): acute inflammation or infection of the external auditory canal; also called *swimmer's ear*

otitis media (ō-TĪ-tĭs MĒ-dē-ă): inflammation or infection of the middle ear

otosclerosis (ō-tō-sklē-RŌ-sĭs): chronic progressive deafness caused by spongy bone formation around the oval window with resulting ankylosis of the stapes

ovarian cyst (ō-VĀ-rē-ăn sĭst): sac of fluid or semisolid mass that grows within the ovary

P

palsy (PAWL-zē): partial or complete loss of motor function resulting in paralysis

pancreatitis (păn-krē-ă-TĪ-tĭs): acute or chronic inflammation of the pancreas

panhypopituitarism (păn-hī-pō-pĭ-TŪ-ĭ-tăr-ĭ-zum): condition resulting from diminished secretion of pituitary hormones; also called *underactive pituitary gland*

papule (PĂP-ūl): small, raised spot or bump on the skin, such as a mole

Parkinson disease (PĂR-kĭn-sŏn dĭ-ZĒZ): progressive, degenerative disorder that results in tremors, gait changes, and occasionally dementia

paronychia (păr-ō-NĬK-ē-ă): acute or chronic infection of the margins of the finger- or toenail, marked by warmth, erythema, edema, pus, throbbing, pain, or tenderness; causes the nail to become discolored and thickened

pathological fracture (păth-ō-LŎJ-ĭk-ăl FRĂK-chūr): breaking of diseased, weakened bone from the stress of normal, everyday activities

pediculosis (pē-dĭk-ū-LŌ-sĭs): infestation of head, body, or pubic lice, marked by itching, the appearance of lice on the body, and eggs (nits) attached to hair shafts

pelvic inflammatory disease (PID) (PĔL-vĭk ĭn-FLĂ-mă-tōr-ē dĭ-ZĒZ): any acute or chronic infection of the female reproductive system, including the uterus, fallopian tubes, and ovaries

peptic ulcer (PĔP-tĭk ŬL-sĕr): inflamed lesion in the gastric or duodenal lining

pericarditis (pĕr-ĭ-kăr-DĪ-tĭs): acute or chronic condition in which the fibrous membrane surrounding the heart becomes inflamed

peripheral artery disease (PAD) (pĕr-ĬF-ĕr-ăl ĂR-tĕr-ē dĭ-ZĒZ): condition of partial or complete obstruction of the arms or legs; similar to peripheral vascular disease (PVD), which includes both arteries and veins

peripheral neuropathy (pĕr-ĬF-ĕr-ăl nū-RŎP-ă-thē): dysfunction of nerves that transmit information to and from the brain and spinal cord, characterized by pain, altered sensation, and muscle weakness

peritonitis (pĕr-ĭ-tō-NĪ-tĭs): inflammation of the organs and structures within the peritoneal cavity

pernicious anemia (pĕr-NĬSH-ŭs ă-NĒ-mē-ă): chronic form of megaloblastic anemia (producing many large, immature, dysfunctional RBCs), caused by a deficit in the absorption of vitamin B_{12}, that reduces the body's ability to produce sufficient numbers of healthy RBCs

petechiae (pē-TĒ-kē-ē): tiny red or purple hemorrhagic spots (singular *petechia*)

phagocytosis (făg-ō-sī-TŌ-sĭs): process in which specialized white blood cells (phagocytes) engulf and destroy microorganisms, foreign antigens, and cell debris

pharyngitis (făr-ĭn-JĪ-tĭs): inflammation of the pharynx; commonly called a *sore throat*

pheochromocytoma (fē-ō-krō-mō-sī-TŌ-mă): tumor of the adrenal medulla (central part of the adrenal gland), usually benign but sometimes causing fluctuation of stress hormones like adrenaline

phimosis (fī-MŌ-sĭs): stenosis or narrowing of the foreskin opening of the penis

photophobia (fō-tō-FŌ-bē-ă): excessive sensitivity to light

pituitary dwarfism (pĭ-TŪ-ĭ-tār-ē DWĂRF-ĭ-zum): type of hypopituitarism in which reduced growth and development occur due to deficiency of growth hormone in childhood

placenta previa (plă-SĔN-tă PRĒ-vē-ă): implantation of the placenta in the lower uterine segment rather than the central or upper portion of the uterine wall, which may cause maternal hemorrhage during labor

plantar fasciitis (PLĂN-tăr făs-ē-Ī-tĭs): painful condition of the supporting structures of the arch of the foot, primarily the plantar fascia, a band of tissue that connects the heel with the toes

pleural effusion (PLOO-răl ĕ-FŪ-zhŭn): excess collection of fluid in the intrapleural space

pleurisy (PLOO-rĭs-ē): condition in which the pleurae become inflamed, causing sharp inspiratory chest pain; also called *pleuritis*

pneumoconiosis (nū-mō-kō-nē-Ō-sĭs): any disease of the respiratory tract caused by chronic or repetitive inhalation of dust particles

pneumonia (nū-MŌ-nē-ă): bacterial or viral infection of the lungs

pneumothorax (nū-mō-THŌ-răks): condition in which air collects in the intrapleural space; categorized as open, closed, spontaneous, or tension, and commonly called *collapsed lung*

poliomyelitis (pōl-ē-ō-mī-ĕl-Ī-tĭs): inflammation of the spinal cord, caused by a virus, which may result in spinal and muscular deformity and paralysis

polycystic kidney disease (PKD) (pŏl-ē-SĬS-tĭk KĬD-nē dĭ-ZĒZ): group of hereditary, progressive disorders in which cysts (small sacs of fluid) form in the kidneys, eventually destroying them

polycythemia vera (pŏl-ē-sī-THĒ-mē-ă VĔ-ră): chronic disorder marked by increased number and mass of all bone marrow cells, especially RBCs, with increased blood viscosity and a tendency to develop blood clots

polydipsia (pŏl-ē-DĬP-sē-ă): much (increased) thirst

polymyositis (PM) (pŏl-ē-mī-ō-SĪ-tĭs): disorder that causes the slow onset of muscle weakness and pain in the muscles of the trunk and progresses to affect muscles of the neck, shoulders, back, hip, and possibly hands and fingers

polyphagia (pŏl-ē-FĀ-jē-ă): much (increased) appetite

polyuria (pŏl-ē-Ū-rē-ă): much (increased) urination

precocious puberty (prē-KŌ-shŭs PŪ-bĕr-tē): premature onset of puberty with the appearance of secondary sex characteristics in young children

premenstrual syndrome (prē-MĔN-stroo-ăl SĬN-drōm): range of symptoms occurring 7 to 14 days before menstruation, including fluid retention, bloating, temporary weight gain, breast tenderness, headaches, depression, irritability, diarrhea, constipation, and appetite changes

presbycusis (prĕz-bĭ-KŪ-sĭs): progressive loss of hearing with aging

presbyopia (prĕz-bē-Ō-pē-ă): permanent loss of accommodation of the lens of the eye that occurs as people enter their 40s, causing a marked inability to maintain focus on near objects

prostatitis (prŏs-tă-TĪ-tĭs): acute or chronic inflammation of the prostate gland

pseudomembranous enterocolitis (soo-dō-MĔM-brān-ŭs ĕn-tĕr-ō-kō-LĪ-tĭs): inflammatory condition of both small and large bowels that results in severe watery diarrhea; also commonly called *C. diff. colitis*

psoriasis (sō-RĪ-ă-sĭs): chronic, inflammatory skin disorder marked by the development of silvery-white scaly plaques or patches with sharply defined borders and reddened skin beneath

pulmonary embolism (PE) (PŬL-mō-nĕ-rē ĔM-bō-lĭ-zum): sudden obstruction of a pulmonary blood vessel by debris, blood clots, or other matter

pulmonary tuberculosis (TB) (PŬL-mō-nĕ-rē tū-bĕr-kū-LŌ-sĭs): contagious infection caused by the *Mycobacterium tuberculosis* organism, primarily affecting the lungs but sometimes also spreading to and affecting other organ systems

puncture (PŬNGK-chūr): hole or wound made by a sharp, pointed instrument

pustule (PŬS-tūl): small, pus-filled blister

pyelonephritis (pī-ĕ-lō-nĕ-FRĪ-tĭs): inflammation and infection caused by bacterial growth in the renal pelvis and kidney

R

Raynaud disease (rĕ-NŌ dĭ-ZĒZ): disorder that affects blood vessels in the fingers, toes, ears, and nose, marked by vessel constriction and reduced blood flow in response to triggers such as cold temperature

renal calculus (RĒ-năl KĂL-kū-lŭs): small stone, composed of mineral salts, that may obstruct portions of the kidneys or a ureter; also called *kidney stone*

renal colic (RĒ-năl KŎL-ĭk): severe, intermittent pain caused by spasms of the ureter

renal failure (RĒ-năl FĀL-yĕr): acute or chronic failure of the kidneys to effectively eliminate fluids or wastes from the body

retinal detachment (RĔT-ĭ-năl dĭ-TACH-mŭnt): separation of the inner sensory layer of the retina from the outer pigment layer, caused by a break in the inner layer that permits vitreous fluid to leak under the retina and lift off its innermost layer; may cause blindness

retinopathy (rĕt-ĭn-ŎP-ă-thē): disease of the retina, often caused by diabetes

Reye syndrome (rī SĬN-drōm): serious disease associated with aspirin use by children with viral illnesses, which may result in permanent brain damage or even death

rheumatic heart disease (roo-MĂT-ĭk hărt dĭ-ZĒZ): complication of rheumatic fever in which inflammation and damage occur to parts of the heart, usually the valves

rheumatoid arthritis (RA) (ROO-mă-toyd ăr-THRĪ-tĭs): autoimmune arthritis that causes progressive joint pain and deformity and may affect organ systems

rhonchi (RŎNG-kī): coarse, gurgling sound heard in the lungs with a stethoscope, caused by secretions in the air passages

rosacea (rō-ZĀ-sē-ă): chronic condition that causes flushing and redness of the face, neck, and chest

rotator cuff tear (rō-TĀ-tōr kŭf tār): traumatic rip of one or more of the muscles or tendons within the rotator cuff of the shoulder

S

salmonellosis (săl-mō-nĕ-LŌ-sĭs): intestinal infection caused by various types of salmonella organisms

scabies (SKĀ-bēz): contagious skin disease transmitted by the itch mite, with symptoms of itching, scaly papules, insect burrows, and secondary infected lesions most prevalent in skin folds at the wrists and elbows, between the fingers, under the arms, in the groin, and under the beltline

scales (skālz): area of skin that is excessively dry and flaky

sciatica (sī-ĂT-ĭ-kă): pain, numbness, weakness, or tingling that is felt from the lower back along the pathway of the sciatic nerve into the legs

scleroderma (sklĕr-ă-DĔR-mă): group of chronic autoimmune diseases that cause inflammatory and fibrotic changes to skin, muscles, joints, tendons, cartilage, and other connective tissues

scoliosis (sko-lē-Ō-sĭs): abnormal S-shaped lateral curvature of the vertebrae

sebaceous cyst (sē-BĀ-shŭs sĭst): small sac or pouch below the skin surface filled with a thick fluid or semisolid oily substance called *sebum*

seborrheic keratosis (sĕ-bō-RĒ-ĭk kĕr-ă-TŌ-sĭs): benign, flat, irregularly shaped skin growths of various colors with a warty, waxy, "stuck-on" appearance

shingles (SHĬNG-gulz): unilateral painful vesicles occurring on the upper body, caused by the herpes zoster virus

shock (shŏk): syndrome of inadequate perfusion (circulation of blood, nutrients, and oxygen through tissues and organs) as a result of hypotension

short bowel syndrome (shōrt BOW-ĕl SĬN-drōm): malabsorption and malnutrition disorder created by the loss of a significant portion of functioning bowel

silicosis (sĭl-ĭ-KŌ-sĭs): respiratory disease caused by chronic or repetitive inhalation of silica (quartz) dust

sinusitis (sī-nŭs-Ī-tĭs): inflammation of the lining of the sinus cavities

Sjögren syndrome (SS) (SHŌ-grĕn SĬN-drōm): autoimmune disorder that causes dysfunction of salivary glands in the mouth and lacrimal glands in the eyes, and affects other areas of the body

small bowel obstruction (SBO) (smăl BOW-ĕl ŏb-STRŬK-shŭn): blockage of normal passage of intestinal contents

spina bifida (SPĪ-nă BĪ-fĭd-ă): incomplete closure of the spinal canal, which may result in protrusion of the spinal cord and meninges at birth and may cause paralysis; also called *neural tube defect*

spinal cord injury (SCI) (SPĪ-năl kord IN-jă-rē): traumatic bruising, crushing, or tearing of the spinal cord

spinal stenosis (SPĪ-năl stĕ-NŌ-sĭs): narrowing of an area of the spine that puts pressure on the spinal cord and spinal nerve roots

sprain (sprān): complete or incomplete tear in the ligaments around a joint

squamous cell carcinoma (SKWĀ-mŭs sĕl kăr-sĭ-NŌ-mă): type of cancer that usually appears in the mouth, esophagus, bronchi, lungs, or cervix, marked by a firm, red nodule or a scaly appearance; may ulcerate

sterility (stĕr-ĬL-ĭ-tē): inability to produce offspring

strabismus (stră-BĬZ-mŭs): deviation or misalignment of eyes that may adversely affect depth perception; types include *exotropia* (eyes turned outward), *esotropia* (eyes turned inward), *hypertropia* (eyes turned upward), and *hypotropia* (eyes turned downward)

strain (strān): trauma to a muscle and sometimes a tendon due to violent contraction or excessive forcible stretching

stress incontinence (strĕs ĭn-KŎNT-ĭn-ĕns): involuntary urine leakage upon physical stress, such as a cough or sneeze

stridor (STRĪ-dōr): high-pitched upper-airway sound heard without a stethoscope, indicating airway obstruction; a medical emergency

stroke (strōk): death of brain cells due to loss of blood supply; also known as *cerebrovascular accident* and *brain attack*

subdural hematoma (sub-DUR-ul hē-mă-TŌ-mă): collection of blood between the dura and the arachnoid (middle or second layer of the meninges)
syphilis (SĬF-ĭ-lĭs): multistage STI caused by the spirochete *Treponema pallidum*, with key Sx including skin lesions; eventually fatal unless treated
systemic lupus erythematosus (SLE) (sĭs-TĔM-ĭk LOO-pŭs ĕr-ĭ-thē-mă-TŌ-sŭs): chronic autoimmune disorder that causes inflammation and degeneration of various connective tissues in the body, such as the skin, lungs, heart, joints, kidneys, blood, or nervous system

T

tendinitis (tĕn-dĭn-Ī-tĭs): condition of inflammation of a tendon due to overuse
tension headache (TĔN-shŭn HED-āk): nonmigraine headache in which pain is felt in all or part of the head
testicular torsion (tĕs-TĬK-ū-lăr TŌR-shŭn): condition in which the testicles become twisted and the spermatic cord, blood vessels, nerves, and vas deferens become strangled
tetanus (TĔT-ă-nŭs): noncontagious illness marked by severe, prolonged spasm of skeletal muscle fibers; also known as *lockjaw*
thoracic outlet syndrome (TOS) (thō-RĂS-ĭk OWT-lĕt SĬN-drōm): group of painful disorders involving compression of the nerves or vessels in the neck and arms
thromboangiitis obliterans (TAO) (thrŏm-bō-ăn-jē-Ī-tĭs ŏb-LĬT-ĕr-ănz): type of vascular disease associated with tobacco use, marked by inflammation and clot formation within small vessels of the hands and feet, which may lead to gangrene and surgical amputation; sometimes called *Buerger disease*
thyrotoxicosis (thī-rō-tŏks-ĭ-KŌ-sĭs): severe episode of worsening symptoms of hyperthyroidism
tinea (TĬ-nē-ă): fungal skin disease occurring on various parts of the body, also called *dermatophytosis* or *ringworm*; forms include tinea capitis (scalp), tinea corporis (trunk), tinea cruris (genital area, also called *jock itch*), tinea nodosa (mustache and beard), tinea pedis (feet, also called *athlete's foot*), and tinea unguium (nails)
tinnitus (tĭn-Ī-tŭs): perception of ringing, buzzing, tinkling, or hissing sound in the ear
toxic shock syndrome (TSS) (TŎKS-ĭk shŏk SĬN-drōm): rare disorder caused by bacterial exotoxins; most commonly occurs in young women who use tampons
transfusion incompatibility reaction (trănz-FŪ-zhŭn ĭn-kŏm-păt-ĭ-BĬL-ĭ-tē rē-ĂK-shŭn): reaction of antibodies present in transfused blood to RBCs in the recipient's blood, or of antibodies in the recipient's blood to RBCs in the transfused blood
transient global amnesia (TGA) (TRĂNZ-ē-ĭnt GLŌ-băl ăm-NĒ-zē-ă): rare disorder, not caused by a neurological event or injury, that causes sudden, temporary loss of recent memory
transient ischemic attack (TIA) (TRĂNZ-ē-ĭnt ĭs-KĒ-mĭk ă-TĂK): temporary strokelike symptoms caused by a brief interruption of blood supply to a part of the brain
transplant rejection (TRĂNZ-plănt rē-JĔK-shŭn): identification of transplanted tissue as foreign by the recipient's immune system, which responds by attacking the tissue
trichomoniasis (trĭk-ō-mō-NĪ-ă-sĭs): STI infestation with *Trichomonas vaginalis* parasites; key Sx include vaginitis, urethritis, and cystitis
trigeminal neuralgia (TN) (trī-JĔM-ĭn-ăl nū-RĂL-jē-ă): neurological disorder that causes severe, episodic facial pain along the pathway of the fifth cranial (trigeminal) nerve; also called *tic douloureux*
tubular necrosis (TŪ-bū-lăr nĕ-KRŌ-sĭs): renal failure caused by acute injury to the renal tubules

U

ulcer (ŬL-sĕr): lesion of the skin or mucous membranes, marked by inflammation, necrosis, and sloughing of damaged tissues
ulcerative colitis (ŬL-sĕr-ā-tĭv kō-LĪ-tĭs): chronic inflammatory disease of the lining of the colon and rectum marked by up to 20 liquid, bloody stools per day
upper respiratory infection (URI) (Ŭ-pĕr rĕs-PĪR-ă-tō-rē ĭn-FĔK-shŭn): infection and inflammation of upper-airway structures, usually caused by a virus; often called the *common cold*
uremia (ū-RĒ-mē-ă): increased level of urea or other wastes in the blood
urgency (UR-jən-sē): need to urinate immediately
urinary retention (Ū-rĭ-nār-ē rĭ-TĔN-shŭn): inability to urinate
urinary tract infection (UTI) (Ū-rĭ-nār-ē trăkt ĭn-FĔK-shŭn): inflammation and infection caused

by bacterial growth in the urinary tract, usually the bladder

uterine fibroids (Ū-tĕr-ĭn FĪ-broyds): benign, smooth tumors made of muscle and fat; also called *leiomyomas*

uterine prolapse (Ū-tĕr-ĭn PRŌ-lăps): downward protrusion of the uterus into the vaginal opening

uveitis (ū-vē-Ī-tĭs): nonspecific term for any intraocular inflammatory disorder, which may affect the iris, ciliary body, choroid, or other parts of the eye

V

varicocele (VĂR-ĭ-kō-sēl): enlargement and dilation of the veins of the spermatic cord that drain the testis

varicose veins (VĂR-ĭ-kōs vānz): bulging, distended veins due to incompetent valves, most commonly in the legs

vertigo (VĔR-tĭ-gō): a feeling of spinning or moving in space

vesicle (VĔS-ĭ-kul): clear, fluid-filled blister

vitiligo (vĭt-ĭl-Ī-gō): chronic skin disease that results in patchy loss of skin pigment; may also affect hair color and cause white patches or streaks

volvulus (VŎL-vū-lŭs): twisting of the bowel upon itself, causing obstruction

W

wart (wōrt): small, benign skin tumor caused by various strains of the human papilloma virus (HPV); appearance varies from tiny to moderate-sized bumps or cauliflower-shaped growths

wheal (hwēl): rounded, temporary elevation in the skin, white in the center with a red-pink periphery and accompanied by itching

wheeze (hwēz): somewhat musical sound heard in the lungs, usually with a stethoscope, caused by partial airway obstruction (such as with asthma)

Wilm tumor (vĭlm TŪ-mor): rapidly growing type of kidney cancer that most commonly affects children; also known as nephroblastoma

APPENDIX C

GLOSSARY OF MEDICAL TERMS

PART I: MEDICAL TO ENGLISH

PREFIXES			
a-	without, not, absence of	hyper-	excessive, above
ab-	away from	hypo-	below, beneath
ad-	toward	in-	without, not, absence of; in, within, inner
ambi-	both, both sides, around, about	infra-	below, beneath
an-	without, not, absence of	inter-	between
anti-	against	intra-	in, within, inner
auto-	self	iso-	same, equal
bi-	two	macro-	large
brady-	slow	mal-	bad, inadequate
circum-	around	micro-	small
con-	together, with	mono-	one, single
contra-	against, opposite	multi-	many, much
di-	twice, two, double	neo-	new
dia-	through, across	oligo-	deficiency
dys-	bad, painful, difficult	pan-	all
ec-	out, outside	para-	beside, near
ecto-	out, outside	peri-	beside, near
en-	in, within, inner	poly-	much, many
end-	in, within, inner	post-	after, following
endo-	in, within, inner	pre-	before
epi-	above, upon	pro-	before, forward
eso-	inward	quadri-	four
eu-	good, normal	re-	behind, back
ex-	away from, outside, external	retro-	behind, back
exo-	away from, outside, external	semi-	half
extra-	away from, outside, external	sub-	below, beneath
hemi-	half	super-	excessive, above

Continued

PREFIXES—cont'd			
supra-	excessive, above	trans-	through, across
tachy-	rapid	tri-	three
tetra-	four	ultra-	beyond
tox-	toxin, poison	uni-	one, single

SUFFIXES			
-ac	pertaining to	-emia	a condition of the blood
-acusia	hearing	-esthesia	sensation
-acusis	hearing	-gen	creating, producing
-al	pertaining to	-genesis	creating, producing
-algesia	pain	-genic	creating, producing
-algesic	pain	-genous	creating, producing
-algia	pain	-gram	record
-ar	pertaining to	-graph	recording instrument
-ary	pertaining to	-graphy	process of recording
-cele	hernia	-gravida	pregnant woman
-centesis	surgical puncture	-ia	condition
-cidal	destroying, killing	-ial	pertaining to
-cide	destroying, killing	-iasis	pathological condition or state
-clasis	to break	-iatrics	field of medicine
-clast	to break	-iatrist	specialist
-constriction	narrowing	-iatry	field of medicine
-cusis	hearing	-ic	pertaining to
-cyte	cell	-ical	pertaining to
-cytic	cell	-ician	specialist
-cytosis	a condition of cells	-ism	condition
-derma	skin	-ist	specialist
-desis	surgical fixation of bone or joint, binding, tying together	-itis	inflammation
-dilation	widening, stretching, expanding	-kinesia	movement
-dipsia	thirst	-kinesis	movement
-dynia	pain	-lepsy	seizure
-eal	pertaining to	-leptic	seizure
-ectasis	dilation, expansion	-lith	stone
-ectomy	excision, surgical removal	-logist	specialist in the study of
-edema	swelling	-logy	study of
-emesis	vomiting	-lysis	destruction

SUFFIXES—cont'd

-malacia	softening	-plastic	pertaining to formation or growth
-megaly	enlargement	-plasty	surgical repair
-meter	measuring instrument	-plegia	paralysis
-metry	measurement	-plegic	pertaining to paralysis
-necrosis	tissue death	-pnea	breathing
-oid	resembling	-prandial	meal
-ole	small	-ptosis	drooping, prolapse
-ologist	specialist in the study of	-rrhage	bursting forth
-ology	study of	-rrhagia	bursting forth
-oma	tumor	-rrhaphy	suture, suturing
-opia	vision, view of	-rrhea	flow, discharge
-opsia	vision, view of	-rrhexis	rupture
-opsis	vision, view of	-salpinx	uterine (fallopian) tube
-opsy	vision, view of	-sclerosis	abnormal condition of hardening
-ory	pertaining to	-scope	viewing instrument
-osis	abnormal condition	-scopy	visual examination
-osmia	smell, odor	-spasm	sudden involuntary contraction
-ous	pertaining to	-stasis	cessation, stopping
-oxia	oxygen	-static	not in motion, at rest
-paresis	slight or partial paralysis	-stenosis	narrowing, stricture
-partum	childbirth, labor	-stomy	mouthlike opening
-pathy	disease	-therapy	treatment
-pause	cessation, stopping	-thorax	chest
-penia	deficiency	-tic	pertaining to
-pepsia	digestion	-tocia	childbirth, labor
-pexy	surgical fixation	-tome	cutting instrument
-phage	eating, swallowing	-tomy	cutting into, incision
-phagia	eating, swallowing	-tous	pertaining to
-phasia	speech	-tripsy	crushing
-phobia	fear	-trophy	nourishment, growth
-phonia	voice	-ule	small
-phoria	feeling	-uresis	urination
-plasia	formation, growth	-uria	urine
-plasm	formation, growth		

COMBINING FORMS

acous/o	hearing	carcin/o	cancer
acr/o	extremities	cardi/o	heart
aden/o	gland	carp/o	carpus
adenoid/o	adenoid	cec/o	cecum
adip/o	fat	cephal/o	head
adren/o	adrenal gland	cerebell/o	cerebellum
adrenal/o	adrenal gland	cerebr/o	brain
aer/o	air	cervic/o	cervix, neck
albino/o	white	cheil/o	lip
alveol/o	alveoli	chol/e	bile, gall
amni/o	amnion (amniotic sac), amniotic fluid	cholangi/o	bile duct
an/o	anus	cholecyst/o	gallbladder
andr/o	male	choledoch/o	common bile duct
angi/o	vessel	chondr/o	cartilage
ankyl/o	stiff joint	chromat/o	color
anter/o	anterior	cirrh/o	yellow
anthrac/o	coal, coal dust	col/o	colon
aort/o	aorta	colon/o	colon
append/o	appendix	colp/o	vagina
appendic/o	appendix	coni/o	dust
arteri/o	artery	conjunctiv/o	conjunctiva
arthr/o	joint	coron/o	heart
articul/o	joint	corne/o	cornea
ather/o	thick, fatty	cost/o	ribs
atri/o	atria	crani/o	cranium
audi/o	hearing	crypt/o	hidden
azot/o	nitrogenous compounds	cutane/o	skin
bacteri/o	bacteria	cyan/o	blue
balan/o	glans penis	cyst/o	bladder
bil/i	bile	cyt/o	cell
blephar/o	eyelid	dacry/o	tear
bronch/o	bronchus	dent/o	teeth
bronchi/o	bronchus	derm/o	skin
bronchiol/o	bronchiole	dermat/o	skin
bucc/o	cheek	diaphragmat/o	diaphragm
burs/o	bursa, sac	dipl/o	double
calc/o	calcium	dist/o	distal

COMBINING FORMS—cont'd			
dors/o	dorsal	hyster/o	uterus
duoden/o	duodenum	idi/o	unknown, peculiar
electr/o	electricity	ile/o	ileum
embry/o	embryo	ili/o	ilium
encephal/o	brain	immun/o	immune
enter/o	small intestine	infer/o	inferior
epididym/o	epididymis	ir/o	iris
epiglott/o	epiglottis	irid/o	iris
episi/o	vulva	jejun/o	jejunum
erythem/o	red	kal/i	potassium
erythr/o	red	kerat/o	keratinized tissue, cornea
esophag/o	esophagus	keton/o	ketone bodies (acids and acetones)
eti/o	cause	kinesi/o	movement
fasci/o	fascia	kyph/o	hump
femor/o	femur	labi/o	lip
fet/o	fetus	lact/o	milk
fibul/o	fibula	lacrim/o	lacrimal gland
galact/o	milk	lamin/o	lamina
gangli/o	ganglion	lapar/o	abdomen, abdominal wall
gastr/o	stomach	laryng/o	larynx
gingiv/o	gums	later/o	lateral
gli/o	glue, gluelike	leuk/o	white
glomerul/o	glomerulus	lex/o	word, phrase
gloss/o	tongue	lingu/o	tongue
gluc/o	glucose, sugar, sweet	lip/o	fat
glucos/o	glucose, sugar, sweet	lith/o	stone
glyc/o	glucose, sugar, sweet	lob/o	lobe
glycos/o	glucose, sugar, sweet	lord/o	bent backward
gonad/o	gonads	lumb/o	lower back
gynec/o	woman, female	lymph/o	lymph
hem/o	blood	lymphaden/o	lymph gland
hemat/o	blood	lymphangi/o	lymphatic vessel
hepat/o	liver	lymphocyt/o	lymph cell
hidr/o	sweat	mamm/o	breast
home/o	same, unchanging	mast/o	breast
humer/o	humerus	meat/o	meatus, opening
hydr/o	water	medi/o	medial

Continued

COMBINING FORMS—cont'd			
melan/o	black	ovari/o	ovary
men/o	menses	ox/i	oxygen
mening/o	meninges	ox/o	oxygen
meningi/o	meninges	pancreat/o	pancreas
menisci/o	meniscus	parathyroid/o	parathyroid
metacarp/o	metacarpus	patell/o	patella
metatars/o	metatarsals	path/o	disease
metr/o	uterus	pelv/i	pelvis
morph/o	shape	pept/o	digestion
muc/o	mucus	perine/o	perineum
muscul/o	muscle	peritone/o	peritoneum
my/o	muscle	phac/o	lens
myc/o	fungus	phag/o	eating, swallowing
myel/o	spinal cord, bone marrow	phak/o	lens
myring/o	tympanic membrane	phalang/o	phalanges
narc/o	sleep, stupor	phall/i	penis
nas/o	nose	pharyng/o	pharynx
nat/o	birth	phas/o	speech
natr/o	sodium	phleb/o	vein
necr/o	dead	phon/o	sound, voice
nephr/o	kidney	pil/o	hair
neur/o	nerve	placent/o	placenta
noct/o	night	pleur/o	pleura
ocul/o	eye	pneum/o	lung, air
odont/o	teeth	pneumon/o	lung, air
olig/o	deficiency	poster/o	posterior
onych/o	nail	presby/o	old age
oophor/o	ovary	proct/o	rectum, anus
ophthalm/o	eye	prostat/o	prostate
optic/o	eye	proxim/o	proximal
or/o	mouth	psych/o	mind
orch/o	testis	pub/o	pubis
orchi/o	testis	pulmon/o	lung
orchid/o	testis	py/o	pus
orth/o	straight	pyel/o	renal pelvis
oste/o	bone	pylor/o	pylorus
ot/o	ear	radi/o	radius
ov/o	ovum	radicul/o	nerve root

COMBINING FORMS—cont'd			
rect/o	rectum	testicul/o	testis
ren/o	kidney	thalam/o	thalamus
retin/o	retina	thorac/o	thorax
rhin/o	nose	thromb/o	thrombus (clot)
rhytid/o	wrinkle	thym/o	thymus
sacr/o	sacrum	thyr/o	thyroid
salping/o	tube (fallopian or eustachian)	thyroid/o	thyroid
scler/o	hardening, sclera	tibi/o	tibia
scoli/o	crooked, bent	tonsill/o	tonsil
seb/o	sebum	ton/o	tension
semin/o	sperm	tox/o	toxin, poison
ser/o	serum	toxic/o	toxin, poison
sial/o	saliva, salivary gland	trache/o	trachea
sigmoid/o	sigmoid colon	trich/o	hair
sinus/o	sinus	tympan/o	tympanic membrane
son/o	sound	uln/o	ulna
sperm/o	sperm	ur/o	urine
spermat/o	sperm	ureter/o	ureter
spin/o	spine	urethr/o	urethra
spir/o	breathing	urin/o	urine
splen/o	spleen	uter/o	uterus
spondyl/o	vertebrae	vagin/o	vagina
steat/o	fat	valv/o	valve
stern/o	sternum	valvul/o	valve
sthen/o	strength	vas/o	vessel
stomat/o	mouth, mouthlike opening	vascul/o	blood vessel
super/o	superior	ven/o	vein
synov/o	synovial membrane	ventr/o	ventral
synovi/o	synovial membrane	ventricul/o	ventricle
tars/o	ankle (tarsal bones)	vertebr/o	vertebrae
ten/o	tendon	vesic/o	bladder
tend/o	tendon	vulv/o	vulva
tendin/o	tendon	xanth/o	yellow
test/o	testis	xer/o	dry

PART II: ENGLISH TO MEDICAL

Term	Prefix	Combining Form	Suffix
abdomen, abdominal wall		lapar/o	
abnormal condition			-osis
abnormal condition of hardening			-sclerosis
about	ambi-		
above	epi-, super-		
above	hyper-, supra-		
absence of	a-, an-, in-		
across	dia-, trans-		
adenoid		adenoid/o	
adrenal gland		adren/o, adrenal/o	
after	post-		
against	anti-, contra-		
air		aer/o, pneum/o, pneumon/o	
all	pan-		
alveoli		alveol/o	
amnion (amniotic sac)		amni/o	
amniotic fluid		amni/o	
ankle (tarsal bones)		tars/o	
anterior		anter/o	
anus		an/o, proct/o	
aorta		aort/o	
appendix		append/o, appendic/o	
around	ambi-, circum-		
artery		arteri/o	
at rest			-static
atria		atri/o	
away from	ab-, ex-, exo-, extra-		
back	re-, retro-		
bacteria		bacteri/o	
bad	dys-, mal-		
before	pre-, pro-		
behind	re-, retro-		
below	hypo-, sub-, infra-		
beneath	hypo-, sub-, infra-		
bent		scoli/o	

Term	Prefix	Combining Form	Suffix
bent backward		lord/o	
beside	para-, peri-		
between	inter-		
beyond	ultra-		
bile		bil/i, chol/e	
bile duct		cholangi/o	
binding			-desis
birth		nat/o	
black		melan/o	
bladder		cyst/o, vesic/o	
blood		hem/o, hemat/o	
blood vessel		vascul/o	
blue		cyan/o	
bone		oste/o	
bone marrow		myel/o	
both, both sides	ambi-		
brain		cerebr/o, encephal/o	
breast		mamm/o, mast/o	
breathing		spir/o	-pnea
bronchiole		bronchiol/o	
bronchus		bronch/o, bronchi/o	
bursa		burs/o	
bursting forth			-rrhage, -rrhagia
calcium		calc/o	
cancer		carcin/o	
carpus		carp/o	
cartilage		chondr/o	
cause		eti/o	
cecum		cec/o	
cell		cyt/o	-cyte, -cytic
cerebellum		cerebell/o	
cervix		cervic/o	
cessation			-pause, -stasis
cheek		bucc/o	
chest			-thorax
childbirth			-partum, -tocia

Continued

Term	Prefix	Combining Form	Suffix
coal, coal dust		anthrac/o	
colon		col/o, colon/o	
color		chromat/o	
common bile duct		choledoch/o	
condition			-ia, -ism
condition of cells			-cytosis
condition of the blood			-emia
conjunctiva		conjunctiv/o	
cornea		corne/o, kerat/o	
cranium		crani/o	
creating, producing			-gen, -genesis, -genic, -genous
crooked		scoli/o	
crushing			-tripsy
cutting instrument			-tome
cutting into			-tomy
dead		necr/o	
deficiency	oligo-	olig/o	-penia
destroying			-cidal, -cide
destruction			-lysis
diaphragm		diaphragmat/o	
difficult	dys-		
digestion		pept/o	-pepsia
dilation			-ectasis
discharge			-rrhea
disease		path/o	-pathy
distal		dist/o	
dorsal		dors/o	
double	di-	dipl/o	
drooping			-ptosis
dry		xer/o	
duodenum		duoden/o	
dust		coni/o	
ear		ot/o	
eating		phag/o	-phage, -phagia
electricity		electr/o	
embryo		embry/o	
enlargement			-megaly

Term	Prefix	Combining Form	Suffix
epididymis		epididym/o	
epiglottis		epiglott/o	
equal	iso-		
esophagus		esophag/o	
excessive	hyper-, super-, supra-		
excision			-ectomy
expanding			-dilation
expansion			-ectasis
external	ex-, exo-, extra-		
extremities		acr/o	
eye		ocul/o, ophthalm/o, optic/o	
eyelid		blephar/o	
fascia		fasci/o	
fat		adip/o, lip/o, steat/o	
fear			-phobia
feeling			-phoria
female		gynec/o	
femur		femor/o	
fetus		fet/o	
fibula		fibul/o	
field of medicine			-iatrics, -iatry
flow			-rrhea
following	post-		
formation			-plasia, -plasm
forward	pro-		
four	quadri-, tetra-		
fungus		myc/o	
gall		chol/e	
gallbladder		cholecyst/o	
ganglion		gangli/o	
gland		aden/o	
glans penis		balan/o	
glomerulus		glomerul/o	
glucose, sugar, sweet		gluc/o, glucos/o, glyc/o, glycos/o	
glue, gluelike		gli/o	
gonads		gonad/o	
good	eu-		

Continued

Term	Prefix	Combining Form	Suffix
growth			-plasia, -plasm, -trophy
gums		gingiv/o	
hair		pil/o, trich/o	
half	hemi-, semi-		
hardening		scler/o	
head		cephal/o	
hearing		acous/o, audi/o	-acusia, -acusis, -cusis
heart		cardi/o, coron/o	
hernia			-cele
hidden		crypt/o	
humerus		humer/o	
hump		kyph/o	
ileum		ile/o	
ilium		ili/o	
immune		immun/o	
in	en-, end-, endo-, in-, intra-		
inadequate	mal-		
incision			-tomy
inferior		infer/o	
inflammation			-itis
inner	en-, end-, endo-, in-, intra-		
inward	eso-		
iris		ir/o, irid/o	
jejunum		jejun/o	
joint		arthr/o, articul/o	
keratinized tissue		kerat/o	
ketone bodies (acids and acetones)		keton/o	
kidney		nephr/o, ren/o	
killing			-cidal, -cide
labor			-partum, -tocia
lacrimal gland		lacrim/o	
lamina		lamin/o	
large	macro-		
larynx		laryng/o	
lateral		later/o	

Term	Prefix	Combining Form	Suffix
lens		phac/o, phak/o	
lip		cheil/o, labi/o	
liver		hepat/o	
lobe		lob/o	
lower back		lumb/o	
lung		pneum/o, pneumon/o, pulmon/o	
lymph		lymph/o	
lymph cell		lymphocyt/o	
lymph gland		lymphaden/o	
lymphatic vessel		lymphangi/o	
male		andr/o	
many	multi-, poly-		
meal			-prandial
measurement			-metry
measuring instrument			-meter
meatus, opening		meat/o	
medial		medi/o	
meninges		mening/o, meningi/o	
meniscus		menisci/o	
menses		men/o	
metacarpus		metacarp/o	
metatarsals		metatars/o	
milk		galact/o, lact/o	
mind		psych/o	
mouth		or/o, stomat/o	
mouthlike opening		stomat/o	-stomy
movement		kinesi/o	-kinesia, -kinesis
much	multi-, poly-		
mucus		muc/o	
muscle		muscul/o, my/o	
nail		onych/o	
narrowing			-constriction, -stenosis
near	para-, peri-		
neck		cervic/o	
nerve		neur/o	
nerve root		radicul/o	
new	neo-		
night		noct/o	

Continued

Term	Prefix	Combining Form	Suffix
nitrogenous compounds		azot/o	
normal	eu-		
nose		nas/o, rhin/o	
not	a-, an-, in-		
not in motion			-static
nourishment			-trophy
odor			-osmia
old age		presby/o	
one	mono-, uni-		
opposite	contra-		
out	ec-, ecto-		
outside	ec-, ecto-, ex-, exo-, extra-		
ovary		oophor/o, ovari/o	
ovum		ov/o	
oxygen		ox/i, ox/o	-oxia
pain			-algesia, -algesic, -algia, -dynia
painful	dys-		
pancreas		pancreat/o	
paralysis			-plegia
parathyroid		parathyroid/o	
patella		patell/o	
pathological condition or state			-iasis
peculiar		idi/o	
pelvis		pelv/i	
penis		phall/i	
perineum		perine/o	
peritoneum		peritone/o	
pertaining to			-ac, -al, -ar, -ary, -eal, -ial, -ic, -ical, -ory, -ous, -tic, -tous
pertaining to formation or growth			-plastic
pertaining to paralysis			-plegic
phalanges		phalang/o	
pharynx		pharyng/o	
phrase		lex/o	

Term	Prefix	Combining Form	Suffix
placenta		placent/o	
pleura		pleur/o	
poison, toxin	tox-	tox/o, toxic/o	
posterior		poster/o	
potassium		kal/i	
pregnant woman			-gravida
process of recording			-graphy
prolapse			-ptosis
prostate		prostat/o	
proximal		proxim/o	
pubis		pub/o	
pus		py/o	
pylorus		pylor/o	
radius		radi/o	
rapid	tachy-		
record			-gram
recording instrument			-graph
rectum		proct/o, rect/o	
red		erythem/o, erythr/o	
renal pelvis		pyel/o	
resembling			-oid
retina		retin/o	
ribs		cost/o	
rupture			-rrhexis
sac		burs/o	
sacrum		sacr/o	
saliva		sial/o	
salivary gland		sial/o	
same	iso-	home/o	
sclera		scler/o	
sebum		seb/o	
seizure			-lepsy, -leptic
self	auto-		
sensation			-esthesia
serum		ser/o	
shape		morph/o	
sigmoid colon		sigmoid/o	
single	mono-, uni-		

Continued

Term	Prefix	Combining Form	Suffix
sinus		sinus/o	
skin		cutane/o, derm/o, dermat/o	-derma
sleep		narc/o	
slight or partial paralysis			-paresis
slow	brady-		
small	micro-		-ole, -ule
small intestine		enter/o	
smell			-osmia
sodium		natr/o	
softening			-malacia
sound		phon/o, son/o	
specialist			-iatrist, -ician, -ist
specialist in the study of			-logist, -ologist
speech		phas/o	-phasia
sperm		semin/o, sperm/o, spermat/o	
spine		spin/o	
spinal cord		myel/o	
spleen		splen/o	
sternum		stern/o	
stiff joint		ankyl/o	
stomach		gastr/o	
stone		lith/o	-lith
stopping			-pause, -stasis
straight		orth/o	
strength		sthen/o	
stretching			-dilation
stricture			-stenosis
study of			-logy, -ology
stupor		narc/o	
sudden involuntary contraction			-spasm
sugar		gluc/o, glyc/o, glycos/o	
superior		super/o	
surgical fixation			-pexy
surgical fixation of bone or joint			-desis
surgical puncture			-centesis

Term	Prefix	Combining Form	Suffix
surgical removal			-ectomy
surgical repair			-plasty
suture, suturing			-rrhaphy
swallowing		phag/o	-phage, -phagia
sweat		hidr/o	
swelling			-edema
synovial membrane		synov/o, synovi/o	
tear		dacry/o	
teeth		dent/o, odont/o	
tendon		ten/o, tend/o, tendin/o	
tension		ton/o	
testis		orch/o, orchi/o, orchid/o, test/o, testicul/o	
thalamus		thalam/o	
thick, fatty		ather/o	
thirst			-dipsia
thorax		thorac/o	
three	tri-		
thrombus (clot)		thromb/o	
through	dia-, trans-		
thymus		thym/o	
thyroid		thyr/o, thyroid/o	
tibia		tibi/o	
tissue death			-necrosis
to break			-clasis, -clast
together	con-		
tongue		gloss/o, lingu/o	
tonsil		tonsill/o	
toward	ad-		
trachea		trache/o	
treatment			-therapy
tube (fallopian or eustachian)		salping/o	
tumor			-oma
twice	di-		
two	bi-, di-		
tying together			-desis

Continued

Term	Prefix	Combining Form	Suffix
tympanic membrane		myring/o, tympan/o	
ulna		uln/o	
unchanging		home/o	
unknown		idi/o	
upon	epi-		
ureter		ureter/o	
urethra		urethr/o	
urination			-uresis
urine		ur/o, urin/o	-uria
uterine (fallopian) tube			-salpinx
uterus		hyster/o, metr/o, uter/o	
vagina		colp/o, vagin/o	
valve		valv/o, valvul/o	
vein		phleb/o, ven/o	
ventral		ventr/o	
ventricle		ventricul/o	
vertebrae		spondyl/o, vertebr/o	
vessel		angi/o, vas/o	
view of			-opia, -opsia, -opsis, -opsy
viewing instrument			-scope
vision			-opia, -opsia, -opsis, -opsy
visual examination			-scopy
voice		phon/o	-phonia
vomiting			-emesis
vulva		episi/o, vulv/o	
water		hydr/o	
white		albin/o, leuk/o	
widening			-dilation
with	con-		
within	en-, end-, endo-, in-, intra-		
without	a-, an-, in-		
woman		gynec/o	
word		lex/o	
wrinkle		rhytid/o	
yellow		cirrh/o, xanth/o	

GLOSSARY OF DIAGNOSTIC TESTS AND PROCEDURES

APPENDIX

D

#

24-hour urine specimen: Total urine excreted over 24 hours, collected for analysis

A

angiography: Diagnostic or therapeutic radiography (radiological imaging) of the heart and blood vessels

arterial blood gases (ABGs): Measurement of O_2 and CO_2 levels and acid-base balance (pH balance) in arterial blood

arthrography: Radiological examination of a joint after injection of a contrast fluid into the joint space

audiometry: Detailed measurement of hearing with an audiometer

automated external defibrillator (AED): Small computer-driven defibrillator that analyzes the patient's rhythm, selects the appropriate energy level, charges the machine, and delivers a shock to the patient

automatic implanted cardioverter defibrillator (AICD): Very small defibrillator, surgically implanted in patients with a high risk for sudden cardiac death, that automatically detects and treats life-threatening arrhythmias

B

barium enema: Enema containing a substance that shows up clearly under x-ray and fluoroscopic examination

barium swallow: X-ray examination of the esophagus after the patient has swallowed a liquid that contains barium

bladder ultrasound (bladder scan): Noninvasive use of a portable ultrasound device to measure the amount of retained urine

blood urea nitrogen (BUN): Lab value used to measure kidney function, based on nitrogen levels in the blood

bone marrow aspiration: Removal of a bone marrow specimen from the cortex of a flat bone for analysis

bone scan: Use of a gamma camera to detect abnormalities in bone density after injection of radioactive material

Botox: Injection of a small amount of botulinum toxin into selected muscles of the face; interferes with muscle contraction, thereby reducing the appearance of wrinkles

bronchoscopy: Visual examination of the airways of the lungs

C

cardiac catheterization: Evaluation of the heart vessels and valves via the injection of dye that shows up under radiology

cardiopulmonary resuscitation (CPR): Emergency procedure that provides manual external cardiac compression and sometimes artificial respiration

cardioversion: Restoration of normal sinus rhythm (NSR) by chemical or electrical means

CD-4 lymphocyte count: Measurement of the number of specialized WBCs sometimes called *helper T cells*, used to identify whether a person's HIV infection is worsening

cerebrospinal fluid (CSF) analysis: Analysis of CSF for blood, bacteria, and other abnormalities

chemical peel: Application of a chemical solution to the skin to improve appearance by removing blemishes, fine wrinkles, uneven pigmentation, scars, and tattoos

chest x-ray (CXR): Radiologic picture of the lungs

cochlear implant: Surgical insertion into the cochlea of a device that receives sound and transmits signals to electrodes implanted within the cochlea, allowing hearing-impaired persons to perceive sound

color vision tests: Use of multicolored charts to evaluate the patient's ability to recognize color

computed tomography (CT) scan: Computerized collection and translation of multiple x-rays into a 3-dimensional picture, creating a more detailed and accurate image than traditional x-rays; study of the brain and spinal cord using radiology and computer analysis

corneal transplant (keratoplasty): Surgical replacement of a diseased cornea with a healthy one from a donor

coronary artery bypass graft (CABG): Surgical creation of an alternate route for blood flow around an area of coronary arterial obstruction

creatine kinase (CK): Test to measure isoenzyme released by skeletal and cardiac muscle into the blood when they are damaged

cryosurgery: Destruction of abnormal tissue by freezing

cryotherapy: Application of cold, such as with ice compresses, to decrease inflammation and pain

culture and sensitivity (C&S): Process of growing microorganisms, then exposing them to antimicrobial drugs to determine which ones kill them most effectively

cystoscopy: Visual examination of the bladder lining with a cystoscope

D

defibrillation: Delivery of an electric shock with the goal of ending ventricular fibrillation and restoring normal sinus rhythm

dermabrasion: Removal of small scars, nevi (moles), tattoos, or fine wrinkles with a wire brush or burr impregnated with diamond particles, leaving a smoother surface

dermaplaning: Removal of small scars, nevi (moles), tattoos, or fine wrinkles with a dermatome (a device resembling an electric razor), leaving a smoother surface

dilation and curettage (D&C): Dilation of the cervix followed by scraping of the endometrial lining

dual-energy x-ray absorptiometry (DXA): Radiological evaluation of bone density to detect osteoporosis

E

echocardiography: Ultrasound procedure used to detect cardiovascular disorders that allows visualization of the size, shape, position, thickness, and movement of all parts of the heart, as well as characteristics of blood flow through the heart

electrocardiography (ECG, EKG): Creation and study of graphic records (electrocardiograms) of electric currents originating in the heart

electroencephalography (EEG): Record of electrical activity of the brain on graph paper; study of electrical activity of the brain

electromyogram (EMG): Record of skeletal muscle electrical activity, used to diagnose neuromuscular disorders

endoscopic retrograde cholangiopancreatography (ERCP): Radiographic examination of vessels that connect the liver, gallbladder, and pancreas to the duodenum after a radiopaque material has been injected through a fiberoptic endoscope

enucleation: Surgical removal of the entire eyeball

enzyme immunosorbent assay (EIA): Rapid enzyme immunochemical method for identifying the presence of antigens, antibodies, or other substances in the blood, used as a primary diagnostic test for many infectious diseases including syphilis and HIV; formerly called *enzyme-linked immunosorbent assay (ELISA)*

erythrocyte sedimentation rate (ESR, sed rate): Test used in the diagnosis and monitoring of many diseases that cause acute or chronic inflammation; measures the rate at which red blood cells settle in plasma or saline located in a tube of unclotted blood; an elevated ESR indicates inflammation

event recorder: Portable monitoring device that transmits heart rhythms by telephone to a central laboratory where dysrhythmias can be detected and analyzed

exercise stress test: Noninvasive test that measures cardiac function during physical activity; also called *treadmill test* or *stress test*

extracorporeal shock wave lithotripsy: Procedure in which shock waves or sound waves crush stones in the kidneys or urinary tract

F

fasting blood glucose (FBG): Test of blood glucose levels after a fast of 8 to 12 hours, used to screen for diabetes; also called *fasting blood sugar (FBS)*

fecal occult blood test (Hemoccult): Test of fecal specimen for presence of hidden blood

finger stick blood sugar (fsbs): Test of blood glucose from a drop of capillary blood obtained by pricking the finger; also called *finger stick blood glucose (fsbg)*

G

gastroccult: Test of gastric contents for pH level and presence of blood

glucose tolerance test (GTT): Measurement of blood glucose levels at specified intervals after ingestion of glucose

glycosylated hemoglobin (Hb A1c): Reflection of the average blood glucose level over the past 3 to 4 months

H

***Helicobacter pylori* test:** Test that detects the presence of antibodies to *Helicobacter pylori*, the most common cause of gastric ulcers

Hemoccult (stool guaiac test): Small sample of feces tested for presence of blood

hemodialysis: Filtration of wastes and fluid from blood as it passes through selectively permeable membranes; also called *dialysis*

Holter monitor: Portable device worn by patient during normal activity that records heart rhythm for up to 24 hours

I

international normalized ratio (INR): Standardized method of checking the prothrombin time (PT); prothrombin is a blood-clotting factor that is used to monitor warfarin (Coumadin) therapy, and warfarin (Coumadin) is an anticoagulant medication that slows the clotting time of blood

intravenous pyelogram (IVP): X-ray examination of the kidneys, ureters, and bladder after injection of a contrast medium

K

KUB: Radiological imaging (x-ray) of the abdomen, specifically the kidneys, ureters, and bladder

L

laparoscopy: Exploration of abdominal contents with a laparoscope

laser-assisted in-situ keratomileusis (LASIK): Procedure in which a laser is used to alter the shape of the deep corneal layer after a top flap in the surface is opened

laser photocoagulation: Destruction of areas of the retina with a laser beam

laser resurfacing: Use of short pulses of light to remove fine lines and damaged skin, and to minimize scars and even out areas of uneven pigmentation; sometimes called a *laser peel*

liver function tests (LFTs): Tests, including aspartate aminotransferase (AST) and alanine aminotransferase (ALT), that determine the liver's ability to perform its many complex functions

lower endoscopy: Visual examination of the GI tract from rectum to cecum; variations include the colonoscopy, sigmoidoscopy, and proctoscopy

lower GI x-ray: X-ray of the large intestine after rectal instillation of barium sulfate

lumbar puncture (LP): Puncture of subarachnoid layer at the fourth intervertebral space to obtain CSF for analysis

M

magnetic resonance imaging (MRI): Use of an electromagnetic field and radio waves to create visual images on a computer screen

mammography: X-ray examination to detect breast cancer

Mantoux test: Intradermal injection of tuberculin purified protein derivative (PPD) just beneath the surface of the skin to identify whether the patient has been exposed to tuberculosis

metered dose inhaler (MDI): Handheld device used to deliver medication to the patient's lower airways

microdermabrasion: Similar to dermabrasion but less invasive, involving multiple treatments of gentle abrasion; useful in reducing fine lines, nevi (moles), age spots, and acne scars

monospot (heterophil): Quick test used to screen for the presence of the heterophil antibody that is present in individuals with Epstein-Barr virus infection

myelography: Radiography of the spinal cord and associated nerves after intrathecal injection (into the spinal canal) of a contrast medium

N

nebulizer: Device that produces a fine spray or mist to deliver medication to a patient's deep airways

needle biopsy: Aspiration of tissue or fluid through a large-gauge needle for analysis

P

pacemaker: Device that can trigger the mechanical contractions of the heart by emitting periodic electrical discharges

Papanicolaou smear: Removal of tissue cells from the cervix for analysis

partial thromboplastin time (PTT): Measure of blood-clotting time, used to monitor heparin therapy; heparin is an anticoagulant medication that slows the clotting time of blood

patch test: Test in which paper or gauze saturated with an allergen is applied to the skin beneath an occlusive dressing and the response is noted

pelvic sonography: Ultrasound imaging of the structures in the female pelvis

percutaneous transluminal coronary angioplasty (PTCA): Method of treating a narrowed coronary artery via inflation and deflation of a balloon on a double-lumen catheter inserted through the right femoral artery

peritoneal dialysis: Filtration of fluid and wastes from the blood using the lining of the patient's peritoneal cavity as a dialyzing membrane

phacoemulsification: Removal of the lens with an ultrasonic device to treat cataracts

pleurodesis: Infusion of a sterile, irritating substance into the pleural space, causing the pleural linings to fuse to one another by developing scar tissue

postural drainage: Placement of the patient in various positions that facilitate drainage of secretions from the lungs, often done along with chest physiotherapy (CPT)

prostate-specific antigen (PSA): Blood test used to screen for prostate cancer

prothrombin time (PT): Procedure that measures the clotting time of blood; used to assess levels of anticoagulation in patients taking warfarin (Coumadin)

pulmonary angiography: Radiographic examination of pulmonary circulation after injection of a contrast dye

pulmonary function tests (PFTs): Group of tests that provide information regarding lung capacity; sometimes called *spirometry*

pulse oximetry: Indirect measurement of arterial-blood O_2 saturation level, also known as the SpO_2; the normal level in a person with healthy lungs is 97% to 99%

R

radial keratotomy: Incision into the outer portion of the cornea to flatten it and help correct nearsightedness

radioactive iodine uptake: Nuclear medicine study that measures how rapidly radioactive iodine is taken up from the blood after oral or intravenous administration

refractive error test: Evaluation of the eye's ability to focus an image

rheumatoid factor: Blood test used to identify rheumatoid arthritis and other disorders

Rinne test: Hearing test that compares bone conduction to air conduction, using a tuning fork

S

scleral buckling: Placement of a band of silicone around the eyeball to stabilize a detached retina

scratch test: Test in which an allergen is placed on a scratched area of the skin and the response is noted

serum creatinine: Lab value used to measure kidney function that is more specific than BUN

slit-lamp microscopy: Examination of the posterior surface of the cornea with a slit lamp

sputum analysis: Examination of mucus or fluid coughed up from the lungs

stool culture: Examination of a fecal specimen for abnormal bacteria and other microorganisms

stress test: Treadmill test that can show if the blood supply is reduced in the arteries that supply the heart

T

thoracentesis: Surgical puncture of the chest wall to remove fluid from the interpleural space; also called *pleurocentesis*

thyroid function test: Reflection of thyroid function by measuring levels of thyroid-stimulating hormone (TSH), triiodothyronine (T3), and thyroxine (T4)

thyroid scan: Radiographic evaluation of the thyroid after a radioactive substance is injected; identifies thyroid size, shape, position, and function

thyroid-stimulating hormone (TSH): Measure of the ability of the thyroid gland to concentrate and retain circulating iodine for synthesis of thyroid hormone

tonometry: Measurement of intraocular pressure or tension to detect glaucoma

total hip replacement (THR): Procedure to replace an arthritic hip with a prosthetic device to restore mobility and function; also referred to as total hip arthroplasty

transcutaneous electrical nerve stimulation (TENS): Delivery of a mild electrical current to a painful area to disrupt transmission of pain signals between the body and brain

transesophageal echocardiography (TEE): Study of the heart via a probe placed in the esophagus

transurethral resection of the prostate (TURP): Removal of tissue from the prostate gland with an endoscope, via the urethra

troponin: Protein released into the body by damaged heart muscle, considered the most accurate blood test to confirm the diagnosis of an MI

tubal ligation: Sterilization procedure in which fallopian tubes are cut and ligated

tympanometry: Procedure for evaluation of the mobility and patency of the eardrum, detection of middle-ear disorders, and evaluation of the patency of the eustachian tube

tympanoplasty: Reconstruction of a perforated tympanic membrane

U

ultrasound: Test in which ultrahigh-frequency sound waves are used to outline the shapes of various body structures

upper endoscopy: Visual examination of the GI tract, from esophagus to duodenum

upper GI x-ray (UGI): X-ray that involves the use of a contrast medium to help visualize abdominal organs, including the stomach and esophagus

urinalysis (UA): Visual and microscopic analysis of a urine specimen

urinary catheterization: Insertion of a tube into the bladder via the urethra to drain urine, obtain a urine specimen, or instill medication

uterine ablation: Procedure that destroys the entire surface of the endometrium and superficial myometrium

V

vasectomy: Sterilization procedure in which a small section of the vas deferens is removed

viral load: Measurement of the number of copies of the human immunodeficiency virus in the blood, used to monitor progression of HIV infection and AIDS

visual acuity test: Examination that identifies the smallest letters, numbers, or objects that can be correctly identified on a standardized Snellen vision chart from 20 feet

vital capacity (VC): Measurement of the volume of air that can be exhaled after maximum inspiration

voiding cystourethrography (VCUG): Radiological examination of the bladder and urethra during urination

W

Weber test: Hearing test that evaluates bone conduction using a tuning fork

APPENDIX

E MEDICAL TERMINOLOGY FAQS

Question: ***How do I decide which word part to use when there is more than one to choose?***

Answer: ***It is often helpful to think of selecting the word part that is the most "user-friendly" to pronounce and that sounds best to the ear.***

Example: Create a term that means "pertaining to the neck."

Choosing a combining form is easy because there is only one, cervic/o, which means "neck." However, there are 12 suffixes that mean "pertaining to." These are listed below with the selected combining form. Try pronouncing each version of the new term listed below. The first one is the easiest to pronounce and sounds best to the ear.

cervical
cervicac
cervicar
cervicary
cerviceal
cervicial
cervicic
cervicical
cervicory
cervicous
cervicotic
cervicotous

Question: ***What if two options seem equally correct and desirable?***

Answer: ***Follow local custom.***

Example: Create a term that means "pain of the neck."

There are two possible options: cervicalgia and cervicodynia. Either one is technically correct, so use the one that conforms to local custom. If you are unsure, make your best guess. The worst that will happen is that someone may be amused at your choice of terms. As you converse with and listen to your fellow health-care professionals, you will quickly learn the preferred local terminology.

Question: ***When a term includes more than one combining form, how do I know what order to put them in?***

Answer: ***If the term refers to a procedure, place the word parts in the order that corresponds with the procedure. If the term pertains to anatomy, move from most proximal to most distal.***

Example: Create a term that means "visual examination of the esophagus, stomach, and duodenum."

As this procedure is performed, the scope first enters the esophagus, then the stomach, and then the duodenum. So when you create the medical term, put the word parts in the same order (with the suffix last): esophag/o, gastr/o, duoden/o, -scopy.

Question: ***I hear some terms pronounced in more than one way. How do I know which pronunciation is correct?***

Answer: ***First, refer to the pronunciation guide in this book. It should guide you in most cases. Second, in some cases more than one pronunciation may be considered acceptable. Third, remember that the most common mistake people make is to emphasize the wrong syllable. When word parts are linked with a combining vowel (usually o), the emphasis is usually on the syllable with the combining vowel.***

Example: The tendency is to pronounce colonoscopy as kō-lŏn-ō-SKŌ-pē. But the correct pronunciation is kō-lŏn-ŎS-kō-pē.

APPENDIX F

DRUGS AND DRUG CLASSIFICATIONS

There are several systems of drug classification. One is based on the body system that is most affected (e.g., respiratory drugs, cardiac drugs); another is based on the therapeutic action (e.g., antihypertensive, antacid); another is based on the chemical action of the drug (e.g., cholinergic, selective serotonin reuptake inhibitor). As the following table indicates, most drugs fall into several different classes.

This table contains a list of the most commonly prescribed medications in the United States. The first column lists the drugs alphabetically according to generic names, followed by the common trade names. The second column lists the drugs' therapeutic classifications, and the third column lists the most common uses of the drugs.

Generic Name (Trade Name)	Therapeutic Classification	Common Use
albuterol (Proventil)	Bronchodilator	Asthma, COPD
alendronate (Fosamax)	Bone resorption inhibitor	Prevention and treatment of osteoporosis
allopurinol (Zyloprim)	Antigout agent, antihyperuricemic	Chronic gout, hyperuricemia
alprazolam (Xanax)	Antianxiety	Anxiety, panic disorder
amantadine (Symmetrel)	Antiviral, antiparkinsonian agent	Parkinson disease, influenza A
amitriptyline (Elavil)	Tricyclic antidepressant	Major depression
amlodipine (Norvasc)	Antianginal, antihypertensive	Chronic stable angina, hypertension, vasospastic angina
amoxicillin (Amoxil)	Anti-infective, antiulcer	Various infections, prevention of bacterial endocarditis, *Helicobacter pylori* (ulcers)
amoxicillin, potassium clavulanate (Augmentin)	Anti-infective	Various infections
aripiprazole (Abilify)	Antipsychotic	Schizophrenia
atenolol (Tenormin)	Antianginal, antihypertensive	Hypertension, angina, prevention of MI
atomoxetine (Straterra)	Agents for attention deficit disorder	ADHD
atorvastatin (Lipitor)	Lipid-lowering agent	Hypercholesterolemia, mixed dyslipidemias, prevention of cardiovascular disease
azelastine (Astelin)	Nasal decongestant	Nasal congestion

Generic Name (Trade Name)	Therapeutic Classification	Common Use
azithromycin (Zithromax)	Anti-infective, atypical mycobacterium agent	Infection
calcitriol (Vitamin D)	Vitamin	Hypocalcemia, hyperparathyroidism
carbidopa, levodopa (Sinemet)	Antiparkinsonian agent	Parkinson disease
carisoprodol (Soma)	Central-acting skeletal muscle relaxant	Muscle spasms associated with acute, painful musculoskeletal disorders
celecoxib (Celebrex)	NSAID, antirheumatic	Rheumatoid arthritis, osteoarthritis, acute pain, dysmenorrhea, ankylosing spondylitis
cephalexin (Keflex)	Anti-infective	Various infections
cetirizine (Zyrtec)	Allergy, cold, and cough remedy, antihistamine	Allergy symptoms, chronic urticaria
ciprofloxacin (Cipro)	Anti-infective	Various infections
citalopram (Celexa)	Antidepressant	Major depressive disorder
clonazepam (Klonopin)	Anticonvulsant	Various types of seizures, panic disorder
clonidine (Catapres)	Antihypertensive	Hypertension, severe cancer pain
clopidogrel (Plavix)	Antiplatelet agent	Prevention of stroke, MI, TIA
conjugated estrogen (Premarin)	Hormone	Menopausal symptoms, estrogen deficiency, prevention of osteoporosis, primary ovarian failure
cyclobenzaprine (Flexeril)	Central-acting skeletal muscle relaxant	Muscle spasms associated with painful musculoskeletal conditions
diazepam (Valium)	Antianxiety, anticonvulsant, sedative-hypnotic, skeletal muscle relaxant	Anxiety, preoperative sedation, status epilepticus, skeletal muscle spasm, alcohol withdrawal
digoxin (Lanoxin)	Antiarrhythmic, inotropic	Atrial arrhythmias, heart failure
diltiazem (Cardizem)	Antiarrhythmic class IV	Hypertension, angina, atrial arrhythmias
docusate sodium (Colace)	Stool softener, laxative, emollient	Prevention or treatment of constipation
donepezil (Aricept)	Anti-Alzheimer agent	Mild to moderate Alzheimer dementia
doxycycline (Vibramycin)	Anti-infective	Various infections
duloxetine (Cymbalta)	Antidepressant	Major depressive disorder, diabetic neuropathic pain

Continued

Generic Name (Trade Name)	Therapeutic Classification	Common Use
enalapril (Vasotec)	Antihypertensive	Hypertension, heart failure
escitalopram (Lexapro)	Antidepressant	Major depressive disorder, general anxiety disorder
esomeprazole (Nexium)	Antiulcer	GERD, erosive esophagitis, duodenal ulcers
eszopiclone (Lunesta)	Sedative-hypnotic	Insomnia
ethinyl estradiol (Ortho Tri-Cyclen Lo)	Hormonal contraceptive	Prevention of pregnancy, regulation of menstrual cycle, acne, emergency contraception
ezetimibe (Zetia)	Lipid-lowering agent	Hypercholesterolemia
famotidine (Pepcid)	Antiulcer	GERD, ulcers
fenofibrate (Tricor)	Lipid-lowering agent	High cholesterol and triglycerides
fexofenadine (Allegra)	Antihistamine	Seasonal allergies, rhinitis, chronic idiopathic urticaria
fluconazole (Diflucan)	Antifungal	Various types of fungal infection
fluoxetine (Prozac)	Antidepressant	Depression, OCD, bulimia nervosa, panic disorder, premenstrual dysphoric disorder
fluticasone (Flonase)	Inhalant corticosteroid	Seasonal allergies, asthma
furosemide (Lasix)	Diuretic	Hypertension, edema caused by heart failure, hepatic impairment, or renal failure
gabapentin (Neurontin)	Anticonvulsant	Seizure disorders, neuropathic pain
glipizide (Glucotrol)	Antidiabetic	Type 2 diabetes
glyburide (Diabeta)	Oral antidiabetic	Type 2 diabetes
hydrochlorothiazide (Hydrodiuril)	Diuretic, antihypertensive	Edema, hypertension, diuresis, heart failure, edema
ibandronate sodium (Boniva)	Bone resorption inhibitor	Osteoporosis
ibuprofen (Motrin)	NSAID, antipyretic, nonopioid analgesic	Mild to moderate pain, rheumatoid arthritis, osteoarthritis, dysmenorrhea, gout, fever, musculoskeletal disorders
infliximab (Remicade)	Antirheumatic DMARD, gastrointestinal anti-inflammatory	Rheumatoid arthritis, Crohn disease, psoriatic arthritis, ankylosing spondylitis, ulcerative colitis, plaque psoriasis
insulin glargine (Lantus)	Antidiabetic, hormone	Type 1 and type 2 diabetes
irbesartan (Avapro)	Antihypertensive	Hypertension
isosorbide dinitrate (Isordil)	Antianginal, vasodilator	Treatment or prevention of chronic unstable angina, esophageal spasms
isotretinoin (Accutane)	Antiacne, retinoid	Severe cystic acne

Generic Name (Trade Name)	Therapeutic Classification	Common Use
lamotrigine (Lamictal)	Anticonvulsant	Various types of seizures, maintenance treatment of bipolar disorder
lansoprazole (Prevacid)	Antiulcer agent	Erosive esophagitis, ulcers, GERD
latanoprost (Xalatan)	Beta-adrenergic blockers	Ocular hypertension, chronic open-angle glaucoma
levofloxacin (Levaquin)	Anti-infective	Various infections
levonorgestrel-releasing intrauterine system (Mirena)	Hormonal contraceptive	Prevention of pregnancy, emergency contraception, regulation of menstrual cycle, acne
levothyroxine (Levothyroid)	Hormone	Hypothyroidism, goiters, thyroid cancer
levothyroxine (Levoxyl)	Hormone	Hypothyroidism, goiters, thyroid cancer
levothyroxine (Synthroid)	Hormone	Hypothyroidism
lisinopril (Prinivil)	Antihypertensive	Hypertension, heart failure
lorazepam (Ativan)	Sedative-hypnotic, antianxiety, anesthetic adjuvant	Anxiety, insomnia, preoperative sedation, status epilepticus
losartan (Cozaar)	Antihypertensive	Hypertension
lovastatin (Mevacor)	Antilipemic	Hypercholesterolemia, atherosclerosis, prevention of coronary artery disease
meclizine (Antivert)	Antiemetic, antihistamine, anticholinergic	Vertigo, motion sickness
meloxicam (Mobic)	NSAID, nonopioid analgesic	Osteoarthritis, rheumatoid arthritis, juvenile arthritis
memantine (Namenda)	Anti-Alzheimer agent	Moderate to severe Alzheimer dementia
metformin (Glucophage)	Oral hypoglycemic	Type 2 diabetes
methylphenidate (Concerta)	Cerebral stimulant	Attention deficit disorder, ADHD, narcolepsy
methylphenidate (Ritalin)	Central nervous system stimulant	Attention deficit disorder, ADHD, narcolepsy
metoprolol (Lopressor)	Antihypertensive, antiangina	Hypertension, MI, angina, heart failure
metoprolol (Toprol-XL)	Antianginal, antihypertensive	Hypertension, angina, prevention of MI
miconazole (Monistat)	Vaginal antifungal	Vaginal, vulval, vulvovaginal candidiasis
mirtazapine (Remeron)	Antidepressant	Major depressive disorder
montelukast (Singulair)	Bronchodilator, allergy, cold, and cough remedy	Asthma, seasonal allergies, rhinitis
morphine (MS Contin)	Opioid analgesic	Moderate to severe pain

Continued

Generic Name (Trade Name)	Therapeutic Classification	Common Use
moxifloxacin (Avelox)	Anti-infective	Various infections
nabumetone (Relafen)	Antirheumatic, NSAID	Rheumatoid arthritis, osteoarthritis
naproxen (Aleve)	NSAID, anti-inflammatory, nonopioid analgesic	Mild to moderate pain, osteoarthritis, rheumatoid arthritis, gouty arthritis, juvenile arthritis, dysmenorrhea
niacin (Niaspan)	Vitamin B_3, antihyperlipidemic	Pellagra, hyperlipidemias, peripheral vascular disease
nitroglycerin (Nitrostat)	Antianginal	Angina, heart failure associated with MI
olanzapine (Zyprexa)	Antipsychotic, mood stabilizer	Psychotic disorders, acute manic episodes associated with bipolar disorder, dementia-related psychotic symptoms
olmesartan medoxomil (Benicar)	Antihypertensive	Hypertension
omeprazole (Prilosec)	Antiulcer agent	GERD, erosive esophagitis
oxcarbazepine (Trileptal)	Anticonvulsant	Seizures
oxycodone (OxyContin)	Opiate analgesic	Moderate to severe pain
oxycodone (Roxicodone)	Opiate analgesic	Moderate to severe pain
pantoprazole (Protonix)	Antiulcer	GERD, ulcers
paroxetine (Paxil)	Antidepressant	Depression, panic disorder, OCD, generalized anxiety disorder, PTSD, social anxiety disorder, premenstrual disorders
penicillin V potassium (Penicillin VK)	Anti-infective	Various infections
pioglitazone (Actos)	Oral antidiabetic	Type 2 diabetes
polyethylene glycol 3350 (MiraLAX)	Laxative	Prevention or treatment of constipation
potassium chloride (Klor-Con)	Electrolyte, mineral replacement	Prevention and treatment of hypokalemia
potassium chloride (Micro-K)	Electrolyte, mineral replacement	Prevention and treatment of hypokalemia
pravastatin (Pravachol)	Lipid-lowering agent	Hypercholesterolemia, prevention of cardiovascular disease
prednisone (Deltasone)	Corticosteroid	Allergies, severe inflammation, neoplasms, multiple sclerosis, collagen disorders, dermatologic disorders
pregabalin (Lyrica)	Anticonvulsant	Neuropathic pain, partial-onset seizures

Generic Name (Trade Name)	Therapeutic Classification	Common Use
promethazine (Phenergan)	Antihistamine, antiemetic, sedative-hypnotic	Nausea, allergies, motion sickness, preoperative sedation, adjunct to anesthesia and analgesia
quetiapine fumarate (Seroquel)	Antipsychotic, mood stabilizer	Schizophrenia, depressive episodes with bipolar disorder, bipolar mania
quinapril (Accupril)	Antihypertensive	Hypertension, CHF
rabeprazole sodium (Aciphex)	Antiulcer	GERD, erosive esophagitis, duodenal ulcers
raloxifene (Evista)	Bone resorption inhibitor	Prevention and treatment of osteoporosis
ramipril (Altace)	Antihypertensive	Hypertension, heart failure, reduction in risk of MI, stroke, and cardiovascular disorders
ranitidine (Zantac)	Antiulcer	GERD, PUD, esophagitis
risperidone (Risperdal)	Antipsychotic, mood stabilizer	Schizophrenia, bipolar mania, irritability associated with autistic disorder
rosuvastatin (Crestor)	Antilipemic	Hypercholesterolemia, hypertriglyceridemia
sertraline (Zoloft)	Antidepressant	Depression, OCD, panic disorder, PTSD, social anxiety disorder, premenstrual dysphoric disorder
sildenafil (Viagra)	Erectile dysfunction agent	Erectile dysfunction
simvastatin (Zocor)	Lipid-lowering agent	High cholesterol and LDL
sitagliptin (Januvia)	Antidiabetic	Type 2 diabetes
spironolactone (Aldactone)	Potassium-sparing diuretic	Edema, hypertension, primary aldosteronism, diuretic-induced hypokalemia
sumatriptan (Imitrex)	Antimigraine agent	Migraine and cluster headaches
tadalafil (Cialis)	Erectile dysfunction agent	Erectile dysfunction
tamsulosin hydrochloride (Flomax)	Peripherally acting antiadrenergic	Benign prostatic hyperplasia
tiotropium (Spiriva)	Bronchodilator	Bronchospasms caused by COPD
tolterodine (Detrol)	Overactive bladder product	Overactive bladder, urinary incontinence
topiramate (Topamax)	Anticonvulsant, mood stabilizer	Seizures, migraine headaches
tramadol (Ultram)	Central-acting analgesic	Moderate pain
trazodone (Desyrel)	Antidepressant	Depression
trimethoprim sulfamethoxazole (Bactrim)	Anti-infective, antiprotozoal	Bacterial and protozoal infections

Continued

Generic Name (Trade Name)	Therapeutic Classification	Common Use
valacyclovir (Valtrex)	Antiviral	Herpes infections
valproic acid (Depakote)	Anticonvulsant	Various types of seizures, bipolar disorder, schizophrenia, migraine prevention
valsartan (Diovan)	Antihypertensive	Hypertension, heart failure
varenicline (Chantix)	Smoking cessation	Quit smoking
venlafaxine (Effexor)	Antidepressant	Major depression, general anxiety disorder, social anxiety disorder
verapamil (Calan)	Antihypertensive, antianginal	Angina, hypertension, dysrhythmias
warfarin (Coumadin)	Anticoagulant	Prevention or treatment of deep vein thrombosis, pulmonary embolism, or other thromboembolic disorders
zolpidem (Ambien)	Miscellaneous sedative-hypnotic	Short-term treatment of insomnia

ADHD, Attention-deficit hyperactivity disorder; *CHF,* congestive heart failure; *COPD,* chronic obstructive pulmonary disease; *DMARD,* disease-modifying antirheumatic drug; *GERD,* gastroesophageal reflux disease; *LDL,* low-density lipoprotein; *MI,* myocardial infarction; *NSAID,* nonsteroidal anti-inflammatory drug; *OCD,* obsessive-compulsive disorder; *PTSD,* post-traumatic stress disorder; *PUD,* peptic ulcer disease; *TIA,* transient ischemic attack.

Commonly Prescribed Combination Products

A number of drugs are marketed in combination form. This table includes some of the most commonly prescribed combination drugs. Some contain two medications, some three, and a few even have four or five. They are listed alphabetically according to their trade name, followed by the actual medications included in the product.

Trade Name	First drug	Second drug	Third drug	Fourth drug
Adderall	amphetamine aspartate	amphetamine sulfate	dextroamphetamine saccharide	dextroamphetamine sulfate
Advair Diskus	fluticasone propionate	salmeterol		
Caduet	amlodipine besylate	atorvastatin calcium		
Combivent	ipratropium bromide	albuterol		
Darvocet-N	acetaminophen	propoxyphene napsylate		
Dyazide	hydrochlorothiazide	triamterene		
Fioricet	butalbital	acetaminophen	caffeine	
Hyzaar	losartan	hydrochlorothiazide		

Trade Name	First drug	Second drug	Third drug	Fourth drug
Kariva	desogestrel	ethinyl estradiol		
Maxzide	triamterene	hydrochlorothiazide		
Norco	hydrocodone bitartrate	acetaminophen		
Nuvaring	etonogestrel	ethinyl estradiol		
Percocet	oxycodone	acetaminophen		
Prempro	conjugated estrogens	medroxyprogesterone acetate		
Septra	trimethoprim	sulfamethoxazole		
Suboxone	buprenorphine	naloxone dihydrate sublingual		
Treximet	sumatriptan	naproxen sodium		
Tussionex	hydrocodone polistirex	chlorpheniramine polistirex		
Tylenol #3	acetaminophen	codeine phosphate		
Ultracet	tramadol	acetaminophen		
Vicodin	acetaminophen	hydrocodone		
Vytorin	ezetimibe	simvastatin		
Yaz	drospirenone	ethinyl estradiol		
Yaz 28, Yasmin	ethinyl estradiol	drospirenone		

For a current list of the most commonly prescribed drugs, see http://www.rxlist.com.

APPENDIX

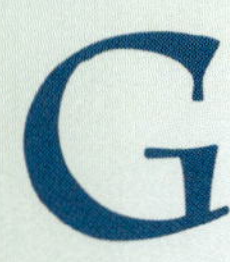

ANSWER KEY: PRACTICE EXERCISES

CHAPTER 1

Matching
Exercise 1

1. b
2. d
3. c
4. f
5. e
6. a

True or False
Exercise 2

1. True
2. True
3. True
4. False
5. True

Multiple Choice
Exercise 3

1. a
2. c
3. c
4. c
5. c
6. c
7. a
8. d
9. d
10. d

True or False
Exercise 4

1. True
2. False
3. False
4. True
5. True

Multiple Choice
Exercise 5

1. b
2. b
3. a
4. c
5. d
6. c
7. c
8. b
9. d
10. b

CHAPTER 2

Fill in the Blanks
Exercise 1

1. Mono-, uni-
2. Oligo-
3. Micro-
4. A-, an-, in-
5. Quadri-, tetra-
6. Hemi-, semi-
7. Ambi-
8. Macro-
9. Poly-
10. Iso-

True or False
Exercise 2

1. False
2. False
3. True
4. False
5. True
6. False
7. True
8. False
9. True
10. True

Fill in the Blanks
Exercise 3

1. Ultra-
2. Ab-
3. Dia-, trans-
4. En-, end-, endo-, in-, intra-
5. Ad-
6. Brady-
7. Epi-
8. Ec-, ecto-
9. Ex-, exo-, extra-
10. Circum-

True or False
Exercise 4

1. True
2. True
3. True
4. False
5. True
6. True
7. False
8. True
9. True
10. False

Fill in the Blanks
Exercise 5

1. Tox-
2. Eu-

3. Neo-
4. Dys-
5. Auto-

True or False
Exercise 6

1. False
2. True
3. False
4. False
5. False

Fill in the Blanks
Exercise 7

1. -Iatrics, iatry
2. -Logist, ologist
3. -Plasty
4. -Cidal, -cide
5. -Graphy
6. Study of
7. Surgical fixation of bone or joint, binding, tying together
8. Excision, surgical removal
9. Measurement
10. Visual examination

True or False
Exercise 8

1. False
2. True
3. True
4. True
5. False
6. False
7. True
8. True
9. False
10. False

Fill in the Blanks
Exercise 9

1. -Acusia, -acusis, -cusis
2. -Opia, -opsia, -opsis, -opsy
3. -Phoria
4. -Osmia
5. -Gen, -genesis, -genic, -genous
6. -Rrhage and -rrhagia
7. -Phage and -phagia
8. -Emesis
9. -Lysis
10. -Rrhexis

True or False
Exercise 10

1. False
2. False
3. True
4. False
5. True
6. True
7. True
8. False
9. False
10. False

Fill in the Blanks
Exercise 11

1. -Gravida
2. -Lith
3. -Lepsy, -leptic
4. -Cele
5. -Malacia
6. -Phonia
7. -Static
8. -Stenosis
9. -Oma
10. -Oid

True or False
Exercise 12

1. False
2. True
3. False
4. False
5. True
6. False
7. False
8. True
9. True
10. True

Fill in the Blanks
Exercise 13

1. -Graph
2. -Tome
3. -Meter
4. -Scope
5. -Cyte, -cytic
6. -Prandial
7. -Ole, -ule
8. -Stomy
9. -Penia
10. -Gram

True or False
Exercise 14

1. True
2. False
3. False
4. False
5. True
6. True
7. False
8. False
9. True
10. True

Deciphering Terms
Exercise 15

1. Two sides
2. Low oxygen
3. Good feeling
4. Absence of hearing
5. Absence of odor
6. Half paralysis
7. Much urination
8. Slow movement
9. After childbirth
10. New growth

Deciphering Terms
Exercise 16

1. Pertaining to poison
2. Recording instrument of self
3. Much fear
4. Absence of sensation
5. Absence of growth
6. Many pregnancies
7. Paralysis of four (limbs)
8. Excessive vomiting
9. After meal
10. Difficult breathing

Multiple Choice
Exercise 17

1. d
2. c
3. c
4. a
5. c
6. b
7. c
8. c
9. d
10. c
11. c
12. a
13. d
14. b
15. a
16. d
17. c
18. c
19. c
20. c
21. d
22. b
23. c
24. d
25. a

CHAPTER 3

Directional Terms
Exercise 1

1. Clockwise from top: Cranial; dorsal; vertebral; abdominopelvic; ventral; thoracic
2. Quadrants, clockwise from top left: Right upper quadrant (RUQ); left upper quadrant (LUQ); left lower quadrant (LLQ); right lower quadrant (RLQ). Regions, clockwise from top left: Right hypochondriac region; epigastric region; left hypochondriac region; left lumbar region; left iliac region; hypogastric region; right iliac region; right lumbar region; umbilical region (center)

Multiple Choice
Exercise 2

1. d
2. b
3. c
4. a
5. b

Locating Body Parts Using Directional Terms
Exercise 3

1. Above right elbow on front of arm
2. Front top of head
3. Lower left arm next to wrist
4. Below umbilicus
5. Below right knee
6. Left front chest
7. Right of umbilicus
8. Next to left knee

Fill in the Blanks
Exercise 4

1. Lateral
2. Apex
3. Upper extremity
4. Supine
5. Right lower quadrant
6. Superficial
7. Posteroanterior
8. Prone
9. Left upper quadrant
10. Base

Multiple Choice
Exercise 5

1. d
2. d
3. d
4. c
5. d

CHAPTER 4

Fill in the Blanks
Exercise 1

1. Albinism
2. Rhytidectomy
3. Xanthoderma
4. Melanoma
5. Cyanosis
6. Etiology
7. Leukorrhea
8. Erythematous
9. Erythrocyte
10. Morphology
11. Pathologist
12. Chromatic
13. Xeroderma
14. Seborrhea
15. Adipoid
16. Sclerosis
17. Lipoma
18. Depilous
19. Hydrotherapy
20. Trichopathy
21. Cutaneous
22. Dermatologist

23. Cytology
24. Keratotomy
25. Dermoplasty
26. Mycosis
27. Necrosis
28. Onychomalacia
29. Cirrhosis
30. Hidrosis
31. Sonogram
32. Idiopathic
33. From top: Cutane/o, dermat/o, derm/o; trich/o, pil/o; kerat/o; adip/o, lip/o

Deciphering Terms
Exercise 2

1. Blue skin
2. Pertaining to hardening
3. Abnormal condition of excessive keratinized tissue
4. Deficiency of white (blood) cells
5. Pertaining to beneath the skin
6. Red (blood) cell
7. Study of the skin
8. Black cell
9. Abnormal condition of hair fungus
10. Excessive nourishment or growth
11. Dry skin
12. Yellow tumor
13. Destruction of fat
14. Abnormal condition of fat
15. Nail tumor

Fill in the Blanks
Exercise 3

1. Abrasion
2. Contusion, ecchymosis
3. Petechia
4. Impetigo
5. Vitiligo
6. Vesicle
7. Pustule
8. Comedo
9. Scabies
10. Papule
11. Alopecia
12. Laceration
13. Fissure
14. Eczema
15. Macule
16. Cellulitis
17. Tinea
18. Scales
19. Cyst
20. Callus

Multiple Choice
Exercise 4

1. b
2. d
3. c
4. d
5. c

Word Building
Exercise 5

1. Adipoid, lipoid
2. Xerodermal
3. Albinism, leukism
4. Xanthosis
5. Dermal
6. Epidermal
7. Dermatomycosis, dermomycosis
8. Erythrocytopenia
9. Cyanosis
10. Scleroderma, dermosclerosis
11. Trichomycosis
12. Keratosis
13. Leukemia
14. Onychomycosis
15. Melanoma
16. Necrotic
17. Hypodermic
18. Lipectomy, adipectomy
19. Adipocyte, lipocyte
20. Xeroderma

True or False
Exercise 6

1. True
2. False
3. True
4. True
5. False
6. False
7. False
8. True
9. True
10. False

Deciphering Terms
Exercise 7

1. Pertaining to sweat
2. Creation or production of shape
3. Pertaining to water
4. Resembling fungus
5. Pertaining to yellowness
6. Record of color
7. Decreased white blood cells
8. Process of recording sound
9. Surgical repair of wrinkles
10. Fear of disease

Multiple Choice
Exercise 8

1. c
2. d
3. b
4. d
5. c

6. d
7. b
8. d
9. d
10. b
11. d
12. b
13. a
14. d
15. d
16. c
17. a
18. d
19. d
20. c

CHAPTER 5

Fill in the Blanks

Exercise 1

1. Cephalalgia
2. Meningioma
3. Thalamotomy
4. Glioma
5. Cerebrovascular
6. Meningitis
7. Ventriculoscopy
8. Cerebellitis
9. Myelography
10. Neurocytoma
11. Tonometer
12. Dyslexia
13. Ganglioma
14. Narcolepsy
15. Radiculopathy
16. Myasthenia
17. Encephalocele
18. Aphasia
19. Spinal stenosis
20. Psychiatry
21. Clockwise from top left: Cerebrum (cerebr/o, encephal/o); corpus callosum; skull; meninges (mening/o, meningi/o); thalamus; cerebellum; cerebrospinal fluid (CSF); spinal cord (myel/o); brainstem (pons, medulla); pituitary gland; hypothalamus

    Clockwise from top right: Spinal cord (myel/o); spine (spin/o); sacral nerves (S1–S5); lumbar nerves (L1–L5); thoracic nerves (T1–T12); cervical nerves (C1–C8)
22. From top: Cell body; dendrites; nucleus; axon; myelin sheath; axon terminal

Deciphering Terms

Exercise 2

1. Pertaining to the brain and spine
2. Disease of the nerves
3. Tumor of bone marrow or the spinal cord
4. Inflammation of the meninges
5. Process of recording the brain (activity)
6. Glue cell
7. Abnormal condition of brain hardening
8. Paralysis of half (of the body)
9. Pertaining to paralysis of two (legs)
10. Partial paralysis of four (extremities)

Fill in the Blanks

Exercise 3

1. Epilepsy
2. Bell palsy
3. Cerebrovascular accident (CVA)
4. Neural tube defect (spina bifida)
5. Transient ischemic attack (TIA)
6. Huntington disease
7. Cerebral contusion
8. Reye syndrome
9. Delirium
10. Epidural hematoma

Multiple Choice

Exercise 4

1. d
2. c
3. a
4. d
5. b

Word Building

Exercise 5

1. Polyneuritis
2. Infraspinal, infraspinous
3. Myelomeningocele
4. Encephalomeningitis
5. Paraspinal, paraspinous
6. Glioma
7. Isoelectric
8. Hemiparesis
9. Quadriplegia
10. Paraplegia

True or False

Exercise 6

1. False
2. True
3. True
4. True
5. False
6. True
7. True
8. True
9. True
10. False

Deciphering Terms

Exercise 7

1. Hernia of the spinal cord and meninges
2. Abnormal condition of hardening of the spinal cord
3. Pertaining to the brain and spine

4. Pertaining to muscle weakness
5. Pertaining to the brain and ventricle
6. Abnormal condition of sleep or stupor
7. Enlargement of the thalamus
8. Record of the spinal cord or bone marrow
9. Cutting into the nerve
10. Pertaining to glue cells

Multiple Choice

Exercise 8

1. d
2. c
3. a
4. d
5. b
6. a
7. a
8. c
9. a
10. b
11. c
12. c
13. d
14. b
15. a
16. c
17. d
18. a
19. d
20. d

CHAPTER 6

Fill in the Blanks

Exercise 1

1. Ventriculostomy
2. Angioedema
3. Tachycardia
4. Valvotomy
5. Electrocardiogram
6. Arteriosclerosis
7. Phleborrhexis
8. Vasorrhaphy
9. Atheroma
10. Hematemesis
11. Valvuloplasty
12. Vasculogenesis
13. Aortostenosis
14. Venostasis
15. Atrioventricular
16. Hemolytic
17. Thrombophlebitis
18. Coronary
19. Clockwise from top right: Aorta (aort/o); left pulmonary artery; left pulmonary veins; left atrium (atri/o); aortic valve; mitral valve; left ventricle (ventricul/o); interventricular septum; right ventricle; inferior vena cava; tricuspid valve; right atrium; pulmonary valve; right pulmonary veins; superior vena cava; right pulmonary artery
20. From top: Lung capillaries; pulmonary circulation; aorta (aort/o); heart (cardi/o); veins (phleb/o, ven/o); arteries (arteri/o); venules; arterioles; tissue capillaries

Deciphering Terms

Exercise 2

1. Condition of a small heart
2. Small vein
3. Record of blood
4. Process of recording a vessel
5. Surgical repair of the aorta
6. Small artery
7. Thick, fatty cell
8. Pain of the atrium
9. Pertaining to electricity
10. Condition of blood in the urine
11. Pertaining to a valve
12. Inflammation of a vein
13. Stopping a vein
14. Disease of a blood vessel
15. Destruction of a clot

Fill in the Blanks

Exercise 3

1. Arrhythmia
2. Bruit
3. Congestive heart failure
4. Each evening
5. Deep vein thrombosis *or* DVT
6. Every 2 hours
7. Myocardial infarction; MI
8. Varicose veins
9. RA, LA
10. RV, LV
11. Blood pressure, hypertension
12. Electrocardiogram
13. Four
14. Each morning
15. Anemia
16. Angina
17. Cardiomyopathy
18. Endocarditis
19. Pericarditis

Multiple Choice

Exercise 4

1. d
2. d
3. c
4. c
5. b

Word Building

Exercise 5

1. Angiogram
2. Aortic
3. Arteriography
4. Atherosclerosis
5. Arteriorrhexis
6. Bradycardia

7. Cardiomegaly
8. Tachycardia
9. Electrocardiogram
10. Hematologist
11. Valvotomy
12. Phlebotomy
13. Phlebitis
14. Thrombocyte
15. Angioplasty
16. Ventriculocele
17. Ventriculometry
18. Microcardia
19. Hemolysis
20. Aortomalacia

True or False

Exercise 6

1. False
2. True
3. True
4. False
5. False
6. False
7. False
8. True
9. True
10. True

Deciphering Terms

Exercise 7

1. Abnormal enlargement of the heart
2. Visual examination of a ventricle
3. Pertaining to vessel tone
4. Widening, stretching, or expanding of a vessel
5. Pain of a vessel
6. Movement of the atria
7. Destruction of a thrombus (clot)
8. Specialist in the study of blood
9. Rupture of an artery
10. Narrowing of a vessel

Multiple Choice

Exercise 8

1. d
2. a
3. d
4. b
5. b
6. b
7. d
8. c
9. b
10. b
11. b
12. b
13. a
14. b
15. d
16. b
17. b
18. b
19. b
20. b

CHAPTER 7

Fill in the Blanks

Exercise 1

1. Lymphadenocele
2. Angiasthenia
3. Toxicogenic
4. Splenomegaly
5. Myeloma
6. Lymphangiecstasis
7. Lymphocytosis
8. Tonsillitis
9. Serous
10. Thymocyte
11. Adenoma
12. Lymphoma
13. Immunopathology
14. Bacteriemia
15. Adenoidectomy
16. Pathophobia
17. Vasorrhaphy
18. Toxoid
19. From top: Tonsil; thymus (thym/o); lymphatic (lymph/o) vessel (angi/o, vas/o); spleen (splen/o); lymph node or gland (aden/o); direction of lymph flow; lymph node; lymphocytes and macrophages

Deciphering Terms

Exercise 2

1. Specialist in the study of disease
2. X-ray of lymph glands
3. Destroying or killing bacteria
4. Process of recording a vessel
5. Study of the immune (system)
6. Pertaining to lymph cell
7. Condition of poison in the blood
8. Produced by bone marrow
9. Pain of the spleen
10. Surgical removal of the tonsils
11. Disease of the lymph glands
12. Suturing of a vessel
13. Study of serum
14. Cutting into or incision of the thymus
15. Pain of a vessel

Fill in the Blanks

Exercise 3

1. Sjögren syndrome
2. Anaphylaxis
3. Epstein-Barr
4. Hodgkin
5. Phagocytosis
6. Scleroderma
7. Non-Hodgkin lymphoma
8. Systemic lupus erythematosus
9. Erythrocyte sedimentation rate
10. CA

11. EBV
12. Lymphatic cancer
13. Chronic fatigue
14. EIA
15. PCP
16. AB, Ab
17. AG, Ag
18. Acquired immunodeficiency syndrome
19. Human immunodeficiency
20. *Pneumocystis carinii* pneumonia

Multiple Choice

Exercise 4

1. a
2. a
3. a
4. a
5. a

Word Building

Exercise 5

1. Angiogram
2. Bacteriology
3. Immunogenic
4. Serous
5. Toxicology
6. Tonsillotomy
7. Pathology
8. Peritonsillar
9. Thymosclerosis
10. Myelogenic
11. Lymphoid
12. Splenomegaly
13. Angioplasty
14. Euthymic
15. Adenopathy

True or False

Exercise 6

1. True
2. True
3. True
4. False
5. False
6. True
7. True
8. True
9. False
10. False

Deciphering Terms

Exercise 7

1. Fatty gland tumor
2. Inflammation of the adenoids
3. Swelling of a vessel
4. Narrowing of a vessel
5. Tumor of the bone marrow
6. Creator or producer of immunity
7. Dilation or expansion of a lymph gland
8. Bursting forth of lymph
9. Tumor of a lymphatic vessel
10. Deficiency of lymph cells

Multiple Choice

Exercise 8

1. c
2. a
3. b
4. c
5. b
6. b
7. a
8. c
9. d
10. a
11. d
12. c
13. d
14. b
15. a
16. b
17. a
18. d
19. b
20. c

CHAPTER 8

Fill in the Blanks

Exercise 1

1. Mucoid
2. Tonsillitis
3. Bronchitis
4. Bronchiectasis
5. Epiglottal
6. Aerophagia
7. Pharyngeal
8. Chondroplasty
9. Orthopnea
10. Nasogastric
11. Carcinoma
12. Oral
13. Anoxia
14. Pneumonia
15. Rhinitis
16. Pleurodynia
17. Pulmonary
18. Sinusoid
19. Thoracentesis
20. Pneumonectomy
21. Tracheotomy
22. Laryngitis
23. Stomatitis
24. Coniosis
25. Lobectomy
26. Alveolitis
27. Anthracosis
28. Diaphragmatocele
29. Bronchiolitis
30. Oximeter
31. Phonograph
32. Spirometer
33. Clockwise from top right: Adenoids; pharynx (pharyng/o); tonsils (tonsill/o); epiglottis (epiglott/o); trachea (trache/o); bronchial tubes (bronch/o, bronchi/o); pleura (pleur/o); pleural space; diaphragm; alveolus (alveol/o); lung (pneumon/o,

pneum/o, pulmon/o); larynx (laryng/o); mouth (or/o, stomat/o); nose (nas/o, rhin/o); frontal sinus (sinus/o)

Deciphering Terms
Exercise 2

1. Pertaining to the larynx
2. Pain of the pleura
3. Pertaining to air or the lungs
4. A condition of the lungs
5. Pertaining to the lungs
6. Cutting into or incision of the sinus
7. Surgical puncture of the thorax
8. Excision or surgical removal of the tonsil
9. Bad, painful, or difficult breathing
10. Blood in the thorax (pleural space)
11. Air in the thorax (pleural space)
12. Good or normal breathing
13. Breathing in the straight position
14. Inflammation of the nose
15. Mouthlike opening in the trachea

Fill in the Blanks
Exercise 3

1. Anthrac/o
2. Chronic obstructive pulmonary disease
3. COPD
4. Purified protein derivative
5. Asthma
6. Coryza
7. Pneumothorax
8. Stridor
9. Stat
10. Upper respiratory infection
11. URI
12. Coryza
13. Cardiopulmonary resuscitation
14. CPR
15. Nosebleed
16. Histoplasmosis
17. Laryngitis
18. Atelectasis
19. Hypercapnia
20. Tonsils, adenoids

Multiple Choice
Exercise 4

1. c
2. a
3. b
4. c
5. a

Word Building
Exercise 5

1. Bronchopulmonary
2. Chondroma
3. Aerogenesis
4. Mucocutaneous
5. Tracheobronchoscopy
6. Tonsillopathy
7. Tracheomalacia
8. Epiglottitis
9. Dyspneic
10. Eupnea
11. Thoracotomy
12. Pharyngomycosis
13. Pleurodynia
14. Pneumopexy, pulmonopexy
15. Pulmonary, pulmonic
16. Sinusoid
17. Tracheostomy
18. Carcinogenic
19. Tachypnea
20. Laryngoscopy

True or False
Exercise 6

1. False
2. False
3. True
4. False
5. True
6. True
7. False
8. False
9. True
10. True

Deciphering Terms
Exercise 7

1. Swallowing air
2. Pertaining to the alveoli
3. Pertaining to the pharynx
4. Record of breathing
5. Pertaining to the nose
6. Resembling coal or coal dust
7. Destruction of mucus
8. Fear of sound or voice
9. Cancerous tumor
10. Pertaining to oxygen

Multiple Choice
Exercise 8

1. a
2. d
3. b
4. a
5. c
6. d
7. b
8. a
9. b
10. a
11. c
12. b
13. a
14. a
15. b
16. c
17. d
18. b
19. b
20. a

CHAPTER 9

Fill in the Blanks
Exercise 1

1. Rectal
2. Laparoscope
3. Oral
4. Pharyngeal
5. Anal
6. Esophagostenosis
7. Cholecystectomy
8. Enteritis
9. Jejunostomy
10. Colonoscopy
11. Sublingual
12. Duodenoscopy
13. Ileotomy
14. Stomatitis
15. Gastralgia
16. Hepatitis
17. Appendectomy
18. Appendicitis
19. Proctoscopy
20. Colectomy
21. Dental
22. Glossospasm
23. Pancreatitis
24. Sigmoidoscope
25. Steatorrhea
26. Biliary
27. Buccogingival
28. Choledocholith
29. Sialolithiasis
30. Cecectomy
31. Cholangiography
32. Cheiloplasty
33. Odontodynia
34. Labiodental
35. Gingivoglossitis
36. Glossokinesthetic
37. Cholecystitis
38. Peptic
39. Phagocyte
40. Pylorostenosis
41. Clockwise from top right: Pharynx (pharyng/o); esophagus (esophag/o); stomach (gastr/o); duodenum (duoden/o); jejunum (jejun/o); small intestine (enter/o); ileum (ile/o); sigmoid colon (sigmoid/o); rectum (rect/o, proct/o); anus (an/o, proct/o); appendix (append/o, appendic/o); cecum (cec/o); abdomen (lapar/o); colon (col/o, colon/o); pancreas (pancreat/o); gallbladder (cholecyst/o); liver (hepat/o); tongue (lingu/o, gloss/o); mouth (or/o, stomat/o); teeth (dent/o)

Deciphering Terms
Exercise 2

1. Excision or surgical removal of the gallbladder
2. Inflammation of the small intestine
3. Visual examination of the anus and rectum
4. Lighted instrument used to view inside the stomach
5. Visual examination of the abdomen
6. Surgical repair of the jejunum
7. Stone in the pancreas
8. Pertaining to below or beneath the tongue
9. Inflammation of the pharynx
10. Specialist in the study of the stomach and small intestine
11. Pertaining to a small stomach
12. Bad, painful, or difficult movement
13. Flow or discharge through
14. Partial paralysis of the stomach
15. Bad, painful, or difficult feeling

Fill in the Blanks
Exercise 3

1. Ascites
2. Diverticulosis
3. Diverticulitis
4. Endoscopic retrograde cholangiopancreatography
5. Emesis
6. c̄
7. Ulcerative colitis
8. Abd
9. Upper gastrointestinal
10. Small bowel obstruction
11. NPO
12. PO
13. PR
14. VS qh
15. Qd
16. Intussusception
17. Jaundice
18. CA
19. BR c̄ BRP
20. Complained of nausea and vomiting

Multiple Choice
Exercise 4

1. c
2. b
3. c
4. c
5. b

Word Building
Exercise 5

1. Hepatopathy
2. Esophagitis
3. Esophagogastroscopy
4. Circumoral
5. Cholecystectomy
6. Gastromegaly
7. Hypercolonic
8. Perianal
9. Pharyngoscopy

10. Hepatoma
11. Appendicitis
12. Appendectomy
13. Ileotomy
14. Hyperemesis
15. Dental
16. Cholecystitis
17. Hypogastric
18. Colonoscopy
19. Cholelith
20. Colonopathy

True or False

Exercise 6

1. False
2. True
3. False
4. True
5. True
6. True
7. False
8. False
9. False
10. True

Deciphering Terms

Exercise 7

1. Absence of nourishment or growth
2. Inflammation of the gums and mouth
3. Study of the rectum and anus
4. Sudden involuntary contraction of the tongue
5. Crushing of a stone
6. Fear of eating or swallowing
7. Bad, painful, or difficult digestion
8. Pertaining to the lips and nose
9. Pain of the mouth
10. Excision or surgical removal of the cecum

Multiple Choice

Exercise 8

1. a
2. b
3. b
4. d
5. a
6. c
7. d
8. a
9. b
10. b
11. d
12. a
13. b
14. c
15. d
16. b
17. a
18. a
19. c
20. b

CHAPTER 10

Fill in the Blanks

Exercise 1

1. Peritoneal
2. Nocturia
3. Vesicocele
4. Glycemia
5. Urethropexy
6. Pyelonephritis
7. Glomerulopathy
8. Cystoscopy
9. Azoturia
10. Nephrologist
11. Ureterostenosis
12. Urology
13. Urinometer
14. Glycosuria
15. Ketonuria
16. Nephrolithiasis
17. Oliguria
18. Pyuria
19. Renal
20. Meatotome
21. Glucogenesis
22. Bacteriuria
23. From top: Left adrenal gland; left kidney (nephr/o, ren/o); left ureter; pelvis (pelv/i); right kidney; right ureter (ureter/o); urinary bladder (cyst/o); urethra (urethr/o)
24. Nephron from top: Efferent arteriole; afferent arteriole; glomerulus (glomerul/o); Bowman capsule; vein; proximal tubule; distal tubule; collecting tubule; peritubular capillaries; loop of Henle. Kidney clockwise from top: Renal cortex; pyramid in renal medulla; renal pelvis (pyel/o); renal artery; renal vein; ureter (ureter/o); kidney (nephr/o, ren/o); calyx; renal capsule

Deciphering Terms

Exercise 2

1. Disease of the kidney
2. Surgical fixation of the urethra
3. Pertaining to beside or near the urethra
4. Excision or surgical removal of the bladder
5. Cutting into or incision of the kidney
6. Mouthlike opening into the ureter
7. Inflammation of the glomerulus and kidney
8. Much thirst
9. Excision or surgical removal of the kidney
10. Urination at night
11. Bacteria in the urine

12. Blood in the urine
13. Kidney stone
14. Pertaining to the absence of urine
15. Enlargement of the bladder

Fill in the Blanks

Exercise 3

1. Glycosuria, glycuria, glucosuria
2. ESRD
3. UTI
4. Enuresis
5. Phimosis
6. Uremia
7. Diuresis
8. Interstitial cystitis
9. Chronic glomerulonephritis
10. Pyelonephritis
11. Urinary retention
12. Stress incontinence
13. Cystoscopy, vesicoscopy
14. Interstitial nephritis
15. Azoturia
16. C&S
17. Bladder ultrasound
18. Voiding cystourethrography
19. I&O
20. Meatometer

Multiple Choice

Exercise 4

1. c
2. d
3. b
4. b
5. c

Word Building

Exercise 5

1. Anuria
2. Polyuria
3. Pyuria
4. Dysuria
5. Oliguria
6. Urethralgia, urethrodynia
7. Cystoscopy
8. Hematuria
9. Nephrolithiasis
10. Nocturia
11. Bacteriuria
12. Ureterectomy
13. Pyelonephritis
14. Cystourethrogram
15. Uric, urinary
16. Cystoplasty
17. Renal
18. Glomerulonephritis
19. Azoturia
20. Urologist

True or False

Exercise 6

1. True
2. False
3. False
4. True
5. False
6. False
7. True
8. True
9. True
10. True

Deciphering Terms

Exercise 7

1. Pertaining to behind the peritoneum
2. Widening, stretching, or expanding an opening
3. Surgical fixation of the bladder and urethra
4. Crushing a stone
5. Creating or producing urine
6. Cessation or stopping of urine
7. Much urination
8. Sudden involuntary contraction of the ureter
9. Hernia of the bladder
10. Enlargement of the kidney

Multiple Choice

Exercise 8

1. a
2. b
3. d
4. c
5. d
6. b
7. b
8. b
9. a
10. b
11. d
12. b
13. d
14. c
15. c
16. a
17. d
18. b
19. b
20. a

CHAPTER 11

Fill in the Blanks

Exercise 1

1. Phalloid
2. Orchiectomy
3. Vasotomy
4. Androgynous
5. Balanitis
6. Spermatogenesis
7. Cryptorchidism
8. Orchidopexy
9. Epididymitis
10. Testomegaly
11. Orchiopathy
12. Prostatoplasty
13. Penoscrotal

14. Aspermia
15. Testicular
16. Seminuria
17. Clockwise from top right: Ureter (ureter/o); bladder (cyst/o); seminal vesicle; rectum; ejaculatory duct; prostate gland (prostat/o); epididymis; testis (test/o, orch/o, orchi/o, orchid/o); scrotum; glans penis (balan/o); prepuce (foreskin); urethra (urethr/o); ductus (vas) deferens (vas/o); pubic symphysis

Fill in the Blanks
Exercise 2

1. Amniocentesis
2. Ovarioptosis
3. Embryonic
4. Cervical
5. Fetotoxic
6. Oophorectomy
7. Galactorrhea
8. Uterine
9. Lactotherapy
10. Colposcopy
11. Gonadectomy
12. Mammoplasty
13. Metrocarcinoma
14. Dysmenorrhea
15. Uterocervical
16. Episiotomy
17. Ovogenesis
18. Vulvodynia
19. Ovarioptosis
20. Hysterotomy
21. Perineoplasty
22. Laparoscopy
23. Placental
24. Salpingitis
25. Sonorous
26. Mastectomy
27. Gynecology
28. Natal
29. Vaginapexy
30. Clockwise from top: Uterus (uter/o, hyster/o); fallopian tube (salping/o); ovary (oophor/o, ovari/o); vagina (vagin/o, colp/o); cervix (cervic/o); ovum

Fill in the Blanks
Exercise 3

1. Gynecology
2. Benign, smooth tumors made of muscle and fat
3. Oral contraceptive
4. A fertilized ovum is implanted outside of the uterus, often in the fallopian tube
5. Transurethral resection of the prostate
6. Endometrial tissue grows in abnormal sites in the lower abdominopelvic area
7. Total abdominal hysterectomy, bilateral salpingo-oophorectomy
8. STI, an infestation with parasite genus trichomonas vaginalis
9. Dilation or expansion of a testis
10. Surgical removal of an ovary and fallopian tube
11. Surgical repair of the glans penis
12. Bad, painful, or difficult formation or growth
13. Pertaining to new formation or growth
14. Process of recording a breast
15. Visual examination of the abdomen

Fill in the Blanks
Exercise 4

1. Ectopic
2. Endometriosis
3. Syphilis
4. Total abdominal hysterectomy, fibroids
5. Obstetrics and gynecology
6. Trichomoniasis
7. OC
8. Papanicolaou
9. Infertility
10. In vitro fertilization
11. TAH-BSO
12. Benign prostatic hypertrophy *or* benign prostatic hyperplasia
13. Transurethral resection of the prostate
14. Impotence
15. Semen in the urine
16. Flow or discharge of milk
17. Creation of an ovum
18. Resembling a penis
19. Failure of one or both testes to descend into the scrotum
20. Full and loud in sound

Multiple Choice
Exercise 5

1. c
2. a
3. c
4. a
5. d

Word Building
Exercise 6

1. Balanitis
2. Episiotomy
3. Anorchidism
4. Orchidopexy
5. Oligospermia
6. Perinatal
7. Dysplasia
8. Neoplasia
9. Retrovaginal
10. Anesthesia
11. Vasostenosis

12. Prostatodynia, prostatalgia
13. Cervicitis
14. Vaginorrhaphy/colporrhaphy
15. Gynecologist
16. Laparoscope
17. Hysterectomy
18. Mammogram
19. Mastopexy/mammopexy
20. Menopause

True or False
Exercise 7

1. True
2. False
3. True
4. False
5. False
6. True
7. True
8. True
9. False
10. False

Deciphering Terms
Exercise 8

1. Suturing of a testis
2. Inflammation of the cervix and vagina
3. Many pregnancies
4. Condition of female breast (enlarged breast on a man)
5. Cessation or stopping of menses
6. Pain of the penis
7. Excessive formation or growth
8. Pertaining to the destruction of sperm
9. Hernia of the prostate
10. Hidden menstrual flow or discharge

Multiple Choice
Exercise 9

1. c
2. c
3. a
4. b
5. a
6. d
7. a
8. a
9. a
10. b
11. c
12. d
13. c
14. b
15. c
16. b
17. a
18. b
19. b
20. d

CHAPTER 12

Fill in the Blanks
Exercise 1

1. Parathyroidectomy
2. Adrenalectomy
3. Adenopathy
4. Toxicologist
5. Hypercalcemia
6. Glucogenesis
7. Hydrolysis
8. Thymoma
9. Glycosuria
10. Adrenal
11. Thyroiditis
12. Pancreatography
13. Acroanesthesia
14. Homeostasis
15. Hyperkalemia
16. Natremia
17. Thyrotoxicosis
18. Clockwise from top right: Pituitary gland; thyroid (throid/o); thymus (thym/o); ovaries (oophor/o, ovari/o); testes (orch/o, orchi/o, orchid/o, test/o); pancreas (pancreat/o); adrenal glands (adren/o, adrenal/o); parathyroid glands (parathyroid/o)

Deciphering Terms
Exercise 2

1. Pertaining to the pancreas
2. Condition of small extremities
3. Treatment (to maintain) sameness
4. Disease of the adrenal gland
5. Condition of excessive potassium in the blood
6. Condition of good or normal blood sugar
7. Pertaining to a bad, painful, or difficult thymus
8. Rupture of the thyroid
9. Disease of a gland
10. Deficiency of glucose
11. Condition of below-normal sugar in the blood
12. Condition of excessive sodium in the blood
13. Sugar in the urine
14. Specialist in the study of poisons
15. Fear of water

Fill in the Blanks
Exercise 3

1. Blood sugar
2. Dwarfism
3. Cancer
4. Calcium
5. T3, T4 *or* triiodothyronine, thyroxine
6. DM
7. Non–insulin-dependent diabetes mellitus
8. Insulin-dependent diabetes mellitus
9. Growth hormone

10. Exophthalmos
11. Giantism
12. Graves disease
13. Cushing disease
14. Myxedema
15. Addison
16. Congenital hypothyroidism
17. Aldosterone
18. Cortisol
19. Glycosylated hemoglobin (Hb A1c)
20. Diabetic ketoacidosis

Multiple Choice
Exercise 4

1. c
2. c
3. b
4. c
5. a

Word Building
Exercise 5

1. Toxicology
2. Adenoma
3. Hypoparathyroid
4. Adrenalopathy
5. Hypercalcemia
6. Glucometer
7. Hydrotherapy
8. Acrocyanosis
9. Hyperkalemia
10. Pancreatitis
11. Euthymic
12. Hyperthyroidism
13. Acrodermatitis
14. Hyponatremia
15. Thymectomy
16. Pancreatocentesis
17. Pancreatoptosis
18. Thymoma
19. Thyromegaly
20. Acrokinesia

True or False
Exercise 6

1. True
2. False
3. False
4. True
5. False
6. False
7. False
8. True
9. True
10. True

Deciphering Terms
Exercise 7

1. Much eating
2. Episode of worsening symptoms of hyperthyroidism
3. Enlargement of the parathyroid
4. Much thirst
5. Destruction of sugar
6. Rupture of the pancreas
7. Creating water
8. Much urination
9. Disease of the pancreas
10. Pertaining to a small thymus

Multiple Choice
Exercise 8

1. c
2. c
3. a
4. d
5. c
6. c
7. a
8. c
9. b
10. c
11. a
12. a
13. c
14. b
15. c
16. d
17. c
18. a
19. b
20. b

CHAPTER 13

Fill in the Blanks
Exercise 1

1. Tibiofibular
2. Phalangitis
3. Vertebroplasty
4. Patellapexy
5. Tenodynia
6. Femorotibial
7. Tendotome
8. Tendinous
9. Myeloplegia
10. Osteolytic
11. Metacarpectomy
12. Humeral
13. Sternocostal
14. Pelvimeter
15. Thoracolumbar
16. Orthopnea
17. Myocardial
18. Arthrocentesis
19. Carpectomy
20. Chondrodysplasia
21. Costochondritis
22. Cervicodynia
23. Craniocerebral
24. Fibular
25. Laminectomy
26. Articular
27. Bursitis
28. Fasciodesis
29. Iliolumbar
30. Lordoscoliosis

31. Kyphosis
32. Musculoskeletal
33. Kinesiology
34. Scoliometer
35. Meniscectomy
36. Sacrodynia
37. Ulnocarpal
38. Lumbodynia
39. Radioulnar
40. Synovectomy
41. Ankylosis
42. Spondylomalacia
43. Pubofemoral
44. Tarsometatarsal
45. Synovioma
46. Metatarsophalangeal
47. Clockwise from top: Cranium (crani/o); sternum (stern/o); ribs (cost/o); costal cartilage (chondr/o); pelvis (pelv/i); carpals (carp/o); metacarpals (metacarp/o); phalanges (phalang/o); tarsals; metatarsals; phalanges (phalang/o); tibia (tibi/o); fibula (fibul/o); patella (patell/o); femur (femor/o); radius; ulna; humerus (humer/o); scapula; clavicle
48. From top: Cervical vertebrae (vertebr/o) (cervic/o), C1, C2, C3–7; lamina (lamin/o); thoracic vertebrae (thorac/o), T1, T2, T3–12; intervertebral disk; lumbar vertebrae (lumb/o), L1, L2–5; sacrum; coccyx
49. Left, from top: Frontalis; temporalis; masseter; biceps brachii; external oblique; rectus femoris; tibialis anterior. Center, from top: Sternocleidomastoid; trapezius; deltoid; pectoralis major; rectus abdominus; latissimus dorsi; sartorius; gluteus maximus; vastus lateralis; gastrocnemius; soleus. Right, from top: Triceps brachii; biceps femoris; tendon (ten/o, tend/o, tendin/o)

Deciphering Terms

Exercise 2

1. Pertaining to beside or near the vertebrae
2. Pertaining to above the tibia
3. Pertaining to the thorax
4. Destruction of a tendon
5. Cutting into or incision of the sternum
6. Pertaining to the phalanges
7. Prolapse of the patella
8. Cutting into or incision of a bone
9. Disease of a muscle
10. Abnormal condition of hardening of the bone marrow or spinal cord
11. Pertaining to the lower back
12. Cutting instrument for a lamina
13. Pain of the femur
14. Surgical repair of the cranium
15. Inflammation of the ribs and cartilage

Fill in the Blanks

Exercise 3

1. Below-the-knee amputation, BKA
2. Scoliosis
3. Osteoarthritis
4. Strain
5. Bursitis
6. C1–C7
7. Crepitation
8. Carpal tunnel syndrome
9. CTS
10. Total hip replacement, total hip arthroplasty
11. S1–S5
12. Straight, upright
13. Fracture, Fx
14. Anteroposterior, AP
15. L1–L5
16. Electromyography
17. Rheumatoid
18. Above-the-knee amputation, AKA
19. Herniated disk

Multiple Choice

Exercise 4

1. d
2. a
3. a
4. b
5. d

Word Building

Exercise 5

1. Costovertebral
2. Osteoarthritis
3. Carpal
4. Paracervical
5. Chondralgia, chondrodynia
6. Laminotome
7. Intercostal
8. Cranioplasty
9. Femoral
10. Humeropathy
11. Orthopedic
12. Lumbodynia, lumbalgia
13. Metacarpitis
14. Myeloma
15. Myoplegia
16. Substernal
17. Osteopathy
18. Patellectomy
19. Pelvimetry
20. Osteopenia

True or False

Exercise 6

1. False
2. True
3. False
4. True
5. True
6. True
7. True
8. False
9. True
10. False

Deciphering Terms

Exercise 7

1. Inflammation of cervix
2. Surgical puncture of a carpus
3. Pain of a joint
4. Breaking of bone
5. Pertaining to outside the tibia
6. Pertaining to the thorax and lower back
7. Measuring instrument for motion
8. Pertaining to a meniscus
9. Pertaining to a muscle
10. Pertaining to the pubis and rectum

Multiple Choice

Exercise 8

1. a
2. b
3. d
4. d
5. a
6. c
7. d
8. c
9. b
10. d
11. a
12. b
13. c
14. d
15. c
16. b
17. c
18. b
19. a
20. d

CHAPTER 14

Fill in the Blanks

Exercise 1

1. Otorrhea
2. Ophthalmorrhexis
3. Oculomycosis
4. Tympanosclerosis
5. Acoustic
6. Audiometry
7. Keratocele
8. Retinopexy
9. Scleral
10. Blepharoptosis
11. Salpingopharyngeal
12. Corneous
13. Diploid
14. Myringoplasty
15. Irotomy
16. Iridectome
17. Phacotoxic
18. Conjunctivitis
19. Lacrimal
20. Dacryopyorrhea
21. Optician
22. Phakolysis
23. Presbycusis
24. Clockwise from center top: Sclera (sclera/o); choroid layer, retina (retin/o); central fovea; optic nerve; optic disk; vitreous body; posterior chamber (vitreous humor); ciliary muscle; ciliary body; anterior chamber (aqueous humor); iris; pupil; lens; cornea (corne/o, kerat/o); canal of Schlemm; conjunctiva
25. Clockwise from center top: Malleus; incus; stapes; semicircular canals; vestibulocochlear nerve; cochlea; vestibule; inner ear: eustachian tube (salping/o); middle ear: round window; external ear: tympanic membrane (tympan/o, myring/o); lobe, external auditory canal; pinna (auricle)

Deciphering Terms

Exercise 2

1. Resembling the cornea or keratinized tissue
2. New formation or growth
3. Abnormal condition of tympanic-membrane fungus
4. Measurement of the tympanic membrane
5. Pertaining to behind the eye
6. Paralysis of the eye
7. Surgical repair of the ear
8. Pertaining to the eye and nose
9. Pertaining to the tympanic membrane
10. Cutting into or incision of the cornea or keratinized tissue
11. Drooping or prolapse of the eyelid
12. Movement of the eye
13. Pertaining to within the eye
14. Cutting instrument for a lacrimal gland
15. Abnormal condition of hardening of the lens

Fill in the Blanks

Exercise 3

1. Eyes, ears, nose, throat
2. Pupils are equal, round, reactive to light and accommodation

3. Astigmatism
4. Anacusis
5. Presbycusis
6. Ménière disease
7. Acute glaucoma
8. Cataracts
9. Diabetic retinopathy
10. Macular degeneration
11. Hordeolum *or* stye
12. Retinal detachment
13. Exotropia
14. Uveitis
15. Astigmatism
16. Conjunctivitis
17. Presbyopia
18. Chalazion
19. Cholesteatoma
20. Nystagmus

Multiple Choice

Exercise 4

1. a
2. b
3. c
4. a
5. d

Word Building

Exercise 5

1. Anacoustic
2. Ocular, ophthalmic
3. Blepharedema
4. Hyperopia
5. Ophthalmology
6. Keratitis
7. Diplopia
8. Myringotomy, tympanotomy
9. Ophthalmoscope, oculoscope
10. Retinopathy
11. Scleroplasty
12. Oculoplasty, ophthalmoplasty
13. Otic
14. Lacrimonasal
15. Phacomalacia
16. Retinosis
17. Conjunctivoma
18. Iridectomy
19. Audiometry
20. Ophthalmoplegia

True or False

Exercise 6

1. False
2. True
3. False
4. False
5. False
6. True
7. False
8. False
9. False
10. True

Deciphering Terms

Exercise 7

1. Flow or discharge of blood in the tears
2. Abnormal condition of the iris
3. Cutting into or incision of the lacrimal gland
4. Resembling the lens
5. Old-age hearing
6. Disease of the retina
7. Pain of the tear gland
8. Sudden involuntary contraction of the eyelid
9. Paralysis of the iris
10. Tumor of the lens

Multiple Choice

Exercise 8

1. a
2. b
3. c
4. d
5. b
6. b
7. b
8. a
9. c
10. d
11. b
12. c
13. c
14. b
15. a
16. a
17. a
18. a
19. a
20. c

INDEX

Page numbers followed by "f" indicate figures; those followed by "t" indicate tables.

A

D

M

N

Q

R

S

T

U

V

W

Y

Z

epi-
ĕp-ĭ

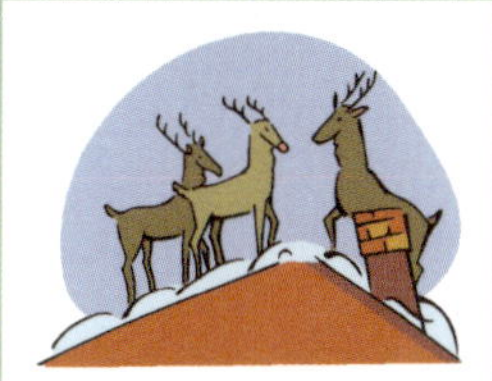

post-
pōst

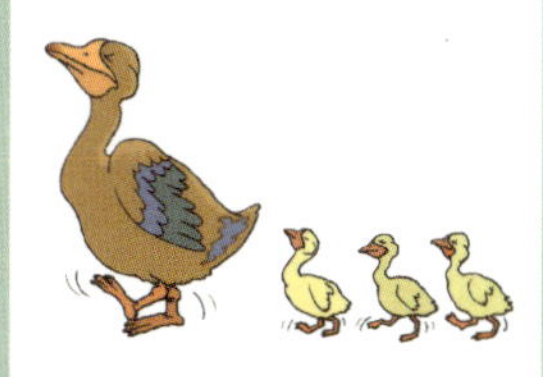

anti- **contra-**
ăn-tē kŏn-tră

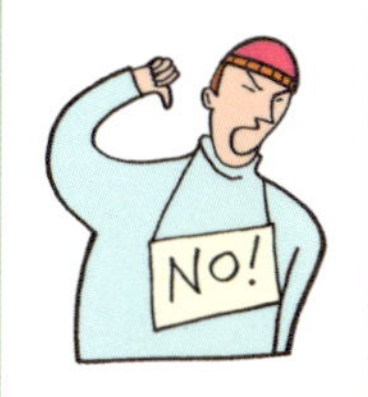

circum-
sĕr-kŭm

ab-
ăb

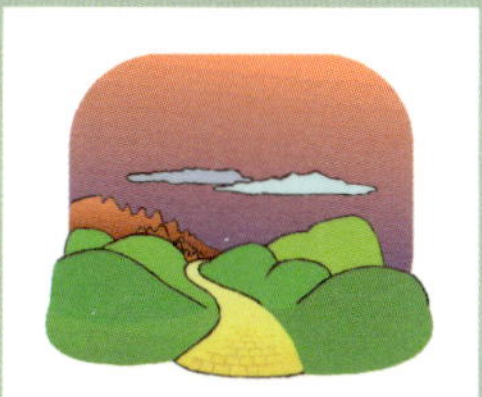

ex- **exo-** **extra-**
ĕks ĕks-ō ĕks-tră

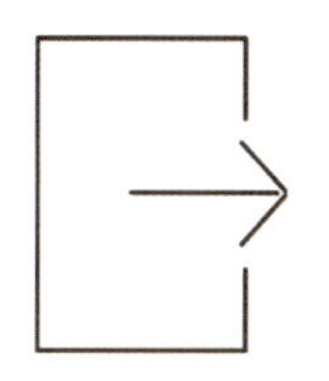

mal-
măl

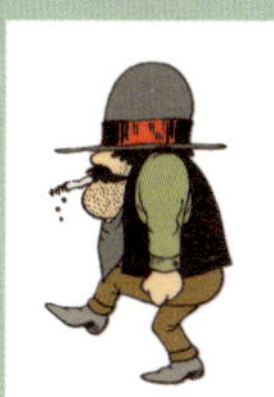

dys-
dĭs

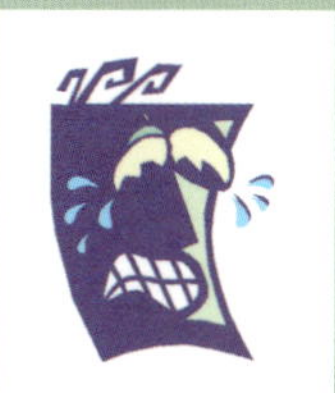

pre-
prē

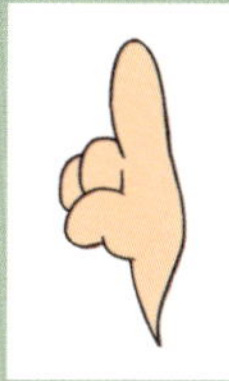

pro-
prō

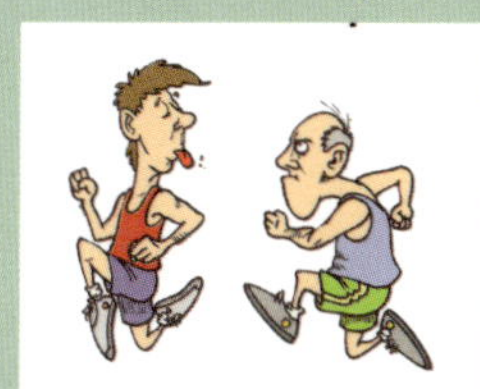

after, following

above, upon

around

against, opposite

away from, outside, external

away from

bad, painful, difficult

bad, inadequate

before, forward

before

re- **retro-**
rē rĕt-rō

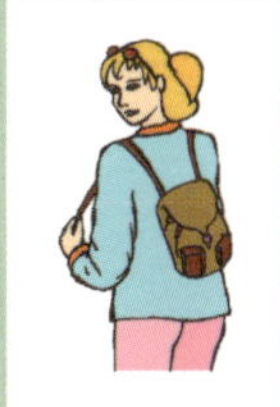

para- **peri-**
păr-ă pĕr-ĭ

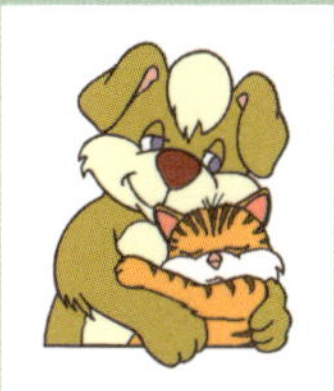

ultra-
ŭl-tră

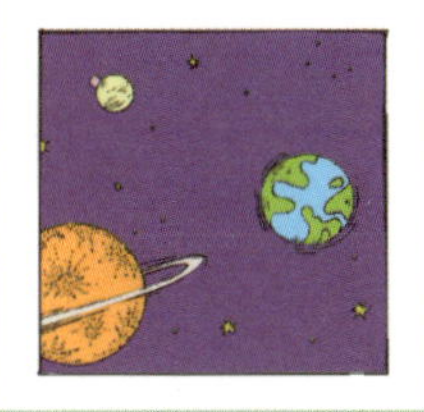

oligo-
ōl-ĭ-gō

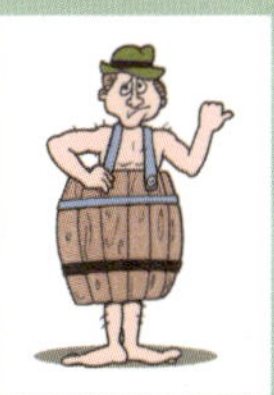

quadri- **tetra-**
kwŏd-rĭ tĕ-tră

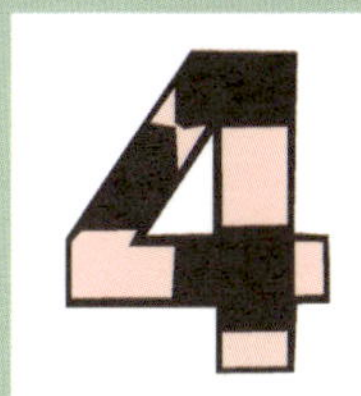

hypo- **sub-** **infra-**
hī-pō sŭb ĭn-fră

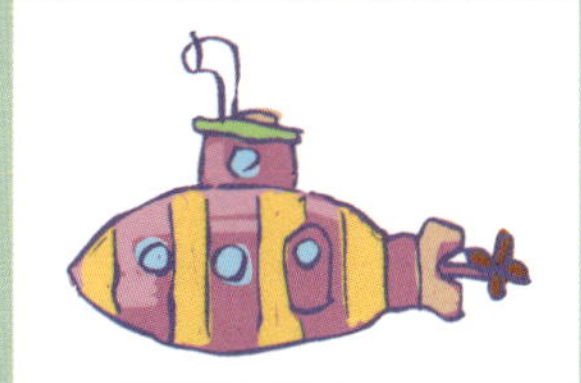

inter-
ĭn-tĕr

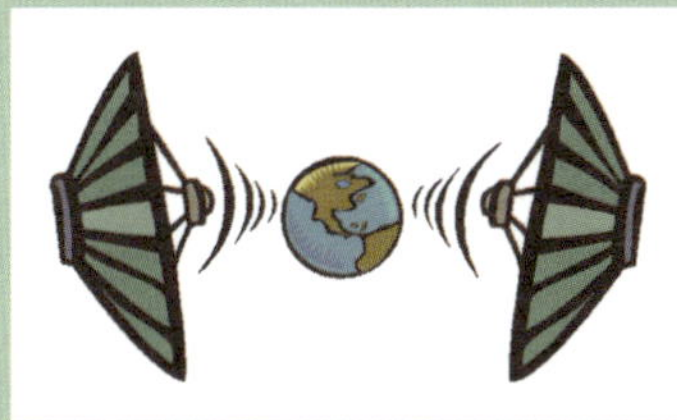

ambi-
ăm-bē

hyper- **super-** **supra-**
hī-pĕr soo-pĕr soo-pră

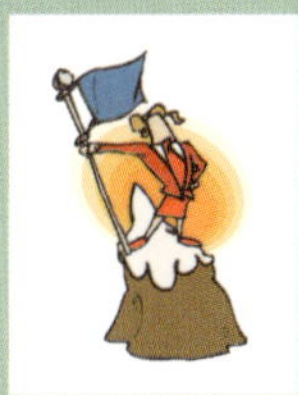

eu-
ū

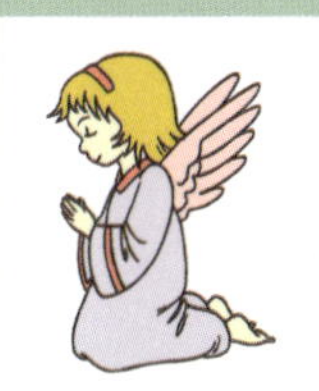

below, beneath

behind, back

between

beside, near

both, both sides, around, about

beyond

excessive, above

deficiency

good, normal

four

hemi- **semi-**
hĕm-ē sĕm-ē

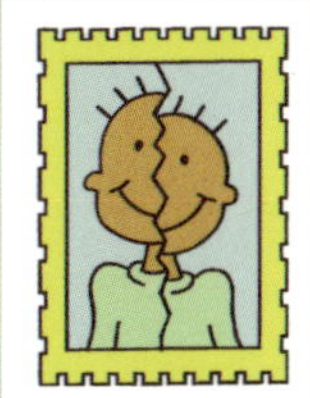

en- **end-** **endo-** **in-** **intra-**
ĕn ĕnd ĕn-dō ĭn ĭn-tră

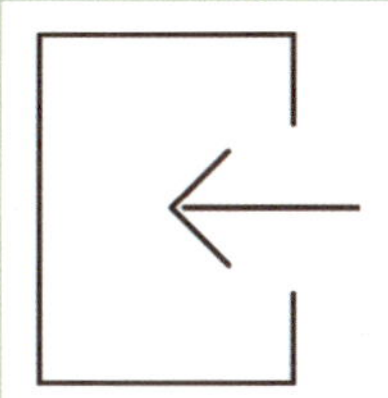

eso-
ĕs-ō

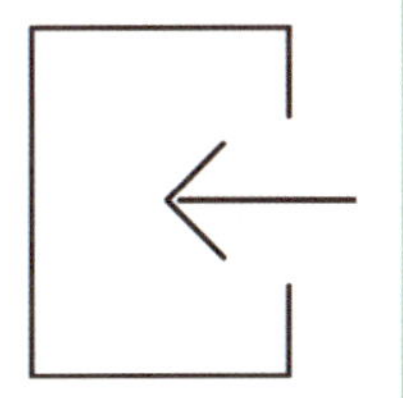

macro-
măk-rō

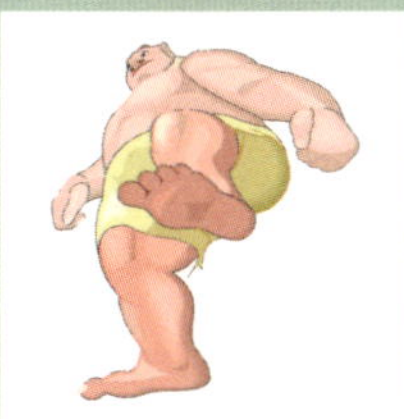

multi- **poly-**
mŭl-tē pŏl-ē

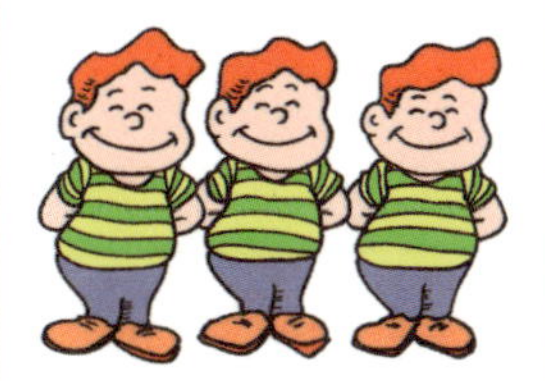

neo-
nē-ō

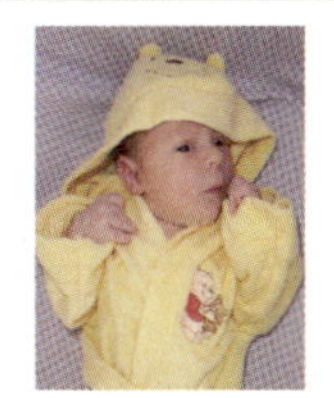

uni- **mono-**
ū-nĭ mŏ-nō

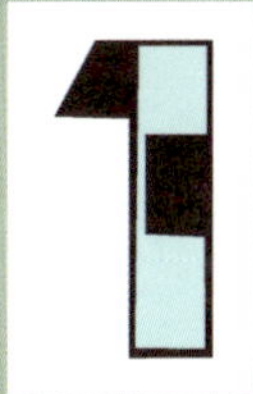

ec- **ecto-**
ĕk ĕk-tō

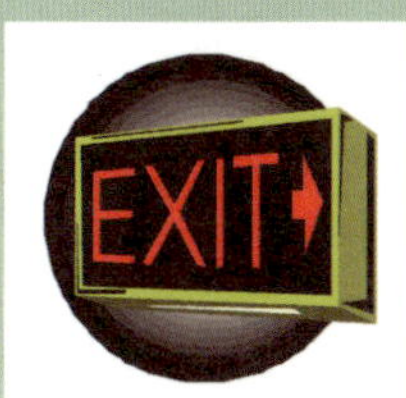

tox-
tŏks

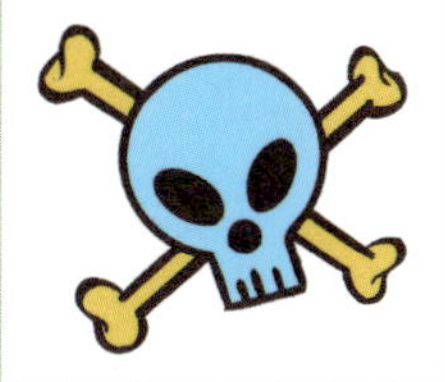

tachy-
tăk-ē

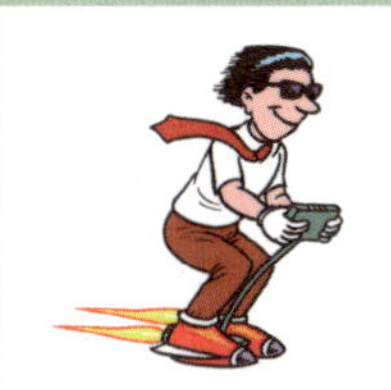

in, within, inner

half

large

inward

new

many, much

out, outside

one, single

rapid

poison, toxin

iso-
ī-sō

auto-
aw-tō

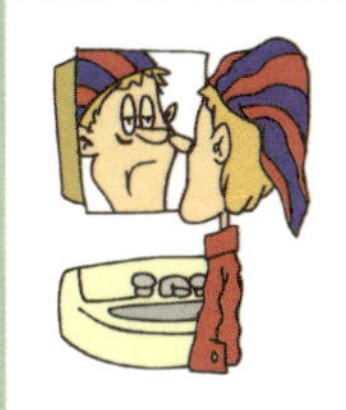

brady-
brăd-ē

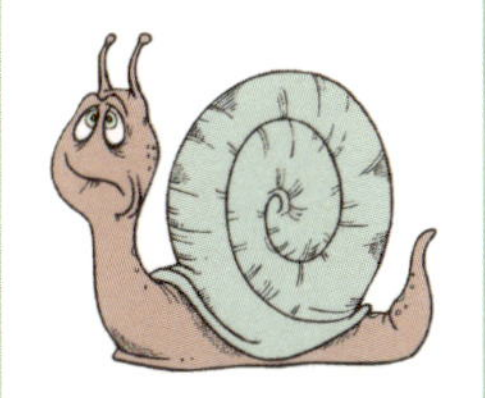

micro-
mī-krō

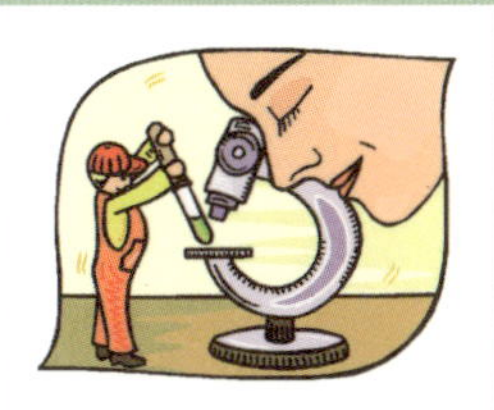

tri-
trī

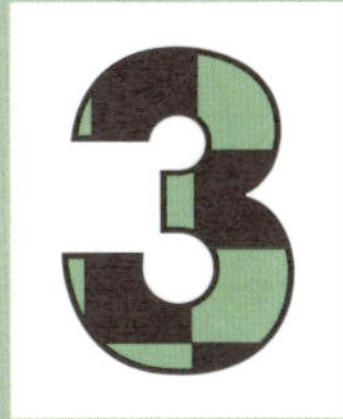

dia- **trans-**
dī-ă trănz

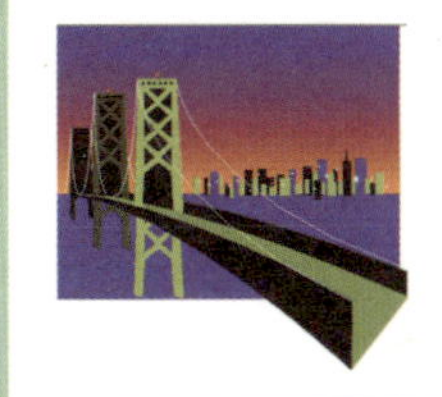

ad-
ăd

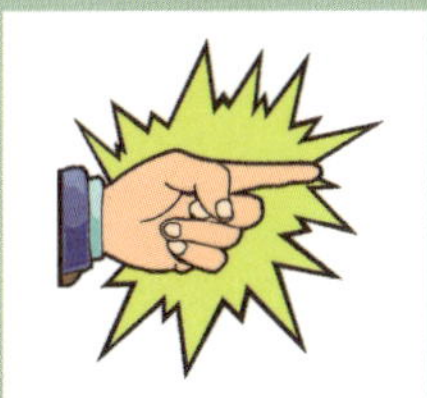

bi- **di-**
bī dī

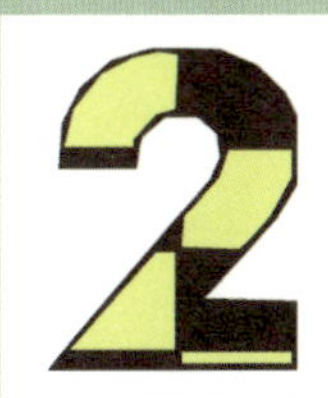

a- **an-** **in-**
ā ăn ĭn

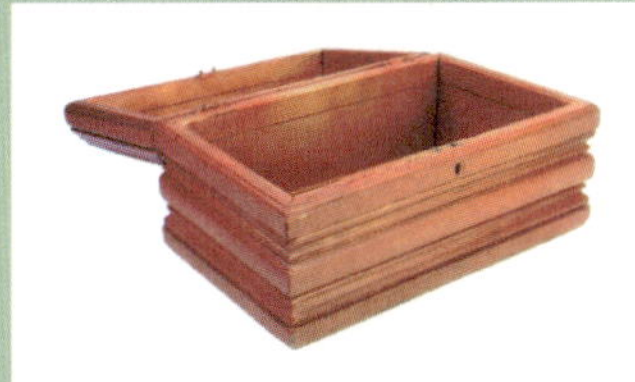

-ac	**-al**	**-ar**	**-ary**	**-eal**	**-ial**
ăk	ăl	ăr	ăr-ē	ē-ăl	ē-ăl
-ic	**-ical**	**-ory**	**-ous**	**-tic**	**-tous**
ĭk	ĭ-kăl	ō-rē	ŭs	tĭk	tŭs

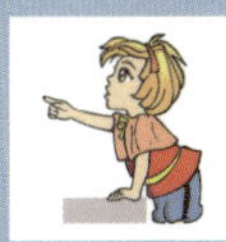

self

same, equal

small

slow

through, across

three

two

toward

pertaining to

without, not, absence of

-algesia ăl-jē-zē-ă **-algesic** ăl-jē-sĭk **-algia** ăl-jē-ă **-dynia** dĭn-ē-ă

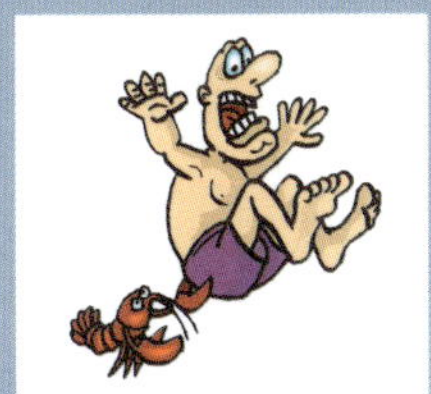

-cele sēl

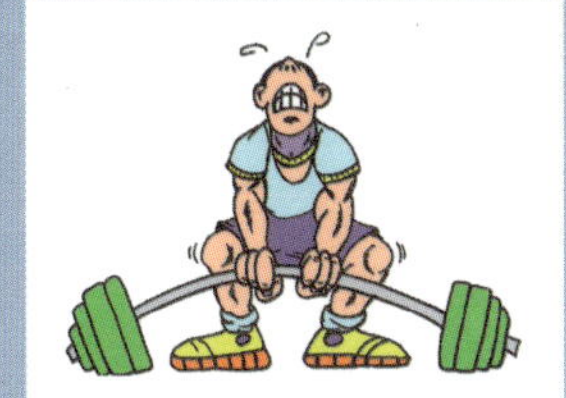

-centesis sĕn-tē-sĭs

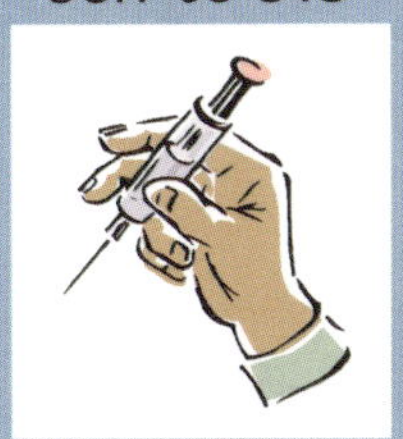

-cidal sĭ-dăl **-cide** sīd

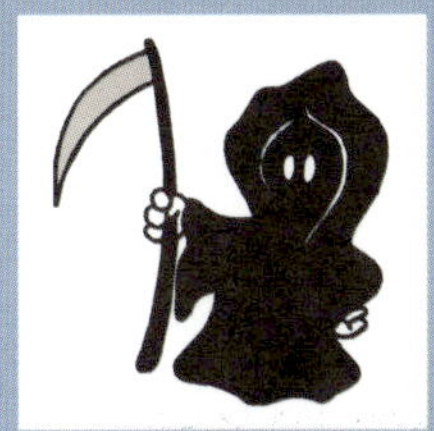

-clasis klă-sĭs **-clast** klăst

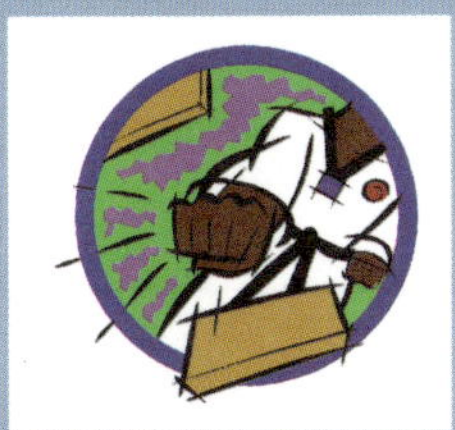

-cyte sīt **-cytic** sīt-ĭk

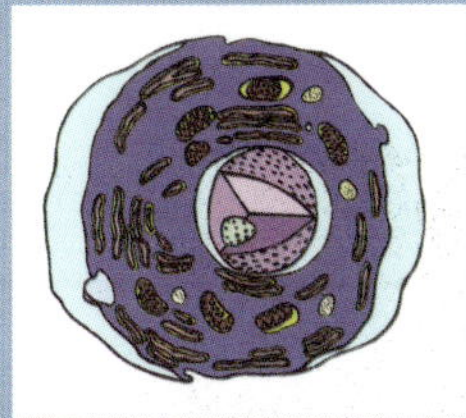

-derma dĕr-mă

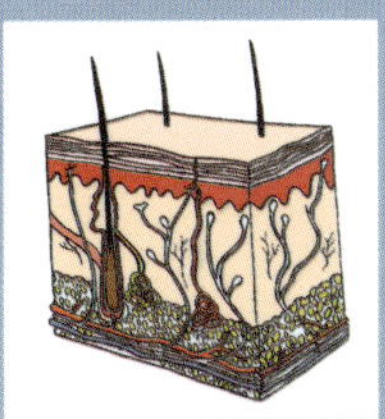

-dipsia dĭp-sē-ă

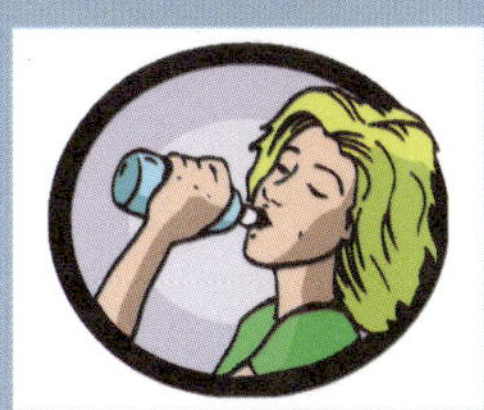

-ectasis ĕk-tă-sĭs

-ectomy ĕk-tō-mē

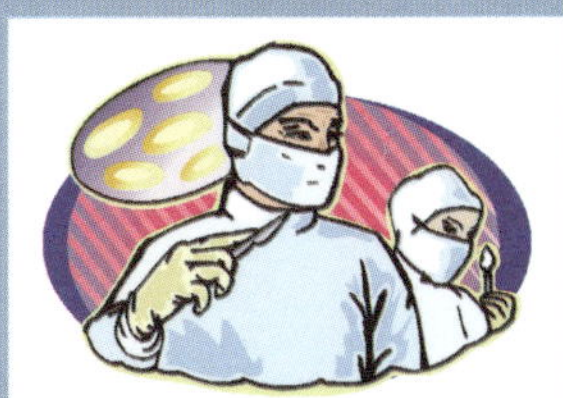

hernia

pain

destroying, killing

surgical puncture

cell

to break

thirst

skin

excision, surgical removal

dilation, expansion

-edema
ĕ-dē-mă

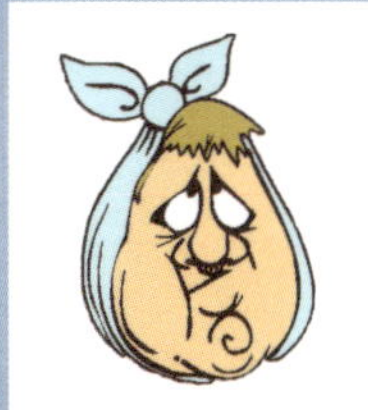

-emia
ē-mē-ă

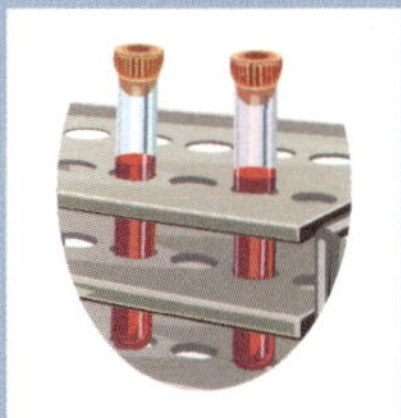

-emesis
ĕm-ĕ-sĭs

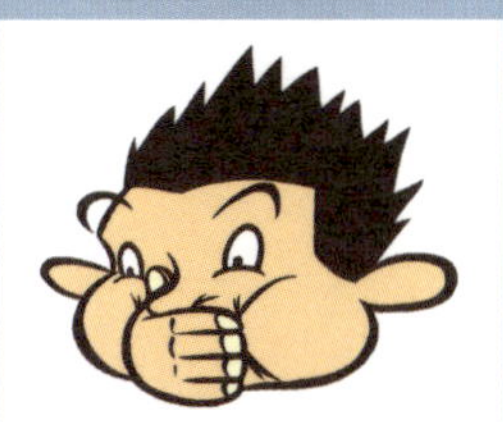

-esthesia
ĕs-thē-zē-ă

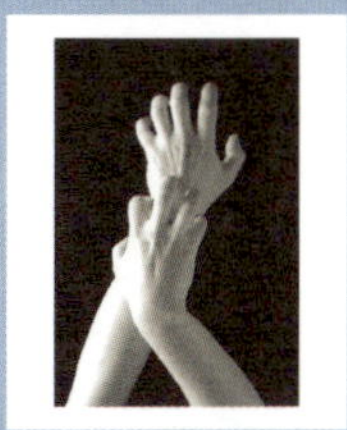

-gen jĕn **-genesis** jĕn-ĕ-sĭs **-genic** jĕn-ĭk **-genous** jĕn-ŭs

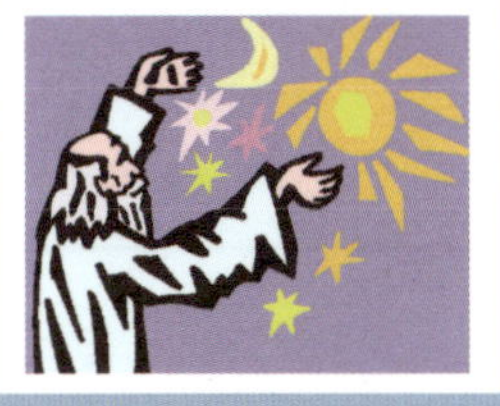

-gram
grăm

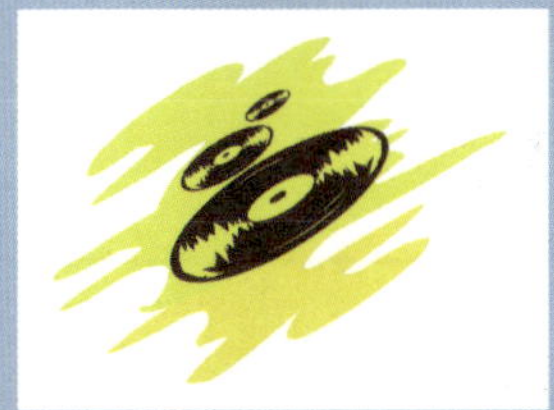

-graph
grăf

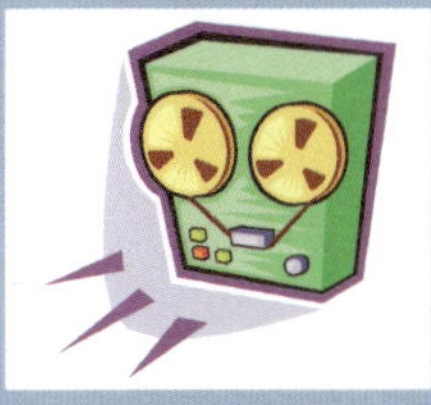

-graphy
gră-fē

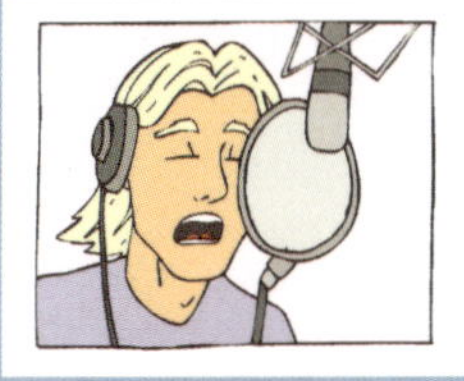

-gravida
grăv-ĭ-dă

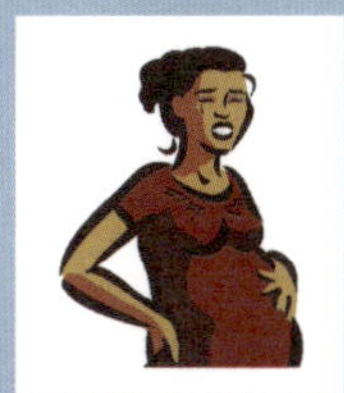

-ia ē-ă **-ism** ĭ-zum

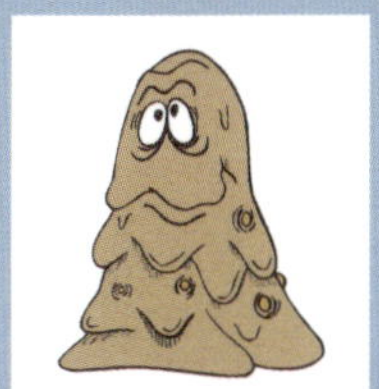

a condition of the blood

swelling

sensation

vomiting

record

creating, producing

process of recording

recording instrument

condition

pregnant woman

-iasis
ī-ă-sĭs

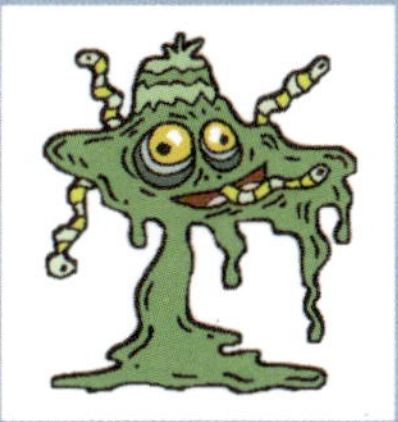

-itis
ī-tĭs

-lith
lĭth

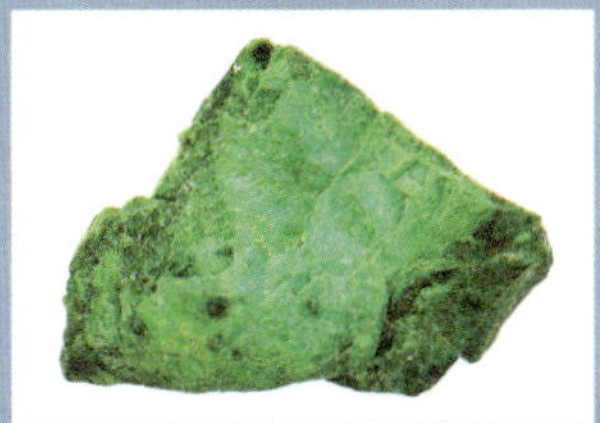

-meter
mĕ-tĕr

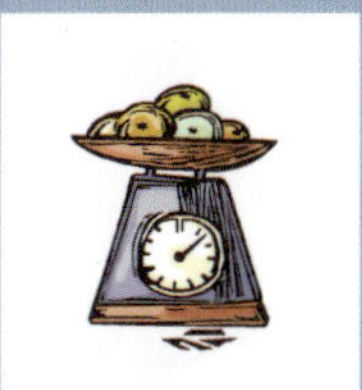

-malacia
mă-lā-sē-ă

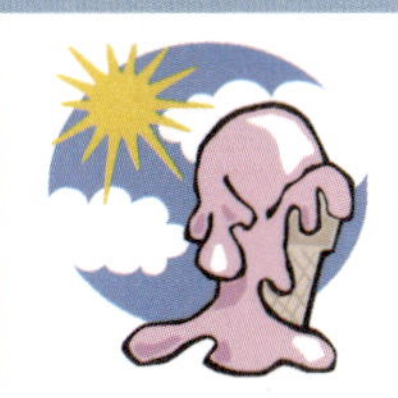

-iatrist **-ician** **-ist** **-logist** **-ologist**
ī-ă-trĭst ĭ-shŭn ĭst lō-jist ŏl-ō-jist

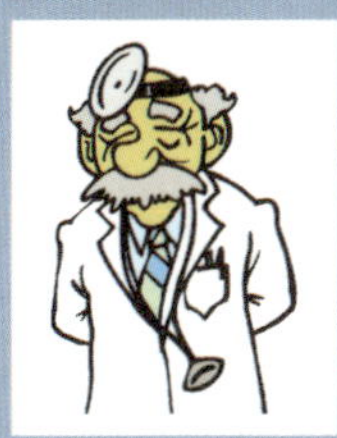

-kinesia **-kinesis**
kī-nē-zē-ă kĭ-nē-sĭs

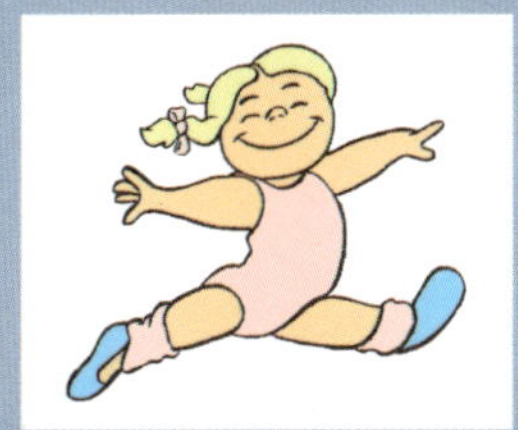

-megaly
mĕg-ă-lē

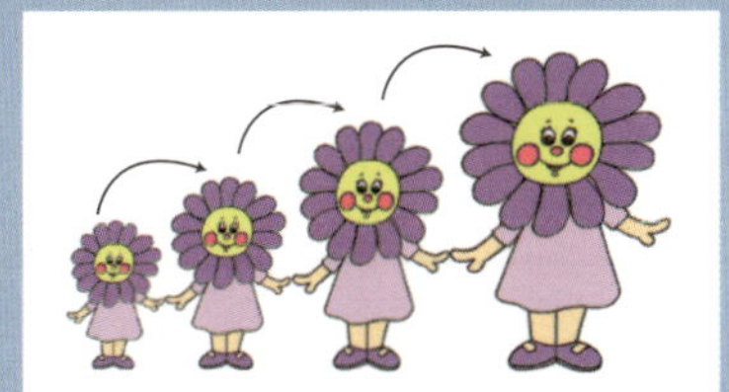

-lysis
lĭ-sĭs

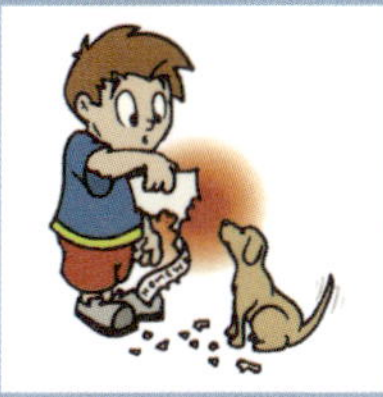

-ole **-ule**
ōl ūl

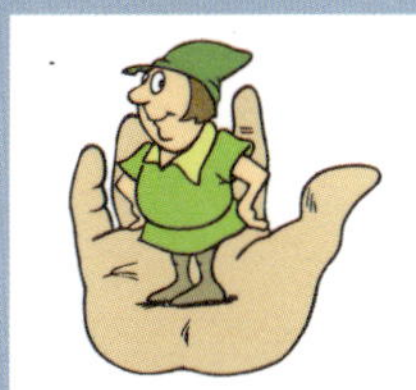

specialist, specialist in the study of

pathological condition or state

movement

inflammation

enlargement

stone

destruction

measuring instrument

small

softening

-oma
ō-mă

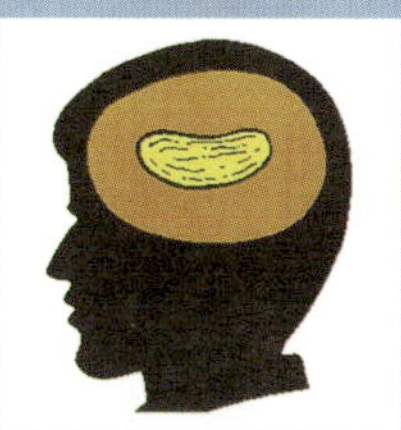

-oid
oyd

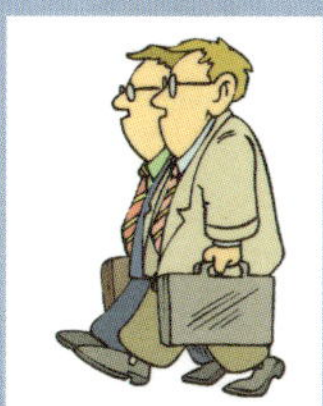

-paresis
păr-ē-sĭs

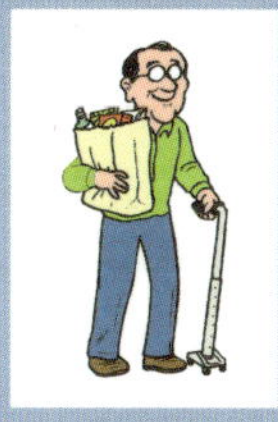

-osis
ō-sĭs

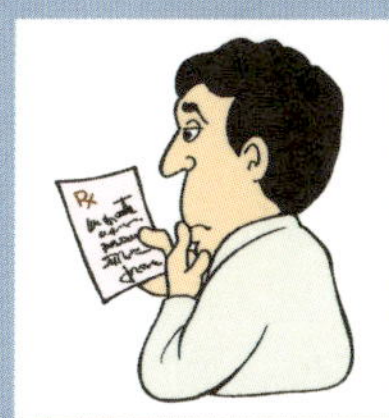

-pepsia
pĕp-sē-ă

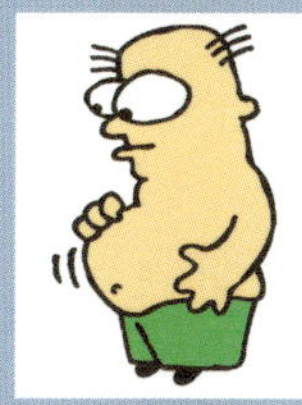

-metry
mĕ-trē

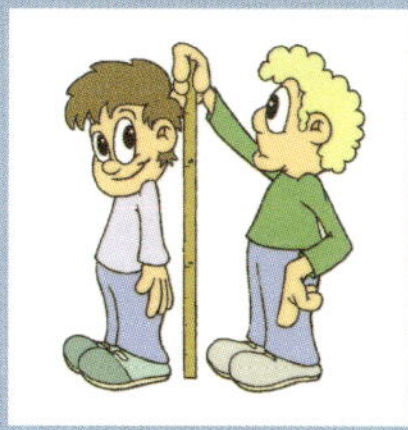

-oxia
ŏk-sē-ă

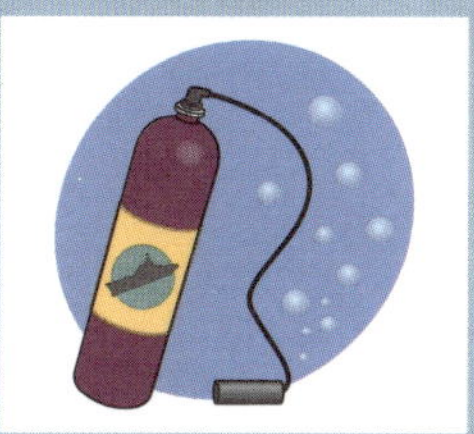

-opia ō-pē-ă

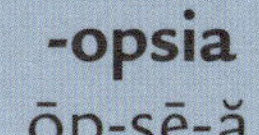

-opsia ōp-sē-ă

-opsis ōp-sis

-opsy ōp-sē

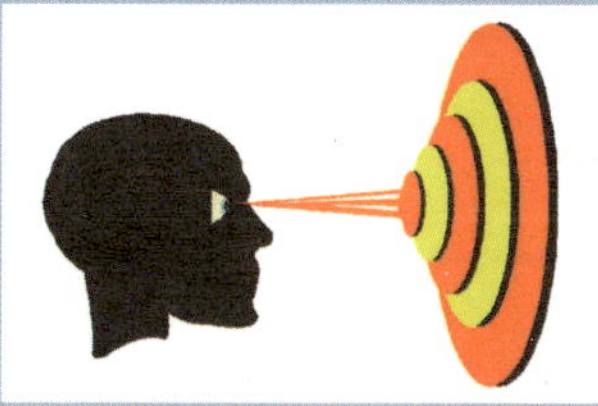

-penia
pē-nē-ă

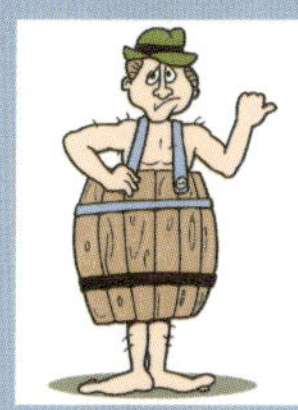

-pathy
pă-thē

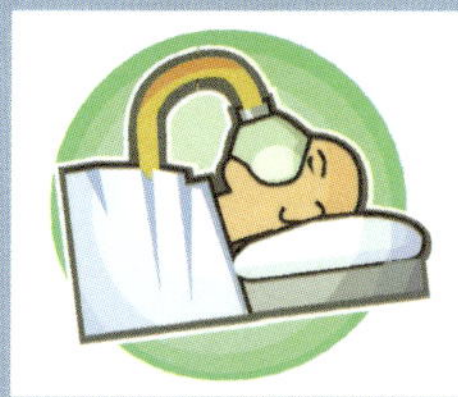

measurement

tumor

oxygen

resembling

vision, view of

slight or partial paralysis

deficiency

abnormal condition

disease

digestion

-pause **-stasis**
pawz stă-sĭs

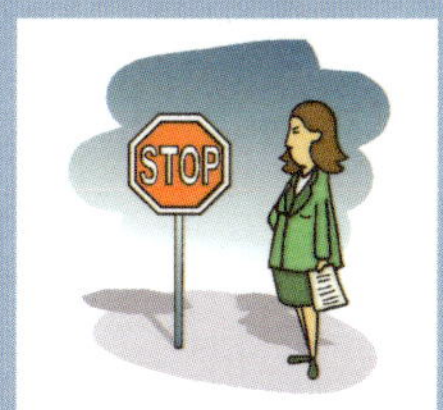

-phasia
fā-zē-ă

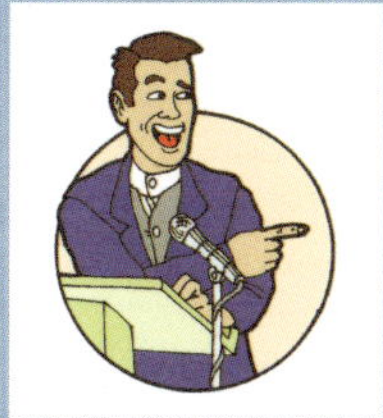

-phobia
fō-bē-ă

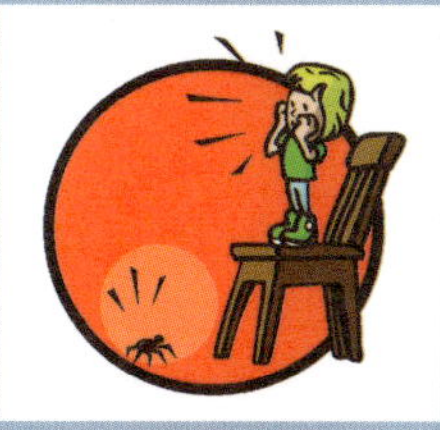

-pexy
pĕk-sē

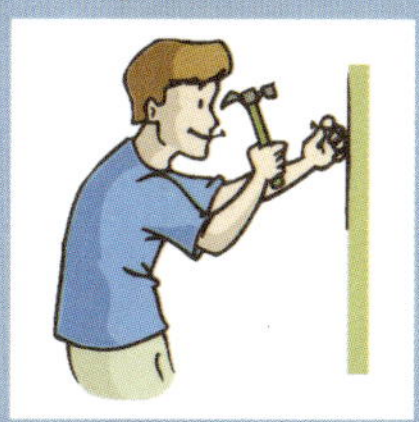

-phage **-phagia**
fāj fā-jē-ă

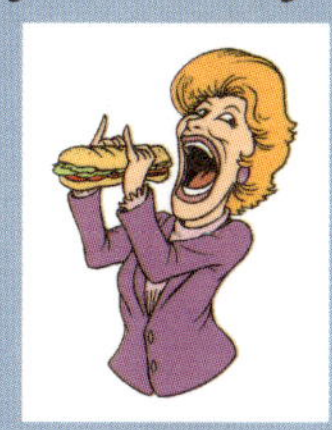

-plasty
plăs-tē

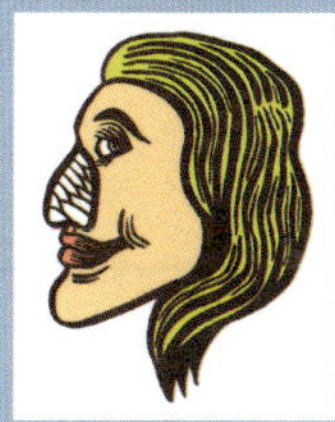

-plegia
plē-jē-ă

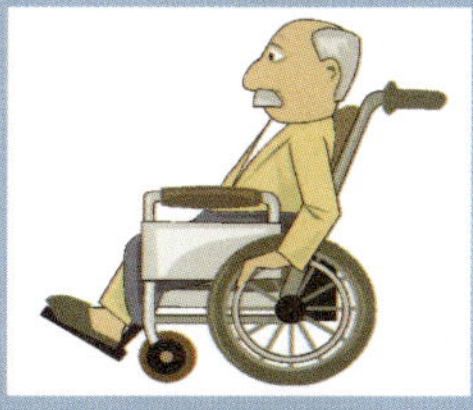

-phoria
fō-rē-ă

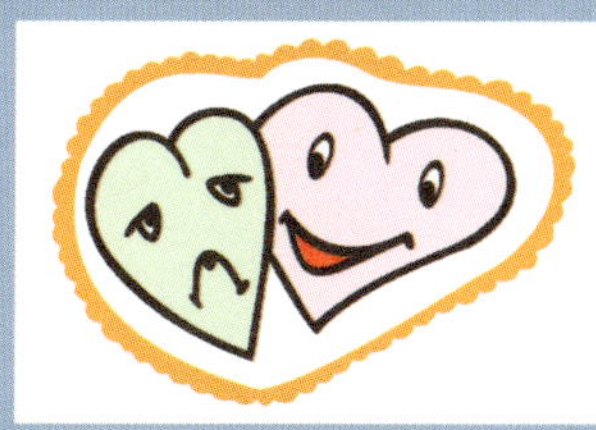

-plasia **-plasm**
plā-zē-ă plă-zum

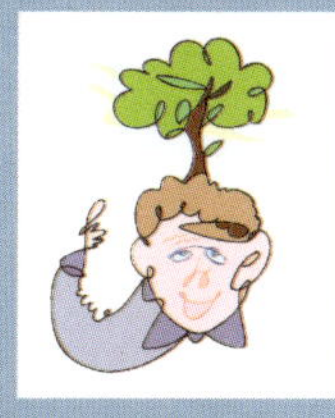

-rrhage **-rrhagia**
rĭj ră-jē-ă

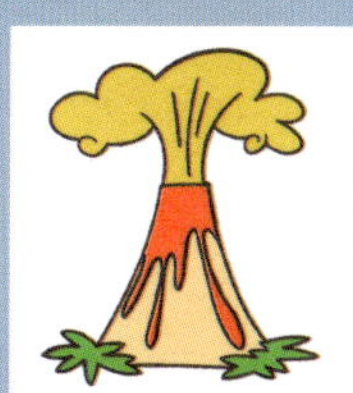

speech

cessation, stopping

surgical fixation

fear

surgical repair

eating, swallowing

feeling

paralysis

bursting forth

formation, growth

-rrhaphy
ră-fē

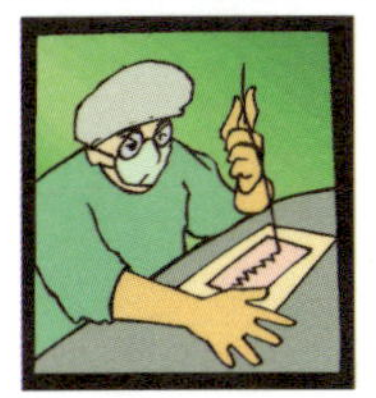

-ptosis
tō-sĭs

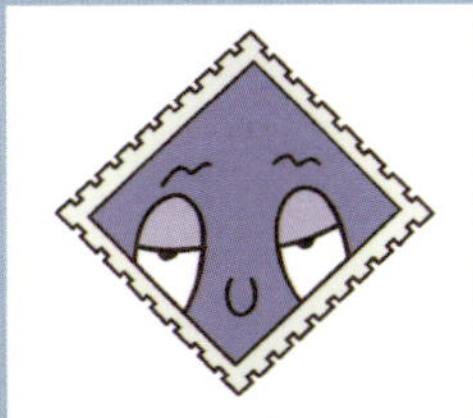

-scopy
skō-pē

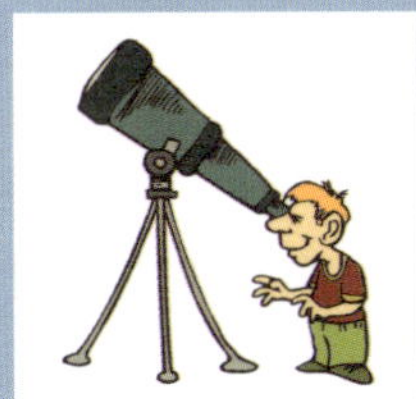

-rrhexis
rĕk-sĭs

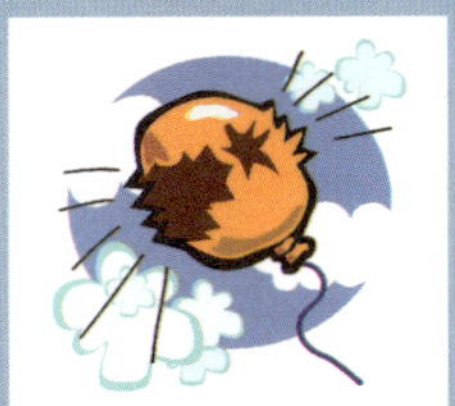

-therapy
thĕr-ă-pē

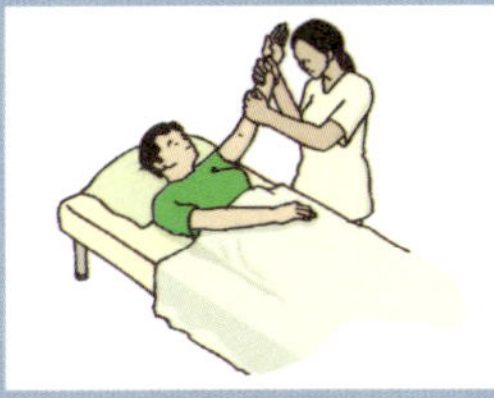

-pnea
nē-ă

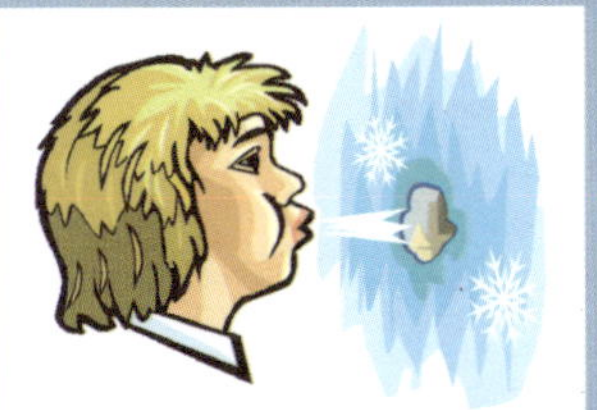

-scope
skōp

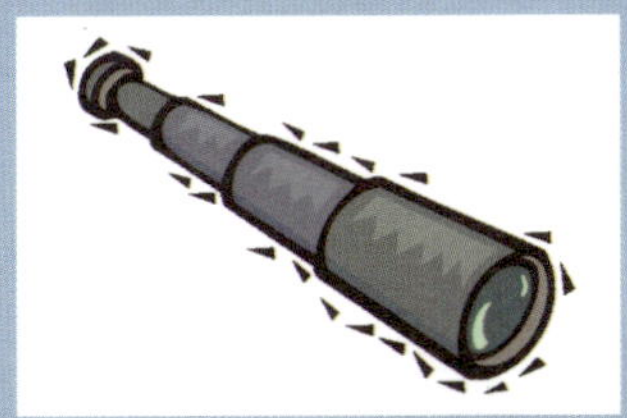

-rrhea
rē-ă

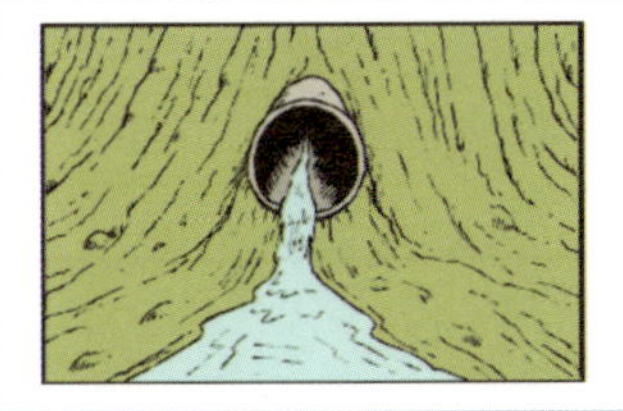

-stomy
stō-mē

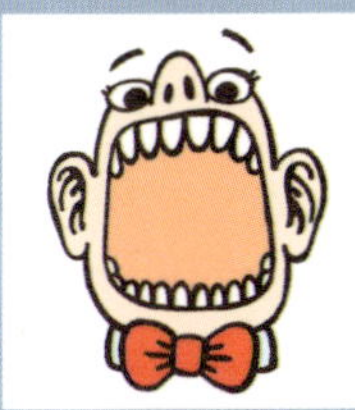

-stenosis
stĕ-nō-sĭs

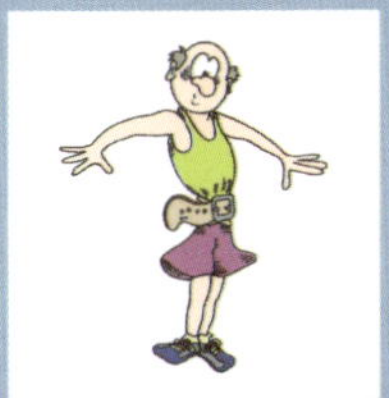

breathing

suture, suturing

viewing instrument

drooping, prolapse

flow, discharge

visual examination

mouthlike opening

rupture

narrowing, stricture

treatment

-tripsy
trĭp-sē

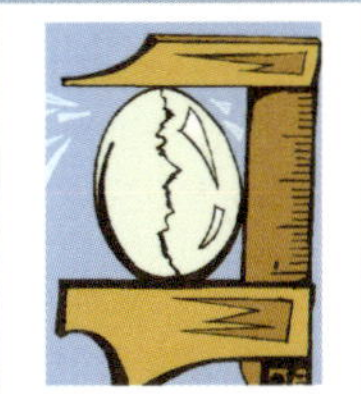

-trophy
trō-fē

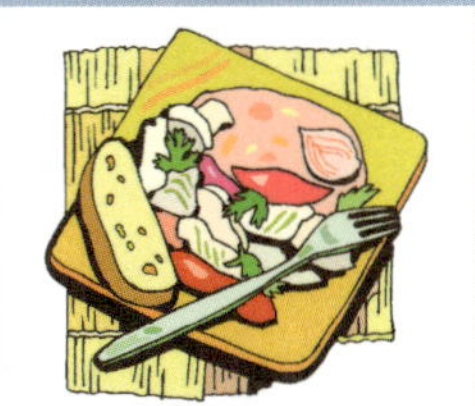

-tome
tōm

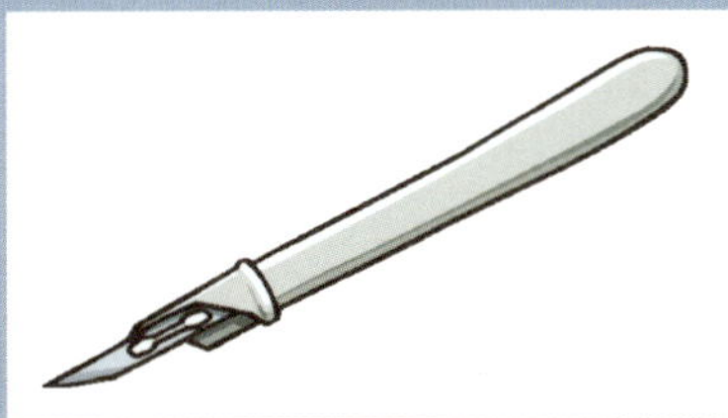

-tomy
tō-mē

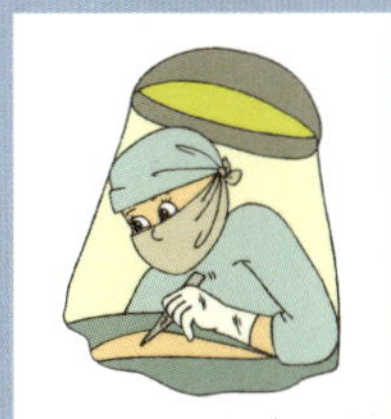

-acusia ă-koo-zē-ă **-acusis** ă-koo-sĭs **-cusis** koo-sĭs

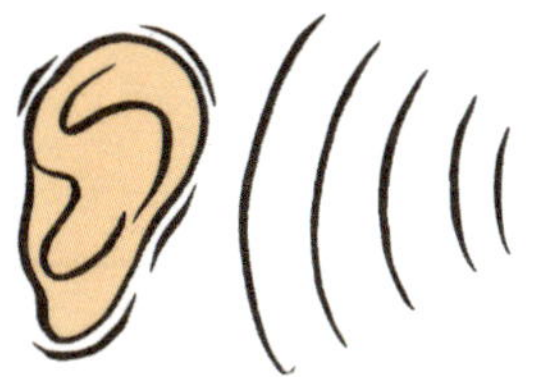

-osmia
ŏz-mē-ă

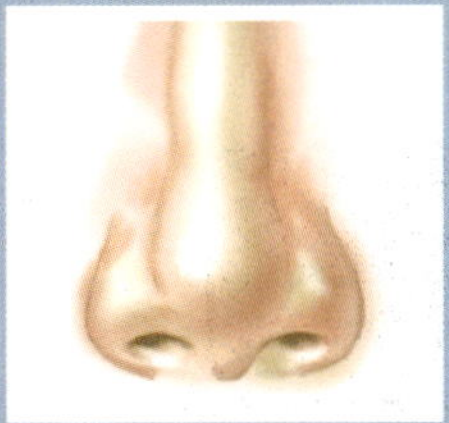

-uria
ū-rē-ă

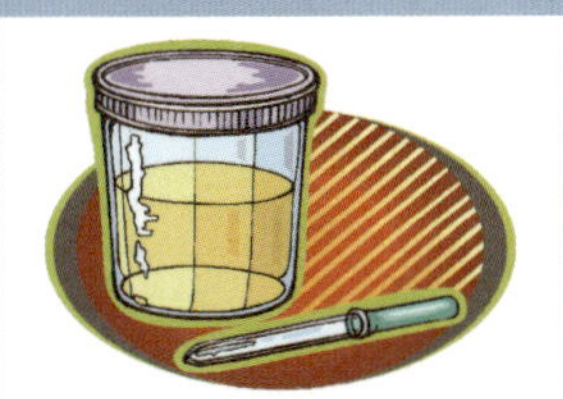

-static
stă-tik

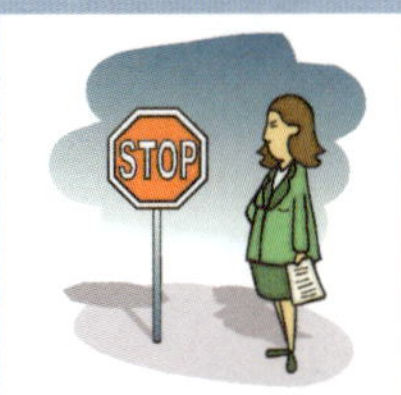

-salpinx
săl-pĭnks

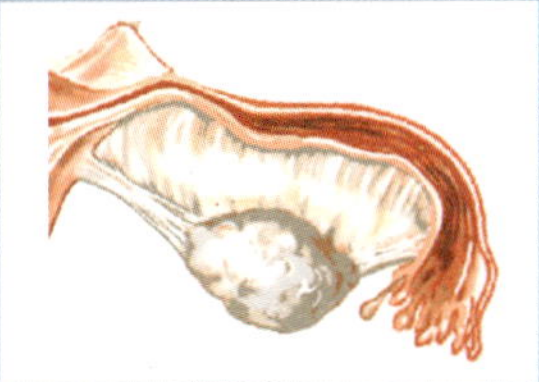

-thorax
thōr-ăks

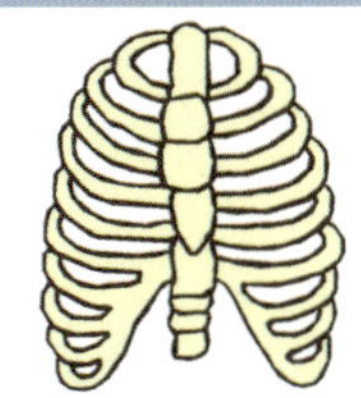

nourishment, growth

crushing

cutting into, incision

cutting instrument

smell, odor

hearing

not in motion, at rest

urine

chest

uterine (fallopian) tube

-lepsy **-leptic**

lĕp-sē lĕp-tĭk

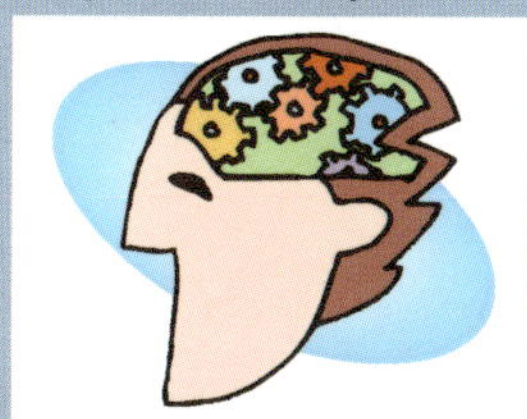

-phonia

fō-nē-ă

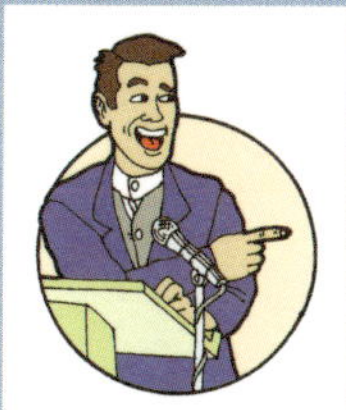

-partum **-tocia**

părt-ŭm tō-sē-ă

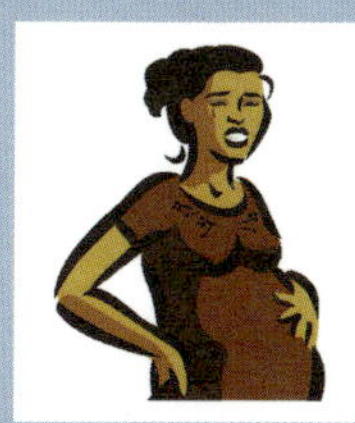

medi/o

mē-dē-ō

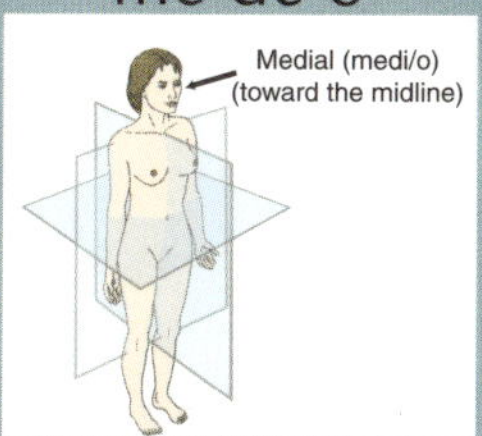

super/o

su-pir-ō

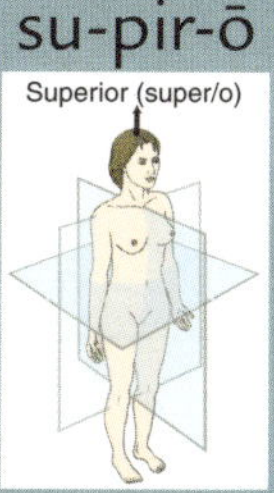

anter/o

an-tir-ō

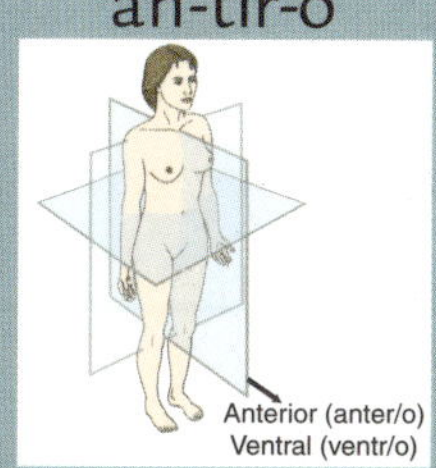

later/o

la-tər-ō

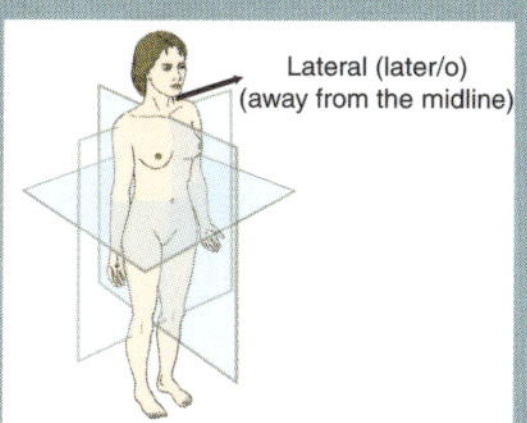

infer/o

in-fir-ō

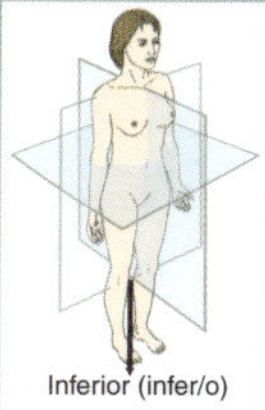

poster/o

pō-stir-ō

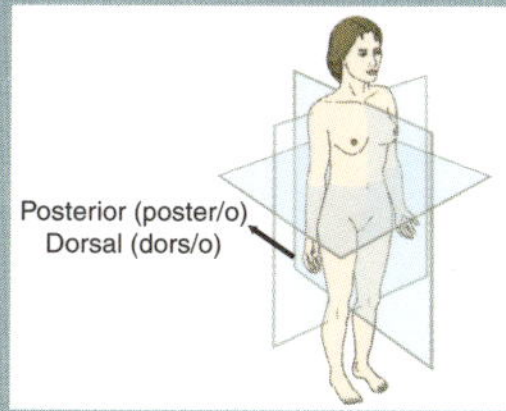

cyt/o

sī-tō

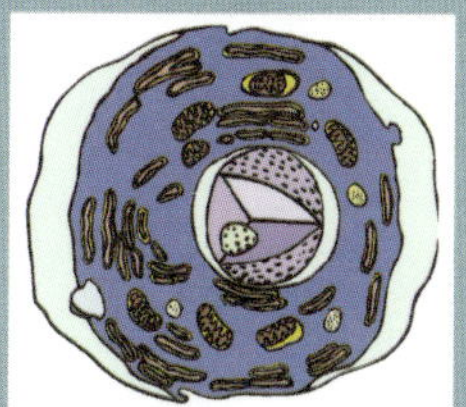

voice

seizure

medial
(toward the midline; nearer to the middle)

childbirth, labor

anterior
(toward or near the front; ventral)

superior
(above or nearer to the head)

inferior
(beneath or nearer to the feet)

lateral
(away from the midline; toward the side)

cell

posterior
(toward or near the back; dorsal)

corne/o **kerat/o**
kōr-nē-ō kĕr-ăt-ō

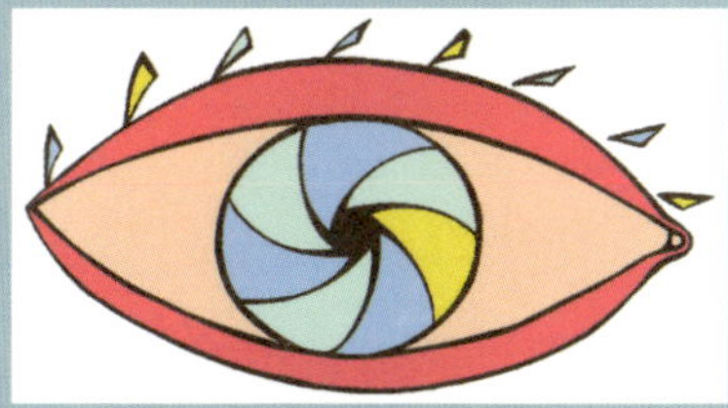

adip/o **lip/o** **steat/o**
ăd-ĭ-pō lĭ-pō stē-ă-tō

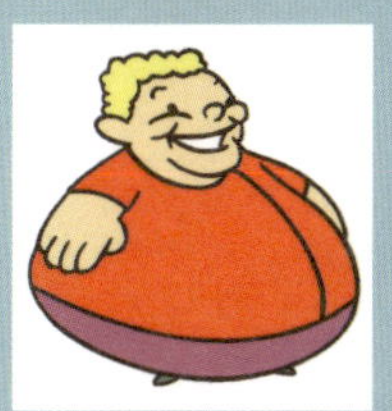

cutane/o **derm/o** **dermat/o**
kū-tā-nē-ō dĕr-mō dĕr-mă-tō

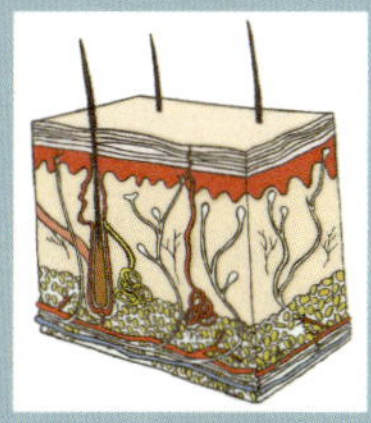

onych/o
ŏn-ĭ-kō

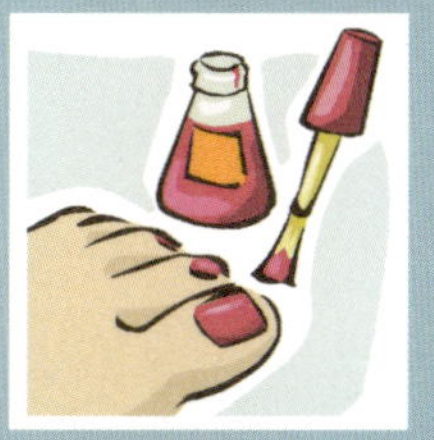

scler/o
sklĕ-rō

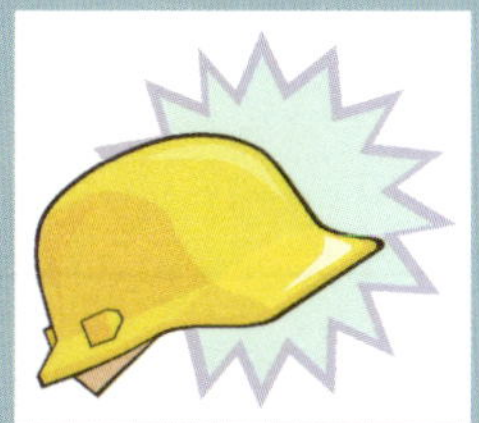

myc/o
mī-kō

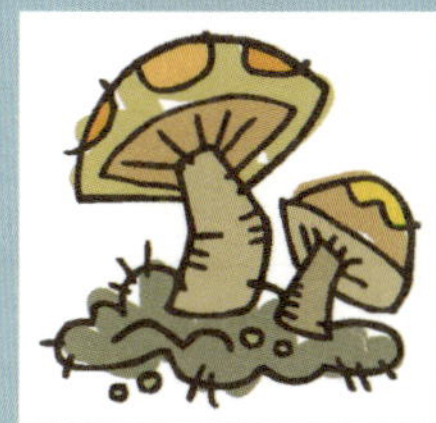

necr/o
nĕ-crō

pil/o **trich/o**
pī-lō trĭ-kō

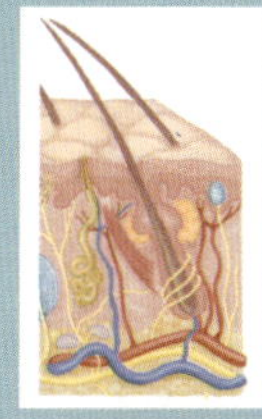

cyan/o
sī-ă-nō

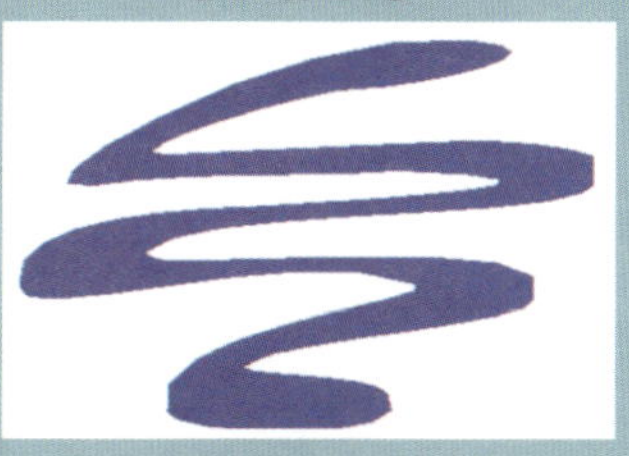

xer/o
zē-rō

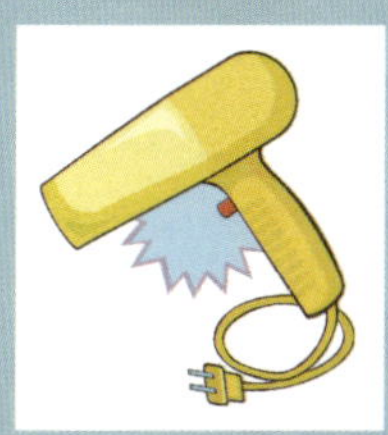

fat

keratinized tissue, cornea

nail

skin

fungus

hardening, sclera

hair

dead

dry

blue

albin/o ăl-bĭ-nō **leuk/o** loo-kō

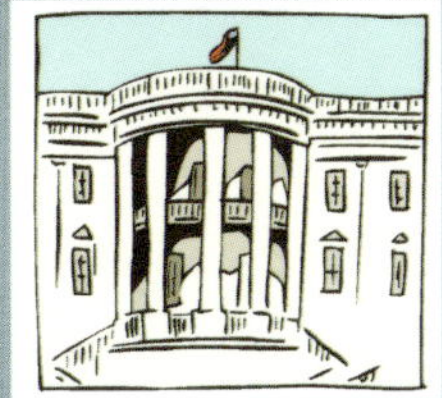

mening/o mĕn-ĭn-jō **meningi/o** mĕn-ĭn-jē-ō

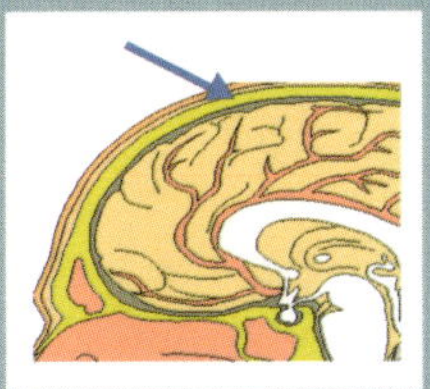

myel/o mī-ĕl-ō

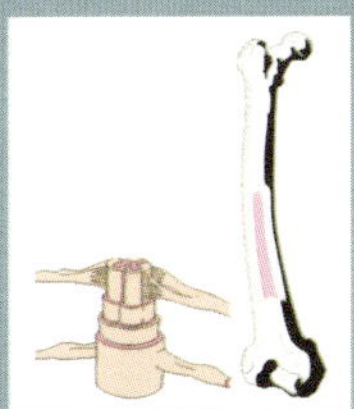

melan/o mĕl-ă-nō

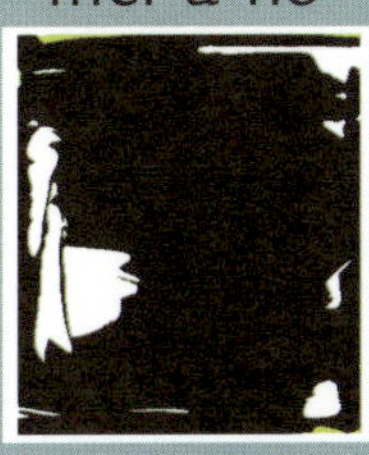

cirrh/o sĭ-rō **xanth/o** zăn-thō

cerebr/o sĕr-ĕ-brō **encephal/o** ĕn-sĕf-ă-lō

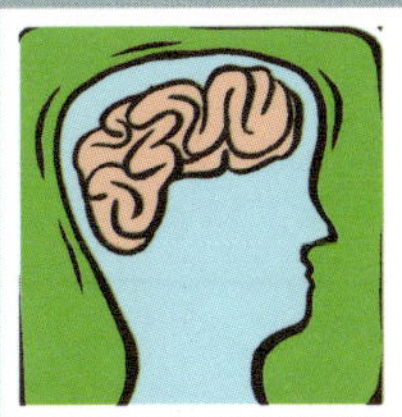

phas/o fā-zō

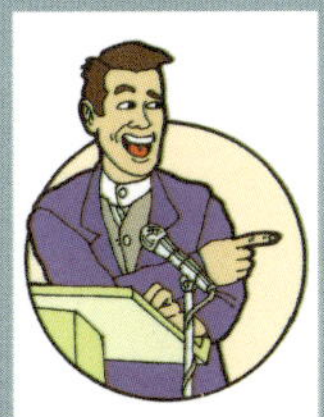

hydr/o hī-drō

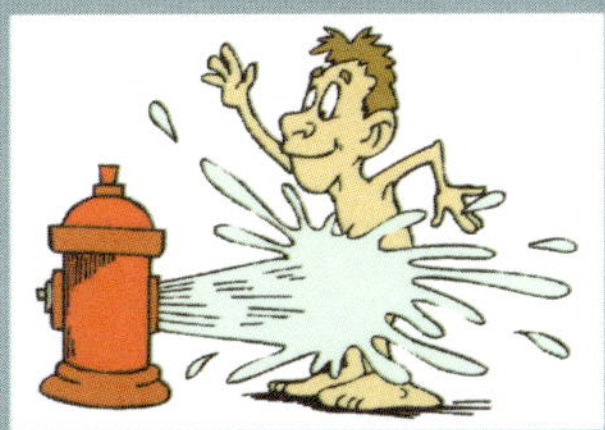

cerebell/o sĕr-ĕ-bĕl-ō

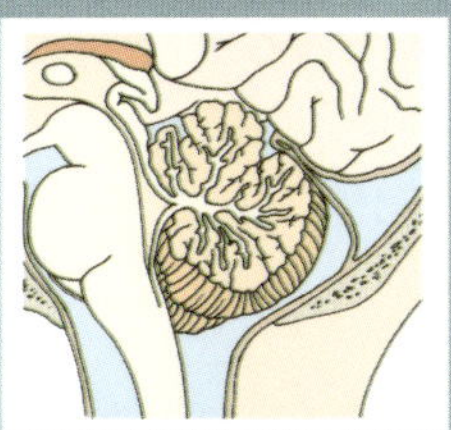

gli/o glī-ō

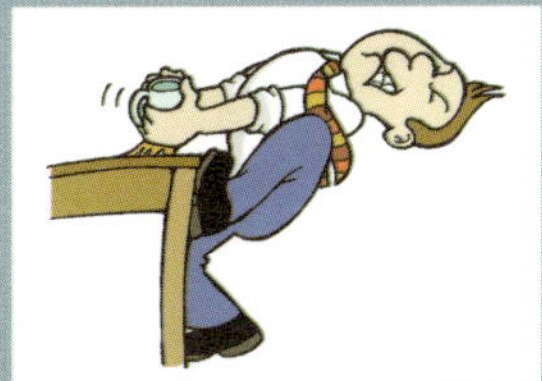

meninges

white

black

spinal cord,
bone marrow

brain

yellow

water

speech

glue, gluelike

cerebellum

neur/o
nū-rō

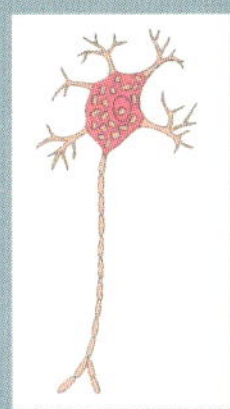

spin/o
spī-nō

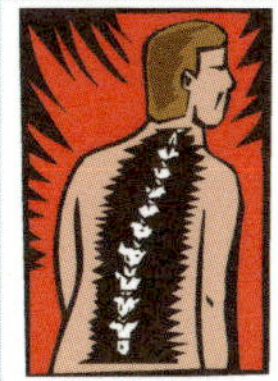

aden/o
ăd-ĕ-nō

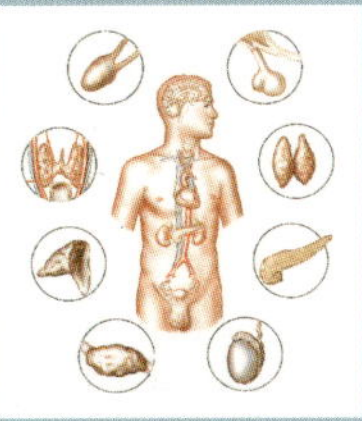

angi/o **vas/o**
ăn-jē-ō văs-ō

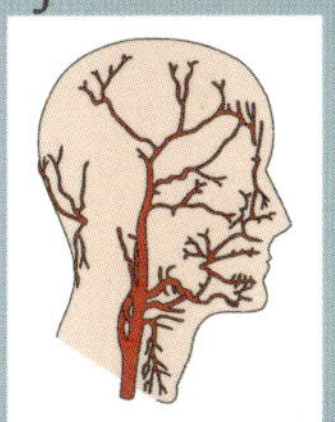

arteri/o
ăr-tē-rē-ō

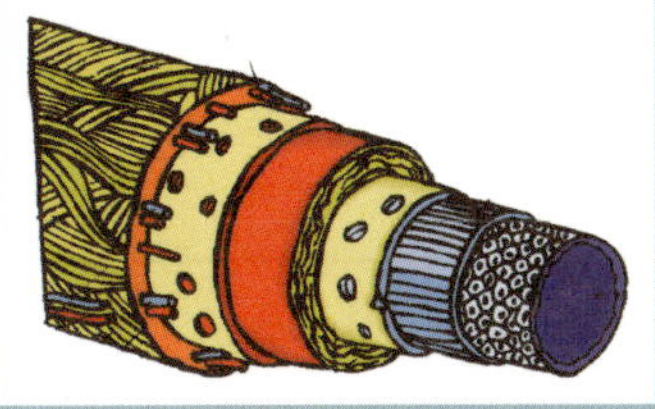

aort/o
ā-ōr-tō

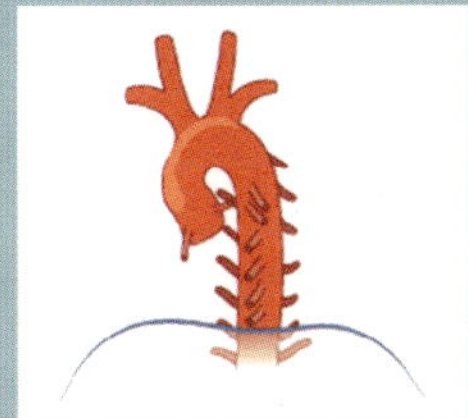

ather/o
ăth-ĕr-ō

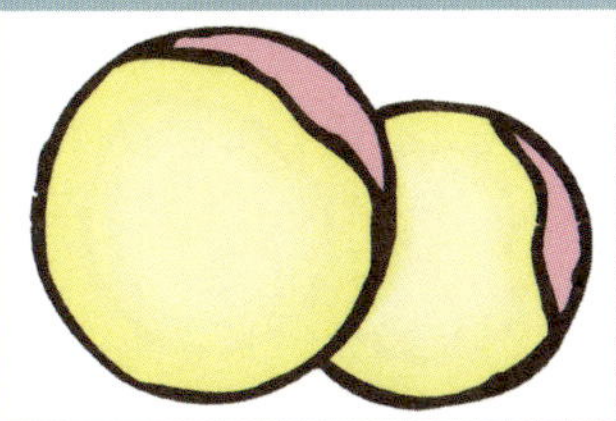

atri/o
ā-trē-ō

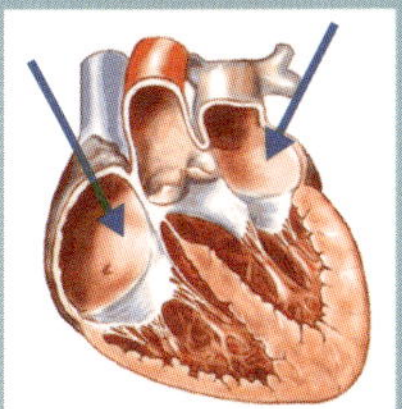

cardi/o **coron/o**
căr-dē-ō kor-ōn-ō

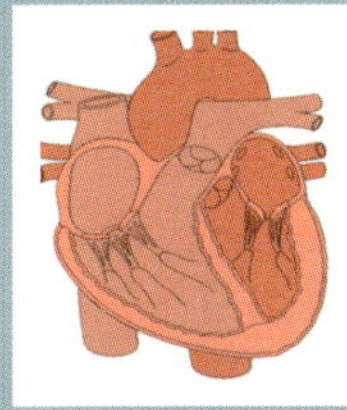

electr/o
ē-lĕk-tr-ō

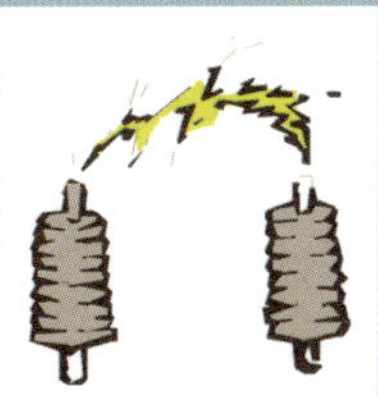

spine

nerve

vessel

gland

aorta

artery

atria

thick, fatty

electricity

heart

hem/o **hemat/o**
hē-mō hĕm-ăt-ō

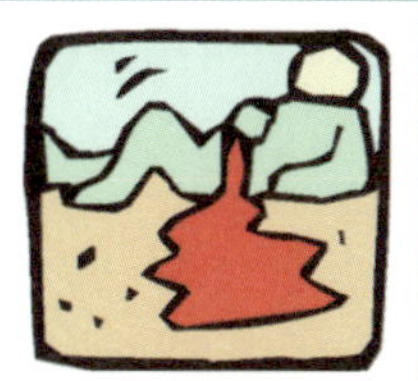

lymph/o
lĭm-fō

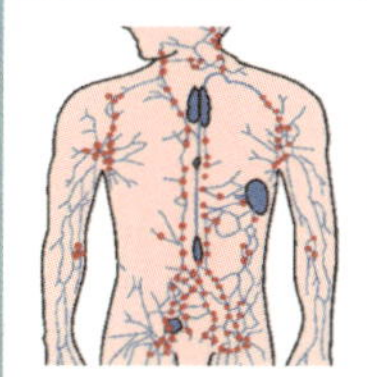

phleb/o **ven/o**
flĕb-ō vē-nō

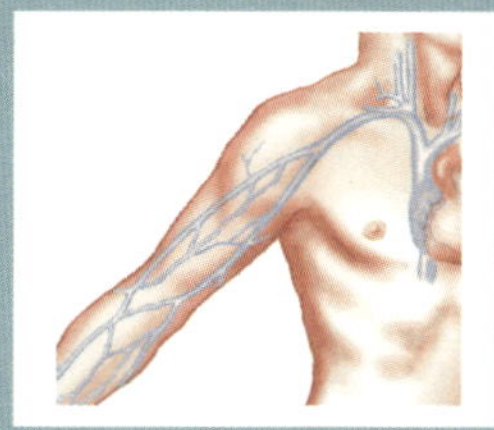

thromb/o
thrŏm-bō

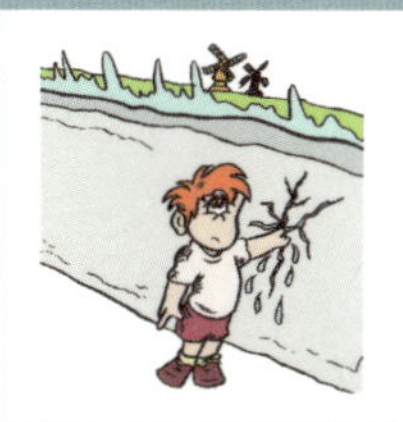

splen/o
splē-nō

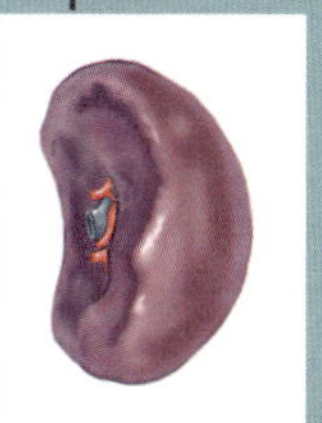

ventricul/o
vĕn-trĭk-ū-lō

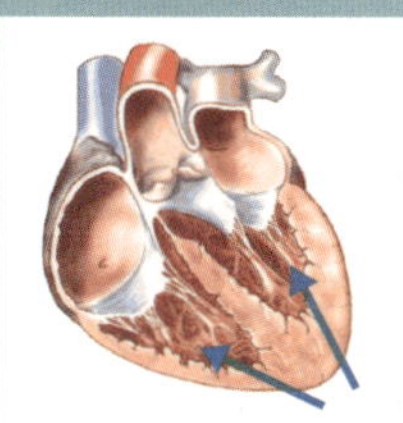

valv/o **valvul/o**
văl-vō văl-vū-lō

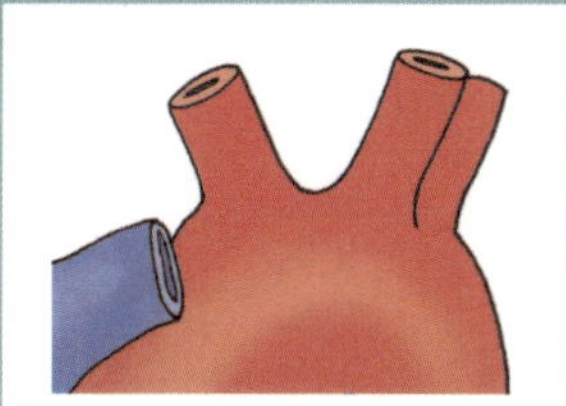

tox/o **toxic/o**
tŏks-ō tŏks-ĭ-kō

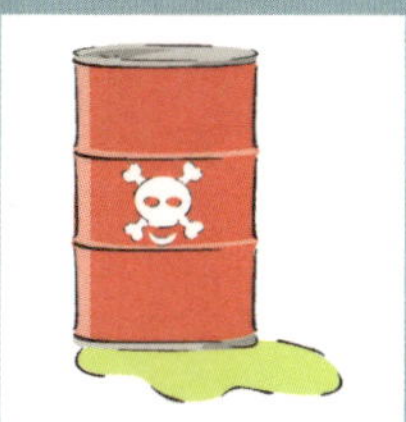

path/o
păth-ō

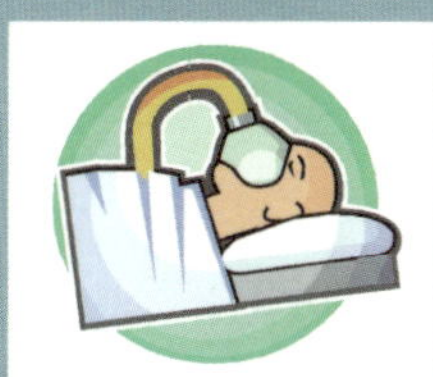

bacteri/o
băk-tē-rē-ō

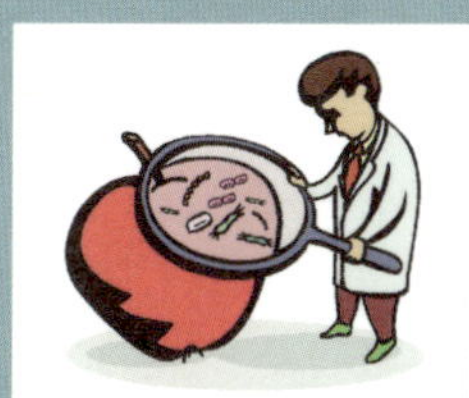

lymph	blood
thrombus (clot)	vein
ventricle	spleen
poison, toxin	valve
bacteria	disease

lymphaden/o
lĭm-făd-ĕ-nō

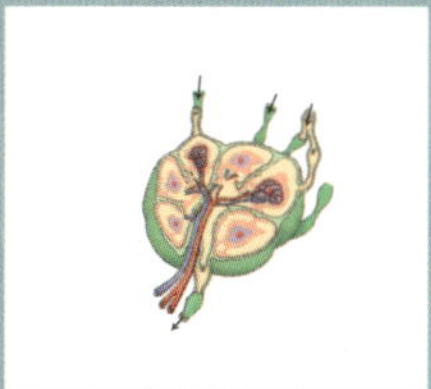

bronch/o **bronchi/o**
brŏng-kō brŏng-kē-ō

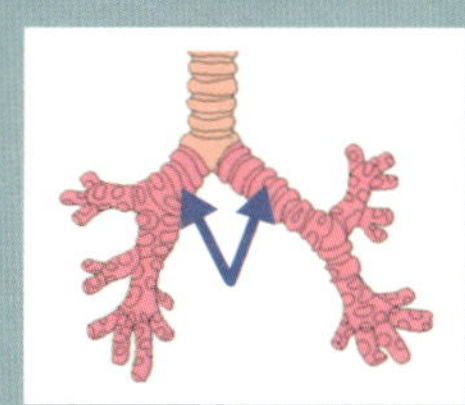

nas/o **rhin/o**
nā-zō rī-nō

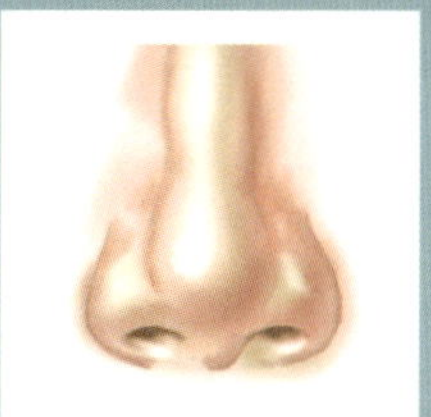

chondr/o
kŏn-drō

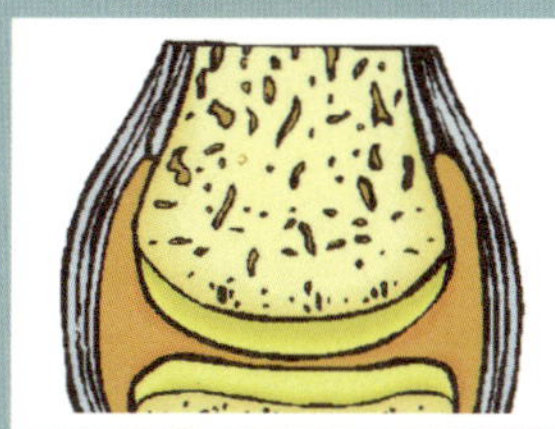

epiglott/o
ĕp-ĭ-glŏt-ō

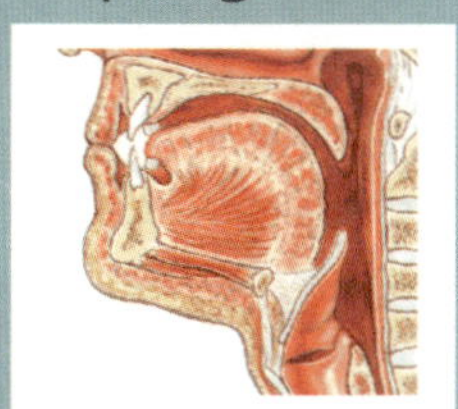

laryng/o
lăr-ĭn-gō

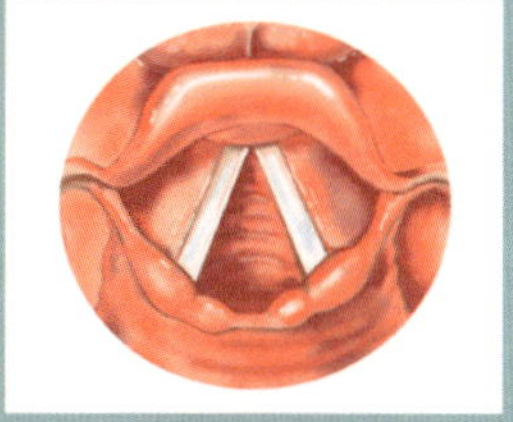

pleur/o
ploo-rō

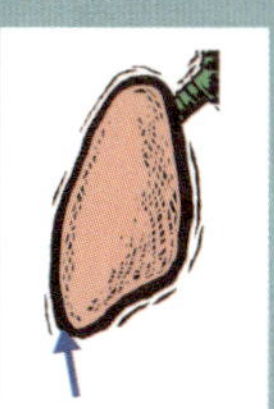

or/o **stomat/o**
ō-rō stō-mă-tō

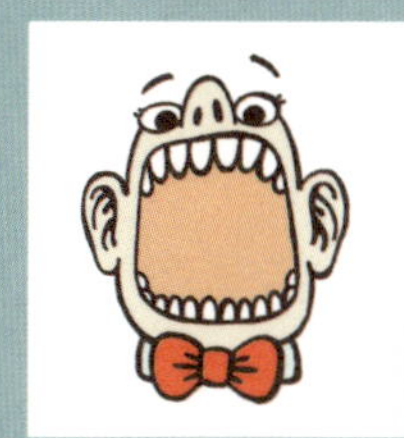

ox/i **ox/o**
ŏk-sē ŏk-sō

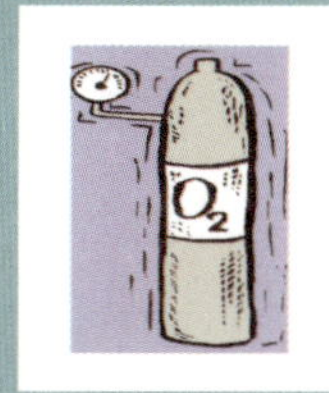

pharyng/o
făr-ĭn-gō

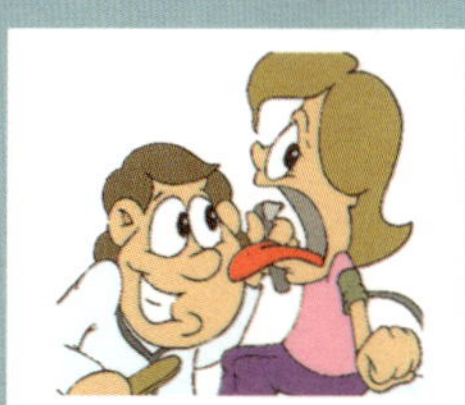

bronchus

lymph gland

cartilage

nose

larynx

epiglottis

mouth, mouthlike opening

pleura

pharynx

oxygen

thorac/o
thō-ră-kō

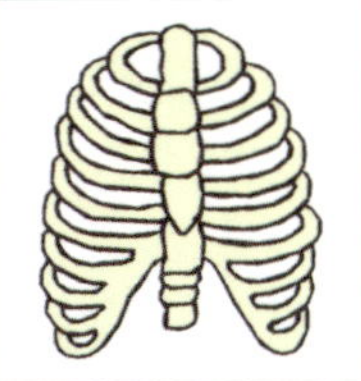

pneum/o **pneumon/o**
nū-mō nū-mŏ-nō

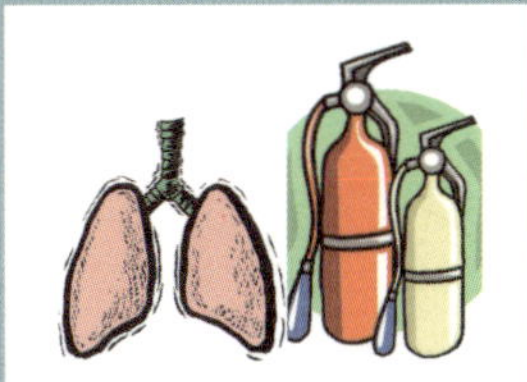

pulmon/o
pŭl-mŏ-nō

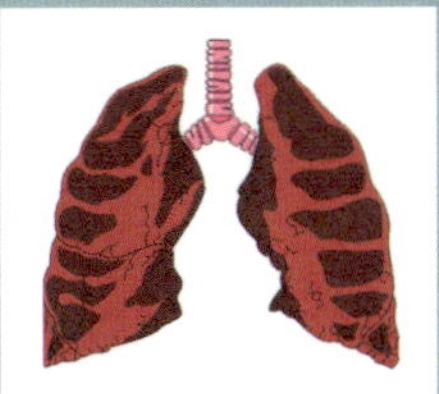

sinus/o
sī-nŭs-ō

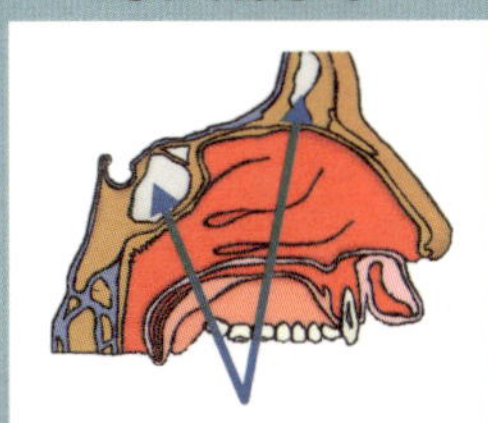

carcin/o
kăr-sĭ-nō

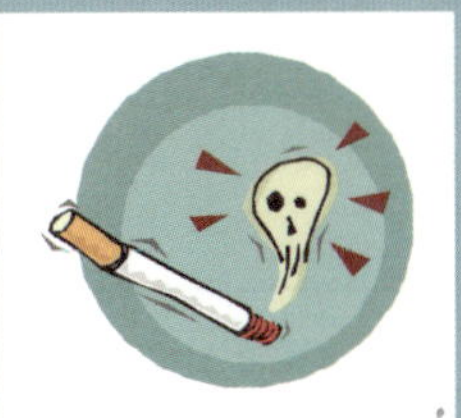

tonsill/o
tŏn-sĭl-ō

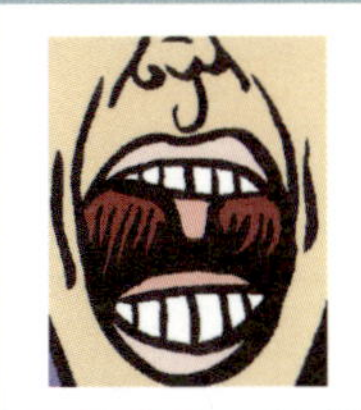

trache/o
trā-kē-ō

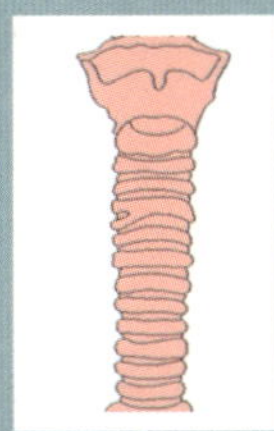

aer/o
ār-ō

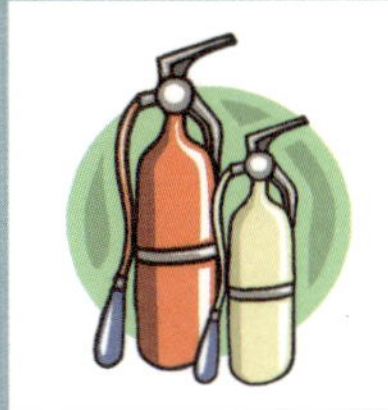

bronchiol/o
brŏng-kē-ō-lō

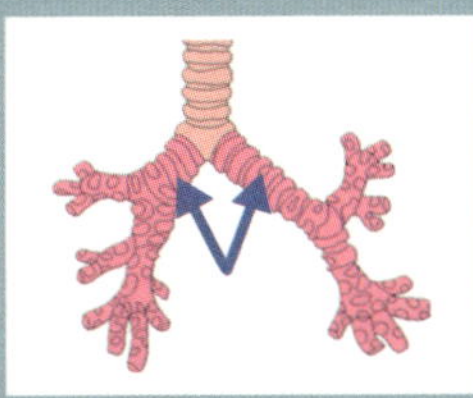

muc/o
mū-kō

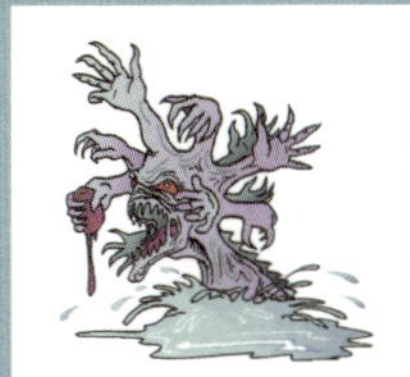

air, lung	thorax
sinus	lung
tonsil	cancer, carcinoma
air	trachea
mucus	bronchiole

orth/o
ōr-thō

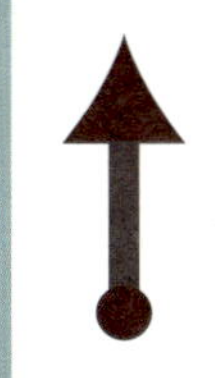

diaphragmat/o
dī-ă-frăg-măt-ō

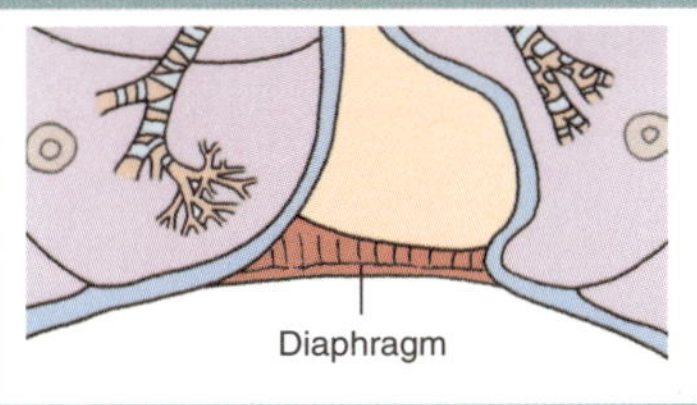

gloss/o **lingu/o**
glŏs-ō ling-gwō

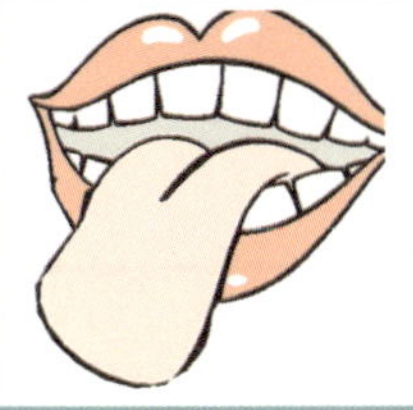

esophag/o
ē-sŏf-ă-gō

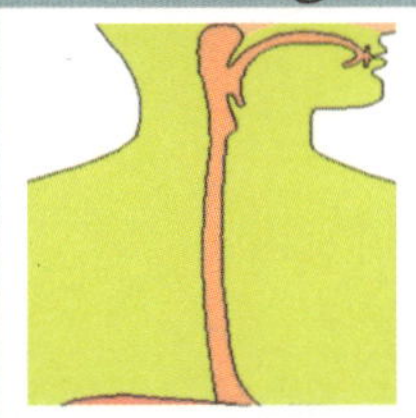

hepat/o
hĕ-pă-tō

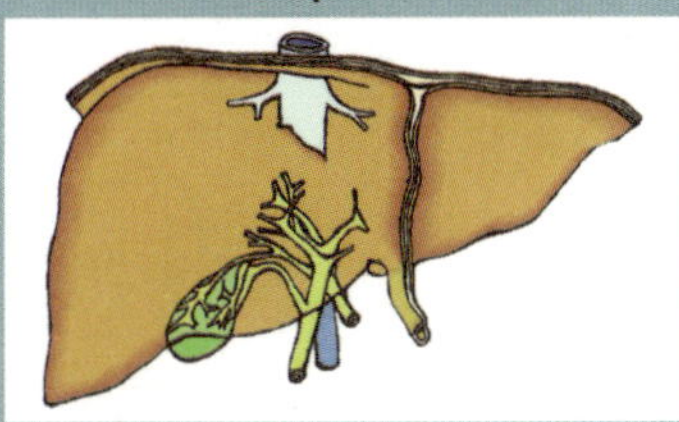

alveol/o
ăl-vē-ō-lō

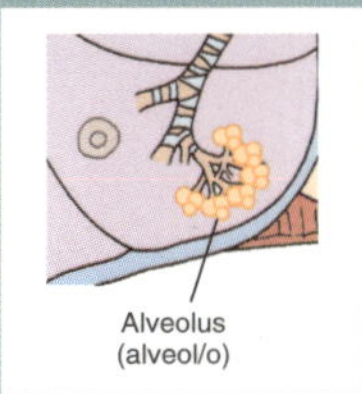

lob/o
lō-bō

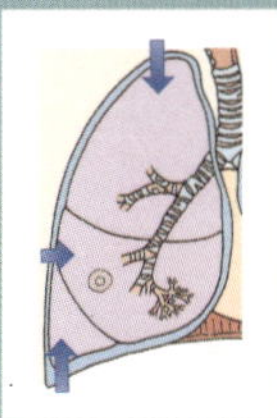

dent/o **odont/o**
dĕn-tō ō-dŏn-tō

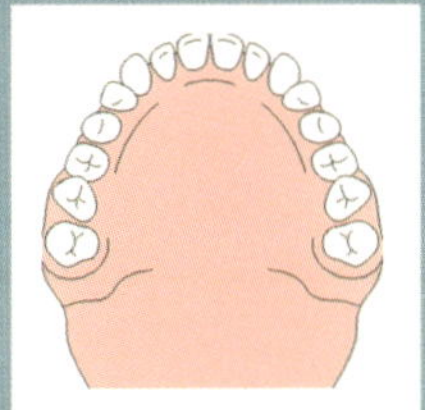

gastr/o
găs-trō

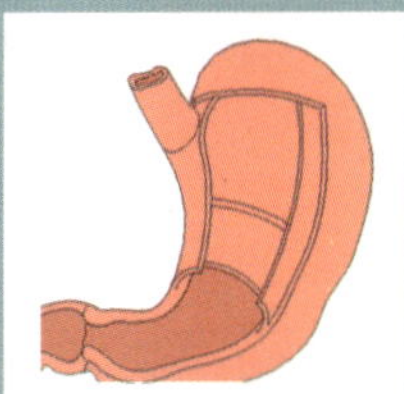

cholecyst/o
kō-lē-sĭs-tō

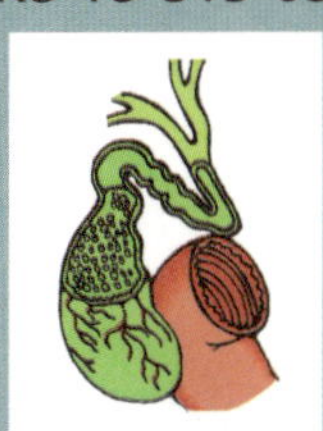

alveoli	straight
lobe	diaphragm
teeth	tongue
stomach	esophagus
gallbladder	liver

pancreat/o
păn-krē-ă-tō

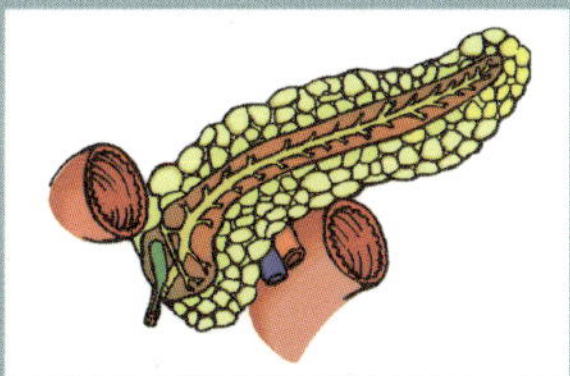

jejun/o
jē-jū-nō

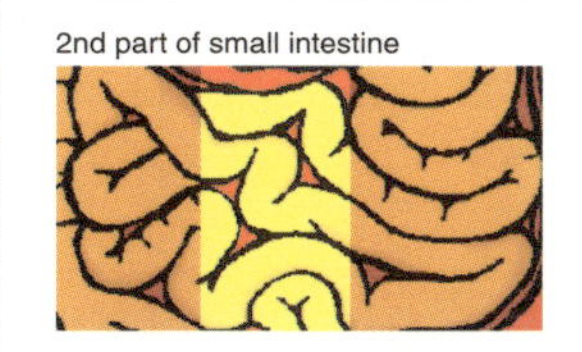

col/o kō-lō

colon/o kō-lŏ-nō

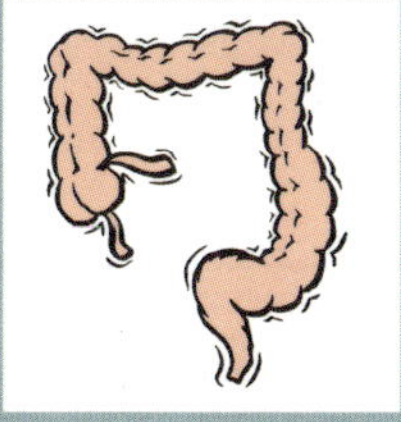

enter/o
ĕn-tĕr-ō

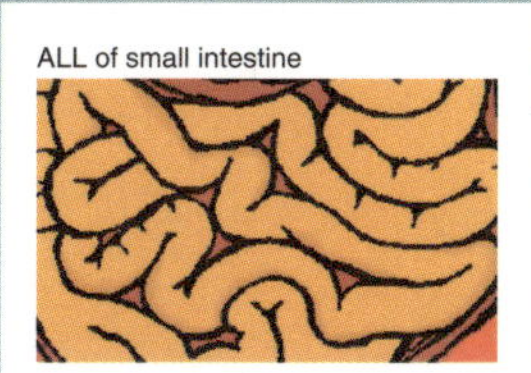

sigmoid/o
sĭg-moyd-ō

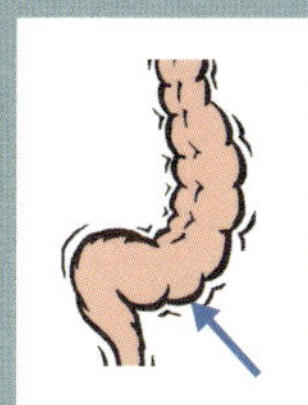

duoden/o
dū-ŏd-ĕn-ō

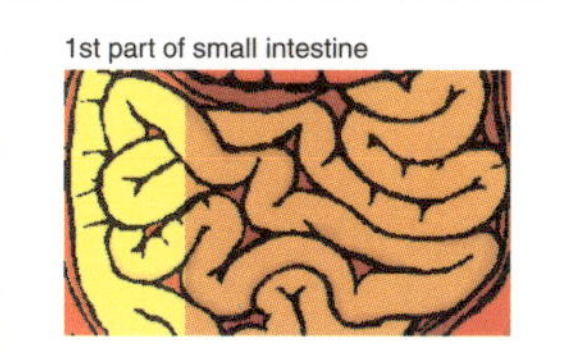

ile/o
ĭl-ē-ō

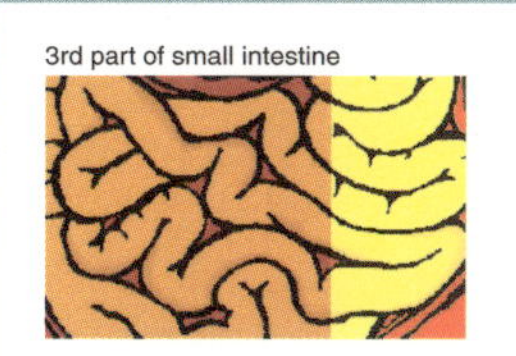

append/o ăp-ĕn-dō

appendic/o ăp-ĕn-d ĭ-kō

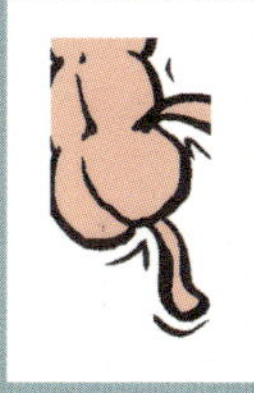

lapar/o
lăp-ăr-ō

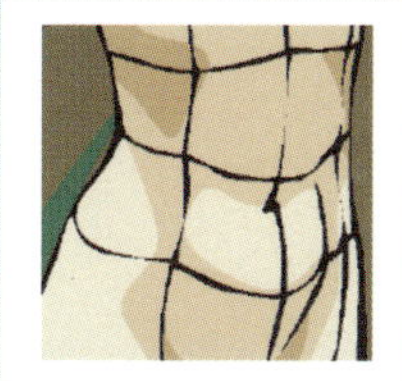

proct/o
prŏk-tō

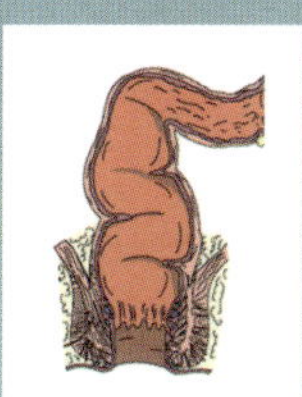

duodenum

pancreas

ileum

jejunum

appendix

colon

abdomen

small intestine

rectum, anus

sigmoid colon

rect/o
rěk-tō

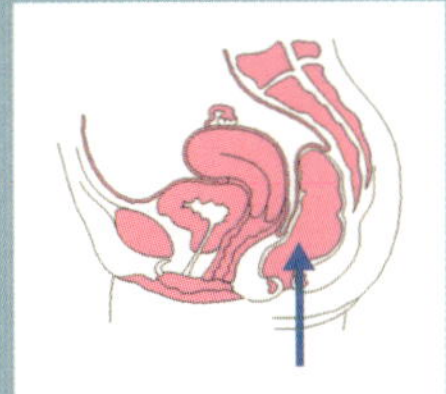

an/o
ā-nō

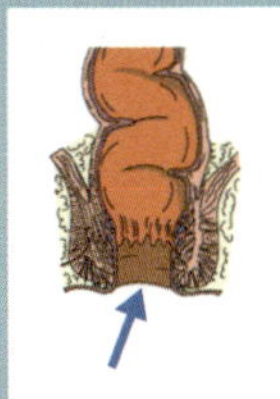

pept/o
pěp-tō

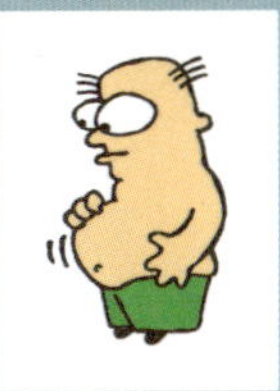

phag/o
făg-ō

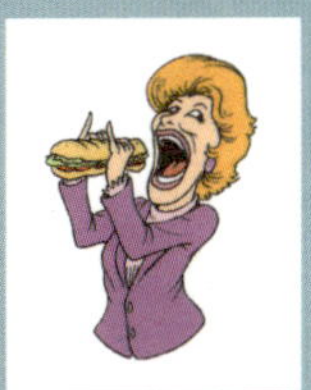

pylor/o
pī-lōr-ō

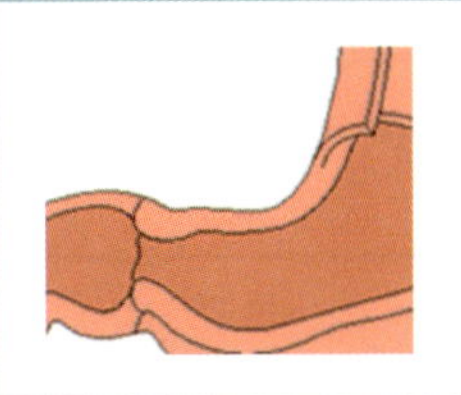

nephr/o **ren/o**
ně-frō rē-nō

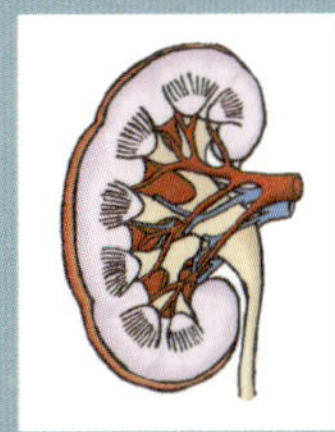

pyel/o
pī-ě-lō

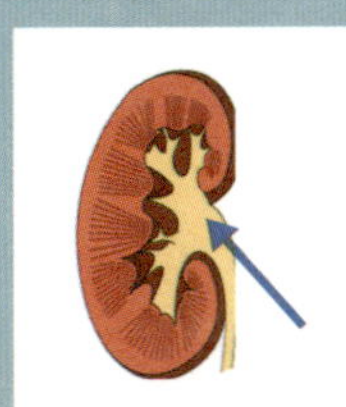

ureter/o
ū-rē-těr-ō

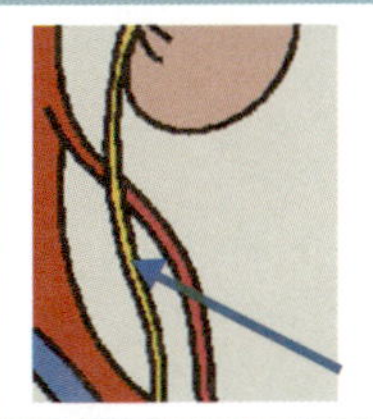

glomerul/o
glō-měr-ū-lō

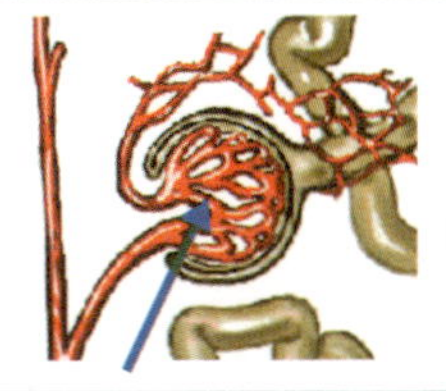

ur/o **urin/o**
ū-rō u-rĭ-nō

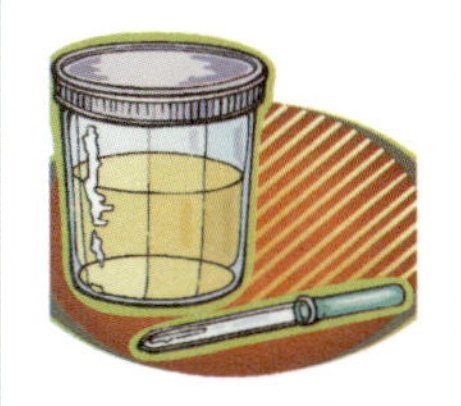

anus

rectum

eating, swallowing

digestion

kidney

pylorus

ureter

renal pelvis

urine

glomerulus

olig/o
ōl-ĭg-ō

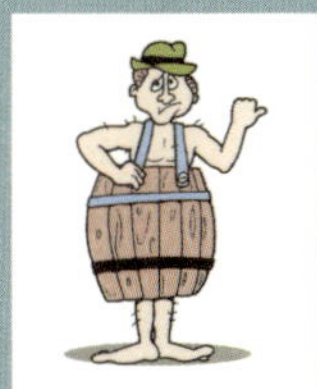

lith/o
lĭth-ō

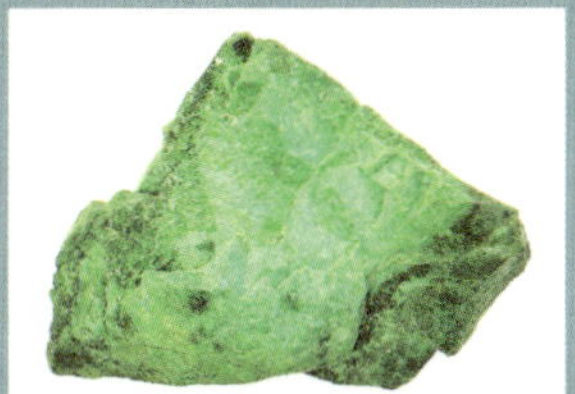

urethr/o
ū-rē-thrō

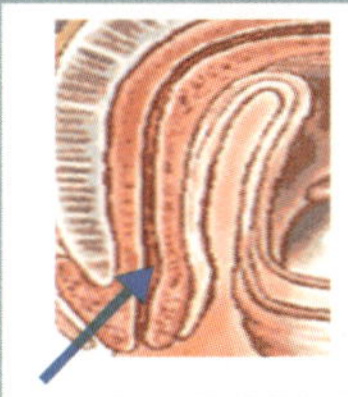

noct/o
nŏk-tō

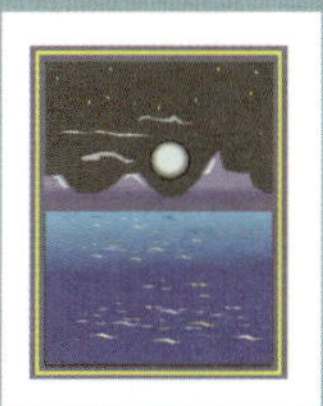

gluc/o gloo-kō **glucos/o** gloo-kōs-ō **glyc/o** glī-kō **glycos/o** glī-kōs-ō

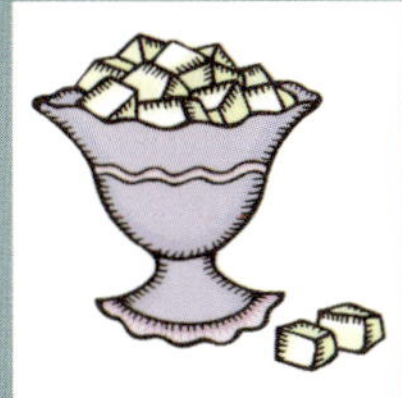

cyst/o sĭs-tō **vesic/o** vĕs-ĭ-kō

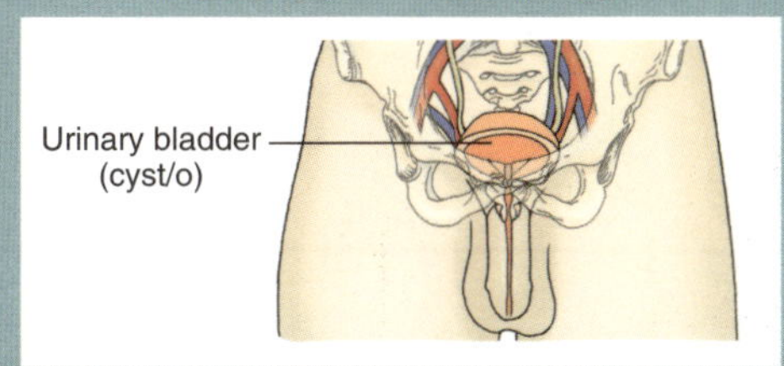

py/o
pī-ō

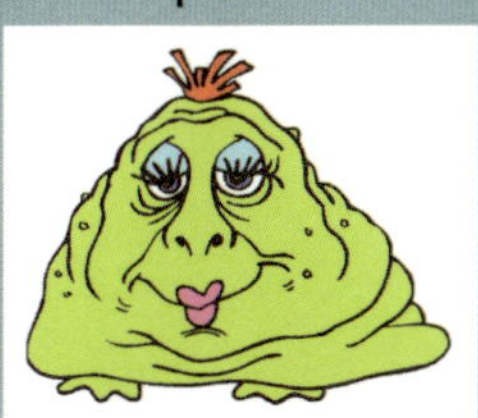

balan/o
băl-ă-nō

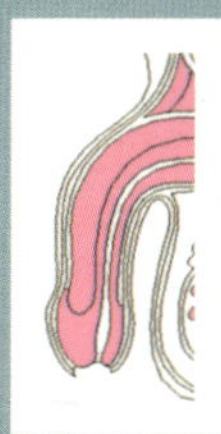

orch/o ŏr-kŏ **orchi/o** ŏr-kē-ō **orchid/o** ŏr-kĭ-dō
test/o tĕs-tō **testicu/o** tĕs-tĭk-ū-lō

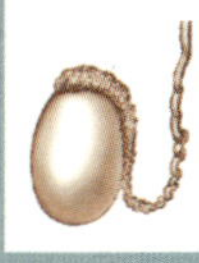

prostat/o
prŏs-tă-tō

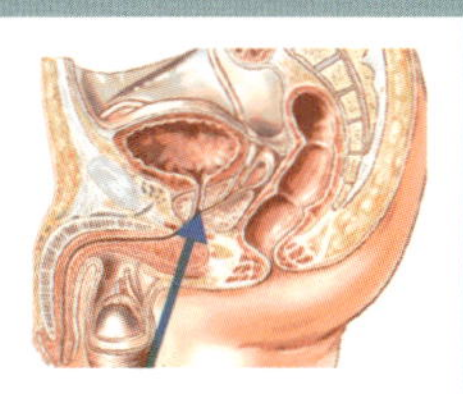

stone

deficiency

night

urethra

bladder

glucose, sugar, sweet

glans penis

pus

prostate

testis

semin/o sĕm-ĭ-nō **sperm/o** spĕr-mō **spermat/o** spĕr-măt-ō

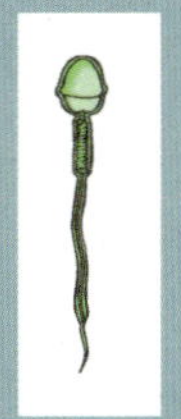

gynec/o gī-nĕ-kō

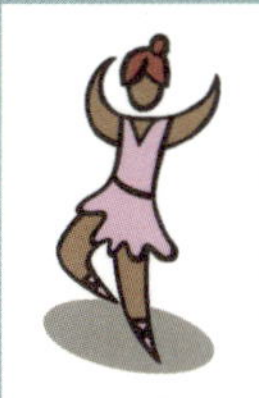

cervic/o sĕr-vĭ-kō

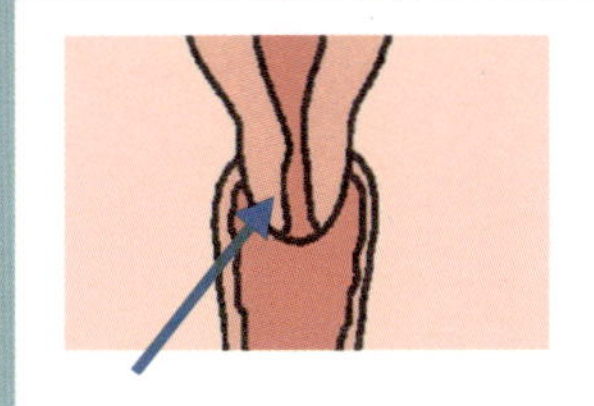

colp/o kŏl-pō **vagin/o** văj-ĭn-ō

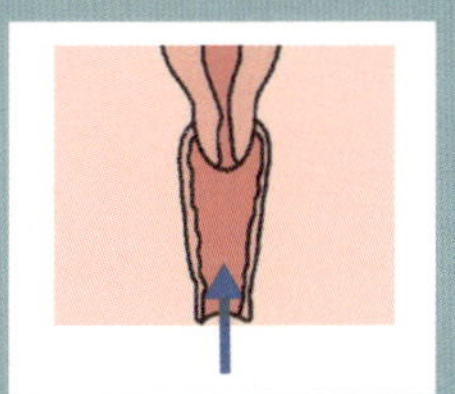

episi/o ĕ-pĭs-ē-ō **vulv/o** vŭlv-ō

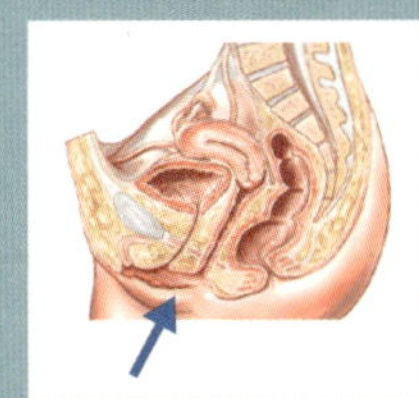

galact/o gă-lăk-tō **lact/o** lăk-tō

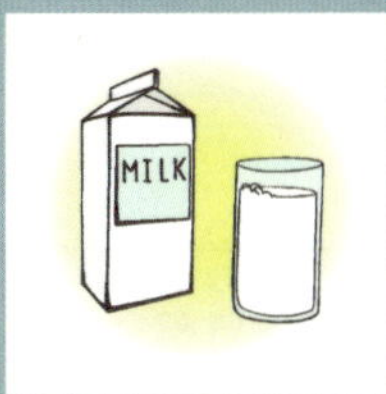

hyster/o hĭs-tĕr-ō **metr/o** mē-trō **uter/o** ū-tĕr-ō

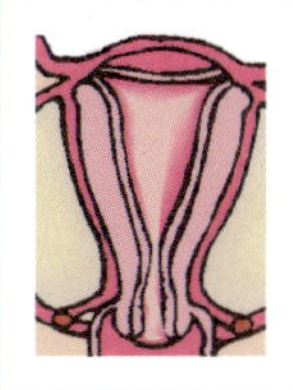

oophor/o ō-ŏf-ō-rō **ovari/o** ō-vă-rē-ō

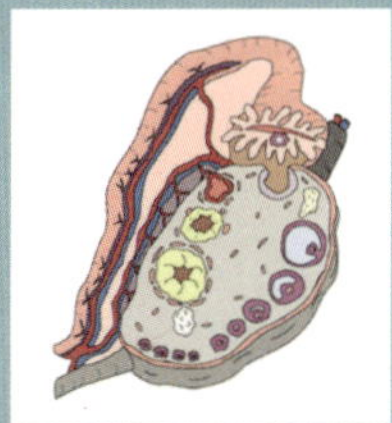

mamm/o măm-ō **mast/o** măs-tō

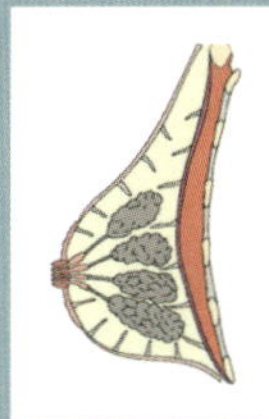

nat/o nā-tō

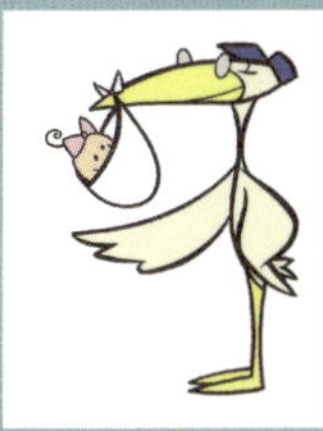

woman, female

sperm

vagina

cervix, neck

milk

vulva

ovary

uterus

birth

breast

salping/o
săl-pĭn-gō

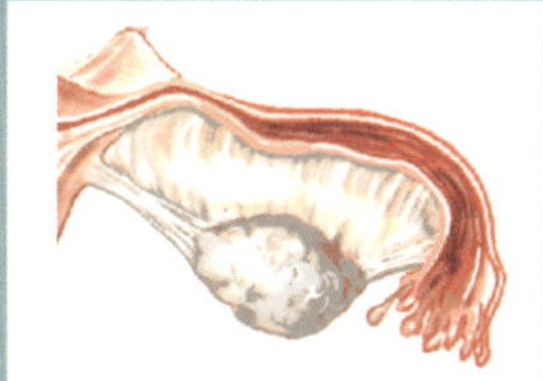

natr/o
nă-trō

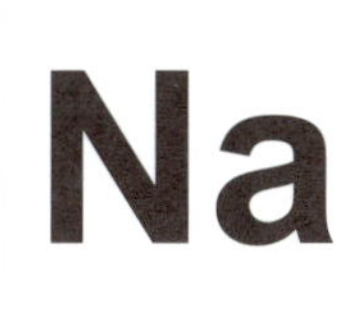

calc/o
kăl-kō

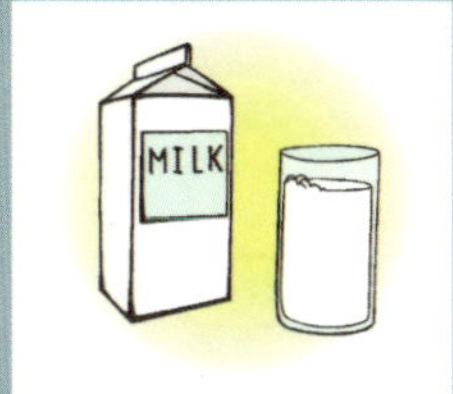

kal/i
kă-lē

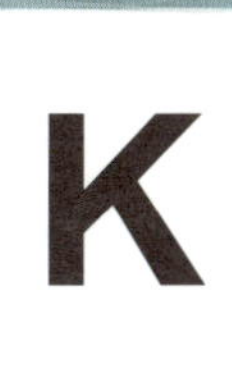

parathyroid/o
păr-ă-thī-royd-ō

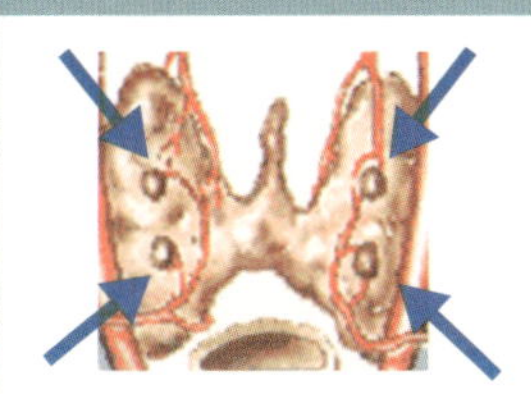

thyr/o **thyroid/o**
thī-rō thī-royd-ō

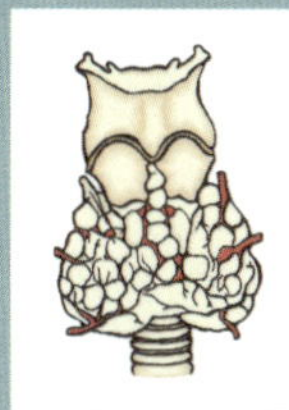

andr/o
ăn-drō

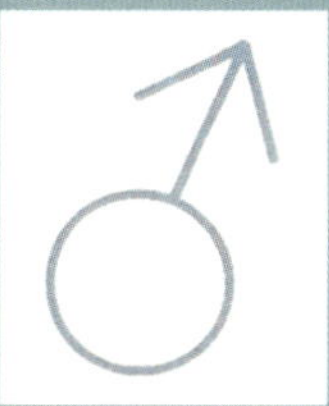

thym/o
thī-mō

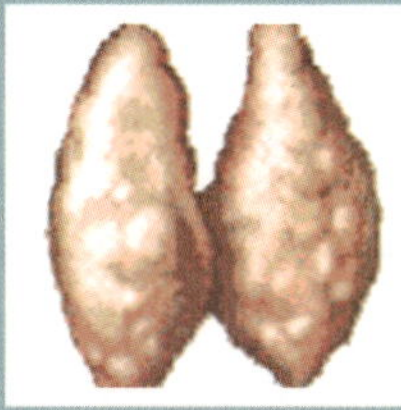

adren/o **adrenal/o**
ăd-rē-nō ăd-rē-năl-ō

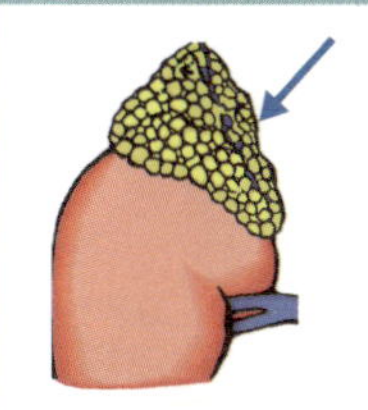

arthr/o **articul/o**
ăr-thrō ăr-tĭk-ū-lō

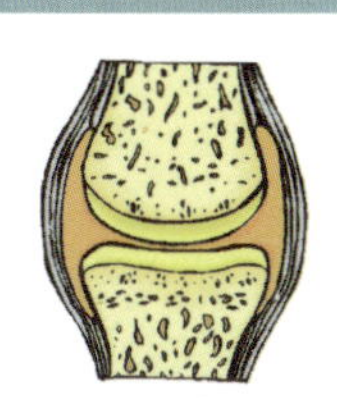

thyroid

tube
(fallopian or eustachian)

male

sodium

thymus
(gland)

calcium

adrenal gland

potassium

joint

parathyroid
(gland)

carp/o
kăr-pō

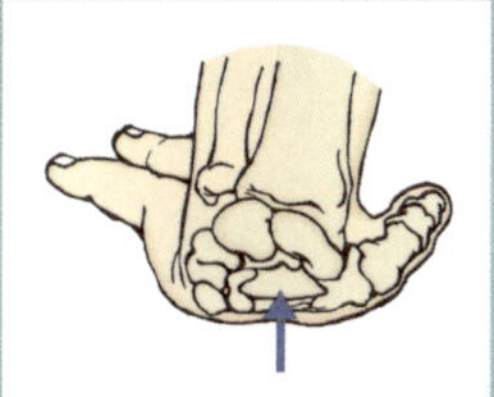

fibul/o
fĭb-ū-lō

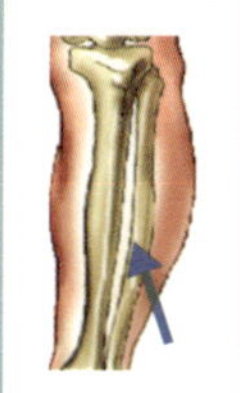

cost/o
kŏs-tō

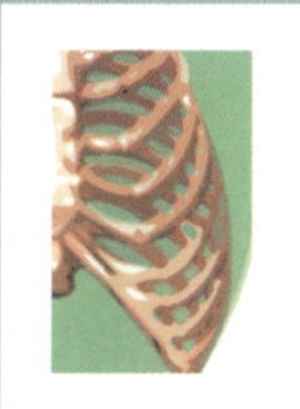

crani/o
krā-nē-ō

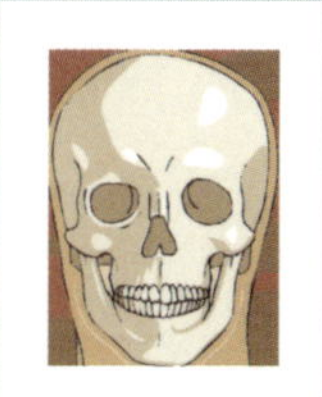

femor/o
fĕm-ō-rō

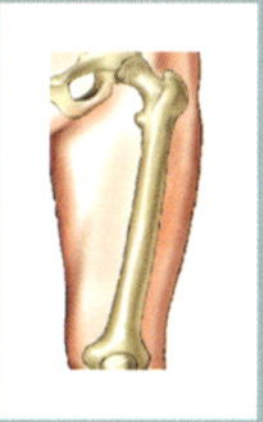

metacarp/o
mĕt-ă-kăr-pō

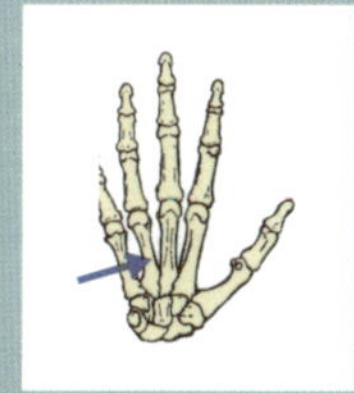

humer/o
hū-mĕr-ō

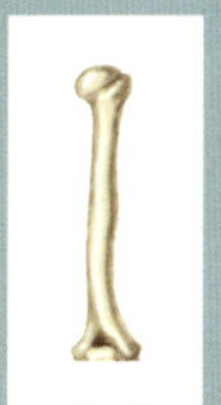

lamin/o
lăm-ĭ-nō

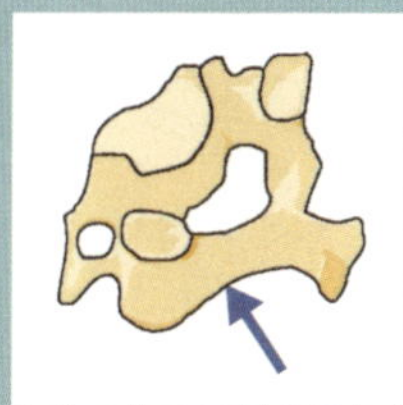

lumb/o
lŭm-bō

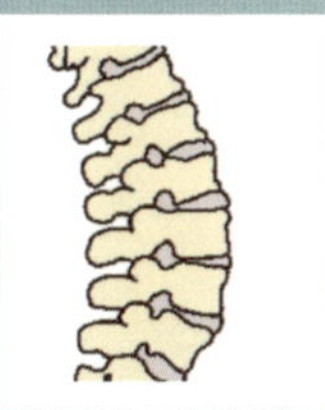

oste/o
ŏs-tē-ō

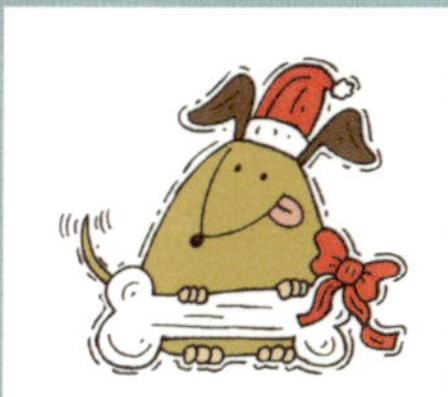

fibula

carpus

cranium

ribs

metacarpus

femur

lamina

humerus

bone

lower back

patell/a **patell/o**
pă-tĕl-ă pă-tĕl-ō

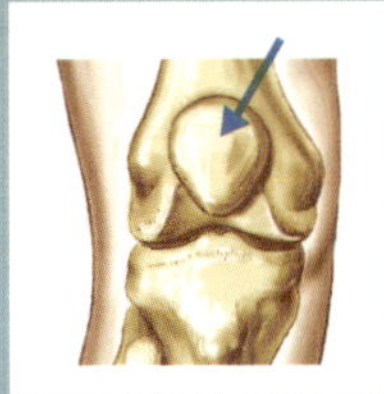

muscul/o **my/o**
mŭs-kū-lō mī-ō

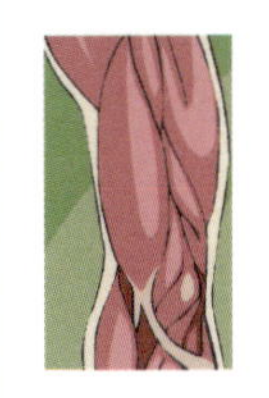

phalang/o
făl-ăn-jō

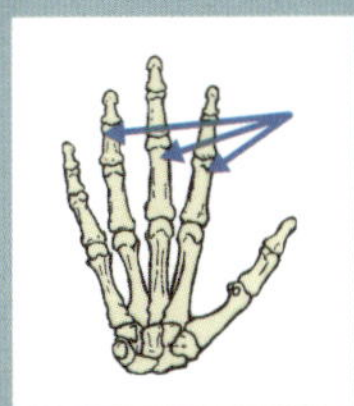

stern/o
stĕr-nō

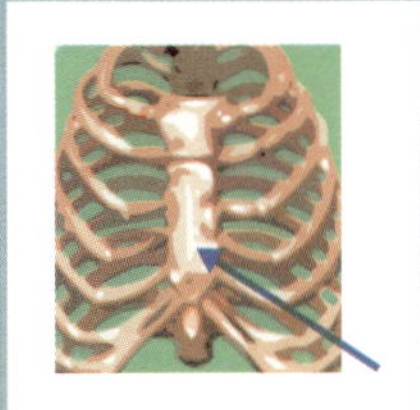

ten/o **tend/o** **tendin/o**
tĕn-ō tĕn-dō tĕn-dĭ-nō

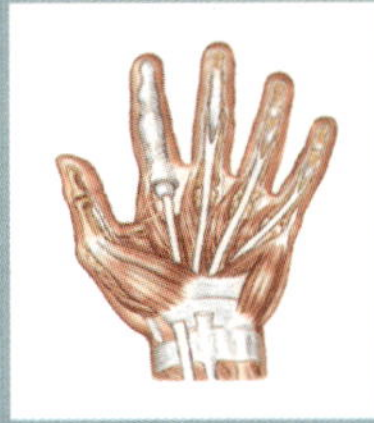

pelv/i
pĕl-vē

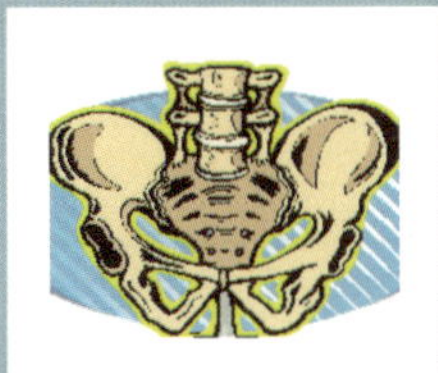

tibi/o
tĭb-ē-ō

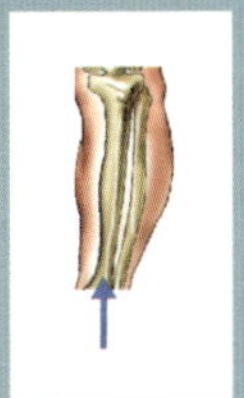

vertebr/o **spondyl/o**
ver-tē-brō spŏn-dĭ-lō

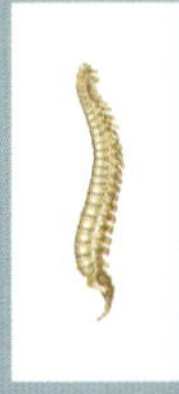

dipl/o
dĭp-lō

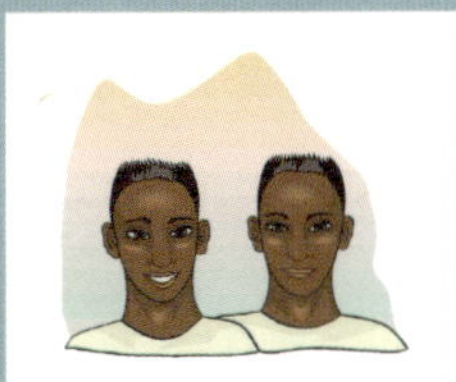

acous/o **audi/o**
ă-koos-ō aw-dē-ō

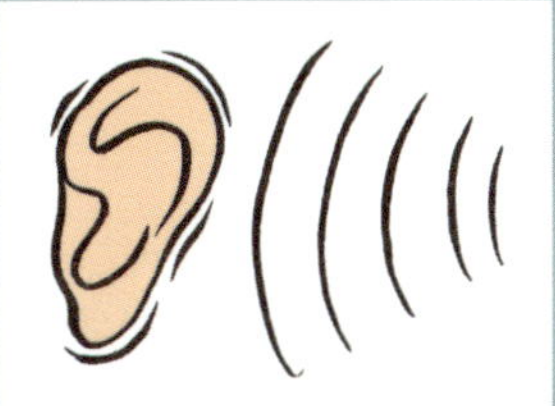

muscle

patella

sternum

phalanges

pelvis

tendon

vertebrae

tibia

hearing

double

blephar/o
blĕf-ă-rō

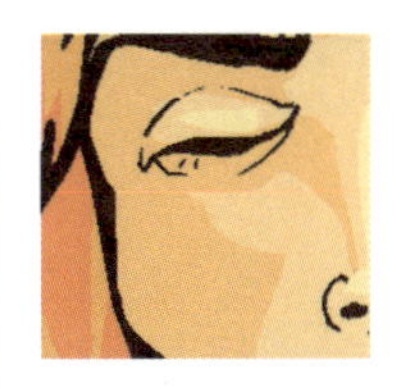

ot/o
ō-tō

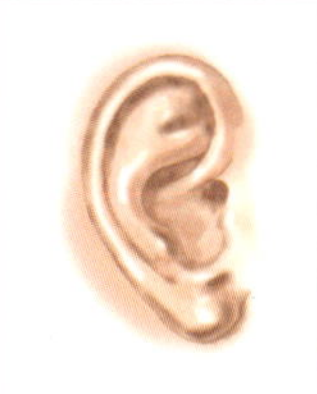

retin/o
rĕt-ĭn-ō

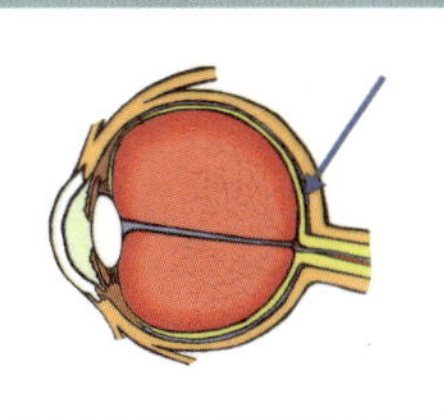

myring/o mĭr-ĭn-gō **tympan/o** tĭm-pă-nō

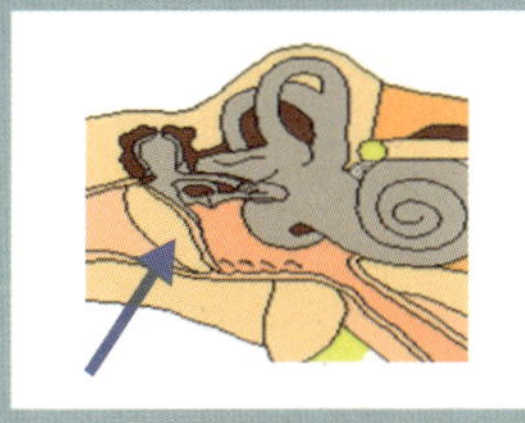

ocul/o ŏk-ū-lō **optic/o** ŏp-tĭ-kō **ophthalm/o** ŏf-thăl-mō

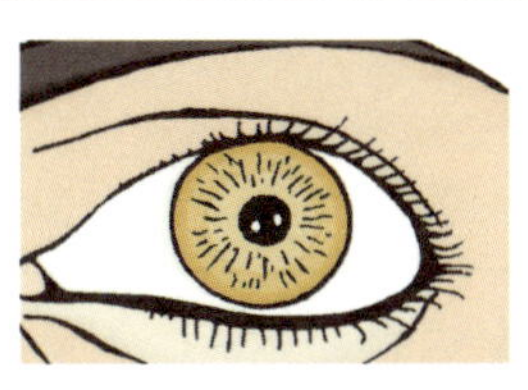

PCP

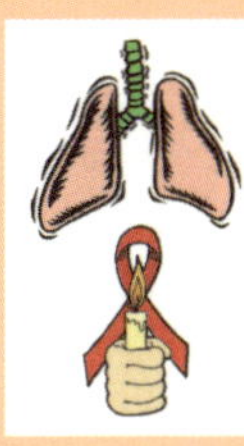

bid

2x

qh

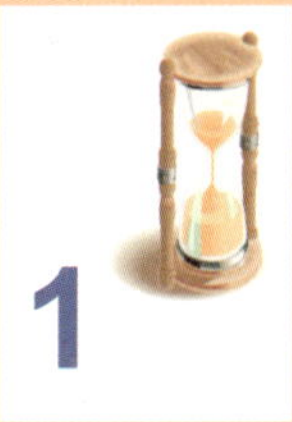

qid

4x

tid

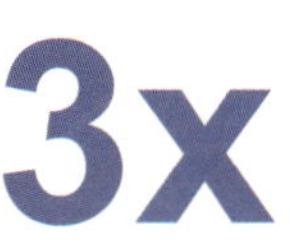

ear

eyelid

tympanic membrane
(eardrum)

retina

Pneumocystis carinii pneumonia

eye

every hour

twice a day

three times a day

four times a day

q2h

qam

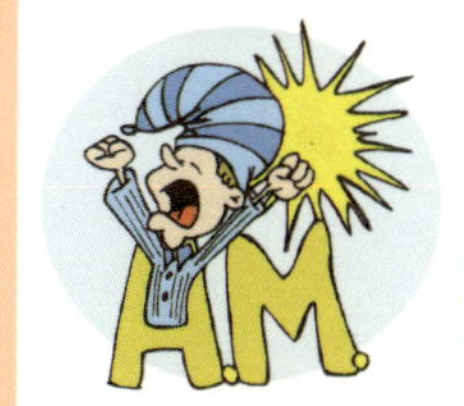

ABGs

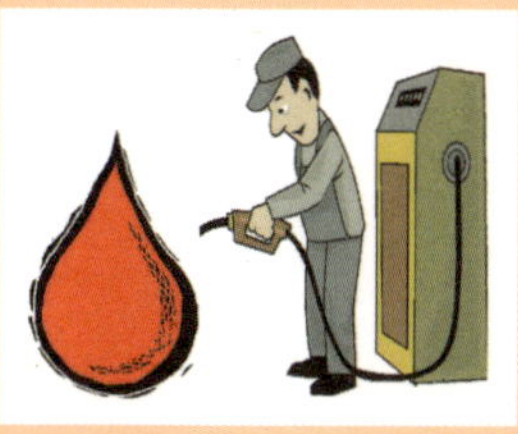

COPD

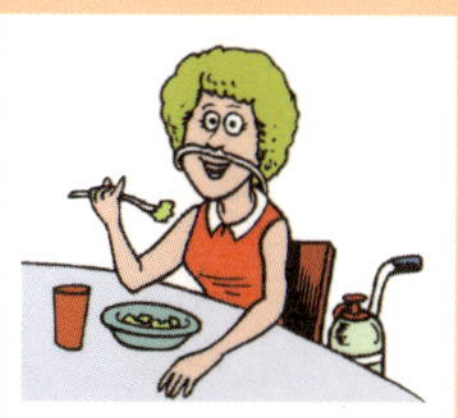

CPR

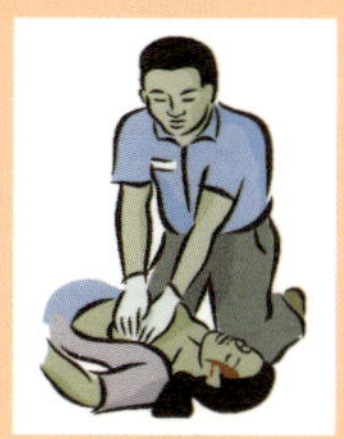

CO_2

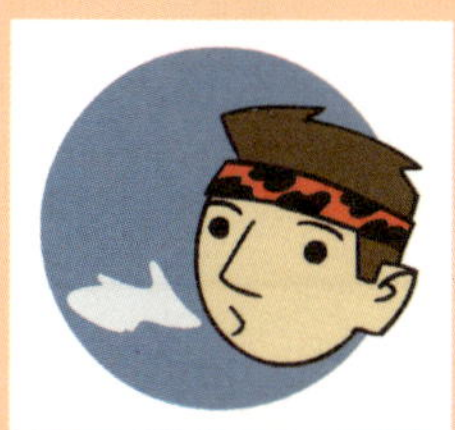

Bx

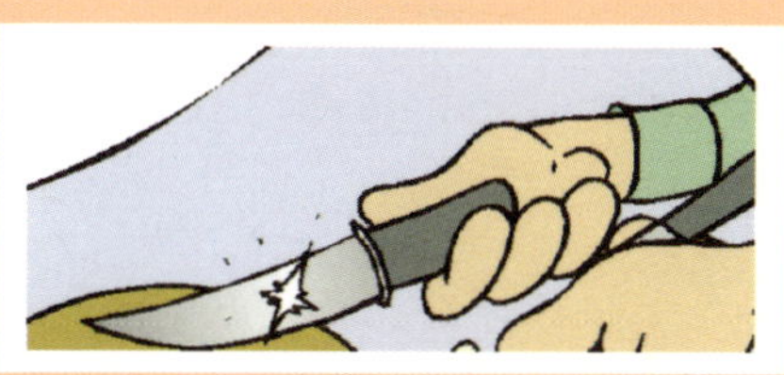

FH

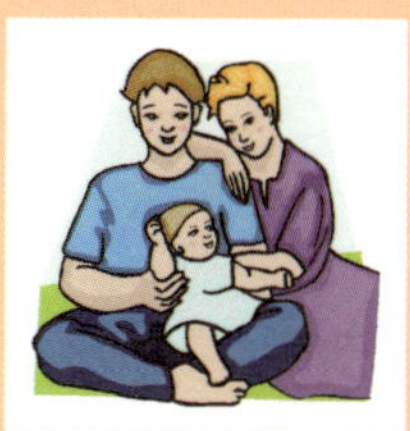

ID

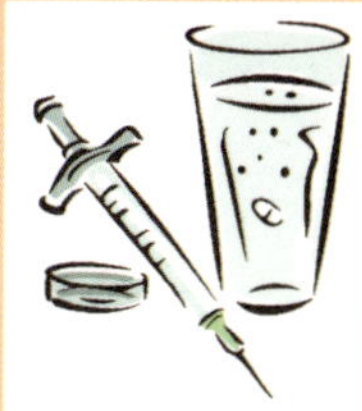

IV

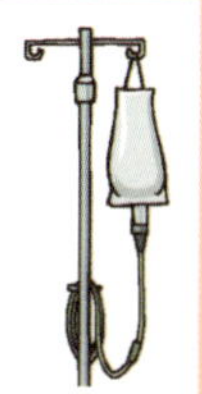

every morning

every two hours

chronic obstructive pulmonary disease

arterial blood gases

carbon dioxide

cardiopulmonary resuscitation

family history

biopsy

intravenous

intradermal (injection)

I&D

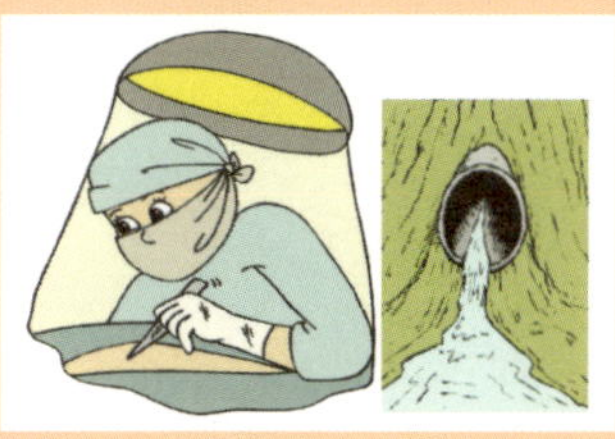

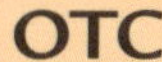

OTC

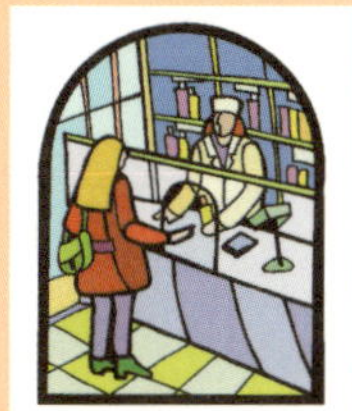

PE

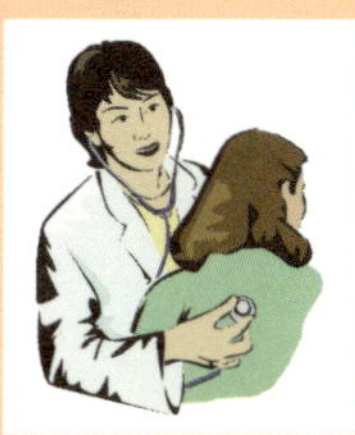

SubQ/Sub-Q

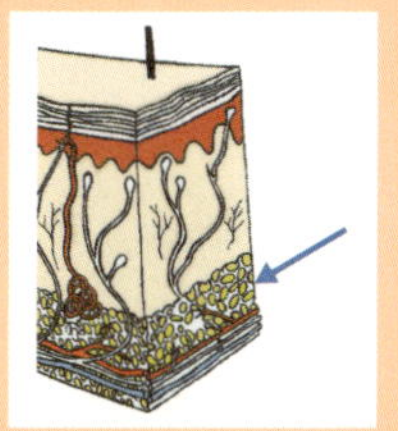

Tx

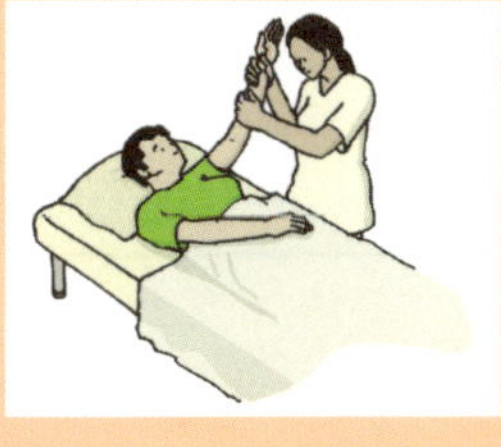

Sx

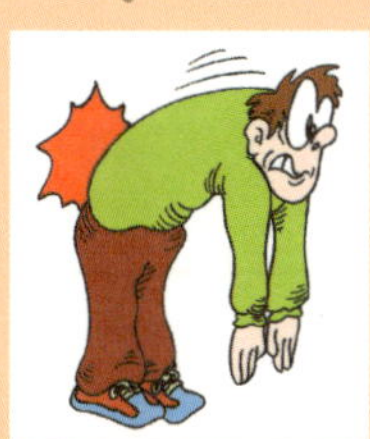

ALS

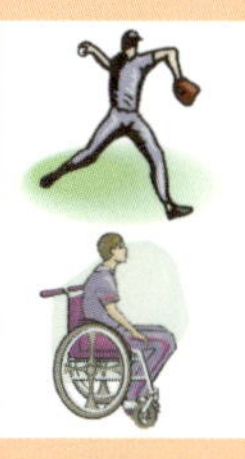

CSF

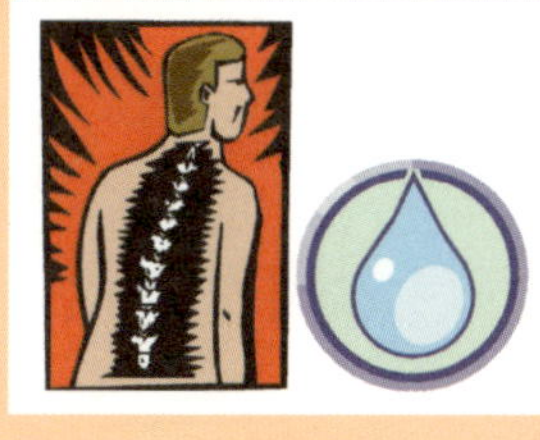

CNS

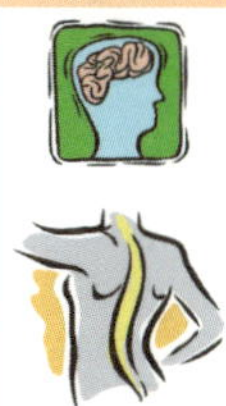

CT

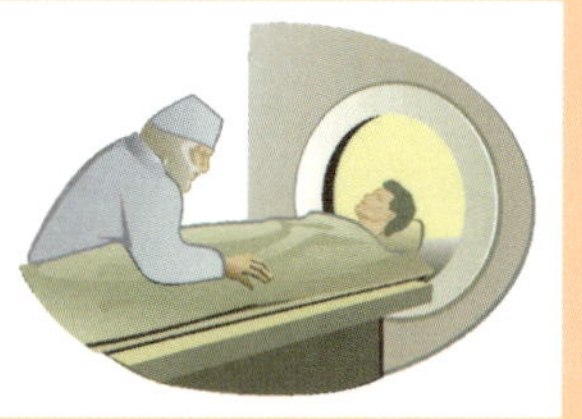

over-the-counter

incision and drainage

subcutaneous

physical examination

symptom(s)

treatment

cerebrospinal fluid

amyotrophic lateral sclerosis (Lou Gehrig disease)

computed tomography

central nervous system

CVA

EEG

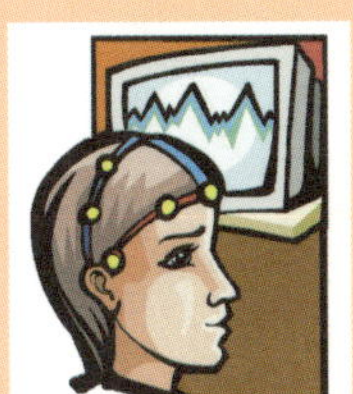

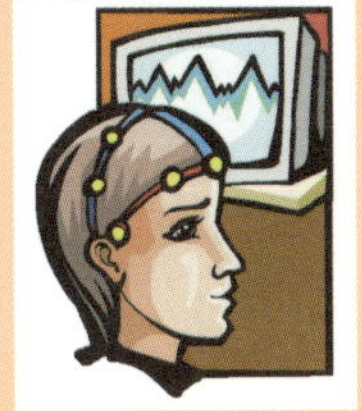

LP

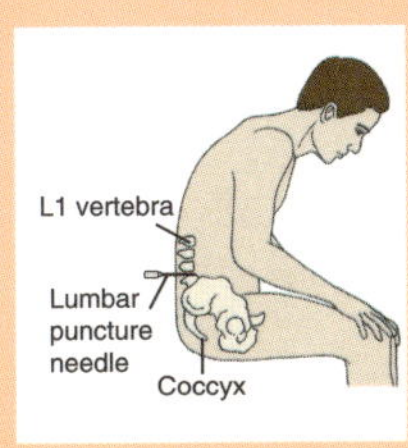

MRI

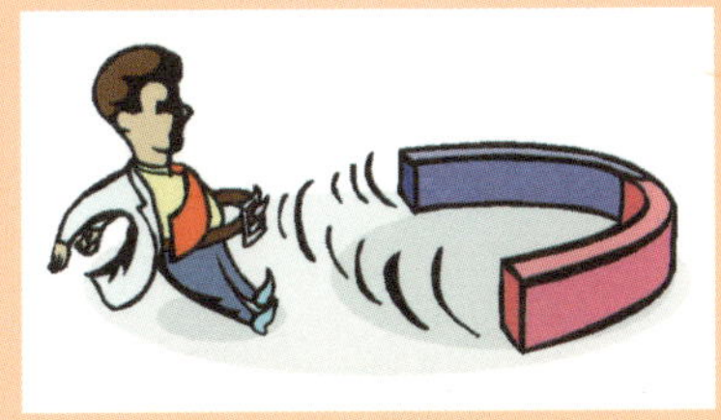

MS

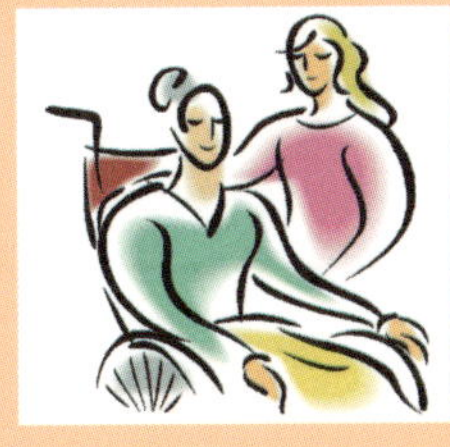

PNS

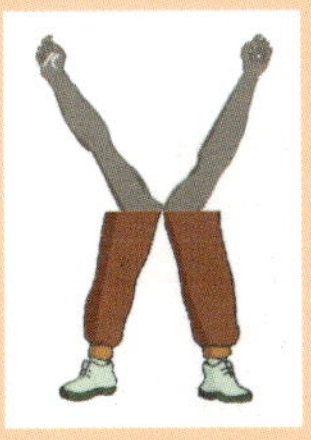

ASHD

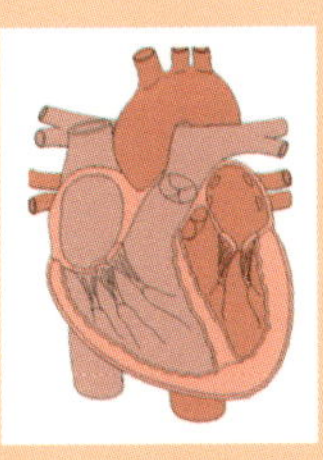

BP

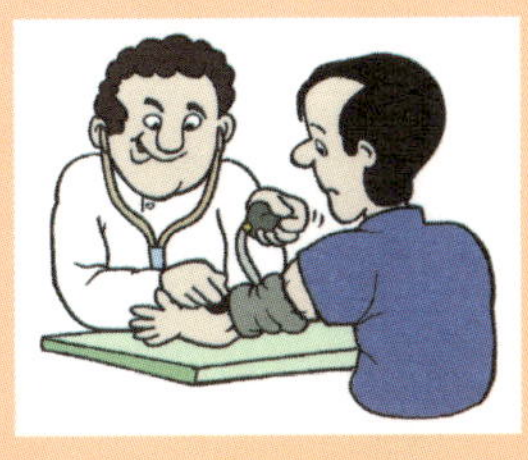

CABG

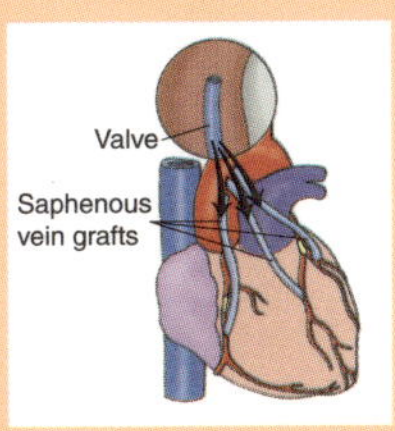

CHF

electroencephalography

cerebrovascular accident (stroke, brain attack)

magnetic resonance imaging

lumbar puncture

peripheral nervous system

multiple sclerosis

blood pressure

arteriosclerotic heart disease

congestive heart failure

coronary artery bypass graft

ECG/EKG

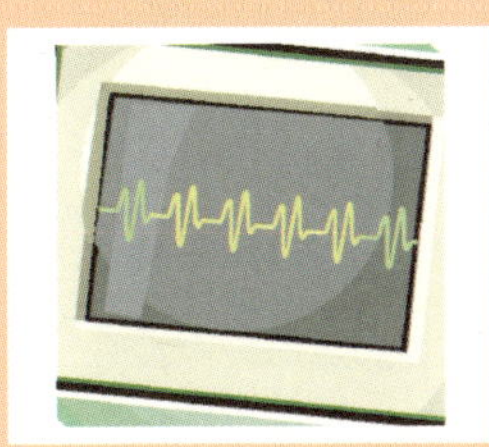

HTN

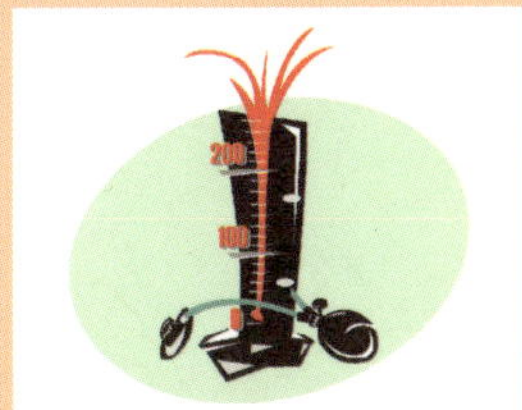

INR

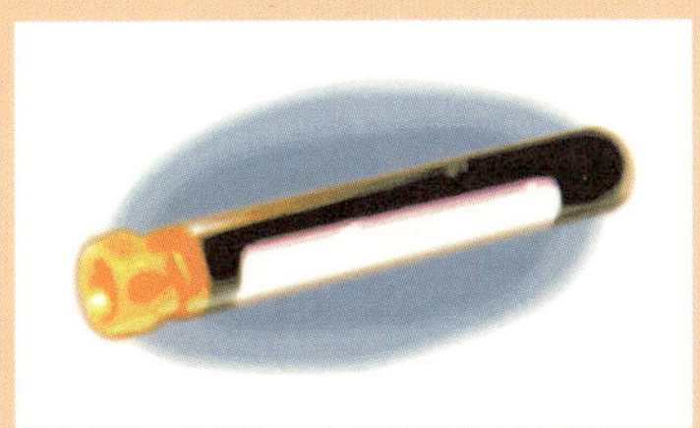

LA

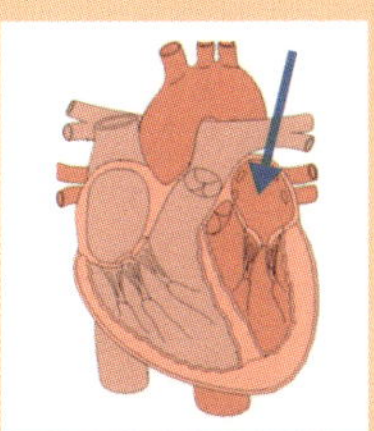

LV

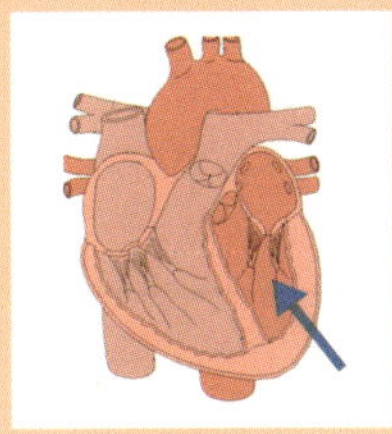

MI

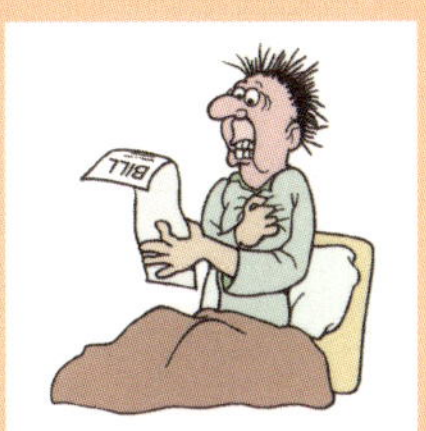

PTCA

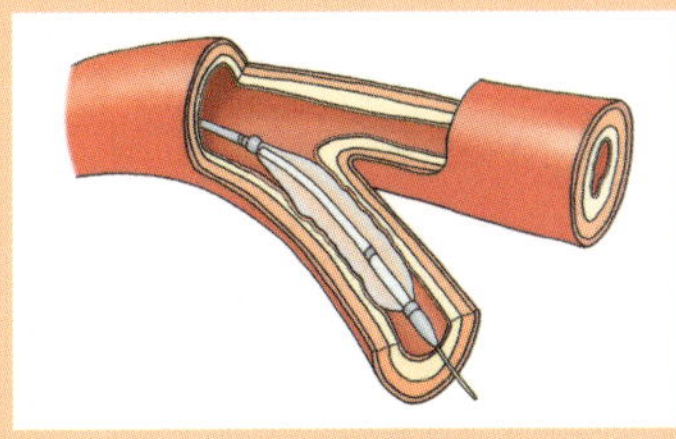

PTT

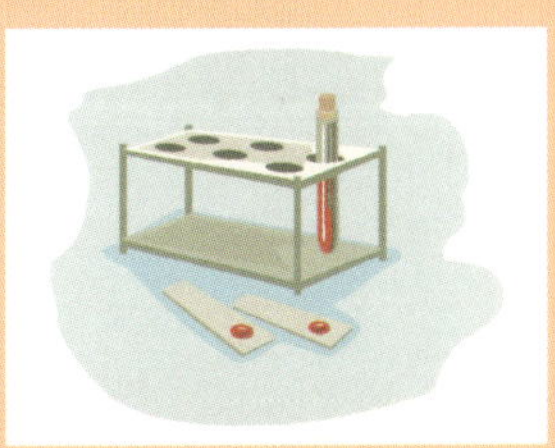

RA

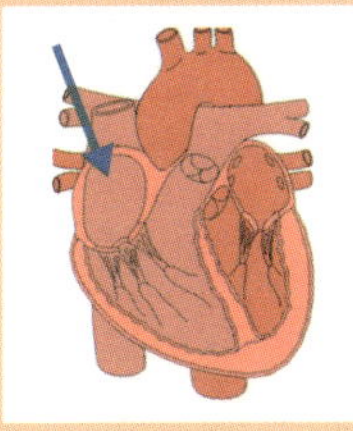

ROM

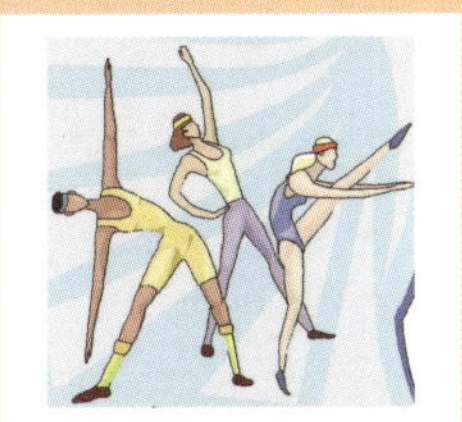

hypertension

electrocardiogram

left atrium

international normalized ratio

myocardial infarction

left ventricle

partial thromboplastin time

percutaneous transluminal coronary angioplasty

range of motion

right atrium